COMPREHENSIVE EXAM REVIEW FOR THE MEDICAL ASSISTANT

ROBYN GOHSMAN

Contributor

CINDY ABEL

Pearson

Boston Columbus Indianapolis New York San Francisco Upper Saddle River
Amsterdam Cape Town Dubai London Madrid Milan Munich Paris
Montreal Toronto Delhi Mexico City Sao Paulo Sydney
Hong Kong Seoul Singapore Taipei Tokyo

Library of Congress Cataloging-in-Publication Data

Comprehensive exam review for the medical assistant / Robyn Gohsman ... [et al.].
p. ; cm.
ISBN-13: 978-0-13-504740-8
ISBN-10: 0-13-504740-4
1. Medical assistants—Examinations, questions, etc. I. Gohsman, Robyn.
[DNLM: 1. Physician Assistants—Examination Questions. W 18.2]
R728.8.C627 2012
610.73'7069076—dc22
2010053190

Publisher: Julie Levin Alexander
Publisher's Assistant: Regina Bruno
Editor-in-Chief: Mark Cohen
Executive Editor: Joan Gill
Associate Editor: Bronwen Glowacki
Editorial Assistant: Mary Ellen Ruitenberg
Director of Marketing: David Gesell
Senior Marketing Manager: Katrin Beacom
Marketing Specialist: Michael Sirinides
Marketing Assistant: Crystal Gonzalez
Managing Production Editor: Patrick Walsh
Production Liaison: Julie Boddorf
Production Editor: Munesh Kumar
Senior Media Editor: Amy Peltier
Media Project Manager: Lorena Cerisano
Manufacturing Manager: Alan Fischer
Senior Art Director: Maria Guglielmo
Cover Designer: Candace Rowley
Cover Photo: Tom Grill/Getty
Composition: Aptara®, Inc.
Printing and Binding: Edwards Brothers
Cover Printer: Lehigh-Phoenix

Credits and acknowledgments borrowed from other sources and reproduced, with permission, in this textbook appear on appropriate page within text.

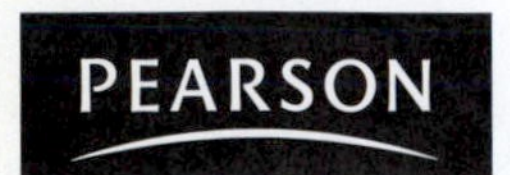

www.pearsonhighered.com

10 9 8 7 6 5 4 3 2 1
ISBN-10: 0-13-504740-4
ISBN-13: 978-0-13-504740-8

Brief Contents

Contents

SECTION 1 General Medical Assisting 1

CHAPTER 8

SECTION 3 Medical Laws, Legal Issues, and Ethical Considerations 127

CHAPTER 9

CHAPTER 22

Preface

Purpose

The purpose of *Pearson's Comprehensive Exam Review for the Medical Assistant* is to prepare and help guide the medical assisting student's review and to do well on the American Association of Medical Assistants (AAMA) Certified Medical Assistant Exam (CMA) and the American Medical Technologists (AMT) Registered Medical Assistant (RMA) and Certified Medical Administrative Specialist (CMAS) Exam(s). The guides used to help develop this textbook are the CMA (AAMA) Certification/Recertification Examination Content Outline, the AMT's Registered Medical Assistant Certification Examination Competencies and Construction Parameters, and the AMT's Certified Medical Administrative Specialist (CMAS) Competencies and Examination Specifications. The questions, answers, and rationales reflect the current knowledge and skills required of the most successful medical assistants working today.

In addition to the general, administrative and clinical knowledge required to successfully complete the CMA (AAMA), RMA (AMT), and CMAS exams, the text provides information regarding preparing for the exam(s) such as study skills, time management, applying for the exam(s), and what to expect the day of the exam.

The text is arranged into the following five sections:

- General Medical Assisting
- Interoffice Relations and Effective Therapeutic Communications
- Medical Laws, Legal Issues, and Ethical Considerations
- Administrative Competencies and Skills
- Clinical Competencies and Skills

Pearson's Comprehensive Exam Review for the Medical Assistant's streamlined approach includes many tables and figures throughout the text. The tables provide information in a very clear and concise format but also provide the opportunity for students to quiz themselves as they move through the chapters. The many figures supporting the text are especially beneficial for those visual learners who need to "see" the ideas/concepts they are reading.

Following each chapter, there are questions that allow the students to test their level of understanding before moving on to the next chapter. The questions were developed using the same format as the questions found on the AAMA and AMT certification exams. Answers to the questions as well as rationales that support the answers are found at the end of the text. At the end of the text is a comprehensive self-evaluation exam with answers and rationales.

Reviewers

Dominica Austin, BSN
Academic Dean
Lincoln College of Technology
Marietta, GA

Deborah J. Bedford, MA, AAS
Program Coordinator/Instructor, retired
North Seattle Community College
Seattle, WA

Michelle Blesi, CMA (AAMA), BA
Program Director/Instructor
Century College
White Bear Lake, MN

Cynthia A. Bloss, AA, RMA, LXMO
Medical Assisting Program Coordinator/Instructor
Keiser Career College
Petersburg, FL

Lou Brown, MT (ASCP) CMA (AAMA)
Program Director, Medical Assisting and Phlebotomy
Wayne Community College
Goldsboro, NC

Minda Brown, RMA, AAS, AA
Registered Medical Assistant
Pima Medical Institute
Colorado Springs, CO

Denise Carsillo, MS, BS, AS, RMA
Associate Dean Allied Health
Lincoln College of Technology
West Palm Beach, FL

Ursula E. Cole, CMA (AAMA), MEd
Medical Program Coordinator
Indiana Business College
Terre Haute, IN

John Conklin, MD
Program Leader, Medical Assisting
Daymar Institute
Clarksville, TN

Bonnie J. Crist, BS, CMA (AAMA)
Medical Program Coordinator
Harrison College
Indianapolis, IN

Eleanor K. Flores, RN, BSN, MEd
Program Director, Medical Assisting
Briarwood College
Southington, CT

Cindy L. Garman, CMA (AAMA)
Director of Career Services/Instructor
Akron Institute of Herzing University
Akron, OH

Alice Macomber, RN, RMA, AHI, RPT, CPI, LMO, AS Nursing, AS Mid-Management
Keiser University Regional Program Director
Keiser University
Port Saint Lucie, FL

Wendi Walker, RN, MSN
Medical Assisting Lead Instructor
Draughons Junior College
Murfreesboro, TN

Sheila M. Williams, AAS, CMA, CET, CCT
MDCA Lead Instructor
Coleman College for Health Sciences
Houston, TX

Section 1 General Medical Assisting

1 Medical Assisting Profession

CONTENTS

According to the Bureau of Labor Statistics, U.S. Department of Labor, *Occupational Outlook Handbook, 2010–2011 Edition* (http://www.bls.gov/oco/ocos164.htm), medical assisting is among the fastest-growing occupations and has a projected growth of 34% between 2008 and 2018. Helping to drive this growth is the fact that medical assistants are multiskilled healthcare professionals who are trained to work both administratively and clinically in ambulatory settings.

Job Responsibilities

The primary job responsibility of the medical assistant is to help physicians provide care for their patients. Depending upon the office setting, medical assistants may divide their time between clinical and administrative tasks, or they may spend the majority of their time working strictly clinically or strictly administratively.

Medical assistants who have graduated from an accredited training program are trained to perform the following tasks:

Administrative tasks

- Receive patients
- Communicate with patients, families, and co-workers
- Answer telephones
- Schedule patients' appointments
- Collect patients' co-pay fees
- Maintain, update, and file patients' records
- Obtain insurance preauthorizations and referrals
- Complete medical insurance forms
- Patient billing
- Bookkeeping
- Correspondence

Clinical tasks (may vary from state to state, depending upon state law)

- Obtaining patients' medical histories and vital signs
- Provide patient education
- Prepare patients for examinations and procedures
- Assist the physician with examinations/procedures
- Provide asepsis and infection control
- Collect and prepare laboratory specimens
- Perform laboratory tests
- Sterilize medical instruments
- Prepare and administer medications
- Perform venipunctures
- Perform electrocardiograms (EKGs or ECGs)
- Remove sutures and change dressings
- Prepare and maintain examination and treatment rooms

In addition to the skills listed above, it is important that those working in the medical assisting profession also have the following intrapersonal skills:

- Exemplary communication skills, both verbal and written
- Neat, well-groomed appearance
- Courteous and pleasant manner
- Empathy
- Integrity
- Discretion
- Thoroughness
- Punctuality
- Confidentiality
- Congeniality
- Competence

Professional Organizations

There are two main professional organizations for medical assistants: the American Medical Technologists (AMT) and the American Association of Medical Assistants (AAMA). Both are national organizations with state and local chapters. Participation in these organizations is not required but is highly recommended, as they provide opportunities for personal and professional growth, networking, and possibly the opportunity to make decisions affecting the future of the profession.

The AMT and AAMA offer continuing medical education (via Continuing Education Units [CEUs]) through their respective organizations. CEUs help medical assistants stay up-to-date on a variety of topics. CEUs may be obtained either through self-study or by participating in local, state, and national seminars.

Certification

Although certification is not required to be able to work as a medical assistant, the Registered Medical Assistant (RMA) (AMT) and Certified Medical Assistant (CMA) (AAMA) certifications indicate that the individual has met certain standards and has obtained a certain level of knowledge and skills. Many employers now require their medical assistants to be certified as either an RMA (AMT) or a CMA (AAMA).

QUALIFICATIONS OF RMA CERTIFICATION

Qualifications

To qualify for RMA certification:

1. Applicant shall be of good moral character.
2. Applicant shall meet one of the following requirements

   A. Applicant shall be a recent graduate of, or scheduled to graduate from:

      1. A medical assistant program that holds programmatic accreditation by (or is in a post-secondary school or college that holds institutional accreditation by) the Accrediting Bureau of Health Education Schools (ABHES) or the Commission on Accreditation of Allied Health Education Programs (CAAHEP).
      2. A medical assistant program in a post-secondary school or college that has institutional accreditation by a Regional Accrediting Commission or by a national accrediting organization approved by the U.S. Department of Education, which program includes a minimum of 720 clock-hours (or equivalent) of training in medical assisting skills (including a clinical externship).
      3. A formal medical services training program of the United States Armed Forces.

   * If you graduated within the last three years, proof of work experience is not required. If you graduated over three years ago, you will be required to show proof of current work experience.

   B. Applicant shall have been employed in the profession of medical assisting for a minimum of five (5) years, no more than two (2) years of which may have been as an instructor in the post-secondary medical assistant program (proof of current work experience and high school education or equivalent is needed). Employment dates must be within the last five (5) years.

   C. The AMT Board of Directors has further determined that applicants who have passed a generalist medical assistant certification examination offered by another medical assisting certification body (provided that the exam has been approved for this purpose by the AMT Board of Directors) and who have been working in the medical assisting field for the past three out of five years and who have met all other AMT training and experience requirements, may be considered for RMA certification without further examination.

If you have any questions, please email AMT at: rma@amt1.com

Source: American Medical Technologists, Rosemont, IL. Reprinted with permission.

RMA (AMT) EXAM

The AMT is a nonprofit certifying body that provides certification examinations for several professions within the medical field, including the RMA exam. The RMA credential is awarded to those individuals who pass the AMT's RMA certification exam and is nationally recognized.

The AMT also offers the Certified Medical Administrative Specialist (CMAS) exam (see page 6). Medical assistants with strong administrative skills are encouraged to apply for and take this exam as well.

Registering for the RMA (AMT) Exam

The RMA (AMT) exam application is available for download from the AMT Web site, http://www.amt1.com. Qualified applicants may choose to take the exam on computer at one of the more than 200 Pearson VUE testing locations in the United States and Canada or they may opt to take the paper-and-pencil exam at another specified location. The computerized exam is available nearly every day of the year except Sundays and holidays. The paper-and-pencil exam must be scheduled in advance and is subject to the availability of the proctor and the facility. Both versions are identical in length, structure, and time allowed for completion.

The nonrefundable application fee for both the computerized and paper-and-pencil versions of the RMA (AMT) exam is $95. Once the completed, signed application and the exam fee are submitted, the AMT will process the application and send an "Authorization to Test" letter to the applicant. For those who opt for the computerized test, the letter will contain information regarding registering to take the exam with Pearson VUE.

Format of the RMA (AMT) Exam

There are 200 to 210 questions on the RMA (AMT) exam, and the minimum passing score is a scaled score of 70. The exam is competency-based and consists of four-option multiple-choice questions. It is important that the single *best* of the four answer options is chosen. The time allowed to complete the exam is two hours.

CERTIFIED MEDICAL ADMINISTRATIVE SPECIALIST (AMT)

Medical Administrative Specialist

A Medical Administrative Specialist serves a key role in medical office, clinic and hospital settings. This multi-skilled practitioner is competent in medical records management, insurance processing, coding and billing, management of practice finances, information processing, and fundamental office management tasks. A Medical Administrative Specialist is very familiar with clinical and technical concepts required to coordinate administrative office functions in the healthcare setting.

Nature of the Work

A Medical Administrative Specialist must have a sincere desire to help people and a willingness to learn the complexities of the health care industry. Medical administrative specialists work most of their time in the "front" office of a physician office, clinic or hospital. A medical administrative specialist must be outgoing, patient, and pay close attention to detail. Also, this individual must be willing to learn new procedures, laws and insurance filing forms. Some of the duties performed by a Medical Administrative Specialist include:

- Set appointment times
- Greet patients
- File and pull charts
- Handle insurance information
- Assist new patients with paperwork
- Know word processing
- Know bookkeeping
- Type medical correspondence
- Transcribe medical dictation
- Understand and know insurance coding information
- Scheduling hospital admissions
- Type case histories
- Fill out and submit insurance medical forms
- Collects and records payments
- Must know medical terminology

Education and Training

A Medical Administrative Specialist must have a high school diploma or G.E.D. with acceptable training. Many colleges, career schools and technical schools offer Medical Administrative Assistant, Medical Office Assistant, or Medical Secretary programs. Graduates from these programs will receive either a certificate or diploma depending on the program. Graduation from a school that is accredited makes it easier to apply for certification.

Certification/Licensing:

Each individual state decides the scope of practice for Medical Administrative Specialists. Most states do not have licensure laws, but many states do have a scope of practice for Medical Administrative Specialists or Medical Assistants.

Certification by a recognized organization enables Medical Administrative Specialists to be promoted faster, [and to] earn higher pay and great respect. Employers prefer to hire experienced workers and many prefer certified applicants who have passed a national examination, indicating that the Medical Administrative Specialist meets certain standards of competence.

Employment

The job outlook for Medical Administrative Specialists is excellent. The field is expected to grow much faster than average, which means an increase in 36% or more between 2000 and 2010. The health services industry is expected to expand because of technological advances in medicine and the aging population.

Salary

Earnings vary depending on experience, education and skill level.
Profession Source: U.S. Bureau of Labor Statistics:

Source: American Medical Technologists, Rosemont, IL. Reprinted with permission.

CONTENT BREAKDOWN FOR THE RMA (AMT) EXAM

Content Area	Approximate Percentage of Total Test
General Medical Assisting	41%
Administrative Medical Assisting	24%
Clinical Medical Assisting	35%

For the computerized version, results are available moments after the exam is completed. If the certification application is complete, a paper certificate and a copy of the results will be provided before the individual leaves the testing center. If the certification application is not complete, the certificate and the results will be made available at a later date.

Maintaining the RMA (AMT) and CMAS Credentials

The AMT states that all RMAs (AMT) and CMAS who were initially certified on or after January 1, 2006, are required to obtain 30 CEUs over a three-year period. At the end of that period, the RMA (AMT) and CMAS must submit a completed and signed Compliance Evaluation Worksheet and an Attestation Form to the AMT. A percentage of the returned worksheets are audited.

CMA (AAMA) EXAM

The AAMA is a key organization in the field of medical assisting, with the main office located in Chicago. The AAMA awards the CMA credential to those individuals who pass the CMA (AAMA) national examination.

Registering for the CMA (AAMA) Exam

The CMA (AAMA) exam application is available for download at the AAMA Web site, http://www.aama-ntl.org/. To register for the exam, the applicant must meet the following criteria:

- Recent graduate from a medical assisting program accredited either by the Commission on Accreditation of Allied Health Programs (CAAHEP) or by the Accrediting Bureau of Health Education Schools (ABHES)
- Nonrecent graduate (graduation date more than 12 months prior to the postmark on the application) from a CAAHEP- or ABHES-accredited medical assisting program
- CMA (AAMA) recertificant

Qualified applicants must complete and sign the CMA (AAMA) exam application and send it to the AAMA along with the exam application fee. The application fee is as follows:

- AAMA members and recent CAAHEP/ABHES graduates pay $125.
- All others pay $250.

Computerized certification exams are available throughout the year. Once the AAMA has received, processed, and approved the completed exam application, a scheduling permit with instructions for scheduling the exam appointment at a Prometric test center will be sent to the applicant.

Format of the CMA (AAMA) Exam

The CMA (AAMA) exam consists of 200 questions divided among general, administrative, and clinical categories. It must be completed in 3 hours and 15 minutes, which includes a 15-minute tutorial. The minimum passing score is 425.

Immediately upon completion of the exam, an unofficial pass/fail result will be provided. An official report, including the scores, will be mailed within 6 to 10 weeks following the exam.

The current exam content outline may be found on the AAMA Web site at http://aama-ntl.org/resources/library/ContentOutline.pdf. Figure 1-1 outlines the general, clinical, and administrative skills of the CMA (AAMA).

Maintaining the CMA (AAMA) Credential

The AAMA requires that all CMAs (AAMA) remain current in their practice. In addition, in order to maintain the credential, they must complete 60 CEUs (30 of which must be AAMA approved) in the five years following certification, which must be distributed as follows: 10 administrative, 10 clinical, and 10 general. The remaining 30 CEUs can be distributed anywhere among the three areas.

If the 60 CEUs are not obtained in the five years following certification, in order to maintain the CMA(AAMA) credential, the individual must recertify by taking the examination.

Preparing for Employment

EXTERNSHIP

One of the requirements of ABHES- and CAAHEP-accredited medical assisting programs is the completion of an externship experience prior to graduation. The externship allows

General, Clinical, and Administrative Skills* of the CMA (AAMA)

General Skills

♦ *Communication*
- Recognize and respect cultural diversity
- Adapt communications to individual's understanding
- Employ professional telephone and interpersonal techniques
- Recognize and respond effectively to verbal, nonverbal, and written communications
- Utilize and apply medical terminology appropriately
- Receive, organize, prioritize, store, and maintain transmittable information utilizing electronic technology
- Serve as "communication liaison" between the physician and patient
- Serve as patient advocate professional and health coach in a team approach in health care
- Identify basics of office emergency preparedness

♦ *Legal Concepts*
- Perform within legal (including federal and state statutes, regulations, opinions, and rulings) and ethical boundaries
- Document patient communication and clinical treatments accurately and appropriately
- Maintain medical records
- Follow employer's established policies dealing with the health care contract
- Comply with established risk management and safety procedures
- Recognize professional credentialing criteria
- Identify and respond to issues of confidentiality

♦ *Instruction*
- Function as a health care advocate to meet individual's needs
- Educate individuals in office policies and procedures
- Educate the patient within the scope of practice and as directed by supervising physician in health maintenance, disease prevention, and compliance with patient's treatment plan
- Identify community resources for health maintenance and disease prevention to meet individual patient needs
- Maintain current list of community resources, including those for emergency preparedness and other patient care needs
- Collaborate with local community resources for emergency preparedness
- Educate patients in their responsibilities relating to third-party reimbursements

♦ *Operational Functions*
- Perform inventory of supplies and equipment
- Perform routine maintenance of administrative and clinical equipment
- Apply computer and other electronic equipment techniques to support office operations
- Perform methods of quality control

Clinical Skills

♦ *Fundamental Principles*
- Identify the roles and responsibilities of the medical assistant in the clinical setting
- Identify the roles and responsibilities of other team members in the medical office
- Apply principles of aseptic technique and infection control
- Practice Standard Precautions, including handwashing and disposal of biohazardous materials
- Perform sterilization techniques
- Comply with quality assurance practices

♦ *Diagnostic Procedures*
- Collect and process specimens
- Perform CLIA-waived tests
- Perform electrocardiography and respiratory testing
- Perform phlebotomy, including venipuncture and capillary puncture
- Utilize knowledge of principles of radiology

♦ *Patient Care*
- Perform initial-response screening following protocols approved by supervising physician
- Obtain, evaluate, and record patient history employing critical thinking skills
- Obtain vital signs
- Prepare and maintain examination and treatment areas
- Prepare patient for examinations, procedures and treatments
- Assist with examinations, procedures, and treatments
- Maintain examination/treatment rooms, including inventory of supplies and equipment
- Prepare and administer oral and parenteral (excluding IV) medications and immunizations *(as directed by supervising physician and as permitted by state law)*
- Utilize knowledge of principles of IV therapy
- Maintain medication and immunization records
- Screen and follow up test results
- Recognize and respond to emergencies

Administrative Skills

♦ *Administrative Procedures*
- Schedule, coordinate, and monitor appointments
- Schedule inpatient/outpatient admissions and procedures
- Apply third-party and managed care policies, procedures, and guidelines
- Establish, organize, and maintain patient medical record
- File medical records appropriately

♦ *Practice Finances*
- Perform procedural and diagnostic coding for reimbursement
- Perform billing and collection procedures
- Perform administrative functions, including bookkeeping and financial procedures
- Prepare submittable ("clean") insurance forms

FIGURE 1-1 General, clinical, and administrative skills of the CMA (AAMA). All skills require decision making based on critical thinking concepts.
Reprinted by permission of the American Association of Medical Assistants (AAMA).

the students to use the skills they acquired in the classroom and to work without payment in a healthcare setting under the supervision of someone at the site.

The externship experience should be treated like a paid position. Although employment is not guaranteed upon completion of the externship, many externship sites use the opportunity to train individuals who may be considered for employment either immediately upon completion of the externship or sometimes months later. The externship experience is often thought of as a "working interview." Even though an externship is not a paid experience, it still needs to be treated as if it were, with students maintaining the utmost professionalism and courtesy while on site.

QUALITIES EMPLOYERS ARE LOOKING FOR

Because every employee is a representative of the physician and the practice, in addition to the skills listed at the beginning of the chapter, employers are looking for the following values and skills:

- Reading and comprehension
- Listening
- Speaking
- Writing
- Problem solving
- Teamwork
- Initiative
- Enthusiasm
- Honesty
- Dependability
- Flexibility
- Promptness

JOB SEARCH

If the externship experience does not result in an offer of employment, you must treat the job search as your new full-time job, which begins by drafting a job search plan.

If you have not already done so, it is advantageous to assess your identified strengths and weaknesses. As you draft your resume, highlight your strengths and work on improving the identified weaknesses. You may want to consider asking your instructors and peers for constructive criticism regarding areas that they perceive may need attention. Often during an interview, the interviewer will ask for one identified weakness and what you are doing to overcome it. Completing the personal assessment early in the job search will provide you time to begin working to overcome identified weaknesses.

Once you have completed the personal assessment and the job search plan, you should begin thinking about where you may want to search for job opportunities.

SOURCES FOR JOB OPPORTUNITIES

Classified Ads	Use local and out-of-town newspapers, professional journals, and trade magazines. Use the local public library's copies of national newspapers.
Employment Agencies	Place your name with agencies and career consultants.
Healthcare Facilities in Your Area	Contact hospitals, veterans' facilities, extended care facilities, and ambulatory care sites.
Internet	Use various Web sites, such as monster.com, careerbuilder.com, or jobs.com.
Local Medical Society	Obtain a list of physicians who are looking for help or a list of all the medical practice offices in your area.
Parents and Friends	Network with your friends and relatives. Make sure they know that you are looking for employment.
Personal Physician	Your own physician may network for you and call his or her colleagues.
Professional Organizations	Use both state and local chapters of any professional associations and allied health groups to which you belong.
Publications	AAMA and other local professional publications.
School Placement Service	One of the best sources, since the staff knows your training and skills well. In many cases, prospective employers will call schools to identify potential new employees.
State Employment Office	After you complete the required application forms, your name will be on file for available positions.

RESUME

Often, the first impression of a job applicant is based upon his or her resume. Attention to detail is critical when drafting a resume. Many employers will not even consider applicants who submit resumes with grammatical, typographic, and spelling errors.

In order to minimize the possibility of error, it is important to proofread your resume at least twice and to ask at least two other individuals to proofread it as well.

Resumes should be one to two pages long, typed on good-quality white or off-white paper measuring 8½ by 11 inches, and contain the following information:

- Name, street address, telephone number, and e-mail address. (Be sure that the voice messages for the telephone number and the e-mail address listed are professional.)
- Career goal
- Educational background, including a summary of the skills learned
- Relevant work experience, including dates of employment and brief summaries of duties performed
- Professional organization memberships
- Certifications obtained
- Reference information

Most employers prefer information within the resume to be presented in a chronological format, with the education, work experience, and achievement sections listing the most recent information first (Figure 1-2).

COVER LETTER

The cover letter is another important tool of the job search and should accompany every resume submitted (Figure 1-3). Like the resume, the cover letter should be error free, formatted correctly, and no more than one page long. Cover letters provide the bridge between the position you are applying for and your resume.

The cover letter should clearly state the position you are applying for, explain what you can do for the prospective employer, and describe why your experience, education, and attributes meet the job requirements of the posted position.

INTERVIEW

Once the resume and cover letter have been submitted, the employer may invite you for an interview. Occasionally, employers will conduct an informal telephone interview before scheduling the more formal face-to-face interview. The informal telephone interview is important and should not be treated lightly. Many times, failure to do well during this interview will prevent the candidate from progressing to the more formal interview.

It is important to research the facilities and practices where you will be interviewing. Note the type of practice, the professional background of the physicians within the practice, and any other important information you can find about the practice. Gathering this information will help you become more familiar with the practice and will allow you to prepare one or two pertinent questions for the interviewer (Box 1-1).

Ralph Taylor
222 East Main Street
Chicago, IL 60601
(312) 555-1212
email address
taylorr@anywhere.com

OBJECTIVE	To obtain a medical assisting position where I am able to utilize my administrative and clinical skills.
EDUCATION	
Associate Degree	Central State College, Hometown, Illinois. Expected date of graduation: June 20XX. Major in Health Science.
Medical Assistant	Central State College, Hometown, Illinois. February 20XX June 20XX. Graduated with honors.
EMPLOYMENT	
Medical Assistant	Dr. Earl Brown, Internal Medicine Externship, 2222 State St., Chicago, IL. Externship duties included: drawing blood, handling medical records, scheduling patients, and patient education. 20XX–20XX.
Nursing Assistant	Jane Young, M.D. Family Practice, 111 Hoyne Ave., Chicago, IL. Duties included taking vital signs, administering EKGs, assisting with well-baby visits and in treatment room. 20XX – 20XX.
PROFESSIONAL ORGANIZATIONS AND MEMBERSHIP	
	American Association of Medical Assistants Central State College Medical Club
CREDENTIALS	
Medical Assistant	Passed certification examination in January 20XX.
CPR	Certified by American Heart Association, December 20XX.
REFERENCES	Furnished upon request.

FIGURE 1-2 Sample chronological resume.

Ralph Taylor
222 East Main St.
Chicago, IL 60601
(312) 555-1212

May 20, 20XX

James Stark, M.D.
1450 N. Devonshire
Chicago, IL 60611

Dear Dr. Stark:

This letter is in response to your recent advertisement in the May 19, 20XX, Chicago Sun News for a certified medical assistant.

I believe that my qualifications are a good match for your position. During my medical assisting program at Central State College in Hometown, Illinois, I maintained a 3.6 GPA on a 4.0 scale.

My medical assisting program at Central State College was completed in December 20XX. I passed the American Association of Medical Assistants' certification examination January 27, 20XX. Currently I am completing an associate degree program at CSC and plan to graduate in June 20XX.

The enclosed résumé includes my experience as a part-time nursing assistant for Dr. Jane Young in her family practice office.

I look forward to meeting you to discuss your position needs and my qualifications.

Thank you for your consideration.

Sincerely,

Ralph Taylor

Ralph Taylor, CMA (AAMA)

FIGURE 1-3 Sample cover letter.
Source: From *Pearson's Comprehensive Medical Assisting Administrative and Clinical Competencies,* 2nd ed., executive ed. J. Gill, Upper Saddle River, NJ: Pearson Education, Inc., 2011, p. 1354. Reprinted with permission.

The most common mistakes made during an interview include the following:

- Inappropriate dress or poor grooming
- Poor posture
- Poor eye contact
- Smoking or chewing gum
- Lack of enthusiasm
- Arriving late
- Using slang or incorrect grammar
- Talking too much
- Speaking critically of previous employers
- Failing to ask questions about the organization

If the interviewer has not provided a business card by the end of the interview, be sure to ask for one. This information will be used when sending your thank-you letter and in any future correspondence.

Immediately following the interview, send a letter thanking the interviewer for his or her time (Figure 1-4). This is a good opportunity to once again express your interest in the position.

Box 1-1 Guidelines for a Successful Interview

1. Learn all you can about the organization. Interviewers are impressed by candidates who indicate knowledge of the facility or organization.
2. Have a specific job in mind when you interview so that you project self-confidence.
3. Know your qualifications for each specific job and task requirement. Rehearse or review possible responses several times before going to the interview. You can role-play with a friend or relative to develop confidence.
4. Prepare responses for the interviewer who asks difficult questions or asks you to describe yourself.
5. Be prepared to discuss where you want to be professionally in five years.
6. Carry extra copies of your resume.
7. Arrive 5 to 10 minutes before your scheduled appointment. You may wish to wait outside the facility if you arrive too early.
8. Dress conservatively to project a well-groomed, professional appearance. Generally, a uniform is not required for an interview.
9. Never ask for permission to smoke during an interview. Do not eat anything during an interview unless the interview takes place during a meal. Chewing gum during the interview is never acceptable.
10. Be alert and prompt in answering the interviewer's questions. Do not offer information that is not requested. Keep your answers concise.
11. Ask questions about the position and the organization. It is generally not a good idea to inquire about benefits at the first interview.
12. Bring a pen, your Social Security number, your driver's license number, extra resumes, and the names of three references with their addresses and telephone numbers.

Ralph Taylor
222 E. Main St.
Chicago, IL 60601
(312) 555-1212

May 30, 20XX

James Stark, M.D.
1450 N. Devonshire
Chicago, IL 60611

Dear Dr. Stark:

Thank you for giving me the opportunity to discuss the medical assisting position that you are seeking to fill in your office. I believe that my skills would be a good match with your needs.

I enjoyed meeting you and your staff today, and I would be very interested in working for you.

Thank you for considering my application. I look forward to hearing from you.

Sincerely,

Ralph Taylor

Ralph Taylor, CMA (AAMA)

FIGURE 1-4 Example of a follow-up letter.

From *Pearson's Comprehensive Medical Assisting Administrative and Clinical Competencies*, 2nd ed., executive ed. J. Gill, Upper Saddle River, NJ: Pearson Education, Inc., 2011, p. 1358. Reprinted with permission.

WORKPLACE LEGALITIES

During the interviewing and hiring process, the employer needs to be mindful of the following:

EMPLOYMENT LAWS

Equal pay Act of 1963	Requires equal pay for men and women doing equal work.
Fair Labor Standards Act of 1938	Provides for the minimum wage and overtime pay and prohibits child labor.
Title VII of the Civil Rights Act of 1964	Prevents employers from discriminating against employees based upon race, color, religion, sex, or national origin. Applies to businesses with 15 or more employees who work 20 or more weeks per year.
Wagner Act of 1935	Prevents employers from discriminating against employees due to union membership or organizing activities.

1 APPLICATION

Directions: Select the best answer for each of the following questions. Check your answers in the Answer Key at the end of the book.

1. The following items should be included in a well-prepared resume:
   a. Career objective
   b. Educational background
   c. References
   d. Relevant work experience
   e. All of the above
2. When interviewing with a prospective employer, it is important to
   a. Maintain proper eye contact
   b. Show enthusiasm
   c. Not be afraid to criticize previous employers
   d. A and C
   e. A and B
3. A person shall be employed for a minimum of _________ years to qualify for RMA certification if he or she has not completed the academic requirements:
   a. three
   b. five
   c. six
   d. four
   e. two

4. Duties performed by a medical administrative specialist may include:
   a. Scheduling appointments
   b. Medical transcription
   c. Performing personal errands for the physician
   d. B and C
   e. A and B

5. __________ is/are good sources for job opportunities:
   a. School placement services
   b. The Internet
   c. Employment agencies
   d. Classified ads
   e. All of the above

6. The RMA credential is awarded by which certifying body?
   a. AMA
   b. CMA
   c. AMT
   d. AAMA
   e. RAMT

7. For individuals who passed the certifying exam in January 2006 or later, in order to maintain the RMA credential, it is necessary to earn __________ CEUs over a three-year period after certification.
   a. 10
   b. 15
   c. 20
   d. 25
   e. 30

8. In order to maintain the CMA credential, a person is required to earn __________ CEUs over a five-year period after certification.
   a. 10
   b. 20
   c. 30
   d. 45
   e. 60

9. According to the Bureau of Labor Statistics, U.S. Department of Labor, *Occupational Outlook Handbook, 2010–2011 Edition,* medical assisting is among the fastest-growing occupations and has a projected growth of __________ % between 2008 and 2018.
   a. 24
   b. 28
   c. 30
   d. 34
   e. 38

10. The cost of the RMA (AMT) exam is:
    a. $75
    b. $95
    c. $100
    d. $125
    e. $250

11. The cost of the CMA (AAMA) exam for someone who graduated more than one year earlier and is not a member of the AAMA is:
    a. $75
    b. $95
    c. $100
    d. $125
    e. $250

12. The minimum passing score for the RMA (AMT) exam is:
    a. 70
    b. 100
    c. 250
    d. 400
    e. 425

13. The minimum passing score for the CMA (AAMA) exam is:
    a. 70
    b. 100
    c. 250
    d. 400
    e. 425

14. Which of the following statements regarding resumes is not true?
    a. Use white or off-white paper.
    b. List all work experience.
    c. Use 8½ by 11 inch paper.
    d. Include your career objective.
    e. Include your educational background.

15. In preparation for and during an interview, you should do all of the following except:
    a. Arrive 5 to 10 minutes early
    b. Ask questions about the organization
    c. Talk about former employers
    d. Show enthusiasm
    e. Dress conservatively

2 Learning Styles, Study Skills, and Test-Taking Strategies

CONTENTS

Taking tests can be one of the most anxiety-ridden processes an individual goes through, and taking tests on information acquired cumulatively over several months can be even more stressful. But if you practice good study skills, plan, and prepare long in advance for the day you take the RMA (AMT), CMAS, and/or CMA (AAMA) exam(s), you will be able to put much of the anxiety aside. Many medical assisting instructors recommend studying for at least 40 hours in preparation for taking the exams.

Learning Styles

If you have not done so already, it is important to know and understand they type of learner you are and adapt your strategy for studying accordingly (Box 2-1).

Study Skills

When you begin making your study plan, be sure to think about your surroundings. Where do you study best? Is it away from home, maybe at the library, where you have peace and quiet? Is it at your desk at home later in the evening once the chores are done and everyone in the house is settling down? It is suggested that you choose a place to study that is comfortable, yet not too comfortable, such as the bed, where you may fall asleep while studying.

Many individuals devise various memory aids to help them while studying, such as rhymes, acronyms, word associations, and flash cards. These memory aids are especially helpful when studying medical terminology, anatomy and physiology, and pharmacology.

Box 2-1 Types of Learners

What Kind of Learner Are You?

To become a successful student, you must evaluate the type of learner you are. Following are the characteristics of the visual, auditory, and tactile learner.

The visual learner

- Tries to envision the word when spelling it out.
- Dislikes listening for long periods of time.
- Becomes distracted by movement when trying to concentrate.
- May not remember names but typically will remember faces.
- Prefers face-to-face meetings.
- Prefers to read descriptions when learning new material.
- Likes to look at pictures when learning new material.

The auditory learner

- Tries to sound out a word when spelling it out.
- Enjoys listening rather than talking.
- Becomes distracted by sounds or noises when trying to concentrate.
- Prefers the telephone to face-to-face meetings.
- Prefers verbal instructions.

The tactile learner

- Writes a word out when learning to spell it.
- Uses gestures and expressive movements when talking.
- Becomes distracted by activity when trying to concentrate.
- Prefers to talk while participating in activities.
- Is not necessarily a good reader; prefers stories that are action oriented.
- Tends to figure things out during the process rather than read directions.

Skill Sets

Once you know the type of learner you are, take steps to use your skills in learning and reviewing material.

The visual learner might try

- Looking at pictures or diagrams when learning new material.
- Studying in a quiet room with no distractions.
- Asking for descriptions or asking instructors to explain how a topic might apply in the real world (e.g., "Would you demonstrate that skill to the class?").

The auditory learner might try

- Reading aloud or taping his or her voice and playing it back to study new material.
- Taping the instructor's lecture and replaying it later to study.
- Studying in a quiet room with no distractions.
- Working with study groups where students discuss the material they've learned.
- Hearing descriptions when learning new material.

The tactile learner might try

- Writing material down several times in order to memorize it.
- Studying in a quiet area with no distractions.
- Asking the instructor to give examples of how a topic is addressed (e.g., "Would you allow the class to role-play that activity so that we can see what it feels like?").
- Practicing activities or skills in order to commit them to memory.

MEMORY AIDS

Rhymes	An example of a rhyme that almost everyone is familiar with is "In 1492, Columbus sailed the ocean blue."
Acronyms	Acronyms can be created for any series of information you must remember and consist of the first letter of each term. For example, the five stages of grief are Denial, Anger, Bargaining, Depression, and Acceptance. You could create the acronym **D** **A** **B** **D** **A** which will help you remember these stages of grief.
Word Associations	An example of a word association is the medical terminology suffix –*malacia,* which means "softening." The word you could associate with this is *lace,* which is soft.
Flash Cards	Create sets of flash cards organized by body system and/or type(s) of medication(s). • Place the term on one side of the card and the definition on the other side. Use pictures or diagrams if possible. • Go through the cards and quiz yourself or work with a partner, separating the terms you define correctly from those you define incorrectly. • Next, go through the terms you didn't define correctly, again separating those answered correctly from those answered incorrectly. • Continue until you are able to define all terms correctly. This is a great study tool you can take anywhere and use anytime.
Teach the Material to Someone Else	It is estimated that when you are required to teach another individual, you retain approximately 90% of what was taught. Share what you are studying/learning with others; this will help you retain information.

Ask others what study tools they use, and be willing to share those you employ.

STUDY GROUPS

Some individuals find it beneficial to participate in a study group, while others find it distracting. If you benefit from study groups, be sure that you are studying with others who are good students and who are either at your level or above it. Some of the benefits of study groups are as follows:

- Participants are able to break down complex ideas into understandable units.
- Group members depend upon your participation, so you are more apt to be prepared.
- You have an opportunity to compare your study notes with those of other members. They may have information you missed and vice versa.
- Studying becomes an interactive activity.
- Group members become a support system.
- You have an opportunity to learn what others do to study and prepare for exams.

TIME MANAGEMENT

Everyone studies and retains information differently. That is why it is important to know what works best for you. Are you a "morning person" or a "night owl"? If you tend to be more alert and productive during the early hours of the day, it is better to get up early and study rather than stay up late at night.

Studies have shown that more information is retained when you study in two or three 30- to 45-minute increments rather than two hours straight. Try studying for 30 to 45 minutes, taking a 15-minute break, studying for 30 to 45 minutes, taking a 15-minute break, and then finishing with another 30 to 45 minutes of studying. During the 15-minute breaks, it is suggested that you get up, walk around, go outside, get something to drink, and then settle back for the next 30- to 45-minute study session. The key is to not get distracted during the breaks and go back to studying at the designated time (Box 2-2).

Box 2-2 Time Management

One of the greatest difficulties for new students is time management and organization of priorities. For students who have trouble in this area, the following steps may help:

- Set aside blocks of time for studying.
- Take periodic breaks when studying; get up and move around, get a drink, or close your eyes for a few moments.
- Prioritize your assignments. Many students find it helpful to write down their assignments and place numbers next to each to indicate the order in which they need to be done.
- Study or read while doing other activities. Students can study or read while exercising at the gym or elsewhere.
- Review study material just prior to class on test day.
- Create "to do" lists.
- Use a daily/weekly/monthly calendar. Write down the dates of upcoming tests or project due dates; then backtrack to add the dates when certain stages of the project should be completed. For example, if a paper is due four weeks from today, add a note to the calendar for one week from today that the outline should be completed, a note for two weeks from today that the rough draft should be completed, and so on.
- Look for study partners for each class. Find study partners who are good students, not those who are not as dedicated as you are to learning the material. Spend time together each week going over the material from the class and studying or preparing for tests or projects.

Students should always be able to consult the course instructor for clarification of subject matter or for verification of course progress. Students must remain aware of their progress in any given class and take an active part in ensuring their own success.

Test-Taking Tips and Strategies

TEST-TAKING TIPS

- Take several practice tests. If you are planning to take the certification exam on the computer, you should take practice tests in this mode; for taking the paper-and-pencil exam, practice taking tests in this format.
- Practice tests help you assess your knowledge and identify areas that you should work on.
- Make sure that you understand *why* the correct answers are correct.
- Do not cram; it does not work.
- Make a list of what you do not know as you review.
- Do not skip from section to section while taking the test.
- Accept the fact that you will not know everything; guess if you do not know the answer but use reasoning (associate and eliminate).
- Don't overanalyze the question or the available answers.
- Eliminate grammatically incorrect answer options.
- Pay particular attention to italicized, capitalized, and underlined options.

TEST-TAKING STRATEGIES

Read the directions and make sure that you understand them. If there is anything you don't understand, ask the exam proctor for clarification. The proctor cannot answer any questions from the exam itself, but he or she can clarify the directions.

MULTIPLE-CHOICE QUESTIONS

All questions on the CMA (AAMA) RMA (AMT) and CMAS exams are multiple choice, with five answers to choose from (A through E). Some questions may appear to have more than one correct answer; you must use reasoning and choose the best answer.

As you begin to work through the questions, keep the following in mind:

- Prior to beginning the exam, take a few slow, deep breaths; this will help relieve any anxiety you might be feeling. Any time you begin to feel anxious, close your eyes, take a few more slow, deep breaths, and resume taking the exam.
- Be sure to read the entire question before answering.
- After you have read the question, come up with the answer mentally and then look for the corresponding answer in the choices presented.
- Don't second-guess yourself. Usually your first instinct is correct.

- If you are unable to answer immediately, don't spend too much time thinking; mark that question and come back to it. Many times the answer to one question can be found in another question.
- Once you have finished the last question, go back and answer any questions you had marked to come back to.
- When working on the questions you had marked to come back to, if you are still unsure of the correct answer, eliminate the choices you know are incorrect and then focus on the remaining options. If you are still unsure, take a guess.
- Prior to submitting the exam, scan your answers and make sure that all questions have been answered.
- Change your answers only if you are positive that you initially answered incorrectly.

TIME MANAGEMENT

It is important to know how many questions are on the exam and how much time you have to answer them.

The CMA (AAMA) exam consists of 200 questions, and you have three hours to complete it. In order to complete the exam within the time allowed, you must answer 67 questions per hour and you must not spend more than an average of 54 seconds on each question.

The RMA (AMT) exam consists of 200 to 210 questions, and you have two hours to complete it. In order to complete the exam within the time allowed, you must answer 105 questions per hour and you must not spend more than an average of 36 seconds on each question.

If you find that you are spending more than the average time allowed on most practice questions, look through the study hints and suggestions above on multiple-choice exams. Continue practicing until you are able to finish within the time allowed.

Exam Day

Make sure that you are well rested and nourished the day of the exam. It is important to get plenty of rest the night prior to the exam and also have something nutritious to eat the day of the exam. You may want to briefly review the topics prior to taking the exam, but this is not the time to cram. This should be done merely for review purposes.

Make sure that you wear comfortable clothing to the exam. It is suggested that you dress in layers that you can add or remove, depending upon the temperature in the exam room. The testing sites are required to keep the testing facilities at a comfortable temperature; however, what is comfortable for one individual may not be comfortable for another.

COMPUTERIZED TESTING

If you are taking the exam at a computerized testing site, consider the following:

- You will receive notification via the U.S. Postal Service that you have been approved to take the exam and may schedule it for a day and time convenient for you.
- Because you can schedule your exam for any day of the week and any time of day, think about when you do your best work. If you are usually tired on Mondays, you may want to schedule the exam for a day later in the week. Also think about whether you are more alert during the early or later portion of the day and schedule the exam for a time that works best for you.
- Know exactly where you are going and allow plenty of time to get there. Consider any possible traffic problems as well.
- Plan to arrive at least 15 minutes prior to the scheduled exam time.
- Have two forms of valid identification, including one containing your photo.
- Once you have presented your identification, you will be fingerprinted and have your picture taken. The fingerprint will allow you to enter and leave the testing room.
- You may not take anything into the exam room except your identification. All purses, backpacks, cell phones, pagers, calculators, and so on must be left outside. Most facilities will provide lockers to store your personal belongings while you are taking the exam.
- Some facilities may "pat you down" before you are allowed to enter the exam room. This is done to ensure that you do not have any of the above-mentioned equipment on your person, as well as any study items that are not allowed.
- No chewing gum, candy or beverages are allowed in the exam room.
- Most facilities have cameras in the exam room and an individual camera placed in each testing booth. Do not let this be a distraction.
- In addition to the camera, there will be a human observer in the exam room.
- Ear plugs may be provided to help reduce any outside noise.

- When you are told to begin, you will read the directions and begin the exam once the preliminary verifications have been completed.
- If you need to use the restroom during the exam, you must raise your hand, wait for the observer to come over, and let him or her know; you must then use your fingerprint to leave the testing room. When you return, you will need to use your fingerprint to enter the room again. The time you are out of the testing room will not be added back to the allowed testing time.
- When you have completed the exam, you must raise your hand and wait for the observer to come over and excuse you. Once again, you will need to use your fingerprint to leave the testing room.

PAPER-AND-PENCIL TESTING (RMA [AMT] AND CMAS ONLY)

If you opt to take your exam using paper and pencil, consider the following:

- You will be notified via the U.S. Postal Service of the date for which the exam has been scheduled and the site where it will be administered.
- Know exactly where you are going and give yourself plenty of time to get there. Consider any possible traffic problems as well.
- Plan to arrive approximately 15 minutes prior to the scheduled exam time.
- Report to the designated area for check-in.
- Have at least one piece of valid photo identification available, such as a driver's license or military identification.
- Verify that the information on the exam roster is correct, including the spelling of your name, your Social Security number, and the address to which the exam results will be mailed.
- Have two #2 sharpened pencils with erasers available.
- You may not have a purse, backpack, cell phone, pager, calculator, and so on with you. All of these items must be left either outside the exam room or in a designated area within the exam room.
- If it is necessary to use the restroom during the exam, you may ask for permission to do so; however, the time spent there will not be added back to the time allowed to complete the exam.

Good luck, and do the best you can!

2 APPLICATION

Directions: Select the best answer for each of the following questions. Check your answers in the Answer Key at the end of the book.

1. Someone who prefers face-to-face meetings is most likely a __________ learner.
   a. Tactile
   b. Visual
   c. Auditory
   d. Manual
   e. Digital
2. Study memory aids include:
   a. Flash cards
   b. Rhymes
   c. Acronyms
   d. Word associations
   e. All of the above
3. Teaching material to another person is an effective study aid because it is estimated that a person retains __________% of the material taught.
   a. 70
   b. 75
   c. 85
   d. 90
   e. 95
4. Benefits of study groups include:
   a. Studying becomes interactive.
   b. One can do less preparation due to the number of people involved.
   c. One prepares more so as not to let the group down.

d. A and B
e. A and C

5. When taking the RMA (AMT) and CMAS exams using paper and pencil, you may not bring ____________into the exam room:
   a. Calculator
   b. Backpack
   c. #2 pencils
   d. Cell phone
   e. A, B, and D

6. Studies have shown that more information is retained when you study in which of the following increments?
   a. Two 30- to 45-minute sessions with a 15-minute break
   b. Three 30- to 45-minute sessions with 15-minute breaks
   c. Four 30- to 45-minute sessions with 15-minute breaks
   d. A and B
   e. B and C

7. The CMA (AAMA) exam consists of how many questions, and how much time do you have to complete it?
   a. 200 questions, two hours to complete
   b. 200 questions, three hours to complete
   c. 200 to 210 questions, two hours to complete
   d. 210 questions, two hours to complete
   e. 210 questions, three hours to complete

8. The RMA (AMT) exam consists of how many questions, and how much time do you have to complete it?
   a. 200 questions, two hours to complete
   b. 200 questions, three hours to complete
   c. 200 to 210 questions, two hours to complete
   d. 210 questions, two hours to complete
   e. 210 questions, three hours to complete

9. When checking in for computerized testing, you may be required to provide which of the following?
   a. Photo identification, current credit card, or other form of identification
   b. Proof of payment for the exam
   c. Fingerprint
   d. A and B
   e. A and C

10. Regarding answering test questions, which of the following series of steps is in the correct sequence?
    a. Read the directions, read the key words in the question, choose the correct answer, and mark the correct answer
    b. Read the directions, read the key words in the question, determine the correct answer mentally, look for the answer in the group of choices, and mark the correct answer
    c. Read the directions, read the entire question, determine the correct answer mentally, look for the answer in the group of choices, and mark the correct answer
    d. Read the directions, read the entire question, determine the correct answer mentally, and look for the answer in the group of choices
    e. Read the directions, read the key words in the question, determine the correct answer mentally, and look for the answer in the group of choices

3 Medical Terminology

CONTENTS

A thorough understanding of medical terminology is one of the most crucial building blocks for success within the medical profession. If you commit to memory and use the medical terms you have learned, you will be able to converse with and understand what others within the medical profession are saying.

Medical terms are made up of three types of word parts: *prefixes, suffixes,* and *root words*. There are some instances in which a vowel is attached to a root word and then called a *combining form*. All word parts work together to form the meaning of the term.

Following is a brief list of some of the most common medical terminology word parts. A medical dictionary or medical terminology textbook should be consulted for a more complete list.

Word Structure

Dividing a word into its root, combining form, prefix, and suffix and understanding each part separately will ultimately help you discover the word's definition. It is important to know that most, but not all, medical terms have literal translations.

A. **Root: the basic meaning of the word.** Root words usually provide information about the body part.

Example: *cardi*ac

cardi = root word

cardi means "heart"

*cardi*ac is defined as pertaining to the heart

***Combining form*: a root word plus a vowel such as *a, e, i, o, u. O* is the most common combining vowel.** Combining forms are used to help make pronunciation easier. Always use the combining form when using two root words next to each other. (Note: In most cases, you would not use the combining form if the suffix also begins with a vowel.)

Example: *cardio*myopathy

cardio = combining form

cardio means "heart"

*cardio*myopathy is defined as disease of the heart muscle

In this example, the combining form is used because the root word *cardi* is being joined with another root word, *my*.

B. **Suffix: the ending of the word.** The suffix usually provides information about a procedure, condition, disorder, or disease; however, there are several suffixes that merely mean "pertaining to."

Example: endocard*itis*

itis = suffix

itis means "inflammation"

endocarditis is defined as inflammation within the heart

C. **Prefix: the first part of the word.** The prefix usually provides information about location, time, number, or status.

Example: *endo*carditis

endo = prefix

endo means "within"

*endo*carditis is defined as inflammation within the heart

At a minimum, you will always find that medical terms have at least one root word. Most medical terms also contain a suffix but not necessarily a prefix.

When trying to define a medical term, always start at the end of the word with the suffix; then go to the prefix (if there is one) and then on to the root word.

ROOT WORDS AND COMBINING FORM DEFINITIONS

COLOR

Root Word	Meaning
albino	white
chromo	color
cyano	blue
erythro	red
leuko	white
melano	black
polio	gray
xantho-	yellow

DIRECTION

Root Word	Meaning
antero	front
disto	away from trunk
dorso	back
latero	away from midline
medio	toward midline
postero	back
proximo	toward trunk
ventro	front

Parts of the Body as Related to Body System

CELLS AND TISSUES

Root Word	Meaning
adeno	gland
cyto	cell
histo	tissue
karyo	nucleus
muco	mucus

CIRCULATORY

Root Word	Meaning
arterio	artery
angio	vessel
aorto	aorta
athero	plaque
cardio	heart
hemato	blood
hemo	blood
phlebo	vein
thrombo	clot
veno	vein

GASTROINTESTINAL

Root Word	Meaning
ano	anus
chole	bile
cholecysto	gallbladder
colono	colon
entero	intestines
esophago	esophagus
gastro	stomach
glosso	tongue
hepato	liver
ictero	jaundice
laparo	abdomen
oro	mouth
pancreato	pancreas
procto	rectum
spleno	spleen
stomato	mouth

INTEGUMENTARY

Root Word	Meaning
cutaneo	skin
dermato	skin
dermo	skin
hidro	sweat glands
kerato	horny layer
lipo	fat
myco	fungus
onycho	nail
rhytido	wrinkle
xero	dry

MUSCULOSKELETAL

Root Word	Meaning
arthro	joint
cephalo	head
cervico	neck
costo	rib
cranio	skull
musculo	muscle
myo	muscle
osteo	bone
tendino	tendon
tendo	tendon
teno	tendon

NERVOUS

Root Word	Meaning
encephalo	brain
meningo	meninges
myelo	marrow, spinal cord
narco	sleep
neuro	nerve
psycho	mind
somno	sleep

REPRODUCTIVE

Root Word	Meaning
cervico	cervix
colpo	vagina
gyneco	female
hystero	uterus
mammo	breast
meno	menstruation
metrio	uterus
oophoro	ovaries
orchid	testicles
orcho	testicles
ovario	ovaries
salpingo	fallopian tube
utero	uterus

RESPIRATORY

Root Word	Meaning
broncho	bronchial tube
laryngo	larynx
naso	nose
pharyngo	pharynx
pneumo	air in the lungs
pulmo	lung
pulmono	lung
rhino	nose
thoraco	chest
tracheo	trachea

URINARY

Root Word	Meaning
cysto	bladder
litho	stone
nephro	kidney
pyelo	renal pelvis
reno	kidney
uretero	ureter
urethra	urethra

SPECIAL SENSES

Root Word	Meaning
audio	hearing
blepharo	eyelid
irido	iris
kerato	cornea
oculo	eye
oto	ear
presbyo	old age
pseudo	false
tympano	eardrum

PATHOLOGY/RADIOLOGY

Root Word	Meaning
carcino	cancer
crypto	hidden
onco	tumor
patho	disease
pyo	pus
pyro	fire

SUFFIXES

DIAGNOSIS AND SYMPTOMS

Suffix	Meaning
-algia	pain
-ase	enzyme
-blast	immature
-cele	swollen sac, protrusion
-cyte	cell
-dynia	pain
-edema	swelling
-emesis	vomiting
-emia	blood condition
-esis	abnormal condition
-itis	inflammation of
-genic	forming
-lith	stone
-lysis	destruction or breaking apart

DIAGNOSIS AND SYMPTOMS (*Continued*)

Suffix	Meaning
-malacia	softening of
-megaly	enlarged
-oid	resembling
-ology	the study of
-ologist	one who studies
-oma	tumor, growth
-opia	vision
-osis	diseased
-pathy	diseased
-penia	deficiency
-phagia	swallowing
-plegia	paralysis
-pnea	breathing
-ptosis	drooping
-rrhagia	excessive or unusual discharge
-rrhea	flowing
-rrhexis	rupture
-sclerosis	abnormal hardening
-stasis	controlling

SURGICAL AND PROCEDURE

Suffix	Meaning
-centesis	surgical puncture to remove fluid
-cide	causing death; killing
-desis	fixing together
-ectomy	excision; removal
-gram	written record
-graph	record
-graphy	process of recording
-meter	instrument used to measure
-metry	to measure
-ostomy	forming an artificial opening
-otomy	incision
-pexy	surgical fixation
-plasty	surgical repair
-rrhaphy	suturing
-scope	instrument for viewing
-scopy	visual examination

PREFIXES

DIRECTION AND POSITION

Prefix	Meaning
ab-	away
ad-	toward
ecto-	outside
endo-	within
epi-	above
exo-	outside
hyper-	above
hypo-	below
inter-	between
intra-	within
para-	beside
peri-	around
retro-	behind, backward
sub-	below
supra-	above
trans-	across or through

AMOUNTS AND TIME

Prefix	Meaning
ante-	before
bi-	two
brady-	slow
hemi-	half
macro-	large
micro-	small
milli-	one-thousandth
multi-	many
nulli-	none
oligo-	scanty
pan-	all
poly-	many
post-	after
pre-	before
quadri-	four
semi-	partial
tachy-	fast
tri-	three
uni-	one

DESCRIPTIVE PREFIXES

Prefix	Meaning
a-	not, negation
anti-	against
auto-	self
dys-	difficult, painful, bad
eu-	normal
homo-	same
homeo-	similar
hetero-	different
mal-	bad
neo-	new
ortho-	straight
pseudo-	false

PLURALS

The following table should serve only as a guide for converting medical terms from the singular form to the plural form. Keep in mind that there are exceptions to the rules listed here.

CONVERTING SINGULAR TO PLURAL

Singular: Term Ends in	Plural	Singular Becomes Plural
a ax ex ix	e ices	vertebra=vertebrae appendix=appendices
is	es	diagnosis=diagnoses
itis	ides	meningitis=meningitides
nx	nges	phalanx=phalanges
on	a	ganglion=ganglia
um	a	ovum=ova
us	i	alvelolus=alveoli

Body Planes, Divisions, Regions, Directions, and Anatomical Position

BODY PLANES

The body is divided into four planes (Figure 3-1):

1. **Frontal (coronal):** divides the body into front and back (anterior and posterior); anterior = ventral, posterior = dorsal
2. **Transverse:** divides the body (at the waist) into upper and lower (superior and inferior)
3. **Sagittal:** divides the body into right and left sides
4. **Midsagittal:** divides the body into equal right and left sides

DIVISIONS

The abdomen is divided into four quadrants, with the umbilicus (navel) as the center (Figure 3-2).

1. **Right upper quadrant (RUQ):** right upper area of the abdomen; contains parts of the liver, gallbladder, and intestines
2. **Left upper quadrant (LUQ):** left upper area of the abdomen; contains parts of the liver, stomach, pancreas, spleen, and intestines
3. **Right lower quadrant (RLQ):** right lower area of the abdomen; contains parts of the intestines, appendix, right ureter, ovary, and fallopian tube
4. **Left lower quadrant (LLQ):** left lower abdominal area; contains parts of the intestines, left ureter, ovary, and fallopian tube

REGIONS

The abdomen is divided like a tic-tac-toe board, with the umbilicus in the center (Figure 3-3).

1. **Top two side squares:** right and left hypochondriac regions
2. **Bottom two side squares:** right and left inguinal (iliac) regions
3. **Top middle square:** epigastric region
4. **Middle two side squares:** right and left lateral regions
5. **Center square:** umbilical region
6. **Lower middle square:** hypogastric region

DIRECTIONS

There are eight directional anatomical terms (Figure 3-4):

1. **Distal:** away from the trunk
2. **Proximal:** toward the trunk
3. **Lateral:** away from the midline
4. **Medial:** midline
5. **Anterior (ventral):** front, in front of
6. **Posterior (dorsal):** back, in back of
7. **Inferior (caudal):** lower, below
8. **Superior (cephalic):** at the head, above

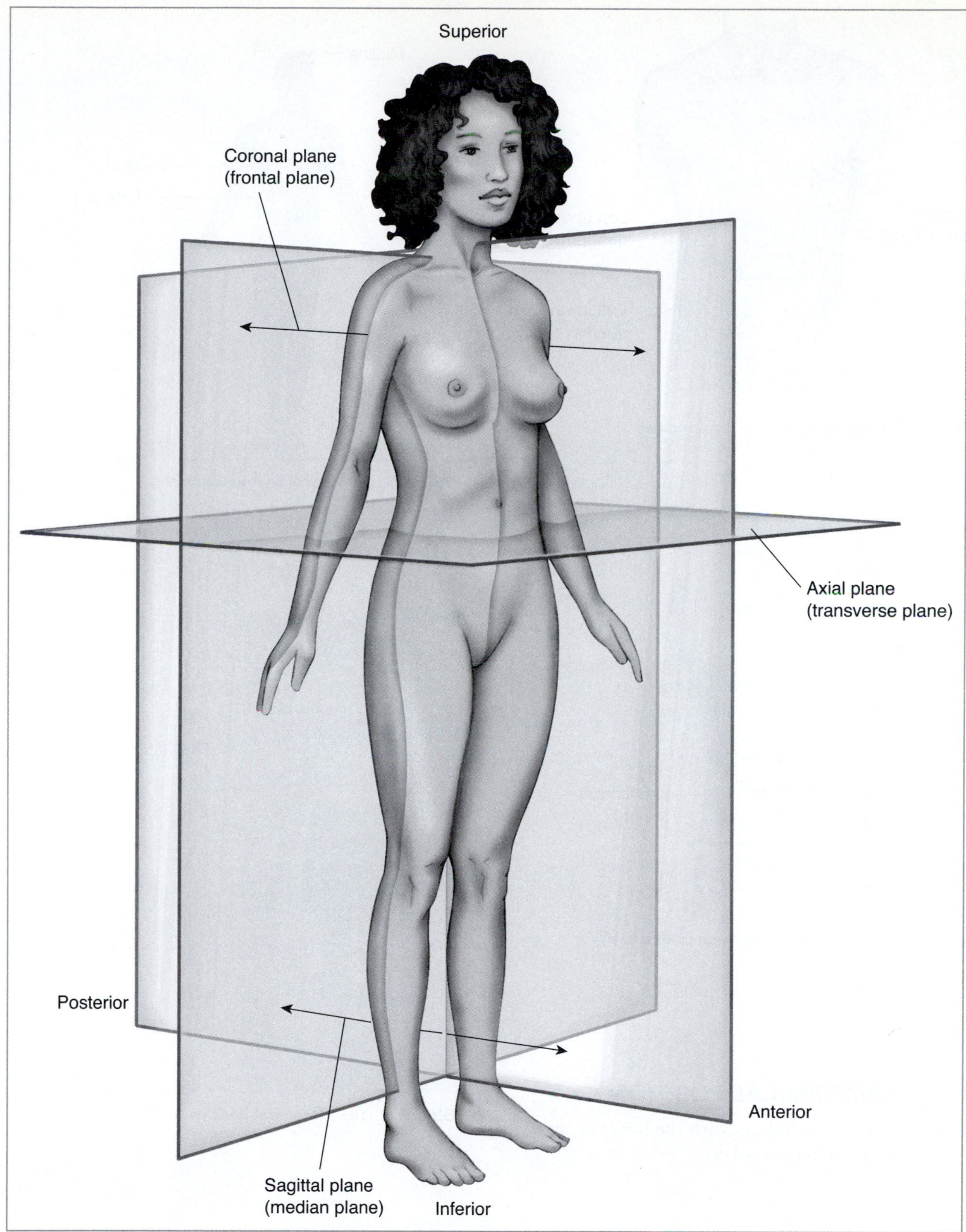

FIGURE 3-1 **Anatomical planes.**

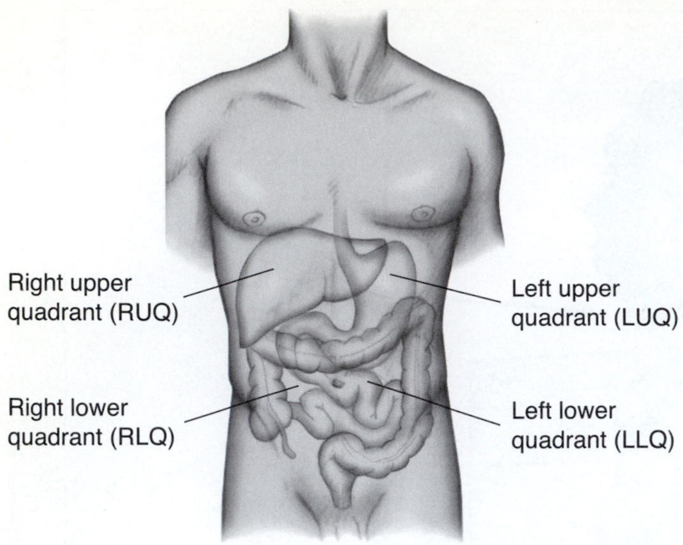

FIGURE 3-2 The four quadrants of the abdomen

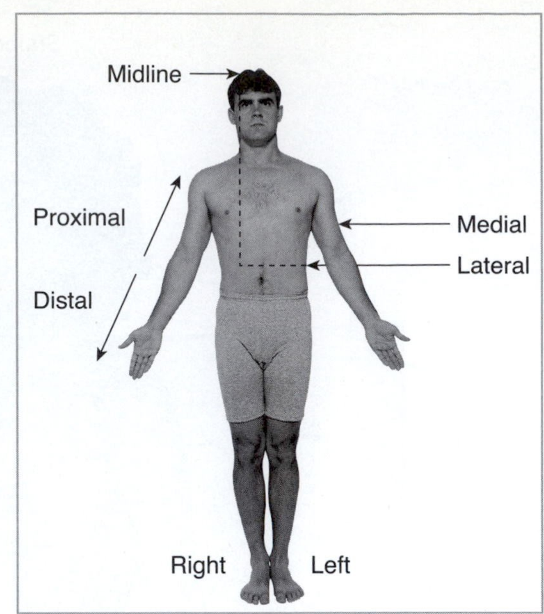

FIGURE 3-4 Directional anatomical terms.

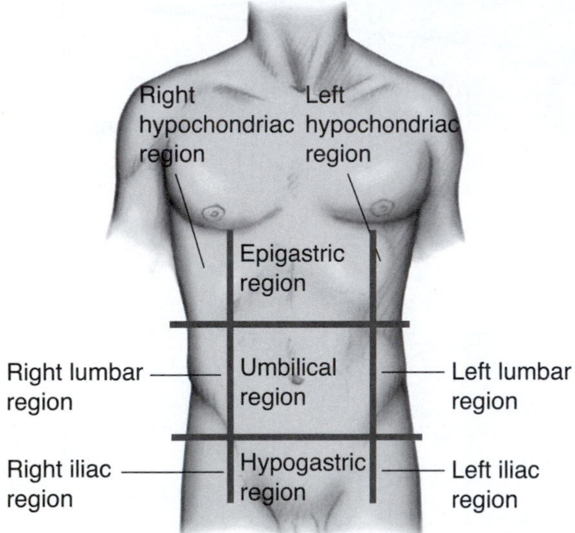

FIGURE 3-3 The regions of the abdominopelvic cavity.

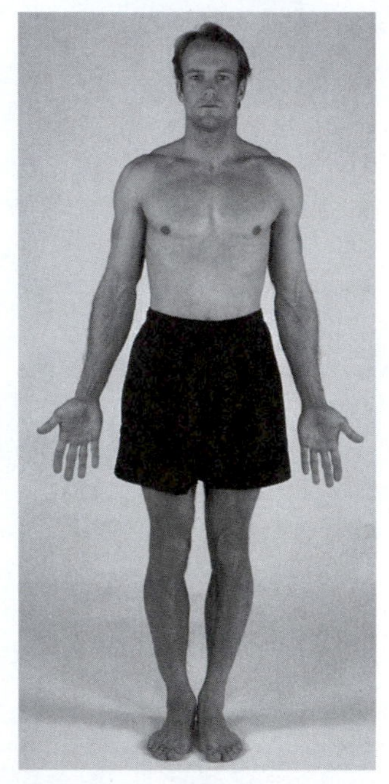

FIGURE 3-5 The anatomical position.

ANATOMICAL POSITION

The body is erect and standing, with the hands at the sides and the palms forward (Figure 3-5).

Abbreviations

Abbreviations are frequently used in medical settings, and as a medical assistant, you will be expected to be familiar with the most common ones. The abbreviations in the following sections are some of the ones most commonly used. Be careful that you do not use any unapproved abbreviations.

ABBREVIATIONS: MEDICATION ADMINISTRATION

Abbreviation	Meaning
a.c.	before meals
ad lib	as desired
b.i.d.	twice a day
gtt.	drops
h	hour
IM	intramuscular
mL	milliliter
NKDA	no known drug allergies
NKA	no known allergies
N.P.O.	nothing by mouth
p.c.	after meals
PO	by mouth
PRN	as needed
q.i.d.	four times a day
stat	immediately
tab	tablet
t.i.d.	three times a day

ABBREVIATIONS: MEDICAL DIAGNOSES

Abbreviation	Meaning
CA	Cancer
CHF	congestive heart failure
COPD	chronic obstructive pulmonary disease
CVA	cerebrovascular accident
DM	diabetes mellitus
IDDM	insulin-dependent diabetes mellitus
MI	myocardial infarction
MS	multiple sclerosis
NIDDM	non-insulin-dependent diabetes mellitus
R.A.	rheumatoid arthritis
TB	tuberculosis
TIA	transient ischemic attack
URI	upper respiratory infection
UTI	urinary tract infection

MISCELLANEOUS ABBREVIATIONS

Abbreviation	Meaning
ADL	activities of daily living
BM	bowel movement
BMI	body mass index
BP	blood pressure
Bx	biopsy
CT	computed tomography
D & C	dilation and curettage
DOA	dead on arrival
DOB	date of birth
DNR	do not resuscitate
Dx	diagnosis
ENT	ear, nose, throat
FU	follow-up
Fx	fracture
HPI	history of present illness
Hx	history
I&D	incision and drainage
K	potassium
MRI	magnetic resonance imaging
N/V	nausea and vomiting
ROS	review of systems
SOB	shortness of breath
Tx	treatment
UA	urinalysis
WNL	within normal limits

Key Concepts

The Joint Commission has determined that some abbreviations should no longer be used because they are easily confused or look like other abbreviations, depending upon someone's writing (Figure 3-6). This information will be determined by your employer's policy.

Medical Specialties

It is important to be familiar with the various medical specialists that patients may be seeing. Often patients are seeing multiple physicians at any given time for specific disease processes. See pages 31 and 32 for lists of common medical and surgical specialties.

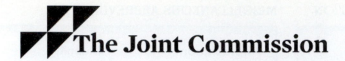

Official "Do Not Use" List[1]

Do Not Use	Potential Problem	Use Instead
U (unit)	Mistaken for "0" (zero), the number "4" (four) or "cc"	Write "unit"
IU (International Unit)	Mistaken for IV (intravenous) or the number 10 (ten)	Write "International Unit"
Q.D., QD, q.d., qd (daily) Q.O.D., QOD, q.o.d, qod (every other day)	Mistaken for each other Period after the Q mistaken for "I" and the "O" mistaken for "I"	Write "daily" Write "every other day"
Trailing zero (X.0 mg)* Lack of leading zero (.X mg)	Decimal point is missed	Write X mg Write 0.X mg
MS MSO_4 and $MgSO_4$	Can mean morphine sulfate or magnesium sulfate Confused for one another	Write "morphine sulfate" Write "magnesium sulfate"

[1] Applies to all orders and all medication-related documentation that is handwritten (including free-text computer entry) or on pre-printed forms.

***Exception:** A "trailing zero" may be used only where required to demonstrate the level of precision of the value being reported, such as for laboratory results, imaging studies that report size of lesions, or catheter/tube sizes. It may not be used in medication orders or other medication-related documentation.

Additional Abbreviations, Acronyms and Symbols
(For possible future inclusion in the Official "Do Not Use" List)

Do Not Use	Potential Problem	Use Instead
> (greater than) < (less than)	Misinterpreted as the number "7" (seven) or the letter "L" Confused for one another	Write "greater than" Write "less than"
Abbreviations for drug names	Misinterpreted due to similar abbreviations for multiple drugs	Write drug names in full
Apothecary units	Unfamiliar to many practitioners Confused with metric units	Use metric units
@	Mistaken for the number "2" (two)	Write "at"
cc	Mistaken for U (units) when poorly written	Write "mL" or "ml" or "milliliters" ("mL" is preferred)
µg	Mistaken for mg (milligrams) resulting in one thousand-fold overdose	Write "mcg" or "micrograms"

Updated 3/5/09

FIGURE 3-6 The Joint Commission's official "Do Not Use" list.
The Joint Commission, 2010. Reprinted with permission.

COMMON MEDICAL SPECIALTIES

Specialty Type	Service(s) Provided
Allergist	Diagnoses and treats allergic conditions
Cardiologist	Diagnoses and treats heart and cardiovascular system conditions
Dermatologist	Diagnoses and treats skin disorders
Emergency Physician	Treats patients with emergent needs, such as in emergency rooms
Endocrinologist	Diagnoses and treats hormone-related disorders
Family Practitioner	Acts as a primary care physician for patients of all ages, treating varied illnesses and performing routine screenings (e.g., physical examinations)
Gastroenterologist	Diagnoses and treats disorders related to the stomach and intestines
General Practitioner	Same as the family practice physician (see preceding), except may not accept child patients
Gerontologist	Diagnoses and treats conditions of the elderly population
Gynecologist	Diagnoses and treats conditions related to the female reproductive system
Hematologist	Diagnoses and treats conditions associated with blood disorders
Infertility Practitioner	Diagnoses and treats disorders related to infertility problems and helps achieve pregnancy via medical means
Intensive Care Physician	Treats patients in the hospital intensive care unit
Internist	Focuses on the prevention and treatment of adult diseases
Neonatologist	Diagnoses and treats newborns
Nephrologist	Diagnoses and treats conditions associated with the kidneys
Neurologist	Diagnoses and treats conditions associated with the nervous system
Obstetrician	Treats pregnant women through the postpartum period
Oncologist	Diagnoses and treats patients with cancerous conditions
Ophthalmologist	Diagnoses and treats eye conditions
Orthopedist	Diagnoses and treats conditions associated with the musculoskeletal system
Otolaryngologist	Diagnoses and treats conditions associated with the ears, nose, and throat
Pediatrician	Treats children
Podiatrist	Diagnoses and treats foot conditions
Proctologist	Diagnoses and treats conditions associated with the colon, rectum, and anus
Psychiatrist	Diagnoses and treats mental disorders
Pulmonologist	Diagnoses and treats conditions associated with the respiratory system
Radiologist	Interprets radiographs (X-rays) and other imaging studies (e.g., ultrasounds or mammograms)
Rheumatologist	Diagnoses and treats conditions associated with arthritis or other joint disorders
Urologist	Diagnoses and treats conditions associated with the urinary system

Source: Medical Assisting: Foundations and Practices by M. S. Frazier, C. Malone, and C. Morgan, Upper Saddle River, NJ: Pearson Education, Inc., 2010, p. 28. Reprinted with permission.

COMMON SURGICAL SPECIALTIES

Surgical Specialty Type	Description
Cardiothoracic	Treats chest diseases and heart and lung conditions
Cosmetic	Repairs or reconstructs body parts, either due to accidents or disease or as elective surgery
General	Treats varied surgical cases
Maxillofacial	Repairs face and mouth disorders
Neurological	Repairs disorders of the neurologic system
Orthopedic	Repairs conditions of the musculoskeletal system
Vascular	Repairs conditions of the blood vessels

Source: Medical Assisting: Foundations and Practices by M. S. Frazier, C. Malone, and C. Morgan, Upper Saddle River, NJ: Pearson Education, Inc., 2010, p. 29. Reprinted with permission.

3 APPLICATION

Directions: Select the best answer for each of the following questions. Check your answers in the Answer Key at the end of the book.

1. The suffix *-pathy* means which of the following?
   a. One who studies disease
   b. Suturing
   c. Surgical repair
   d. Diseased
   e. Recording
2. The prefix *ortho-* means which of the following?
   a. Teeth
   b. Fixation
   c. Straight
   d. Repair
   e. Outside
3. The most common combining vowel is
   a. *u*
   b. *o*
   c. *i*
   d. *e*
   e. *a*
4. A suffix usually provides information about
   a. A procedure
   b. Location
   c. Disease
   d. A and B
   e. A and C
5. The root word *chromo* means which of the following?
   a. Yellow
   b. Blue
   c. Red
   d. Color
   e. Gray
6. The combining form *histo* means which of the following?
   a. Tissue
   b. Cell
   c. History
   d. Hysterectomy
   e. Nucleus
7. The correct word part for vein is which of the following?
   a. *veno*
   b. *hemo*
   c. *phlebo*
   d. A and B
   e. A and C
8. The root word *antero* means the same thing as which of the following?
   a. *disto*
   b. *dorso*
   c. *postero*
   d. *latero*
   e. *ventro*

9. Blepharitis is defined as:
   a. Inflammation of the eyelid
   b. Inflammation of the iris
   c. Inflammation of the nail
   d. Inflammation of the eye
   e. Inflammation of the ear

10. Ureterolithotomy is defined as:
   a. Removal of a tumor in the urethra
   b. Removal of a stone in the ureter
   c. Removal of a tumor in the ureter
   d. Removal of a stone in the urethra
   e. Creation of an opening in the ureter

11. The correct suffix for pain is which of the following?
   a. *-dynia*
   b. *-esis*
   c. *-lysis*
   d. *-pathy*
   e. none of the above

12. Softening of the bone is known as:
   a. Osteopathy
   b. Osteophage
   c. Osteonecrosis
   d. Osteomalacia
   e. Osteodynia

13. Colposcope is defined as which of the following?
   a. Visual examination of the colon
   b. Instrument used to view the colon
   c. Visual examination of the vagina
   d. Instrument used to view the vagina
   e. None of the above

14. A sagittal plane slices the body into which of the following?
   a. Front and back
   b. Left and right
   c. Ventral and dorsal
   d. Superior and inferior
   e. Top and bottom

15. The directional term meaning "toward the trunk" is which of the following?
   a. *medial*
   b. *distal*
   c. *proximal*
   d. *midline*
   e. *lateral*

16. The suffix meaning "rupture" is which of the following?
   a. *-rrhaphy*
   b. *-rrhexis*
   c. *-rrhagia*
   d. *-rrhea*
   e. *-rrhectomy*

17. The correct medical term for "slow heartbeat" is which of the following?
   a. *pericardium*
   b. *tachycardia*
   c. *bradycardia*
   d. *myocardia*
   e. *endocardium*

18. The prefix meaning "within" is which of the following?
   a. *endo-*
   b. *inter-*
   c. *intra-*
   d. A and B
   e. A and C

19. The medical term *oligouria* is defined as which of the following?
   a. Excessive urine
   b. Scanty urine
   c. Large ureters
   d. Yellow urine
   e. Small ureters

20. A physician who diagnoses and treats conditions of the elderly population is known as a (an):
   a. Rheumatologist
   b. Intensivist
   c. Gerontologist
   d. Nephrologist
   e. Oncologist

21. A physician who diagnoses and treats conditions related to the stomach and intestines is known as a (an):
   a. Intensivist
   b. Rheumatologist
   c. Gynecologist
   d. Oncologist
   e. Gastroenterologist

22. When a singular term ends in *ax,* you convert it to plural by changing *ax* to which of the following?
   a. *ex*
   b. *ix*
   c. *ices*
   d. *axes*
   e. *ixes*

23. The right upper quadrant (RUQ) contains which of the following organs?
   a. Part of the liver, stomach, pancreas, spleen, and intestines
   b. Part of the liver, gallbladder, and intestines
   c. Intestines, appendix, right ureter, ovary, and fallopian tube
   d. Liver, intestines, gallbladder, and right ureter
   e. Liver, pancreas, gallbladder, and intestines

24. The correct abbreviation for "as needed" is which of the following?
   a. t.i.d.
   b. a.c.
   c. b.i.d.
   d. gtt
   e. PRN

25. Which of the following medical terms is defined as fungus of the nail?
   a. *onychotomy*
   b. *onychitis*
   c. *onycholysis*
   d. *onychomycosis*
   e. *onychorrhexis*

26. Which of the following medical terms is defined as removal of the ovaries?
   a. *salpingectomy*
   b. *orchidectomy*
   c. *hysterectomy*
   d. *oophorectomy*
   e. *prostatectomy*

27. Dyspnea is defined as which of the following?
   a. Abnormality in the color of the skin
   b. Difficulty swallowing
   c. Disturbance of the normal sleep pattern
   d. Difficulty urinating
   e. Difficulty breathing

28. Hemostasis is defined as which of the following?
   a. Controlled bleeding
   b. Breakdown of blood
   c. Disease of the blood
   d. Blood in the chest cavity
   e. Circulation of the blood

29. A prefix usually provides information about:
   a. Location
   b. Number
   c. Time
   d. Status
   e. All of the above

30. Which of the following root words is defined as "yellow"?
   a. *cyano*
   b. *melano*
   c. *polio*
   d. *xantho*
   e. *xero*

4 Basic Anatomy and Physiology

CONTENTS

Reproductive System

Anatomy and Physiology of the Reproductive System

Anatomy and Physiology of the Female and Male Reproductive Organs

Endocrine System

Anatomy and Physiology of the Endocrine System

Anatomy and Physiology of the Endocrine Glands

Reproductive Glands

Anatomy and Physiology Defined

Anatomy is the study of the structures of the body. *Physiology* is the study of the functions of the structures.

Levels of Organization

The human body is composed of several systems, organs, tissues, and cells (Figure 4-1).

CELLS

The cell is the smallest and most basic unit of all living things. Cells vary in size and function and are capable of replicating. Some cells are very specialized. Every cell has three basic components (Figure 4-2):

Cell membrane: The outer covering of the cell, which has the capability of allowing some substances to pass through the membrane while keeping others out. This selectivity allows cells to receive nutrition and dispose of waste. It also helps cells to maintain their shape.

Cytoplasm: A jellylike substance found between the cell membrane and the nucleus. It consists of 80% water and is usually clear (i.e., colorless). Organelles are found within the cytoplasm and have a specific function: to maintain the viability of the cell.

Nucleus: Control system of the cell that is responsible for the cell's metabolism, growth, and reproduction.

- Chromosomes are found within the nucleus of the cell and carry the genes responsible for determining hereditary characteristics. There are 46 chromosomes in all human cells. Chromosomes are long, coiled molecules of DNA (deoxyribonucleic acid).

TISSUES

When similar or like cells come together to perform a specific function, they form what is known as *tissue.* There are four basic types of tissue (Figure 4-3):

Epithelial tissue: Found in the skin and lining of the respiratory, intestinal, and urinary tracts. These tissues protect, absorb, secrete, and excrete.

- **Epithelium:** Specialized tissue that forms the epidermis of the skin and mucous membranes.
- **Endothelium:** Specialized tissue lining blood and lymph vessels, body cavities, glands, and organs.

Connective tissue: Connects and supports various body structures. Blood, adipose tissue, and osseous tissue are types of connective tissue. Blood is the only liquid tissue in the body.

- **Adipose tissue:** Also known as *fat.* Provides cushioning and insulation.

CELLULAR ORGANELLES AND THEIR FUNCTIONS

Organelle	Function
Endoplasmic Reticulum	A tubular network that is attached to the nuclear membrane. Rough endoplasmic reticulum has ribosomes embedded within it; smooth endoplasmic reticulum does not.
Ribosomes	Location for the production of protein that is essential to the vitality of the cell.
Golgi Apparatus	A saclike membranous structure that sorts, modifies, and transports various proteins throughout the cell.
Mitochondria	Considered the powerhouse of the cell, they are responsible for the production of adenosine triphosphate (ATP), a form of cellular energy.
Lysosome	Sometimes considered the stomach of the cell, they are the sites of digestion of proteins, lipids, and carbohydrates. Anything that is not digested by the lysosome is sent to the cellular membrane for removal from the cell.
Centrioles	These paired organelles lie at 90 degree angles near the nucleus. They are involved in cellular division.

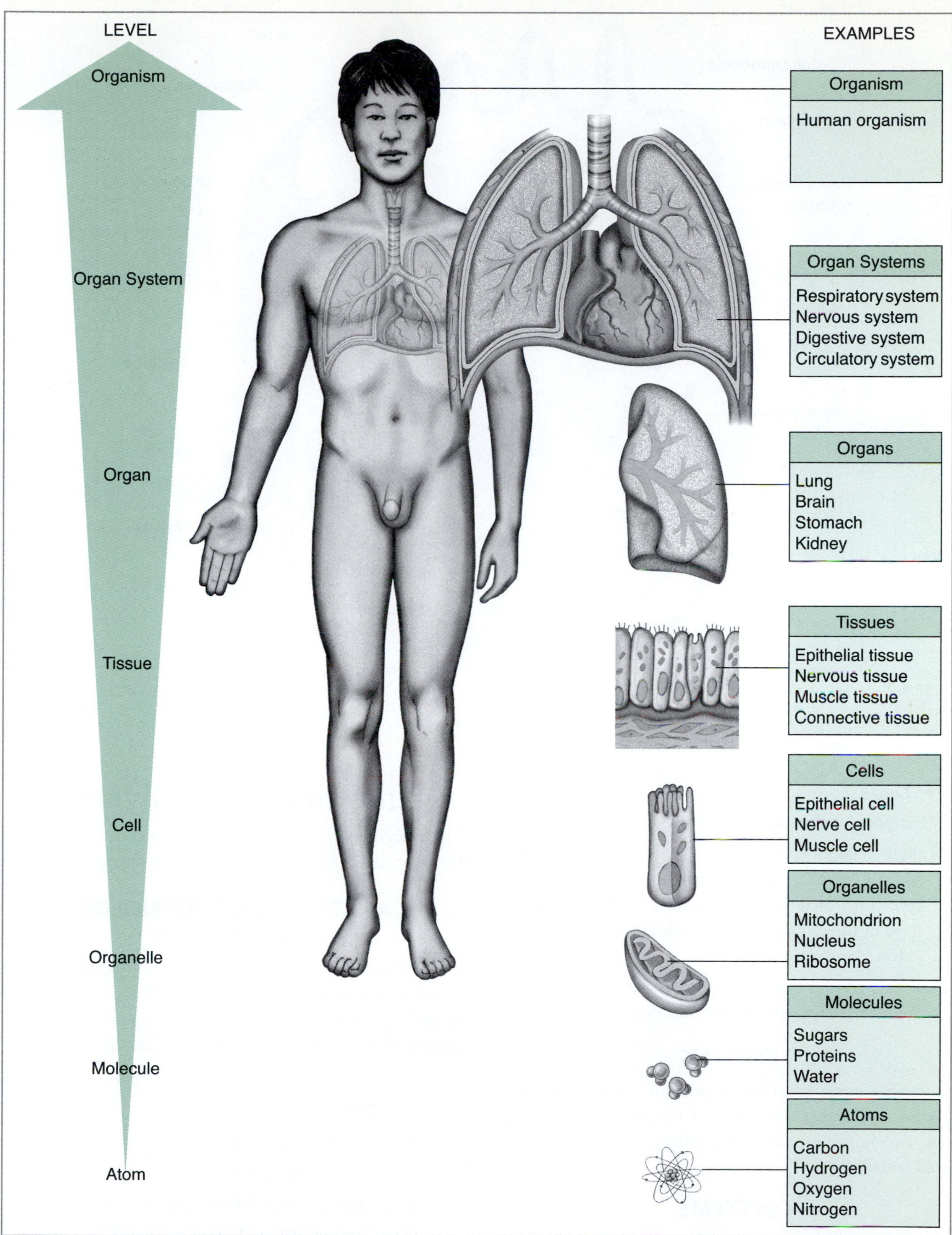
LEVEL
EXAMPLES
Organism
Organ System
Organ
Tissue
Cell
Organelle
Molecule
Atom
Organism
Human organism
Organ Systems
Respiratory system
Nervous system
Digestive system
Circulatory system
Organs
Lung
Brain
Stomach
Kidney
Tissues
Epithelial tissue
Nervous tissue
Muscle tissue
Connective tissue
Cells
Epithelial cell
Nerve cell
Muscle cell
Organelles
Mitochondrion
Nucleus
Ribosome
Molecules
Sugars
Proteins
Water
Atoms
Carbon
Hydrogen
Oxygen
Nitrogen

FIGURE 4-1 Organization of the human body.

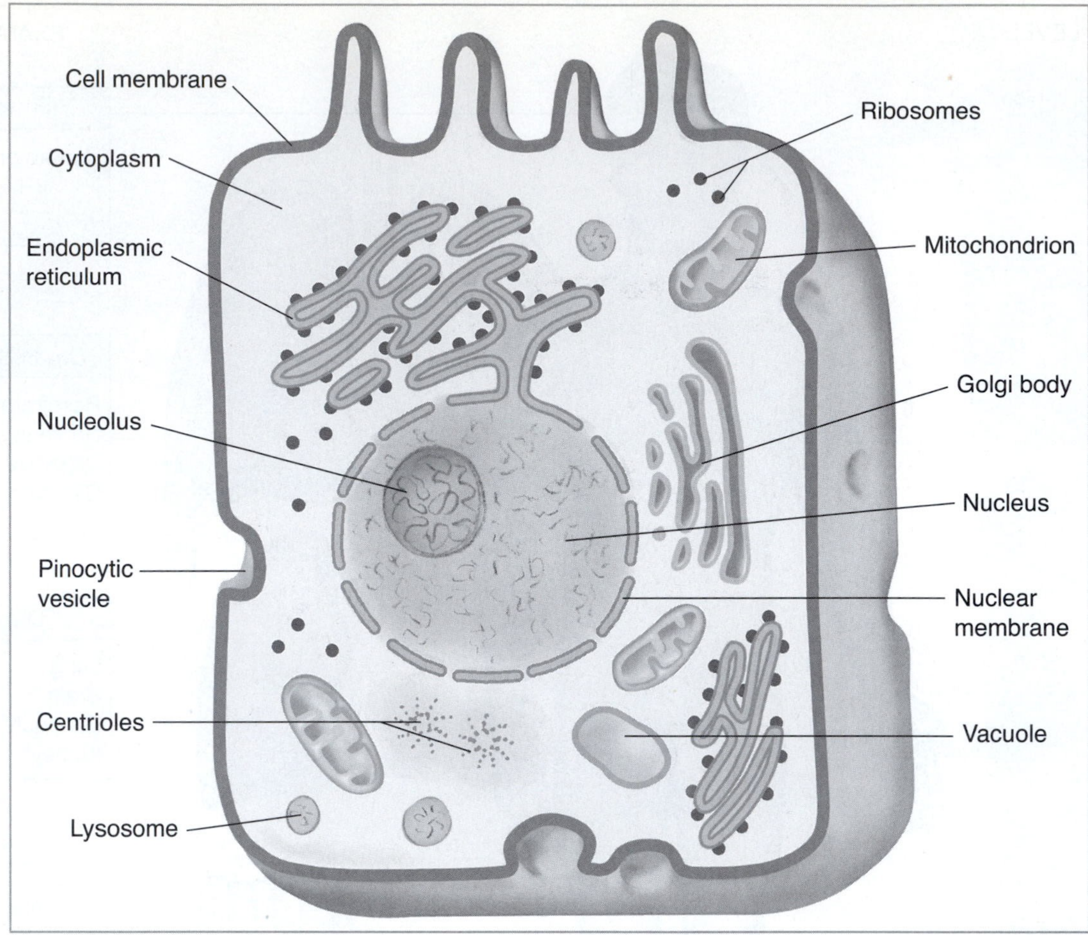

FIGURE 4-2 Major components of the cell.

- **Loose connective tissue:** Surrounds organs and supports nerve cells and blood vessels.

Muscle tissue: Has the ability to contract and relax and, in turn, produces movement. There are three types of muscle tissue: skeletal, smooth, and cardiac. Each of these types of tissue is discussed in the section "Muscular System."

Nervous tissue: Sends impulses to and from the brain. Found in brain, spinal cord, and nerves.

ORGANS

Tissues that come together to perform a specific function are known as *organs*. Examples of organs are the kidneys, heart, and lungs, among many others, which will be discussed below.

SYSTEMS

Organs that work together to perform a specific function are known as a *system*.

Integumentary System

The integumentary system protects organs from the environment and helps regulate body temperature.

ANATOMY AND PHYSIOLOGY OF THE SKIN

The integumentary system consists of the skin and the glands found within the skin, hair, and nails. The function of the skin is to protect, regulate temperature, serve as a sensory receptor, and secrete sweat and sebum.

- The skin can reveal information about the patient. Examples:

  Warmth: inflammation or fever

  Coolness: lack of circulation

  Erythema (redness): inflammation

  Cyanosis (pale, blue): lack of oxygen

  Elasticity and fullness: skin hydration

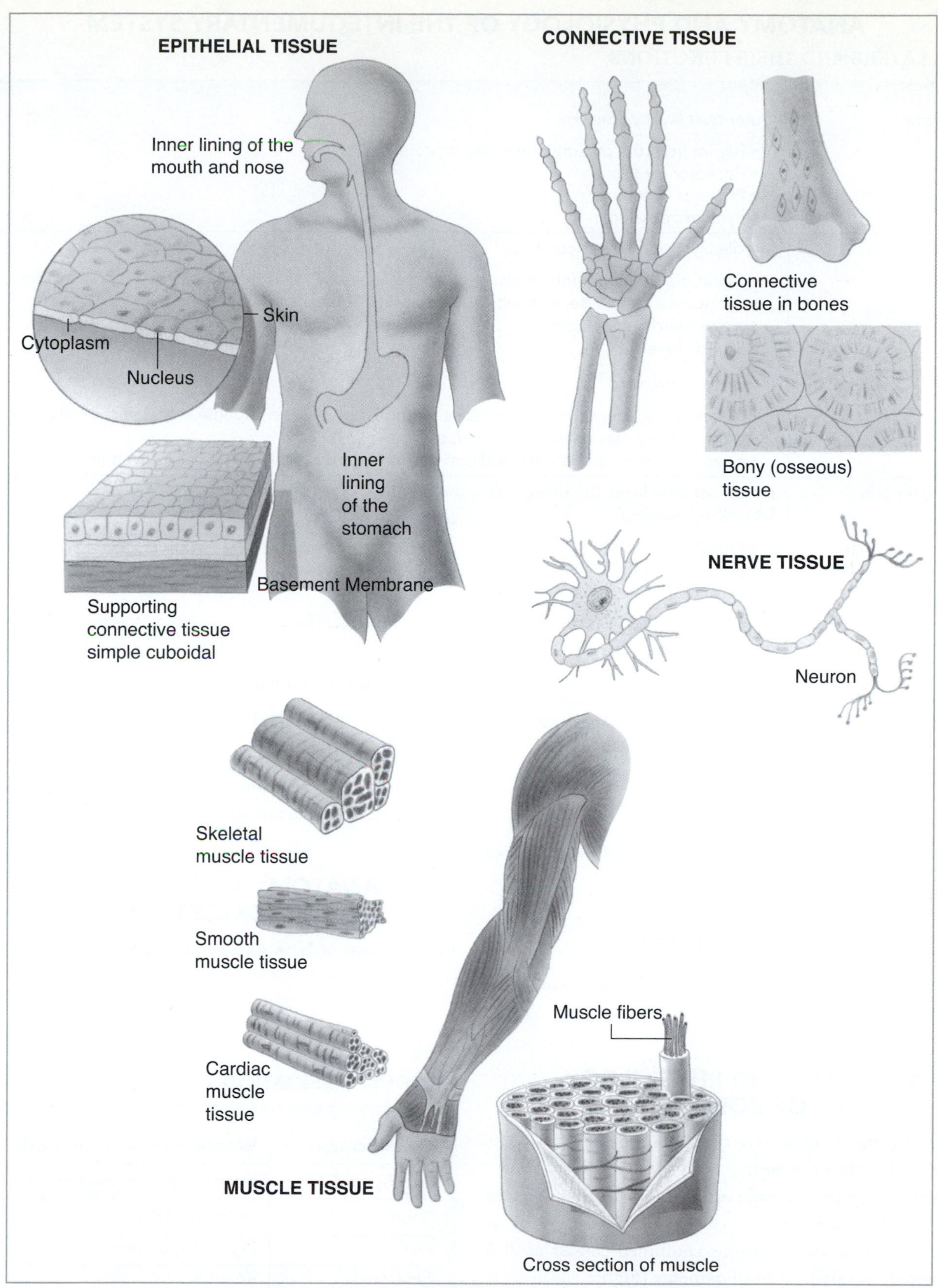
EPITHELIAL TISSUE
CONNECTIVE TISSUE
Inner lining of the mouth and nose
Skin
Cytoplasm
Nucleus
Inner lining of the stomach
Basement Membrane
Supporting connective tissue simple cuboidal
Connective tissue in bones
Bony (osseous) tissue
NERVE TISSUE
Neuron
Skeletal muscle tissue
Smooth muscle tissue
Cardiac muscle tissue
MUSCLE TISSUE
Muscle fibers
Cross section of muscle

FIGURE 4-3 Types of tissue in the human body.

ANATOMY AND PHYSIOLOGY OF THE INTEGUMENTARY SYSTEM

TISSUE LAYERS AND THEIR FUNCTIONS

Epidermis	Outermost layer of the skin • Barrier from the outside; therefore, is protective • Receptor for touch • Prevents water loss • Synthesizes vitamin D
Dermis	Middle layer of the skin; contains • Sweat glands (sudoriferous glands): secrete sweat • Sebaceous glands: secrete sebum, an oily, fatty substance • Nerves and nerve endings • Blood vessels Does the following: • Regulates temperature: heat escapes through blood vessel expansion and release of sweat through the pores to cool body surfaces • Keeps skin oiled and elastic, and prevents dry hair and scalp by producing sebum
Subcutaneous Tissue	Innermost fatty layer, the tissue below the dermis Does the following: • Provides body fuel • Retains heat • Cushions inner tissues

TERMS USED TO DESCRIBE SKIN

Erythema	Reddened skin
Cyanosis	Blue skin
Jaundice	Yellow skin

Skeletal System

The skeletal system supports the body's framework and provides shape.

ANATOMY AND PHYSIOLOGY OF BONES

Bones are a form of connective tissue and one of the hardest tissues found within the body.

The skeletal system is made up of different types of bones and has two divisions, the axial skeleton and the appendicular skeleton. These two divisions combined consist of 206 bones, as well as cartilage and ligaments (Figure 4-4).

Bones provide the following:

- Shape, support, and a framework for the body
- Support and protection for the internal organs
- Storage for minerals, calcium, and phosphorus
- A place for blood cells to form in the bone marrow (hematopoiesis)
- Assistance with movement by providing a place for skeletal muscle to attach

ANATOMY AND PHYSIOLOGY OF THE SKELETAL SYSTEM

Bones consist of 50% water and are classified by their shape (Figure 4-5).

BONE CLASSIFICATIONS

Classification	Where Found in the Body
See Figure 4-6	Upper and lower extremities
Short	Wrist and ankle
Flat	Skull, ribs, breastbone
Sesamoid	Kneecap
Irregular	Spine and hip
Sutural	Skull

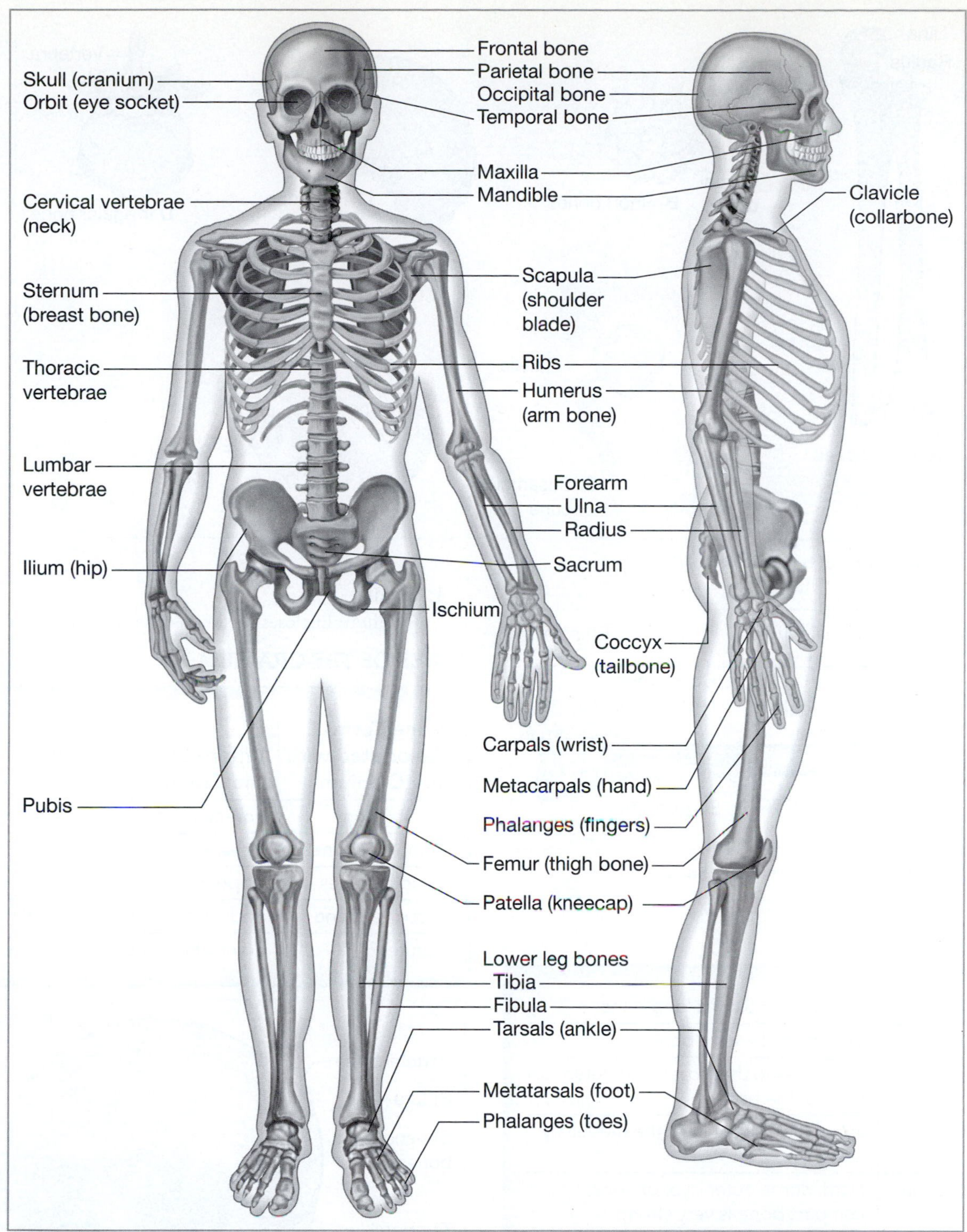

FIGURE 4-4 The skeletal system.

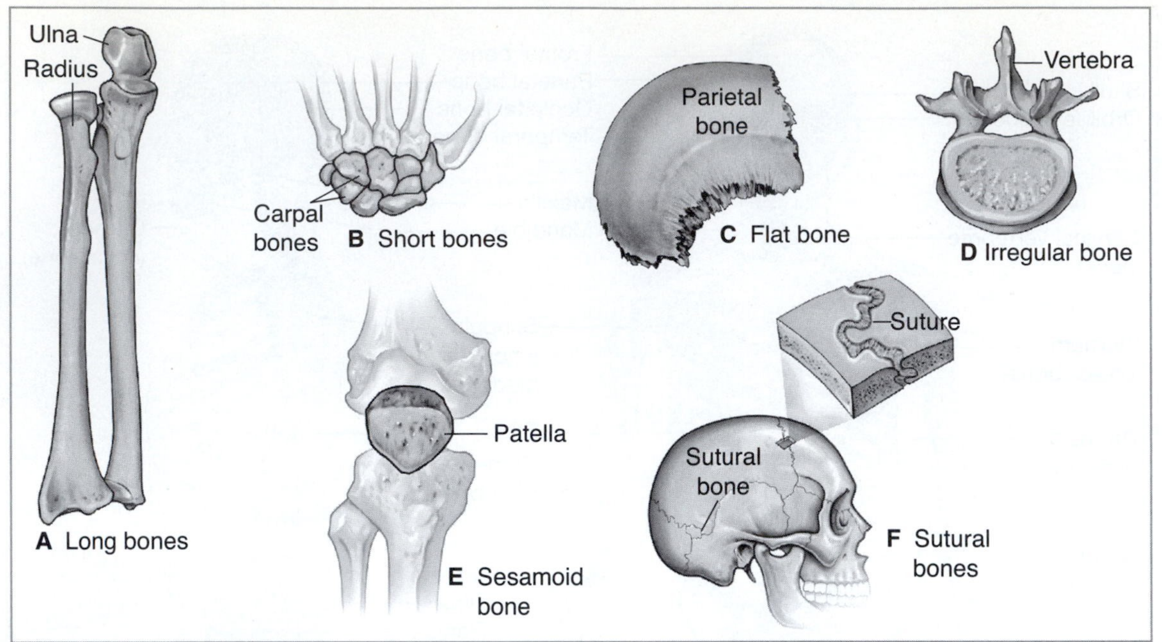

FIGURE 4-5 Classification of bones by shape.

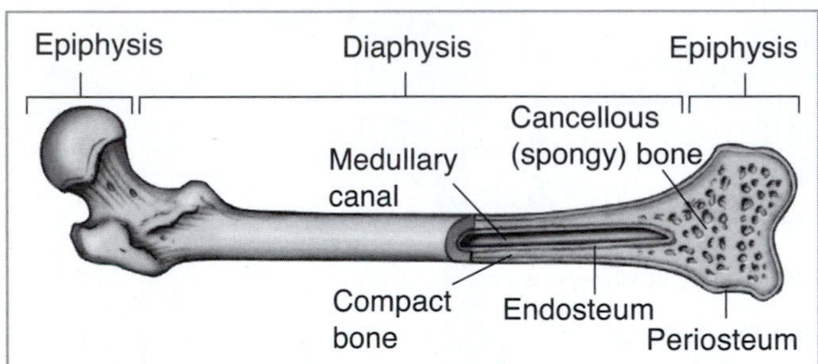

FIGURE 4-6 The features found in a long bone.

STRUCTURE OF BONE

Epiphysis	The wide ends of a long bone
Diaphysis	The shaft of a long bone
Periosteum	Tough tissue that covers the outermost layer of the bone
Endosteum	Tough tissue that lines the medullary cavity
Compact Bone	Hard, dense outer layer of bone; compact bone is very strong
Spongy Bone	Found in the ends and inner portions of long bones
Foramen	An opening in a bone where blood vessels, nerves, and ligaments pass through
Process	A projection on a bone that allows muscles and tendons to attach to the bone
Ligaments	Attach bone to bone
Tendons	Attach bone to muscle

1. **Skull**

   Cranium: Encloses the brain (Figure 4-7).

BONES OF THE CRANIUM

Bone/Terms Associated with the Cranium	Where Located within the Cranium
Frontal Bone	Forehead and eye sockets
Temporal Bones	Sides and base of the cranium
Parietal Bones	Upper side of the cranium
Occipital Bone	Back of the head and base of the skull
Sutures	Point where two bones are joined

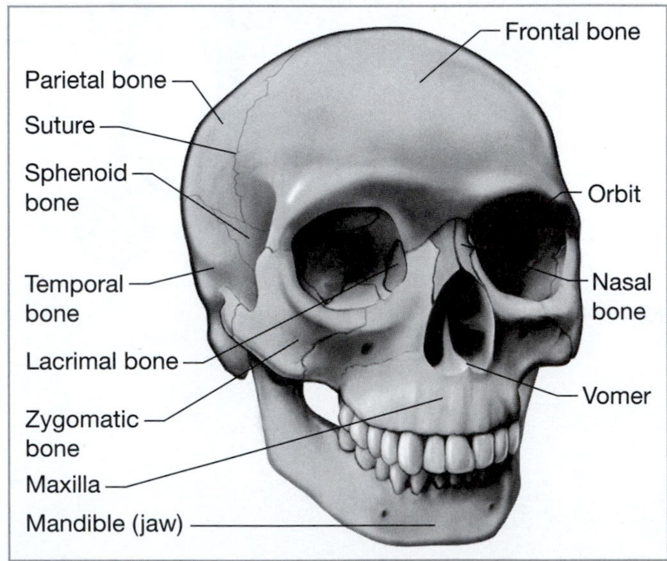

FIGURE 4-7 The cranial and facial bones.

2. **Extremities**

BONES OF THE UPPER EXTREMITIES

Bone/Upper Extremity	Where Located
Humerus	Upper arm
Radius	Lower arm, on the thumb side
Ulna	Lower arm, on the little finger side
Metacarpals	Hand
Carpals	Wrist
Phalanges	Fingers and toes

BONES OF THE LOWER EXTREMITIES

Bone/Lower Extremity	Where Located
Ilium	Upper portion of the hip; wing-shaped
Ischium	Lower portion of the hip
Pubis	Front portion of the hips
Femur	Upper leg; longest and strongest of the bones
Patella	Knee
Tibia	Lower leg; larger of the two lower leg bones (shin bone)
Fibula	Lower leg; smaller of the two lower leg bones
Tarsals	Ankle
Calcaneus	Heel
Metatarsals	Foot; forms the arch of the foot
Phalanges	Toes and fingers

3. **Torso**

BONES IN THE TORSO

Bone/Torso	Where Located
Scapula	Upper back (shoulder blade)
Clavicle	Anterior shoulder bone (collar bone)
Sternum	Middle of the front of the rib cage Ribs connect to the sternum; CPR chest compression is done there The xiphoid process, cartilage that is found at the lower portion of the sternum

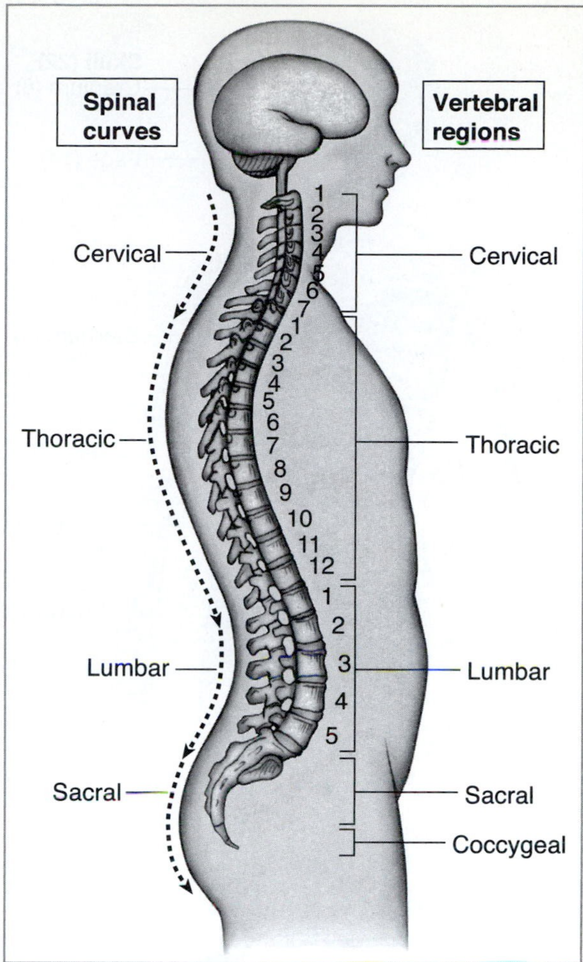

FIGURE 4-8 Vertebral regions showing the four spinal curves.

4. **Vertebrae (Figure 4-8)**

TYPES OF VERTEBRAE

Type of Vertebra	Number of Bones and Direction of Curve
Cervical	7 bones that curve inward; the atlas is the top bone
Thoracic	12 bones that curve outward
Lumbar	5 bones that curve inward
Sacral	5 fused bones that curve outward
Coccygeal	4 fused bones; also known as the *tailbone*

DIVISIONS WITHIN THE SKELETAL SYSTEM

1. **Axial skeleton:** consists of 80 bones found in the skull, spinal column, sternum, and ribs (Figure 4-9).

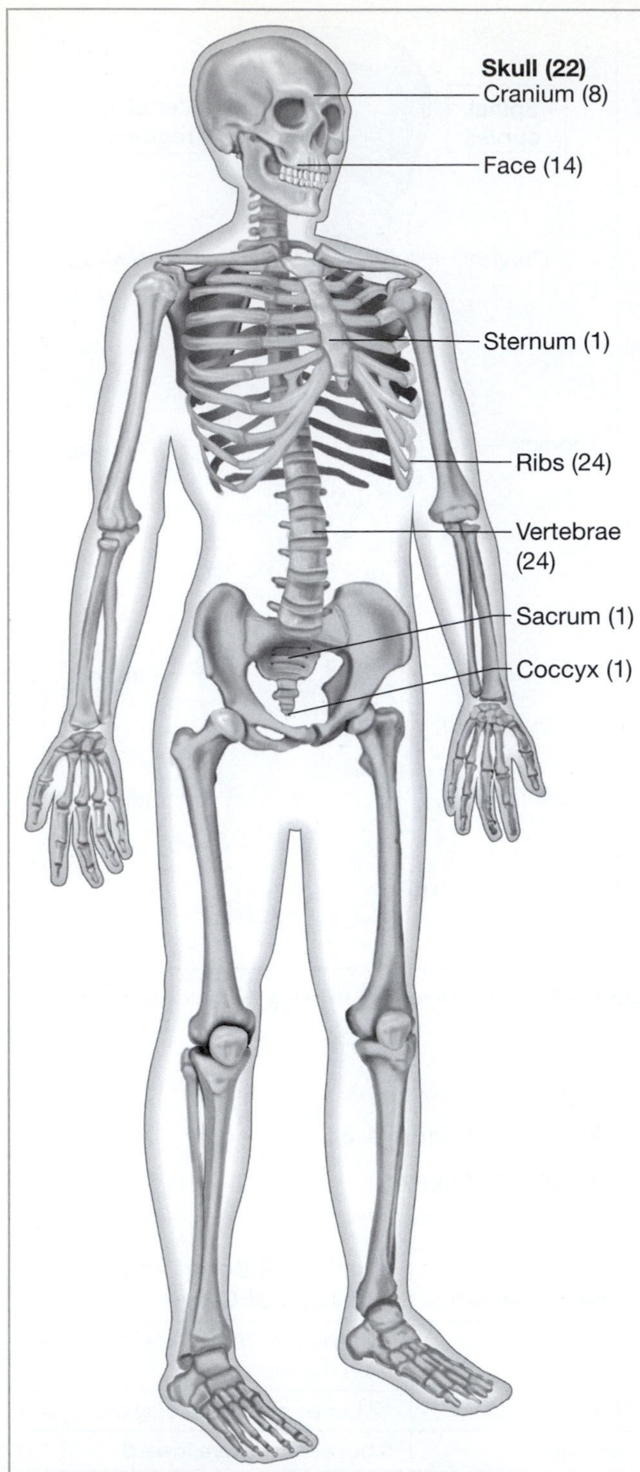

FIGURE 4-9 The axial skeleton.

2. **Appendicular skeleton:** Consists of 126 bones found in the upper extremities (shoulders, arms, forearms, wrists, and hands) and lower extremities (hips, thighs, legs, ankles, and feet).

JOINTS

The place where two bones connect is called a *joint* or an *articulation*.

JOINT CLASSIFICATIONS

Synarthrotic Sutures	Bones join and form a joint that does not produce movement. *Example*: coronal and sagittal sutures of the skull
Amphiarthrotic Symphyses	Also known as a *cartilaginous joint* Produce very slight movement Where two bones join and are firmly held together by cartilage *Example*: pubic symphysis
Diarthrotic Synovial	Allow free movement in several directions • *Ball and socket joints*: allow wide range of motion in many directions Example: hips and shoulders • *Gliding joints*: allow sliding or twisting Example: joints between the bones of the wrist and ankle • *Hinge joints*: allow movement primarily in one direction Example: knees and elbows • *Pivot*: allows rotation around an axis Example: joint between the radius and ulna

Muscular System

The muscular system allows movement and vital functions to occur. This system consists of several types of muscle that are made up of fibers and fascia connected to bones by tendons.

The functions of the muscular system are as follows:

- Make movement possible
- Hold the body erect
- Protect internal organs
- Generate heat to keep the body warm
- Move food through the digestive tract
- Assist in the return of blood to the heart
- Move fluids through other body systems

ANATOMY AND PHYSIOLOGY OF MUSCLES

There are more than 600 muscles in the human body, and these muscles make up about 42% of body weight. Muscles consist of about 75% water and 20% protein. This composition does not vary with different muscle types.

TYPES OF MUSCLE TISSUE

Type of Muscle	Appearance and Function
Skeletal	Also known as *voluntary muscle* Striated (striped) Attached to bones and make motion possible
Smooth	Also known as *involuntary muscle* Unstriated (no stripes) Found in walls of internal organs in the digestive tract, blood vessels, and urinary bladder
Cardiac	Striated (striped) Found within the muscular walls of the heart Also known as *myocardial muscle*

STRUCTURE OF SKELETAL MUSCLES

Muscle Fibers	Threadlike structures that are held together by connective tissue
Fascia	A sheet of connective tissue that covers, supports, and separates muscle tissues
Tendons	Connective tissue that attaches muscle to bone
Aponeurosis	Fibrous connective tissue that attaches muscle to bone or to other muscles

ATTACHMENTS TO SKELETAL MUSCLES

Origin	Muscle attachment to bone at the point that is a more fixed part of the skeleton
Insertion	Muscle attachment to bone at the point that moves
Antagonist	Muscles that work in opposition to each other
Prime Mover	The muscle that produces movement when the muscles contract
Synergist	The muscle that works together with another muscle to produce movement

RANGE OF MOTION

The movement caused by muscle contraction may result in one of the actions shown in Figure 4-10.

MAJOR SKELETAL MUSCLES Muscles (Figure 4-11) are typically named for one of the following:

	Example
Origin and Insertion	Sternocleidomastoid Originates near the sternum and is inserted into the mastoid process
Action	*Flexor* carpi Makes flexion of the wrist possible
Location	Vastus *lateralis* Muscle on the outer portion of the thigh
Fiber Direction	External abdominal *oblique* Abdominal muscle that runs on an angle (oblique)
Number of Divisions	*Biceps* brachii Biceps have two divisions.
Size	Gluteus *maximus* Largest muscles of the buttock
Shape	*Deltoid* Shaped like an inverted triangle or the Greek letter delta

MUSCLES OF THE HEAD

Sternocleidomastoid	Pulls the head from side to side and pulls the head to the chest
Frontalis	Raises the eyebrows
Orbicularis Oris	Allows the lips to pucker
Orbicularis Oculi	Allows the eyes to close
Zygomaticus	Pulls the corners of the mouth up
Masseter and Temporalis	Close the jaw

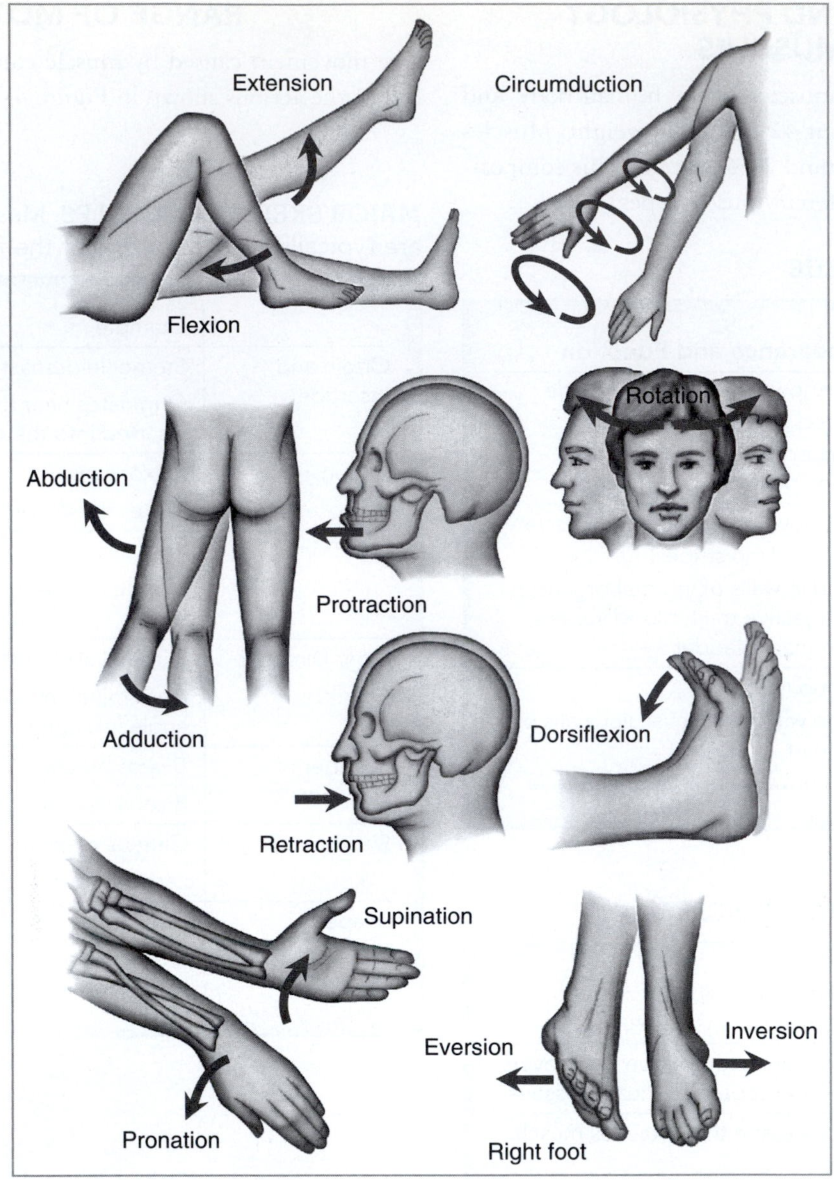

FIGURE 4-10 **Types of body movement.**

MUSCLES OF THE ARM, WRIST, AND HAND

Muscle	Action
Pectoralis Major	Pulls the arm across the chest Rotates and adducts the arms
Latissimus Dorsi	Extension, adduction, and rotation of the arm inward
Deltoid	Adduction and extension of the arm at the shoulder
Biceps Brachii	Flexes the arm at the elbow and rotates the hand laterally
Brachialis	Flexes the arm at the elbow
Triceps Brachii	Extends the arm at the elbow
Flexor Carpi Radialis and Ulnaris	Flex and abduct the wrist
Extensor Digitorum	Extends the fingers but not the thumb

RESPIRATORY MUSCLES

Muscle	Action
Diaphragm	Contraction causes inspiration.
External and Internal Intercostals	Expand and lower the ribs during breathing

ABDOMINAL MUSCLES

Muscle	Action
External and Internal Obliques	Compress the abdominal wall
Transverse Abdominis	Compresses the abdominal wall
Rectus Abdominis	Flexes the vertebral column and compresses the abdominal wall

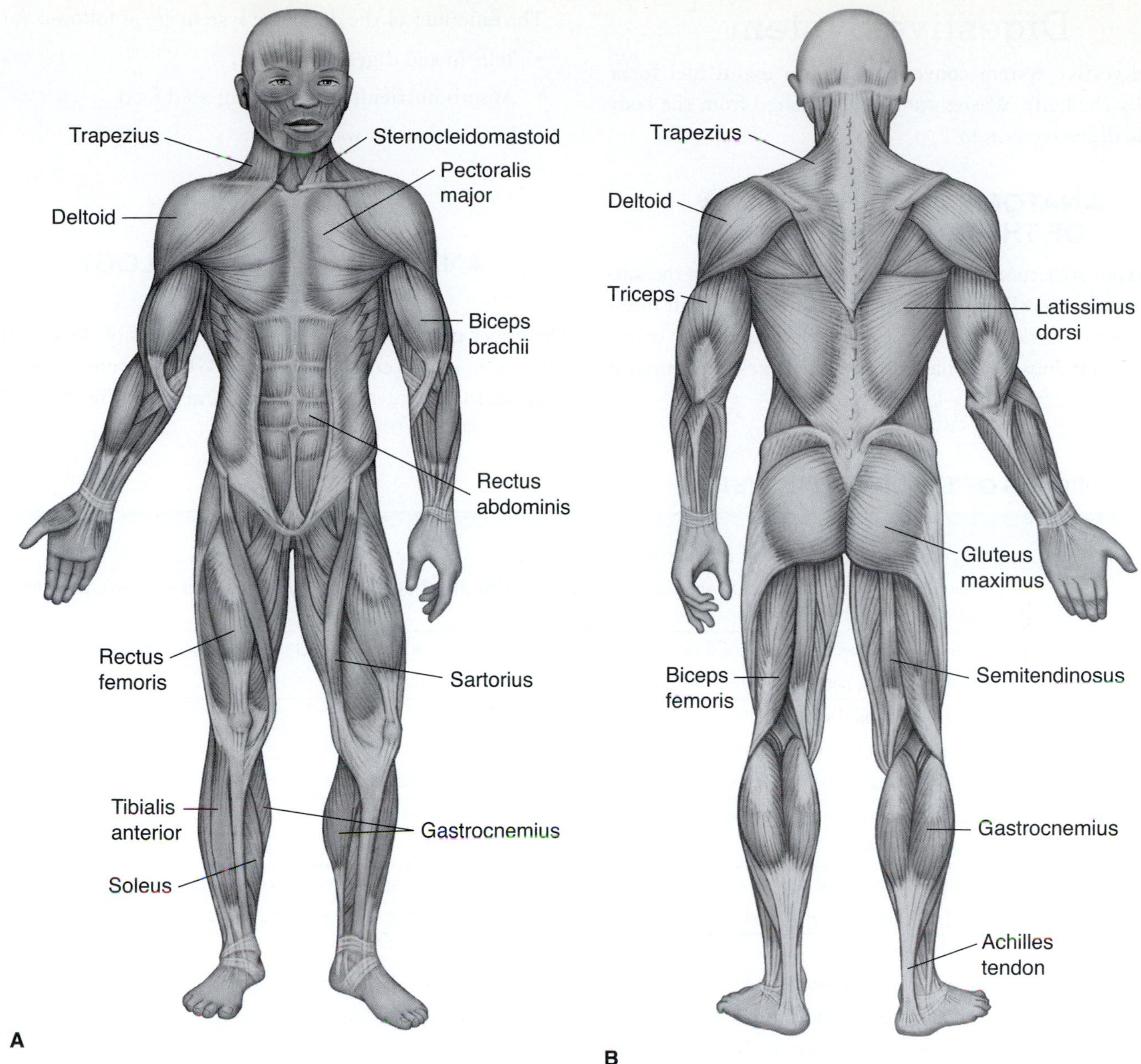

FIGURE 4-11 (A) Selected skeletal muscles (anterior view). (B) Selected skeletal muscles (and the Achilles tendon [posterior view]).

MUSCLES OF THE TORSO

Trapezius	Raises the arms and pulls the shoulders downward
Pectoralis Minor	Pulls the scapula downward and raises the ribs

MUSCLES OF THE LEG, ANKLE, AND FOOT

Psoas Major	Flexes the thigh
Iliacus	Flexes the thigh
Gluteus Maximus	Extends the thigh
Gastrocnemius	Flexes the foot and aids in pushing the body forward
Tibialis Anterior	Causes dorsiflexion and inversion of the foot

Digestive System

The digestive system converts food into useful fuel to be used by the body. Wastes are also eliminated from the body via the digestive system.

ANATOMY AND PHYSIOLOGY OF THE DIGESTIVE SYSTEM

The major structures of the digestive system include the salivary glands, mouth, throat, esophagus, stomach, small intestines, large intestines, liver, gallbladder, pancreas, colon, rectum, and anus. The main part of the digestive system is the digestive tract.

The functions of the digestive system are as follows:

- Take in and digest food
- Absorb nutrients from the digested food
- Eliminate solid waste products

ANATOMY AND PHYSIOLOGY OF DIGESTION

The upper gastrointestinal (GI) tract consists of the mouth, esophagus, and stomach. The lower GI tract consists of the small and large intestines, rectum, and anus (Figure 4-12).

MAJOR ORGANS OF THE DIGESTIVE SYSTEM

Mouth	Digestion begins in the mouth with mastication (chewing). Saliva is secreted via the salivary glands and mixed with the chewed food, which causes a chemical breakdown of the food.
Teeth	There are two sets of teeth: 28 deciduous teeth (baby teeth), which are replaced by 32 permanent teeth. Each tooth consists of three main portions: crown, root, and neck.
Pharynx	Also known as the *throat* It is shared with the respiratory system. Food passes from the mouth through the pharynx to the esophagus.
Esophagus	Collapsible tube that passes food from the pharynx to the stomach Muscular contractions cause the food to move through the esophagus to the stomach.
Stomach	Saclike organ that acts as a holding tank for food while the digestive process continues Hydrochloric acid and gastric juices within the stomach convert the chewed food into a semiliquid (chime).
Small Intestine	It is 21 feet long. Chime is passed from the stomach into the small intestine, where bile from the liver and pancreas is added. Digestion and absorption of most nutrients occur in the small intestine. Fats are broken down in the small intestine.
Large Intestine	It is 5 feet long. Digestion and absorption are completed in the large intestine. Vitamin K is produced in the large intestine.

SMALL INTESTINE (FIGURE 4-13)

Duodenum	First portion of the small intestine Extends from the pylorus to the jejunum
Jejunum	Middle portion of the small intestine Extends from the duodenum to the ileum
Ileum	Last portion of the small intestine Extends from the jejunum to the large intestine

LARGE INTESTINE (FIGURE 4-14)

Cecum	A pouch on the right side of the abdomen Extends from the ileum (small intestine) to the colon Appendix is found in the lower portion of the cecum
Colon	Divided into four parts: • *Ascending colon*: extends upward from the cecum under the liver • *Transverse colon*: extends from right to left toward the spleen • *Descending colon*: extends downward from the spleen to the sigmoid colon • *Sigmoid colon*: extends from the descending colon to the rectum
Rectum	Extends from the colon to the anus
Anus	Sphincter muscle at the end of the digestive tract

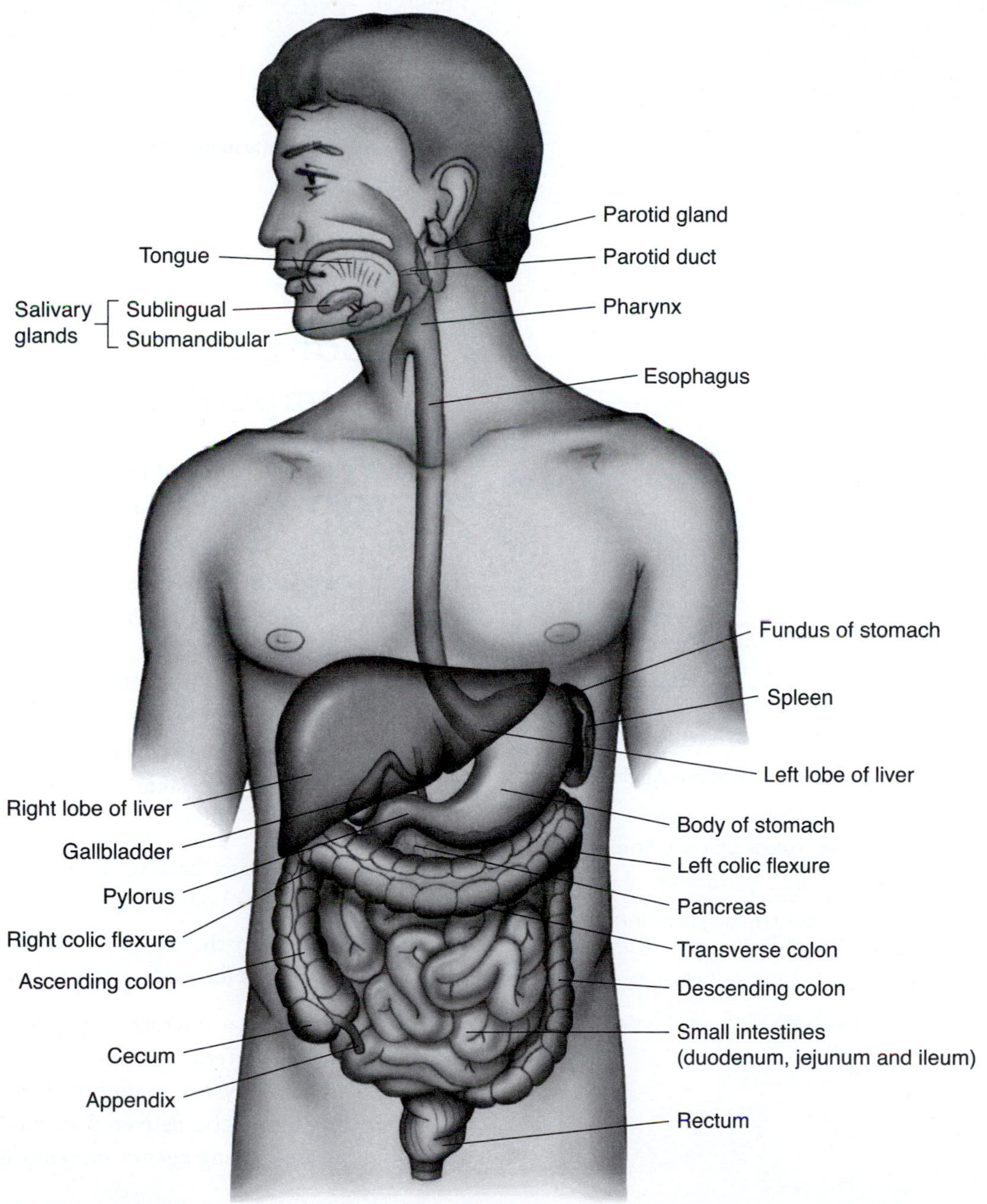

FIGURE 4-12 The digestive system.

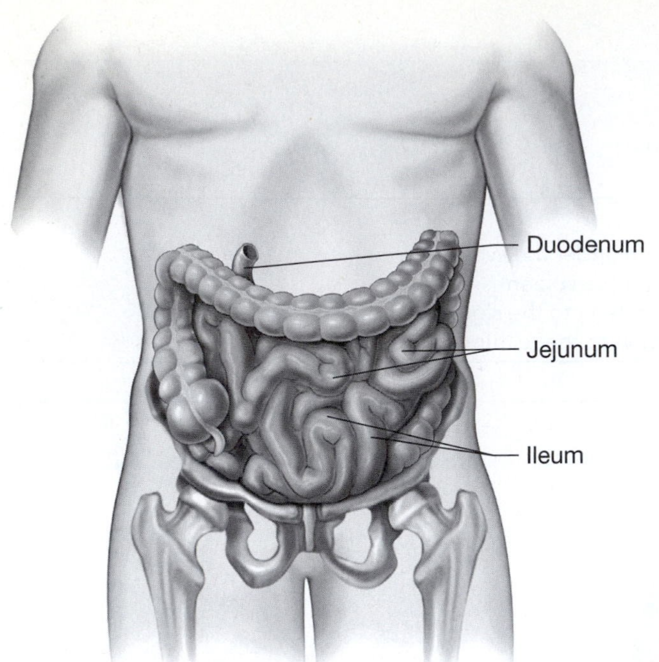

FIGURE 4-13 Small intestine.

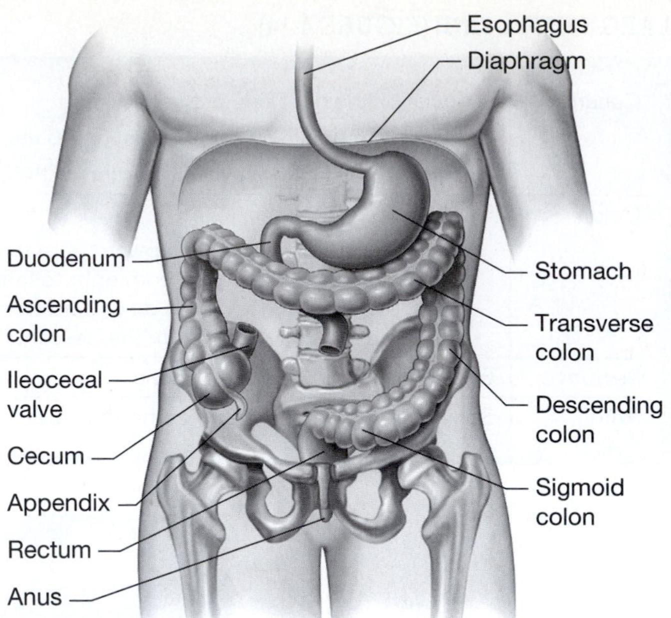

FIGURE 4-14 Large intestine (colon).

ACCESSORY ORGANS OF THE DIGESTIVE SYSTEM

Salivary Glands	Located in the mouth Produce saliva as a response to various sights, smells, tastes, or mental images of food Three pairs of salivary glands: • Parotid • Submandibular • Sublingual
Gallbladder	Bile is stored and concentrated in the gallbladder.
Liver	Produces bile, which breaks down fats Stores proteins Removes excess glucose from blood Destroys old erythrocytes
Pancreas	Secretes pancreatic juices into the small intestine Secretes insulin and glucagons

Cardiovascular and Lymphatic Systems

ANATOMY AND PHYSIOLOGY OF THE CARDIOVASCULAR AND LYMPHATIC SYSTEMS

The cardiovascular system consists mainly of the heart, blood vessels, and blood. The lymphatic system consists of the thymus, spleen, and lymph.

The main function of the cardiovascular system is to pump blood, oxygen, and nutrients to the tissues throughout the body. The cardiovascular system works in conjunction with the lymphatic system to carry out the following functions:

- Carry cellular waste back to the appropriate organs for removal from the body
- Absorb fats from the digestive system and distribute them to the cells for use

The cardiovascular and lymphatic systems aid in homeostasis by fighting bacteria, viruses, cancer cells, and other invaders. These two systems combined allow oxygenated blood and nutrients to be delivered to vital organs, while wastes and disease-causing agents are removed.

ANATOMY AND PHYSIOLOGY OF THE HEART, BLOOD VESSELS, BLOOD, THYMUS, AND SPLEEN

The heart is a pump that consists mostly of cardiac muscle, is about the size of a fist, and is located to the left of midline of the chest.

LININGS OF THE HEART (FIGURE 4-15)

Pericardium	Outer layer
Myocardium	Also known as the *heart muscle* Middle layer; the thickest layer.
Endocardium	Inner layer

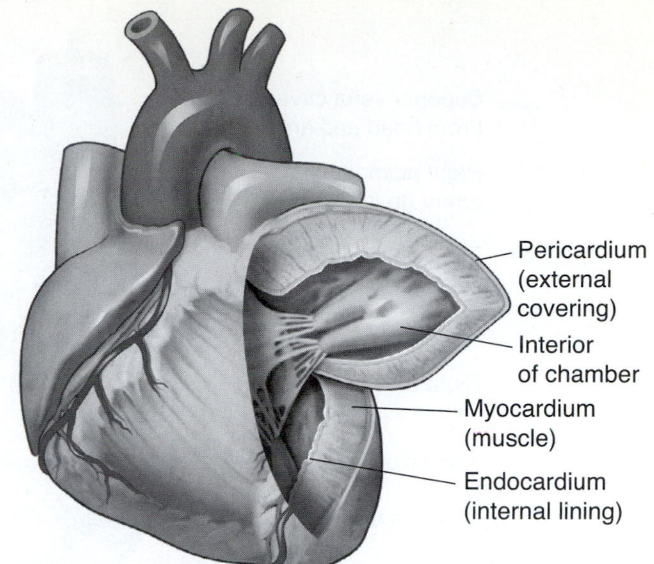

FIGURE 4-15 Linings of the heart.

The chambers within the heart consist of two atria and two ventricles. The atria receive blood and the ventricles pump blood out. The right side of the heart works to move incoming *oxygen-poor* blood to the lungs for oxygenation. The left side of the heart works to move incoming *oxygen-rich* blood to the body.

CHAMBERS WITHIN THE HEART

Right Atrium	Receives oxygen-poor blood from tissues
Right Ventricle	Pumps oxygen-poor blood to the pulmonary artery and then out to the lungs
Left Atrium	Receives oxygen-rich blood from the lungs
Left Ventricle	Pumps oxygen-rich blood from the left atrium through the aorta and then out to the body Very muscular; when it contracts, it must send blood out to the farthest point within the body

HEART VALVES The function of the heart valves is to keep blood from "back flowing" (Figure 4-16).

Tricuspid	Controls the opening between the right atrium and right ventricle
Bicuspid	Also known as the *mitral valve* Controls the opening between the left atrium and left ventricle
Pulmonary Semilunar	Controls the opening between the right ventricle and the pulmonary artery

CONTRACTION OF HEART MUSCLES AND CLOSING OF VALVES (RESULTING IN A HEARTBEAT)

Sinoatrial Node	Also known as the *SA node* and/or the *pacemaker* Responsible for initiating and establishing the rhythm of the heartbeat Located in the upper wall of the right atrium
Atrioventricular Node	Also known as the *AV node* Receives the impulse from the SA node and transmits that impulse to the bundle of His Located beneath the endocardium of the right atrium
Bundle of His	Receives the impulse from the AV node and transmits it to the right and left ventricles Extends from the AV node into the intraventricular septum, which branches out into each ventricle
Purkinje Fibers	Specialized fibers located within the ventricular muscles that cause the ventricles to contract

- Systole = the contraction phase.
- Diastole = the relaxation phase.

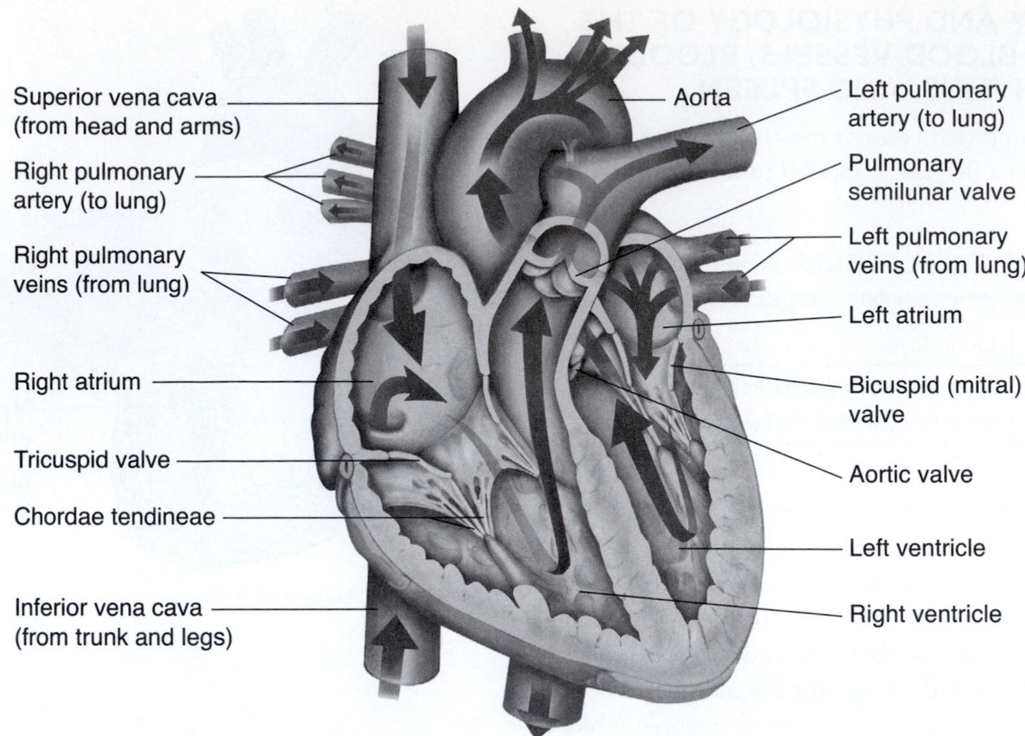

FIGURE 4-16 The flow of blood through the heart.

BLOOD VESSELS

Aorta	Main trunk of the arterial system; largest artery in the body
Arteries	Carry oxygenated blood away from the heart
Arterioles	Thinner, smaller branches of arteries
Veins	Return blood from locations throughout the body back to the heart
Venules	Small veins that join together and form veins
Capillaries	Microscopic blood vessels that connect arteries and veins where nutrients and oxygen diffuse into cells and wastes diffuse back into the venous system

ARTERIES COMMONLY USED TO PALPATE PULSES

Radial	Proximal to the thumb; found in the wrist
Brachial	Found in the antecubital space
Carotid	Found bilaterally just lateral of mid-line
Temporal	Found bilaterally in the area of the temple(s) on the skull
Femoral	Found bilaterally in the groin area
Popliteal	Found bilaterally behind the knee
Dorsalis Pedis	Found bilaterally on the upper portion of the foot
Anterior Tibial	Found bilaterally on the interior side of the ankle

COMPONENTS OF BLOOD

Erythrocytes	Also known as *red blood cells* (*RBCs*) Mature red blood cells without a nucleus Contain hemoglobin, which transports oxygen
Leukocytes	Also known as *white blood cells* (*WBCs*) Larger than RBCs Protect against invaders such as bacteria
Thrombocytes	Also known as *platelets* Important element in clotting blood
Plasma	Straw-colored fluid 90% water

BLOOD TYPES

Blood Type	**Antigen Found on Surface of the RBC**	**Antibody Found in the Plasma**	**Donor Types**
A	A	Anti-B	O and A
B	B	Anti-A	O and B
AB	A and B	Neither A nor B	O, A, B, and AB
O	Neither anti-A nor anti-B	Anti-A and anti-B	O

DONATING AND RECEIVING BLOOD

Universal Donor	Blood type O
Universal Recipient	Blood type AB

STRUCTURES OF THE LYMPHATIC SYSTEM

Lymph Fluid	Located within the arteries and tissues Carries food, oxygen, and hormones to cells and carries waste back to the circulatory system
Lymph Nodes	Located throughout the body Filter and trap bacteria, viruses, cancer cells, and other invaders
Tonsils	Located in the upper portion of the throat
Spleen	Located in the left upper quadrant of the abdominal cavity Helps fight infection by killing or weakening bacteria, viruses, cancer cells and other invaders Destroys damaged RBCs
Thymus	Located just above the heart Filters and traps bacteria, viruses, cancer cells, and other invaders

Respiratory System

The respiratory system allows the exchange of gases to occur within the body.

ANATOMY AND PHYSIOLOGY OF THE RESPIRATORY SYSTEM

The respiratory system consists of the upper and lower respiratory tracts.

The functions of the respiratory system are as follows:

- Supply oxygen to the blood so that the blood can deliver it to the rest of the body
- Expel carbon dioxide from the body via the lungs
- Produce movement of air through the larynx, allowing speech to occur.

UPPER RESPIRATORY TRACT

Nose	Passageway for air to move through Warms and moistens inhaled air Traps dust and pollen Organ of smell
Nasal Septum	Cartilage that divides the nose into two equal right and left sections
Mucous Membranes	Tissue that lines the nose, mouth, and respiratory system
Sinuses	Air-filled cavities that are lined with mucous membranes Help produce sound Produce mucus
Mouth	Shared by the digestive system Another passageway for air to move through
Pharynx	Shared with the digestive system Commonly known as the *throat* A passageway for air and food to move through Tonsils located in the pharynx Divided into three parts: • *Nasopharynx*: connects with the nose and is posterior to the nasal cavity • *Oropharynx*: connects with the back of the mouth and is visible when the mouth is open • *Laryngopharynx*: continues to the esophagus and trachea
Epiglottis	Located at the base of the tongue Closes the laryngopharynx when swallowing and prevents food from entering the trachea and lungs
Larynx	Also known as the *voice box* Located between the pharynx and trachea Contains the vocal cords
Trachea	Also known as the *windpipe* Extends between the larynx and the bronchi

LOWER RESPIRATORY TRACT

Bronchi	Two main branches of the trachea that serve as an air passageway from the trachea to the right and left lungs
Bronchial Tree	Bronchi and their branching structures
Bronchioles	Smallest branches of the bronchi
Alveoli	Small air sacs found at the end of each bronchiole Where oxygen and carbon dioxide exchange occurs
Lungs	Large, cone-shaped organs found in the chest Supply oxygen, remove wastes, and defend against intruders. Right lung has three lobes Left lung has two lobes
Pleura	Membrane that surrounds each lung and the inside of the thoracic cavity
Surfactant	Lubricating fluid that prevents friction between the lungs and thoracic cavity during inhalation and exhalation
Diaphragm	Muscle that separates the thoracic cavity from the abdomen As the diaphragm contracts during inhalation, the thoracic cavity expands, allowing oxygen into the lungs. As the diaphragm relaxes during exhalation, it recoils and pushes carbon dioxide out of the lungs.

ANATOMY AND PHYSIOLOGY OF THE LUNGS AND ASSOCIATED STRUCTURES

PARANASAL SINUSES

Maxillary Sinuses	Largest of the paranasal sinuses Located in the maxillary bones, which are found beneath the cheeks and above the teeth
Ethmoid Sinuses	Located within the ethmoid bone, which is found between the eye sockets and above the nose
Frontal Sinuses	Located just above the eyebrows in the frontal bone
Sphenoid Sinuses	Located deep within the skull behind the ethmoid sinuses

RESPIRATION

Inhalation	Also known as *inspiration.* Contraction of the diaphragm causes elevation of the ribs and increases the size of the thorax, causing a decrease in pressure and allowing air to enter more easily.
Exhalation	Also known as *expiration.* Relaxation of the diaphragm and decrease in the size of the thorax causes pressure to increase and forces air out of the lungs.
Internal Respiration	Exchange of gases at the cellular level between blood and tissues
External Respiration	Exchange of gases within the lungs

Nervous System and Special Senses

The nervous system is the command center for all bodily activities, while the special senses allow us to feel, smell, taste, hear, and see.

ANATOMY AND PHYSIOLOGY OF THE NERVOUS SYSTEM

The nervous system consists mainly of the brain, spinal cord, nerves, and sensory organs and is divided into the central, peripheral, and autonomic nervous systems.

The functions of the nervous system are as follows:

- Receives and interprets sensory information
- Carries out functions based upon the information received

The functions of the special senses are as follows:

- Receive and transmit visual images, sound, and sensations of touch and taste to the brain

NERVOUS SYSTEM DIVISIONS

Divisions	Organs within the Division
Central Nervous System (CNS)	Brain Spinal cord Cerebrospinal fluid
Peripheral Nervous System (PNS)	Cranial nerves (12 pair) Spinal nerves (31 pair)
Autonomic Nervous System (ANS)	Sympathetic nervous system Parasympathetic nervous system

BASIC STRUCTURES OF THE NERVOUS SYSTEM

Neurons	Structural and functional unit of the nervous system Parts of the neuron (Figure 4-17): • *Dendrites*: receive impulses and send them throughout the cell body • *Axon*: sends the impulse away from the body • *Myelin*: fatty insulating substance that covers most axons Neurons that conduct impulses: • *Efferent neurons*: carry impulses away from the brain and spinal cord • *Afferent neurons*: carry impulses toward the brain and spinal cord
Nerve Fibers	The axon and dendrites of the neuron
Nerves	Bundle of nerve fibers found outside of the brain and spinal cord
Tracts	Groups of nerve fibers within the CNS
Nerve Impulses	Excitement transmitted through nerve fibers and neurons
Synapse	Space between two neurons

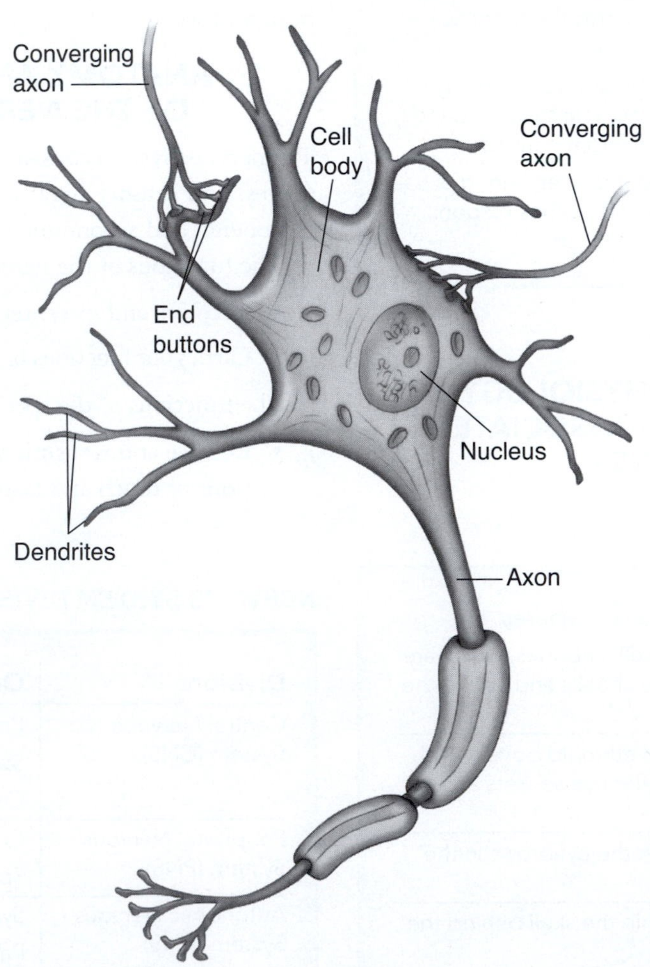

FIGURE 4-17 A neuron (nerve cell) with converging axons.

CENTRAL NERVOUS SYSTEM (CNS)

BRAIN

Meninges	Three-layer connective tissue that encloses the brain and spinal cord. Layers: • *Dura mater*: thick outermost layer • *Arachnoid membrane*: second layer; resembles a spider web • *Pia mater*: inner layer; located closest to the brain and spinal cord
Cerebrospinal Fluid	Also known as *CSF* Flows throughout the brain and around the spinal cord Nourishes, cushions, and cools
Cerebrum	Largest and uppermost part of the brain Consists of four lobes: • *Frontal lobe*: controls motor functions, reasoning, planning, emotion, and speech • *Parietal lobe*: receives and interprets nerve impulses related to touch, pressure, pain, and temperature • *Occipital lobe*: controls eyesight • *Temporal lobe*: controls hearing and smell
Thalamus	Located below the cerebrum The relay station in the brain, directing where within the brain the impulses should go
Hypothalamus	Located below the thalamus Regulates the following: • Autonomic nervous activity related to behavior and emotions • Hormones • Body temperature • Hunger sensations • Thirst • Sleep-wake cycles
Cerebellum	Located at the back of the head Second largest part of the brain Coordinates voluntary muscle activity
Brainstem	Looks like a branch Connects cerebral hemispheres with the spinal cord Consists of the following: • *Midbrain*: sends/receives information from eyes and ears • *Pons*: where nerve cells cross from the right side of the body to the left side of the body and vice versa; helps regulate rate and depth of breathing • *Medulla oblongata*: connects the brain and spinal cord and controls the muscles associated with breathing, heart rate, and blood pressure
Spinal Cord	Contains the nerves that send impulses to the limbs and lower part of the body

PERIPHERAL NERVOUS SYSTEM (PNS)

The nerves in the PNS connect the CNS with sensory organs, muscles, blood vessels, and glands.

COMPONENTS OF THE PERIPHERAL NERVOUS SYSTEM

Somatic Nervous System	Part of the PNS that connects nerves with skin and skeletal muscles.
Cranial Nerves	12 pair Named for the function they serve Originate from the brainstem
Spinal Nerves	31 pair Originate from the spinal cord Send/receive impulses from the arms, legs, neck, and trunk Not individually named, but grouped together as follows: • *Cervical nerves*: 8 pair (C1–C8) • *Thoracic nerves*: 12 pair (T1–T12) • *Lumbar nerves*: 5 pair (L1–L5) • *Sacral nerves*: 5 pair (S1–S5) • *Coccygeal nerves*: 1 pair

THE 12 PAIRS OF CRANIAL NERVES

Sympathetic Nervous System	Causes the response and energy required for stressful situations Sympathetic response: • Increased respiration rate • Increased heart rate • Increased blood flow to muscles • Dilated pupils • Dilated bronchioles Works with the parasympathetic nervous system. Fight-or-flight
Parasympathetic Nervous System	Parasympathetic response follows a sympathetic response and causes organs to return to their normal state Parasympathetic response: • Decreased heart rate • Decreased blood pressure • Constriction of pupils • Contraction of bronchioles • Stimulation of salivary glands Works with the sympathetic nervous system

AUTONOMIC NERVOUS SYSTEM (ANS)

The autonomic nervous system controls involuntary actions of the body and adjusts body functions in response to stress.

STRUCTURES OF THE SPECIAL SENSES

TASTE AND SMELL Taste and smell work together.

Taste Buds	Located on the tongue, on the roof of the mouth, and in the throat (Figure 4-18) Function as taste receptors
Olfactory Cells	Located in the roof of the nasal cavity Send impulse to olfactory nerves within the brain

Touch

- The sense of touch is found throughout the body.
- The sense of touch originates in the dermis, which is filled with receptors also known as *nerve endings*.
- Some areas of the body have more receptors than others; therefore, they are more sensitive.
- Receptors send a message to the spinal cord, which in turn sends the message to the brain.

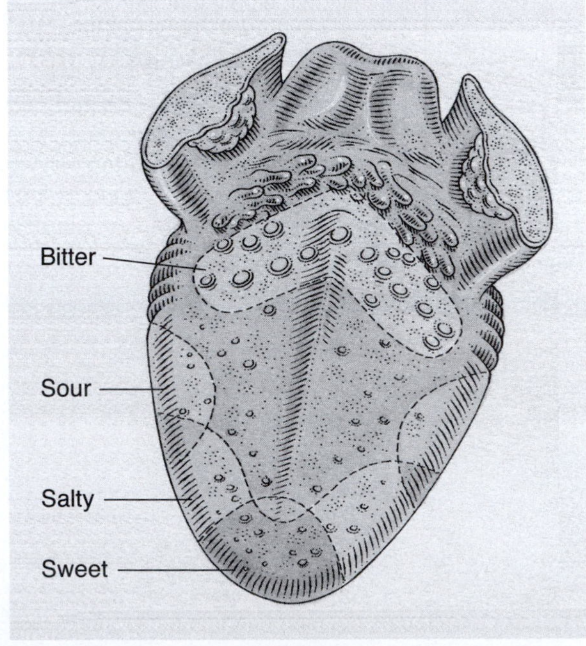

FIGURE 4-18 Tongue and taste buds.

SIGHT

Orbit	Also known as the *eye socket* Cavity within the skull that houses the eyeball
Eye Muscles	Six muscles make eye movement possible. Muscles of the right and left eyes work together.
Eyelids	Protect the eye from excess light and foreign material Help keep the eye moist
Conjunctiva	Mucous membrane that lines the eyelid and anterior portion of the eyeball Protects the surface of the eyeball
Lacrimal Apparatus	Also known as the *tear apparatus* Produces, stores, and removes tears • *Lacrimal gland*: located above the outer corner of each eye; secretes tears • *Lacrimal sac*: also known as the *tear sac* • *Lacrimal duct*: drains tears into the nasal passage
Eyeball	Consists of three layers: • *Sclera*: white of the eye; maintains the shape of the eye • *Cornea*: window of the eye; allows light to enter and provides the most optical power • *Choroid*: absorbs excess light
Iris	Provides the color of the eye
Pupil	Black opening of the eye in the middle of the iris Controls the amount of light that enters the eye
Lens	Focuses images on the retina
Retina	Light-sensitive inner layer containing specialized cells Specialized cells: • *Rods*: black and white receptors • *Cones*: color receptors for red, blue, and green
Aqueous Humor	Clear, watery fluid that nourishes structures of the eye

HEARING

Outer Ear	The visible portion of the ear Outer ear consists of the following: • *Pinna*: also known as the *auricle*; external portion of the ear that collects and funnels sound down into the external auditory canal • *External auditory canal*: transmits sounds from the auricle to the tympanic membrane • *Tympanic membrane*: separates the outer ear from the middle ear; transmits sound waves by vibrating
Middle Ear	Function is to transmit sound waves and assist in equalizing pressure on both sides of the tympanic membrane. Middle ear consists of three small bones: • *Malleus*: also known as the *hammer* • *Incus*: also known as the *anvil* • *Stapes*: also known as the *stirrup* These bones transmit the sound waves from the tympanic membrane to the inner ear. • *Eustachian tube*: joins the middle ear and nasopharynx.

(continued)

(Continued)

Inner Ear	Contains receptors for hearing and balance Inner ear consists of the following: • *Cochlea*: spiral-shaped structure that looks like a snail shell • *Semicircular canals*: three curved passages that contain hair-like cells; assist with maintaining equilibrium and hearing

Urinary System

The urinary system is responsible for producing and excreting urine from the body.

ANATOMY AND PHYSIOLOGY OF THE URINARY SYSTEM

The kidneys, ureters, bladder, and urethra are responsible for maintaining the proper balance of salts and water within the body. The urinary system maintains this balance by filtering blood and removing wastes. Once in the kidneys, these wastes are converted to urine, which is eventually expelled from the body via urination.

The functions of the urinary system are as follows:

- Maintain homeostasis within the body by removing urea (waste) from the blood and keeping chemicals and water in balance.
- Urea is converted to urine within the kidney and then transferred to the urinary bladder until it is expelled.

ANATOMY AND PHYSIOLOGY OF THE KIDNEYS AND ASSOCIATED STRUCTURES

Kidneys (Figure 4-19)	Primary organs of the urinary system Located behind the peritoneum
Renal Pelvis	Funnels urine from within the kidney into the ureter
Nephrons	Functional units of the kidneys Remove waste from blood plasma and help maintain fluid balance within the body
Glomerulus	Capillaries within the nephron that filter
Ureters	Two tubes that allow urine to flow from the kidneys down to the urinary bladder
Urinary Bladder	An expandable muscular organ that serves as a reservoir for urine until it is expelled from the body
Urethra	Tube that leads from the urinary bladder to the outside of the body

Reproductive System

Male and female reproductive organs share some similarities in that their main purpose is to promote continuation of the species through reproduction; however, most organs differ significantly between the sexes.

ANATOMY AND PHYSIOLOGY OF THE REPRODUCTIVE SYSTEM

The primary organs of the male reproductive system are the penis, urethra, scrotum, testicles, and prostate gland. Some of the organs are shared with the urinary system. The primary organs of the female reproductive system are the uterus, fallopian tubes, ovaries, vagina, and breasts.

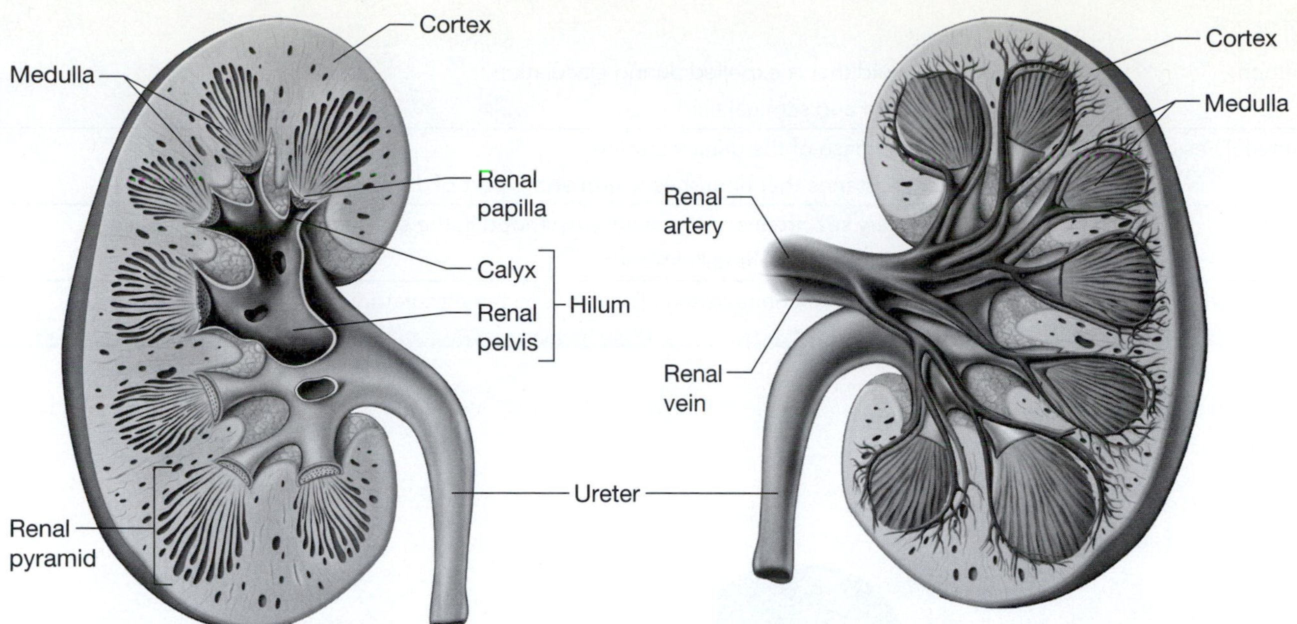

FIGURE 4-19 **(A) Sectioned kidney. (B) Renal artery and vein.**

The primary functions of the male reproductive system are as follows:

- Produce sperm and deliver them to an ovum, where fertilization can occur.

The primary functions of the female reproductive system are as follows:

- Produce ova for fertilization by sperm.
- Provide support for the developing fetus during pregnancy.
- Produce milk to feed the newborn following delivery.

ANATOMY AND PHYSIOLOGY OF THE FEMALE AND MALE REPRODUCTIVE ORGANS

MALE REPRODUCTIVE ORGANS (FIGURE 4-20)

Bulbourethral Glands	Also known as *Cowper's glands* Located on either side of the urethra Secretes a thick mucus (known as *preejaculate*) that acts as a lubricant during sexual arousal
Ejaculatory Duct	A passageway within the prostate that is formed by the junction of the vas deferens and the seminal vesicle duct Point at which semen enters the urethra
Epididymis	A long, coiled tube located on the upper part of each testicle and running the length of the testicle Where sperm mature and are stored until transported to the vas deferens
Glans Penis	Also known as the *head* of the penis The soft, sensitive bulbous part of the penis
Penis	Male organ of copulation/urination Becomes erect during arousal
Prostate Gland	Muscular secreting tissue surrounding the urethra Contracts during ejaculation and secretes part of the seminal fluid
Scrotum	A pouch-looking organ that hangs behind the penis and contains the testes Provides protection for the testes

(continued)

(Continued)

Semen	Thick white fluid that is expelled during ejaculation Contains sperm and seminal fluid
Seminal Vesicle	Located at the base of the urinary bladder Secretes a substance that nourishes sperm and is part of the seminal fluid
Testes	The two primary sex organs of the male; suspended in the scrotum Produce sperm and secrete testosterone
Vas Deferens	The passageway that connects the epididymis to the ejaculatory duct

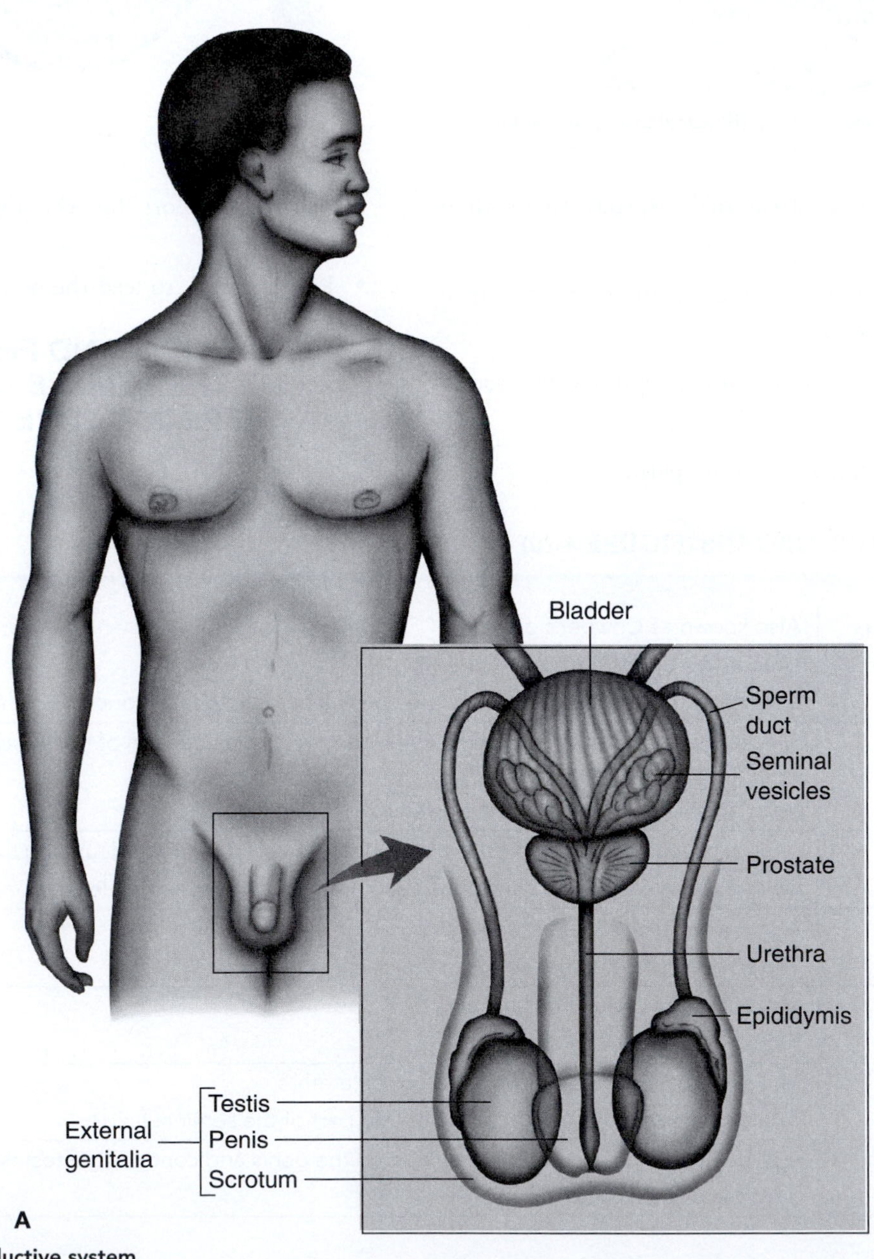

FIGURE 4-20 Male reproductive system.

FEMALE REPRODUCTIVE ORGANS (FIGURE 4-21)

Areola	Dark-pigmented area surrounding the nipple
Breasts	Also known as *mammary glands* Produce milk after childbirth
Cervix	The narrow lower portion of the uterus that extends to the vagina
Corpus Luteum	A small mass of cells that form following ovulation
Endometrium	The inner lining of the uterus Builds up to prepare for implantation of a fertilized ovum or for shedding, as occurs with menstruation
Fallopian Tubes	Located on either side of the uterus next to the ovaries Passageway for released ova to travel from the ovary to the uterus; also carry sperm up from the vagina and uterus
Fetus	The result of conception from the end of the eighth week to birth
Ovaries (two)	Primary female reproductive organs Where ova develop and estrogen is secreted
Ovulation	Occurs every month in women of reproductive age when an ovum is released from the ovary
Ovum	A mature single egg (also known as a *gamete*)
Perineum	The area between the vagina and the rectum
Progesterone	Female hormone that prepares the endometrium for implantation and helps to sustain pregnancy
Uterus	In the nonpregnant female, a normally hollow pear-shaped muscular organ that sheds the endometrial lining every month unless pregnancy occurs During pregnancy, the uterus expands and provides nourishment and protection for the developing fetus inside.
Vagina	Muscular tube that opens from the outside of the body and connects to the cervix
Vulva	Organs that make up the external genitalia: • *Mons pubis*: fat pad located over the symphysis pubis; covered by hair after puberty • *Labia majora*: two fat lip-like folds located on either side of the vagina • *Labia minora*: Two thin lip-like folds located on either side of the vagina and within the labia majora • *Clitoris*: erectile tissue located in front of the vagina

PREGNANCY-ASSOCIATED TERMS

Abortus	Product of an abortion, whether induced or spontaneous
Antepartum	Time preceding childbirth
Eclampsia	Pregnancy-related hypertension that causes seizures
Ectopic Pregnancy	Implantation of a fertilized ovum somewhere other than the uterus, usually within the fallopian tube
Gestation	Period of development during pregnancy from conception to delivery Lasts approximately 280 days
Placenta Previa	The placenta attaches low in the uterus and blocks the birth canal.
Preeclampsia	Also known as *toxemia* Complication during pregnancy producing hypertension, edema. and proteinuria
Premature Birth	Birth of a child prior to 37 weeks' gestation
Neonatal	Pertaining to the newborn period (first four weeks) of life.
Episiotomy	Surgical incision of the perineum and vagina to aid in the vaginal delivery of a baby

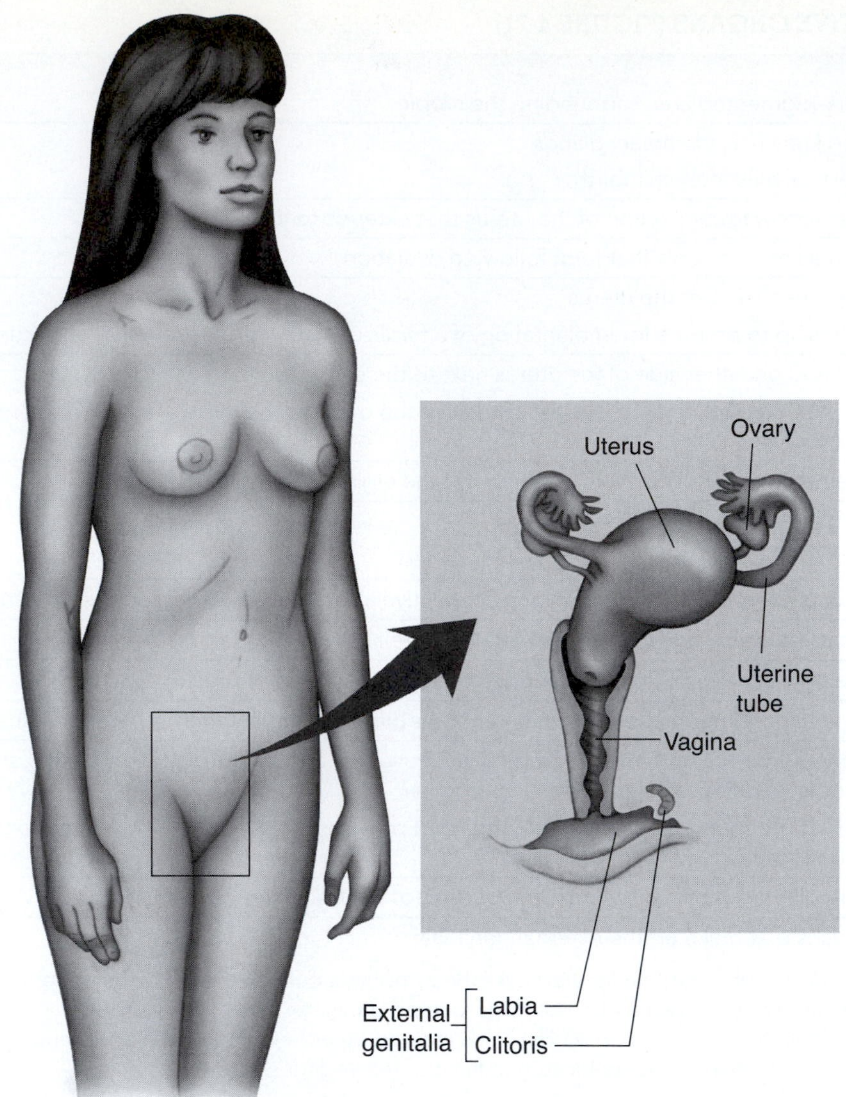

FIGURE 4-21 Female reproductive system.

Endocrine System

The endocrine system is a series of ductless glands that are responsible for producing and regulating hormones.

ANATOMY AND PHYSIOLOGY OF THE ENDOCRINE SYSTEM

The primary glands of the endocrine system are the pituitary, thyroid, parathyroid, adrenal, pancreas, thymus, and pineal glands. In addition, the ovaries and testes of the reproductive system play an important role in the endocrine system.

The primary function of the endocrine system is as follows:

- Work closely with the nervous system to maintain homeostasis.

ANATOMY AND PHYSIOLOGY OF THE ENDOCRINE GLANDS

The pituitary gland (Figure 4-22), called the *master gland*, is located at the base of the brain. Its secretions are controlled by the hypothalamus.

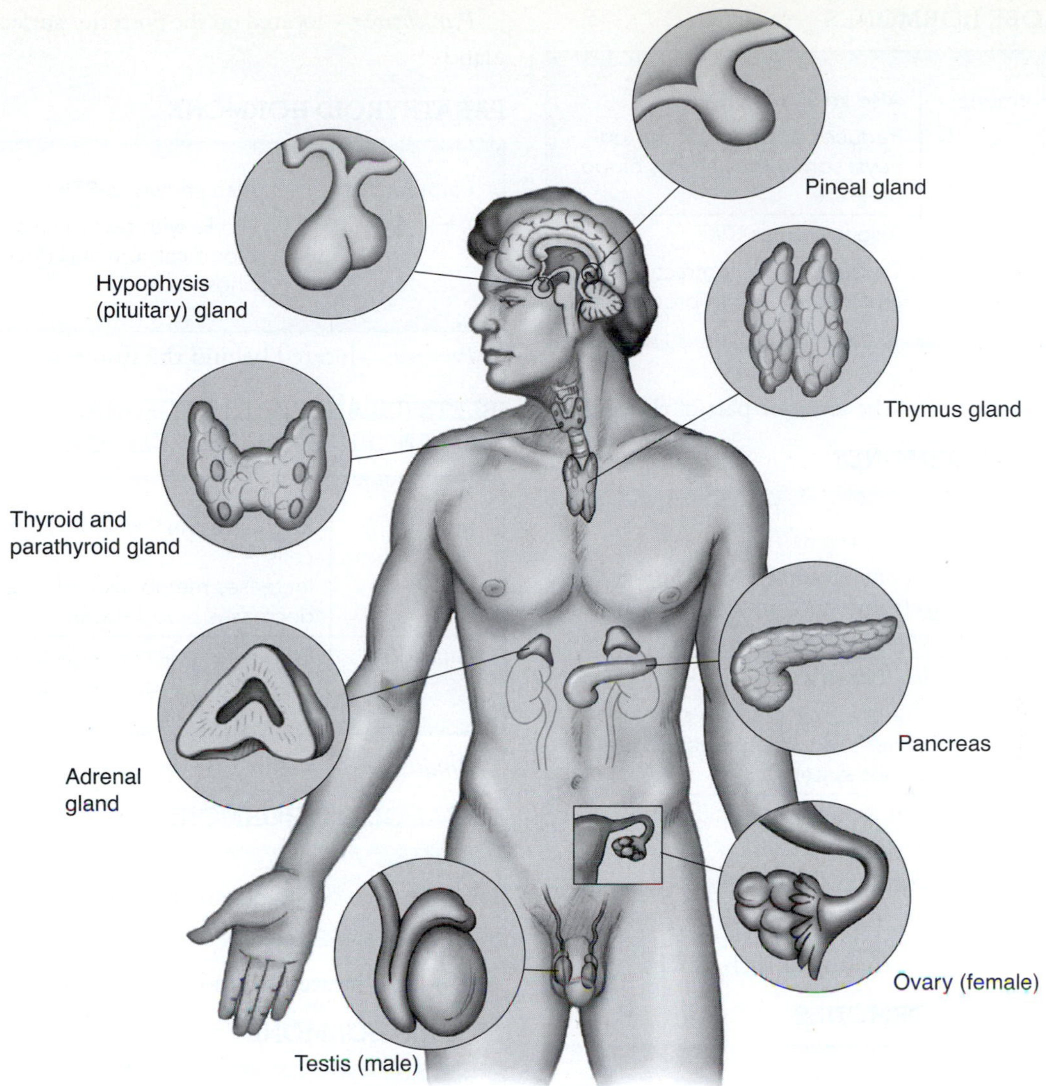

FIGURE 4-22 The primary glands of the endocrine system.

ANTERIOR LOBE HORMONES

Growth Hormone	Stimulates cell growth and reproduction
Prolactin	Promotes female breast development and milk production following childbirth Stimulates male sex hormone production
Thyroid-Stimulating Hormone	Also known as *TSH* Controls secretion of the thyroid gland's hormones
Adrenocorticotropic Hormone	Also known as *ACTH* Controls secretion of certain hormones from the adrenal cortex
Follicle-Stimulating Hormone	Also known as *FSH* Influences the reproductive organs In females, stimulates secretion of estrogen In males, stimulates production of sperm
Luteinizing Hormone	Also known as *LH* Stimulates ovulation in females Stimulates testosterone secretion in males

POSTERIOR LOBE HORMONES

Antidiuretic Hormone	Also known as *ADH* Reduces excretion of the kidneys; sometimes affects blood pressure
Oxytocin	Also known as *OXT* Causes uterine contractions and influences milk production

Thyroid gland—located in the anterior part of the neck

THYROID GLAND HORMONES

Thyroxine	Also known as *T4* Influences metabolism, protein synthesis, and maturation of the nervous system
Triiodothyronine	Also known as *T3* Influences metabolism, protein synthesis, and maturation of the nervous system
Calcitonin	Decreases blood calcium and phosphate levels

Adrenal gland—located at the top of each kidney

ADRENAL MEDULLA HORMONES

Epinephrine	Stimulates the sympathetic nervous system and increases the heart rate; is a vasoconstrictor and thus increases blood pressure; relaxes bronchioles
Norepinephrine	Stimulates the sympathetic nervous system

ADRENAL CORTEX HORMONES

Aldosterone	Helps conserve sodium and water in the kidneys and decreases potassium reabsorption
Glucocorticoids/ Cortisol	Influence protein, fat, and glucose metabolism, therefore influencing the blood glucose level; also has anti-inflammatory properties
Androgens (Sex Hormones)	Promote sex characteristics and functions

Parathyroid—located on the posterior surface of the thyroid gland

PARATHYROID HORMONE

Parathormone	Also known as *PTH* Works with calcitonin and increases blood calcium and decreases blood phosphate

Pancreas—located behind the stomach

ISLETS (ISLANDS) OF LANGERHANS: FOUND WITHIN THE PANCREAS AND SECRETE VARIOUS HORMONES

Insulin	Regulates the transport of glucose to the cells Increases metabolism of carbohydrates; decreases blood sugar
Glucagon	Stimulates release of glycogen from the liver, promoting increased blood sugar

Pineal gland—located in the third ventricle of the brain

PINEAL GLAND HORMONE

Melatonin	Regulates sleep–wake cycles

Thymus—located behind the sternum

THYMUS HORMONE

Thymosin	Affects lymphocyte production

REPRODUCTIVE GLANDS

Ovaries—located in the female pelvis

OVARIAN HORMONES

Estrogen	Promotes secondary sexual characteristics and regulates the menstrual cycle
Progesterone	Promotes secondary sexual characteristics and prepares the uterus for possible pregnancy

Testes—located in the male scrotum

TESTICULAR HORMONES

Testosterone	Promote secondary sexual characteristics and functions in males

4 APPLICATION

Directions: Select the best answer for each of the following questions. Check your answers in the Answer Key at the end of the book.

1. Which part of the brain coordinates voluntary muscle activity?
   a. Brainstem
   b. Cerebellum
   c. Hypothalamus
   d. Thalamus
   e. Cerebrum
2. Which of the following are examples of molecules?
   a. Sugar
   b. Proteins
   c. Water
   d. All of the above
   e. None of the above
3. The maxilla and mandible bones are found in which of the following?
   a. Upper leg
   b. Lower leg
   c. Upper arm
   d. Lower arm
   e. Cranium
4. Which of the following is the considered to be the "thigh bone"?
   a. Tibia
   b. Fibula
   c. Ulna
   d. Femur
   e. Radius
5. Which of the following is the correct sequence for organization within the human body from smallest to largest?
   a. Atom → Cell → Molecule → Organelle → Tissue → Organ → Organ System → Organism
   b. Atom → Molecule → Organelle → Cell → Tissue → Organ → Organ System → Organism
   c. Atom → Cell → Tissue → Organelle → Organ → Organ System → Organism
   d. Atom → Cell → Organelle → Tissue → Organ → Organism → Organ System
   e. Atom → Cell → Organelle → Tissue → Organ → Organism → Organ System
6. The act of straightening a flexed limb (increasing the angle) is known as:
   a. Flexion
   b. Extension
   c. Retraction
   d. Inversion
   e. Eversion
7. The anterior neck muscle that allows movement of the head to the chest is which of the following?
   a. Trapezius
   b. Biceps brachii
   c. Pectoralis major
   d. Latissimus dorsi
   e. Sternocleidomastoid
8. Which of the following is part of the large intestine?
   a. Duodenum
   b. Jejunum
   c. Ileum
   d. All of the above
   e. None of the above
9. Which of the following hormones causes uterine contractions and influences milk production?
   a. Thyroxine
   b. Oxytocin
   c. Calcitonin
   d. Prolactin
   e. Estrogen
10. The tip of the tongue has taste receptors that are sensitive to which of the following?
    a. Sweet
    b. Salty
    c. Sour
    d. Bitter
    e. Hot and cold
11. Where are the adrenal glands located?
    a. Behind the nasal cavity
    b. Within the throat

c. On top of the kidneys
d. Within the testes
e. At the base of the brain

12. The movement of a body part away from midline is known as:
a. Supination
b. Rotation
c. Inversion
d. Abduction
e. Adduction

13. An example of a sesamoid bone is which of the following?
a. Patella
b. Parietal bone
c. Vertebra
d. Ulna
e. Radius

14. Which of the following is also known as the *mitral valve*?
a. Tricuspid valve
b. Bicuspid valve
c. Aortic valve
d. A and B
e. None of the above

15. The fingerlike projections of a nerve cell are known as which of the following?
a. Axon
b. Converging axon
c. End buttons
d. Myelin sheath
e. Dendrites

16. Blood is an example of what type of tissue?
a. Epithelial
b. Connective
c. Muscle
d. Nervous
e. None of the above

17. The epidermis is responsible for all of the following except:
a. Provides a barrier from the outside: therefore, it is protective
b. Keeps skin oiled and elastic and prevents dry hair and scalp by producing sebum
c. Prevents water loss
d. Synthesizes vitamin D
e. Receptor for touch

18. How many bones are found in the human body?
a. 204
b. 205
c. 206
d. 207
e. 208

19. An opening in a bone where blood vessels, nerves, and ligaments pass through is known as:
a. Foramen
b. Process
c. Endosteum
d. Periosteum
e. Diaphysis

20. The appendicular skeleton consists of those bones found in which of the following?
a. Upper extremities
b. Lower extremities
c. Skull
d. A and B
e. None of the above

21. Cranial nerve number 7 is also known as the
a. Optic nerve
b. Olfactory nerve
c. Facial nerve
d. Trigeminal nerve
e. Vagus nerve

22. Muscle tissue that is striated is found in which of the following types of muscle?
a. Cardiac
b. Smooth
c. Skeletal
d. A and C
e. A and B

23. Short bones are found in which part of the body?
a. Upper and lower extremities
b. Wrist and ankle
c. Kneecap
d. Spine and hip
e. Skull

24. Muscle attachment to bone at the point that is more fixed is called:
a. Prime mover
b. Origin
c. Insertion
d. Antagonist
e. Synergist

25. Vitamin K is produced in which of the following?
a. Large intestine
b. Small intestine
c. Stomach
d. Pancreas
e. Liver

26. Tissues that absorb, protect, secrete, and excrete are which of the following types of tissue?
    a. Epithelial
    b. Connective
    c. Muscle
    d. Nervous
    e. None of the above

27. Which of the following organs stores proteins?
    a. Pancreas
    b. Gallbladder
    c. Stomach
    d. Liver
    e. None of the above

28. Which of the following is responsible for receiving oxygen-rich blood from the lungs?
    a. Left atrium
    b. Left ventricle
    c. Right atrium
    d. Right ventricle
    e. Aorta

29. Which of the following is a wing-shaped bone found in the upper portion of the hip?
    a. Illium
    b. Ischium
    c. Pubis
    d. Femur
    e. Coccyx

30. The sinoatrial node is responsible for which of the following?
    a. Initiating and establishing the rhythm of the heartbeat
    b. Transmitting an impulse to the bundle of His
    c. Transmitting an impulse to the right and left ventricles
    d. Causing the ventricles to contract
    e. Controlling the opening between the right ventricle and the pulmonary artery

31. Which of the following are the bones of the wrist?
    a. Carpals
    b. Metacarpals
    c. Tarsals
    d. Metatarsals
    e. Phalanges

32. This component of blood is also known as *platelets:*
    a. Erythrocytes
    b. Leukocytes
    c. Thrombocytes
    d. Plasma
    e. Serum

33. Which of the following structures within the lymphatic system helps fight infection by killing or weakening bacteria, viruses, cancer cells, and other invaders?
    a. Thymus
    b. Tonsils
    c. Lymph nodes
    d. Pancreas
    e. Spleen

34. The exchange of gases at the cellular level between blood and tissues is known as:
    a. Inhalation
    b. Exhalation
    c. Internal respiration
    d. External respiration
    e. All of the above

35. The central nervous system consists of all of the following except:
    a. Hypothalamus
    b. Spinal nerves
    c. Brainstem
    d. Cerebrospinal fluid
    e. Cerebellum

36. Which part of the brain regulates hormones, body temperature, hunger sensations, thirst, and sleep-wake cycles?
    a. Brainstem
    b. Cerebellum
    c. Hypothalamus
    d. Thalamus
    e. Cerebrum

37. All of the following are considered a sympathetic response except:
    a. Increased respiration rate
    b. Increased heart rate
    c. Increased blood flow to muscles
    d. Constricted pupils
    e. Dilated bronchioles

38. The number of vertebrae within the thoracic region is:
    a. 5
    b. 7
    c. 10
    d. 12
    e. 24

39. Which of the following is a sheet of connective tissue that covers, supports, and separates muscle tissues?
    a. Fascia
    b. Tendons
    c. Muscle fibers
    d. Aponeurosis
    e. Tendons

40. Which of the following provides the color of the eye?
   a. Conjunctiva
   b. Lacrimal apparatus
   c. Pupil
   d. Lens
   e. Iris

41. Which of the following separates the outer ear from the middle ear?
   a. Tympanic membrane
   b. Maleus
   c. Eustachian tube
   d. Cochlea
   e. Auricle

42. The tube that allows urine to flow from the kidneys to the urinary bladder is which of the following?
   a. Urethra
   b. Ureter
   c. Glomerulus
   d. Renal pelvis
   e. Nephron

43. The bulbous portion of the penis is known as which of the following?
   a. Prostate gland
   b. Cowper's gland
   c. Epididymis
   d. Glans penis
   e. Vas deferens

44. Which of the following best describes preeclampsia?
   a. The newborn period
   b. The placenta attaches low in the uterus and blocks the birth canal
   c. Pregnancy-related hypertension that causes seizures
   d. Complication during pregnancy producing hypertension, edema, and proteinuria
   e. Implantation of a fertilized ovum somewhere other than the uterus

45. Which of the following hormones promotes female breast development and milk production following childbirth?
   a. Estrogen
   b. Progesterone
   c. Testosterone
   d. Prolactin
   e. Follicle-stimulating hormone

46. The posterior calf muscles are which of the following?
   a. Rectus femoris
   b. Gastrocnemius
   c. Tibialis anterior
   d. Trapezius
   e. Biceps femoris

47. Which of the following hormones influences the reproductive organs in both males and females?
   a. Estrogen
   b. Progesterone
   c. Testosterone
   d. Prolactin
   e. Follicle-stimulating hormone

48. A popliteal pulse may be palpated:
   a. In the wrist
   b. In the antecubital space.
   c. On the upper portion of the foot
   d. On the interior side of the ankle
   e. Behind the knee

49. Insulin performs which of the following functions within the body?
   a. Stimulates release of glycogen from the liver
   b. Influences protein, fat, and glucose metabolism, therefore influencing blood glucose level
   c. Decreases blood sugar and phosphate levels
   d. Regulates the transport of glucose to the cells and increases metabolism of carbohydrates
   e. Helps conserve glycogen and water in the kidneys

50. Which of the following is found at the end of a long bone?
   a. Medullary canal
   b. Endosteum
   c. Periosteum
   d. Diaphysis
   e. Epiphysis

51. A small mass of cells that form following ovulation is known as:
   a. Areola
   b. Corpus luteum
   c. Ova
   d. Pregnancy
   e. Ovarian cys

5 Basic Pathophysiology of the Body Systems and Diagnostic Procedures and Treatments

CONTENTS

Common Diseases and Conditions of the Special Senses

Diagnostic Procedures and Treatments Related to the Nervous System and Special Senses

Pathophysiology of the Urinary System

Common Diseases and Conditions of the Urinary System

Diagnostic Procedures and Treatments Related to the Urinary System

Pathophysiology of the Reproductive System

Common Diseases and Conditions of the Male Reproductive System

Common Diseases and Conditions of the Female Reproductive System

Sexually Transmitted Infections (STIs)

Diagnostic Procedures and Treatments Related to the Reproductive System

Pathophysiology of the Endocrine System

Common Diseases and Conditions of the Endocrine System

Diagnostic Procedures and Treatments Related to the Endocrine System

Pathophysiology Defined

Pathophysiology is the study of the changes that happen to the structures and functions of the body and in turn lead to disease.

Neoplasia

Neoplasia is defined as growth of cells that may be either benign (not progressive and noncancerous) or malignant (invasive and cancerous).

TERMS ASSOCIATED WITH NEOPLASIA

Cancer	Cells that do not appear or behave as normal cells and that grow and spread rapidly
Carcinoma	Malignant tumor that typically metastasizes (spreads) through the lymphatic system or the bloodstream
Carcinoma in Situ	Malignant tumor that has not extended beyond the original site
Hyperplasia	Excessive growth of cells that may result in a tumor
Metastasis	Process in which cancer cells break away from the original tumor and travel to other areas of the body, where they form new tumors
Sarcoma	Neoplasm of the connective tissue

Pathophysiology of the Integumentary System

COMMON DISEASES AND CONDITIONS OF THE SKIN

Acne Vulgaris	Bacterial infection of the hair follicles and sebaceous glands Typically begins at puberty
Cellulitis	Acute infection of cells or connective tissue Caused by either staphylococcus or streptococcus bacteria via a cut or lesion on the skin
Decubitus Ulcer	Also known as *bed sore* or *pressure ulcer* Caused by lack of blood flow to a bony prominence when a patient lies in the same position for too long
Dermatitis/ Eczema	Any acute or chronic skin inflammation No known cause May be hereditary
Herpes Simplex	Also known as *cold sores* and *fever blisters* Highly contagious viral infection Transferred via skin-to-skin contact
Impetigo	Contagious skin infection usually caused by streptococcus or staphylococcus Transferred via skin-to-skin contact and by handling contaminated objects
Measles	Caused by virus Contagious Spread by airborne and droplet nuclei
Neoplasm	Abnormal tissue that grows more rapidly than normal Can be either benign (noncancerous) or malignant (cancerous) Not contagious
Pediculosis	Also known as *lice* Caused by a highly contagious parasite Typically found in hair
Petechiae	Pinpoint hemorrhages found on the skin
Psoriasis	Chronic red, raised areas of the skin that are scaly and itchy; may progress to silver-yellow scales Hereditary

Ringworm	Fungus affecting the scalp, feet, groin, or the body in general Contagious Transferred via skin-to-skin contact
Rosacea	Chronic inflammatory disorder that affects the face Not contagious
Scabies	Infection caused by a mite that burrows under the skin, causing itching Contagious
Shingles	Also known as *herpes zoster* Occurs as a result of reactivation of the herpes zoster virus when the immune system becomes weakened; this is the same virus that causes chickenpox Contagious for those who have not had chickenpox
Urticaria	Hives or raised wheals caused by an allergic reaction or stress
Varicella	Also known as *chickenpox* Highly contagious; caused by varicella-zoster virus
Vitiligo	White patches of the skin Not contagious

DIAGNOSTIC PROCEDURES AND TREATMENTS RELATED TO THE INTEGUMENTARY SYSTEM

Biopsy is the removal of a small piece of living tissue for diagnostic examination.

TYPES OF BIOPSIES

Incisional Biopsy	A piece of a tumor or lesion is removed.
Excisional Biopsy	The entire tumor or lesion is removed.
Needle Biopsy	A hollow needle is used to remove tissue.

TREATMENT PROCEDURES

Cauterization	Destruction of tissue by burning either with chemicals or electricity
Cryosurgery	Destruction or elimination of abnormal tissue through extremely cold applications, usually liquid nitrogen
Debridement	Removal of damaged tissue and debris from a wound
Incision and Drainage (I&D)	Incision of a lesion and drainage of the contents

Pathophysiology of the Skeletal System

COMMON DISEASES AND CONDITIONS OF THE SKELETAL SYSTEM

Ankylosing Spondylitis	Inflammatory disease that leads to calcification and fusion of the joints between vertebrae Can lead to loss of movement of the joints and kyphosis (humpback)
Arthritis	Inflammation of one or more joints Caused by various disease processes including wear and tear, autoimmune disorders, and injury
Bursitis	Also known as *tennis elbow* Inflammation of the bursa (the small sac of fluid that lubricates the area where two bones form a joint)
Carpal Tunnel Syndrome	Pressure on the median nerve causing pain, numbness, and hand weakness
Gout	Inflammation of the joints Caused by formation of crystals in the joints
Osteomalacia	Softening of the bone
Osteoporosis	Progressive bone density loss and thinning of bone tissue

ABNORMAL CURVATURES OF THE SPINE

Kyphosis	Also known as *humpback* Exaggerated outward curvature of the spine
Lordosis	Also known as *swayback* Exaggerated inward curvature of the spine
Scoliosis	Abnormal lateral curvature of the spine

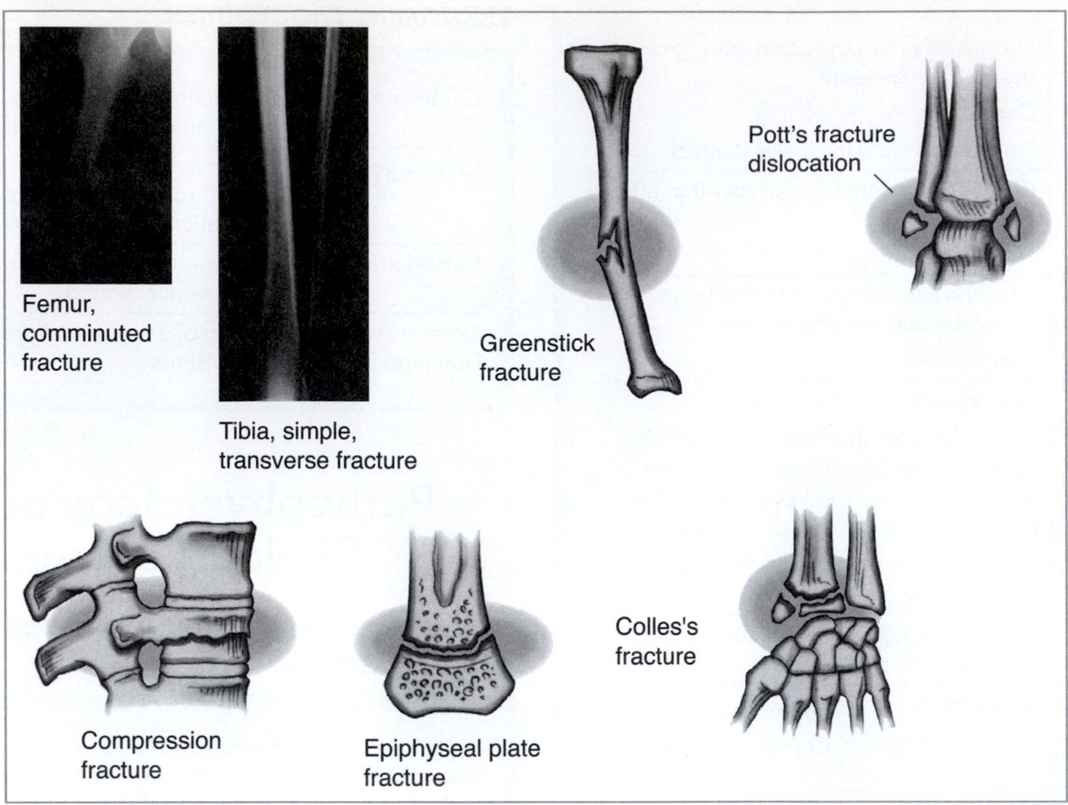

FIGURE 5-1 Types of fractures.

TYPES OF FRACTURES (FIGURE 5-1)

Closed	Also known as a *simple* or *complete fracture* Does not break the skin
Colles	A break in the distal portion of the radius Typically the result of trying to break a fall
Comminuted	Crushing of part of the bone
Compression	Occurs in the vertebrae and causes the bones to be pressed together Usually a result of a fall resulting in sitting down with a significant amount of force
Epiphyseal	Occurs in the epiphysis Most common in children
Greenstick	Also known as an *incomplete fracture* Most common in young children One side of the long bone is broken. The fracture does not go all the way through the bone.
Oblique	Fracture that is at an angle
Open	Also known as a *compound fracture* The broken bone protrudes through the skin.
Pott's	Occurs in the ankle and affects the tibia and fibula
Spiral	Occurs when the bone is twisted apart Usually due to a sports injury
Transverse	Fracture that is straight across the bone

DIAGNOSTIC PROCEDURES AND TREATMENTS RELATED TO THE SKELETAL SYSTEM

Magnetic Resonance Imaging	Also known as *MRI* Used to image interior of joints and spinal disorders
Radiography	Also known as an *X-ray* Used to visualize bones
Manipulation	Also known as *closed reduction* Attempt to realign bone(s) involved in a fracture or joint dislocation
Traction	Attempt to return a bone or joint to normal alignment by pulling in the distal direction
Immobilization	Holding, suturing, or fastening a bone in a fixed position A cast is typically used to immobilize.
External Fixation	Treatment of a fracture in which pins are placed through the skin in order to hold the fractured bone in place during healing
Internal Fixation	Pins or plates placed directly into the bone to hold the bone pieces in place to promote proper healing of a fracture

Pathophysiology of the Muscular System

COMMON DISEASES AND CONDITIONS OF THE MUSCULOSKELETAL SYSTEM

Atrophy	Wasting away of muscles as a result of poor nutrition, lack of use, or lack of nerve impulses
Epicondylitis	Inflammation of the tendon in the forearm
Fibromyalgia	Chronic inflammatory disease that affects muscle and surrounding connective tissue May develop after emotional trauma, infection, or change in climate
Muscular Dystrophy	Progressive atrophy of skeletal muscle that causes loss of strength, disability, and deformity Genetic cause
Myasthenia Gravis	Chronic disease that causes various degrees of weakness of the skeletal muscle
Paraplegia	Paralysis of both legs and the lower part of the body Caused by a spinal cord injury
Quadriplegia	Paralysis of all four extremities Caused by a spinal cord injury
Sprain	Overstretching or tearing of ligaments that support a joint
Strain	Twisting or pulling a muscle or tendon
Tendonitis	Inflammation and irritation of the tendon
Torticollis	Shortening of the muscle in the neck

DIAGNOSTIC PROCEDURES AND TREATMENTS RELATED TO THE MUSCULAR SYSTEM

Deep Tendon Reflexes (DTRs)	A reflex hammer is used to strike tendons, and then the reaction is observed.
Electromyography	Also known as *EMG* Strength of muscle contractions is recorded following electrical stimulation.
Physical Therapy	Also known as *PT* Treatment used to prevent disability and restore function by exercise, stretching, massage, and heat.
Range-of-Motion (ROM) Testing	Used to evaluate join mobility and muscle strength.

Pathophysiology of the Digestive System

COMMON DISEASES AND CONDITIONS OF THE DIGESTIVE SYSTEM

Crohn's Disease	Inflammation of the GI tract, usually the small intestine
Cirrhosis	Chronic liver cell destruction
Hepatitis	Inflammation of the liver; skin may be jaundiced
Colitis	Inflammation of the colon
Esophagitis	Inflammation of the esophagus caused by acid reflux
Gastroenteritis	Inflammation of the stomach and intestines
Hemorrhoids	Dilated, inflamed veins of the rectal mucosa
Hernia	Protrusion of an organ through the wall of the cavity that contains it
Hiatal Hernia	Upward protrusion of the stomach into the mediastinal cavity
Intussusception	Telescoping or sliding of one part of the intestine into another
Pyloric Stenosis	Narrowing of the pyloric sphincter, which may prevent emptying of the contents of the stomach into the duodenum
Ulcers	Deterioration of the mucous membrane lining

DIAGNOSTIC PROCEDURES AND TREATMENTS RELATED TO THE DIGESTIVE SYSTEM

Cholecystography	X-ray study of the gallbladder
Upper GI Series	Series of X-rays of the upper GI tract Barium swallow required as preparation for the series
Lower GI Series	Series of X-rays of the lower GI tract Barium enema required as preparation for the series
Colonoscopy	Viewing of the colon to detect problems using a colonoscope
Sigmoidoscopy	Viewing of the sigmoid colon to detect problems using a sigmoidoscope
Gastroscopy	Viewing of the stomach to detect problems
Proctoscopy	Viewing of the rectum to detect problems using a proctoscope
Hemorrhoidectomy	Excision of hemorrhoids

Pathophysiology of the Cardiovascular and Lymphatic Systems

COMMON DISEASES AND CONDITIONS OF THE CARDIOVASCULAR AND LYMPHATIC SYSTEMS

Anemia	Abnormally low numbers of healthy red blood cells, resulting in low levels of hemoglobin
Aneurysm	Weakening of the wall of a blood vessel, usually an artery
Angina Pectoris	Spasm of the heart muscle due to decreased oxygen to the myocardium, causing pain and later ischemia Usually results from stress or physical activity

Arteriosclerosis	Thickening and hardening of the walls of the arteries
Atherosclerosis	A form of arteriosclerosis caused by a reduction of blood flow to the heart muscle in the myocardium due to a buildup of fatty plaques in the coronary arteries
Bradycardia	Heart rate less than 60 beats per minute
Cerebrovascular Accident	Blood flow to the brain is reduced or a hemorrhage has occurred within the brain Commonly known as *stroke* or *CVA*
Congestive Heart Failure	Decreased pumping action of the heart as a result of reduced blood flow Commonly known as *CHF*
Coronary Artery Disease	Narrowing of the coronary arteries, which prevents adequate blood flow to the myocardium Commonly known as *CAD*
Hypertension	Blood pressure of 140/90 or greater
Hypotension	Blood pressure below 90/60
Leukemia	Malignant cancer of the bone marrow and white blood cells
Lymphadenitis	Inflamed lymph nodes resulting in swollen glands
Lymphedema	Accumulation of fluid in the legs and ankles due to improper draining
Lymphoma	Malignant tumor of the lymph nodes and tissue
Mitral Valve Prolapse	Protrusion of the mitral valve, which prevents a complete seal, causing blood to leak around it.
Mononucleosis	Increased number of mononuclear leukocytes in the blood Caused by Epstein-Barr virus
Myocardial Infarction	Also known as a *heart attack* or *MI* Partial or complete closure (occlusion) of the coronary artery resulting in deoxygenation and destruction of heart muscle
Rheumatic Heart Disease	Disease of the heart valves May develop following an upper respiratory streptococcal infection Causes damage to the lining of the heart and the heart valves
Sickle Cell Anemia	Sickle-shaped red blood cells Life-threatening inherited form of anemia May be a carrier without having the disease Occurs most often in African Americans
Splenomegaly	Enlargement of the spleen
Tachycardia	Heart rate more than 100 beats per minute
Varicose Veins	Dilation and engorgement of veins when the valves within the veins do not function properly Most common in the legs

DIAGNOSTIC PROCEDURES AND TREATMENTS RELATED TO THE CARDIOVASCULAR AND LYMPHATIC SYSTEMS

Angiography	X-ray study of the blood vessels after a contrast medium is injected into a vessel
Arteriogram	X-ray record of arterial blood vessels after a contrast medium has been injected
Cardiac Catheterization	Inserting a catheter through a vein or artery and guiding it into the heart Allows visualization of the heart's activity and measures pressures within the heart's chambers
Cardiopulmonary Resuscitation	Also known as *CPR* Emergency form of life support Performed using chest compressions and artificial respiration

(*continued*)

(Continued)

Coronary Artery Bypass Graft	Also known as *CABG* Surgical procedure used to bypass blockage of the coronary artery A piece of vein from the leg is removed and implanted within the heart to create a bypass around the blockage
Defibrillation	Electrical shock used to restore the normal heart rhythm
Echocardiogram	Ultrasound procedure used to evaluate the structures and activity of the heart
Electrocardiogram	Also known as *EKG or ECG* A record showing a tracing of the heart's electrical activity and rhythm
Holter Monitor	Electrodes attached to measure and record the heart rate and rhythm for at least 24 hours
Lymphangiogram	Injection of a contrast medium into the lymphatic system to allow better visualization of the lymphatic vessels and nodes
Pacemaker	An electronic device that is either attached externally or implanted under the skin and connected to the heart Used to regulate the heart rhythm
Pulse Oximetry	A monitor attached to a finger, which allows measurement of the oxygen level in the blood
Stress Testing	Measures heart activity under controlled physical activity conditions
Transesophageal Echocardiogram	Also known as *TEE* Ultrasound procedure that allows viewing of the heart from within the esophagus

Pathophysiology of the Respiratory System

COMMON DISEASES AND CONDITIONS OF THE RESPIRATORY SYSTEM

Allergic Rhinitis	Also known as *hay fever* Seasonal allergies cause inflammation of the mucous membranes in the eyes and nose
Asbestosis	Disease of the lung caused by chronic inhalation of asbestos
Asthma	Chronic inflammatory disease Usually caused by allergens or other irritants May result in temporary swelling of the lining of the airways, muscle tightening around the airways, and production of thick mucus
Bronchitis	Inflammation of the bronchial walls that causes temporary swelling of the mucous membranes within the bronchi Usually caused by an infection but may be a result of irritants May be acute or chronic
Chronic Obstructive Pulmonary Disease	Also known as *COPD* General term for a group of respiratory conditions, mainly chronic bronchitis and emphysema Results in chronic obstruction of air flow to and from the lungs
Common Cold	Viral infection of the upper respiratory tract Highly contagious Spread mostly via hand-to-hand contact
Cystic Fibrosis	Inherited genetic disorder Thick, dry, sticky mucus clogs organs, mainly the lungs
Diphtheria	Acute infection of the throat and upper respiratory tract caused by bacteria Potentially fatal childhood disease
Emphysema	Long-term progressive disease that causes shortness of breath Decrease in the number of alveoli; those that are left are enlarged and unable to function properly
Influenza	Acute viral infection of the respiratory tract Highly contagious Spread by droplet nuclei via coughing, sneezing, and hand-to-hand contact

Laryngitis	Inflammation of the larynx Usually results in temporary loss of voice
Legionnaire's Disease	Type of bacterial pneumonia Spread by contaminated cooling systems and showers in hotels
Pharyngitis	Also known as *sore throat* Inflammation of the pharynx
Pleurisy	Inflammation of the lining around the lungs (pleura)
Pneumoconiosis	Disease of the lung caused by chronic inhalation of dust
Pneumonia	Inflammation of the lungs caused by bacteria, viruses, fungi, or chemical irritants
Pneumothorax	Air in the pleural space that causes the lung to collapse
Pulmonary Edema	Accumulation of fluid in the lungs Usually a result of a defect in the left ventricle
Pulmonary Embolism	Blood clot in the lung
Severe Acute Respiratory Syndrome	Also known as *SARS* Viral infection of the upper respiratory tract Spread through contact, coughing, and sneezing
Sinusitis	Inflammation of the mucous membranes that line the sinuses
Tachypnea	Rapid rate of respiration Usually more than 20 breaths per minute
Tuberculosis	Also known as *TB* Bacterial infection spread by coughing, sneezing, talking, and laughing
Whooping Cough	Also known as *pertussis* Infectious disease of the upper respiratory tract caused by bacteria Contagious

DIAGNOSTIC PROCEDURES AND TREATMENTS RELATED TO THE RESPIRATORY SYSTEM

Bronchoscopy	Visual examination of the bronchi using a bronchoscope
Chest X-Ray	Radiographic imaging of the structures within the chest Used for diagnosing pneumonia, lung tumors, pneumothorax, and tuberculosis
Endotracheal Intubation	Establishing an airway by passing a tube through the nose or mouth into the trachea
Postural Drainage	Positioning the patient at different angles in order to promote drainage of lung secretions
Pulmonary Function Tests	Also known as *PFTs* Tests used to measure lung capacity as well as the capability to move air into and out of the lungs
Spirometry	Measurement of the volume of air inhaled and exhaled, as well as the length of each breath, using a spirometer
Tuberculin Skin Testing	Screening test to detect exposure to tuberculosis; most often done via PPD (purified protein derivative)
Septoplasty	Surgical reconstruction of the nasal septum
Thoracentesis	Surgical puncture of the chest wall with a needle; used to obtain fluid and/or air from the pleural cavity
Tracheostomy	Creation of an opening and passing of a tube within the trachea to enable air passage or removal of secretions
Tracheotomy	Emergency procedure performed to obtain an airway
Ventilator	Mechanical device used for artificial respiration

Pathophysiology of the Nervous System and Special Senses

COMMON DISEASES AND CONDITIONS OF THE NERVOUS SYSTEM

Alzheimer's Disease	Progressive degenerative disorder of the brain affecting the ability to carry out activities of daily living
Amyotrophic Lateral Sclerosis	Also known as *ALS* and *Lou Gehrig's disease* Degenerative disease of neurons resulting in progressive weakness
Bell's Palsy	Damage to a facial nerve resulting in paralysis and drooping on one side of the face
Cerebral Palsy	Brain damage before or during birth resulting in poor muscle control and spasticity
Cerebrovascular Accident	Also known as *CVA* and *stroke* Decrease of the blood supply to the brain caused by a clot or a hemorrhage
Encephalitis	Severe inflammation of the brain; most commonly caused by a virus
Epilepsy	Abnormal electrical impulses within the brain that cause bursts of excitement and may result in seizures
Hydrocephalus	Excessive fluid within the brain
Meningitis	Inflammation of the covering of the brain and spinal cord
Multiple Sclerosis	Also known as *MS* Autoimmune disorder that causes destruction of the myelin sheath, resulting in episodic tremors, weakness, mood swings, and vision changes
Neuralgia	Nerve pain caused by an irritated or damaged nerve
Paraplegia	Paralysis from the waist down Usually the result of damage to the spinal cord
Parkinson's Disease	Degeneration of nerve cells in the brain that control movement, resulting in tremors
Quadriplegia	Paralysis from the shoulders down Usually the result of damage to the spinal cord
Sciatica	Inflammation of the sciatic nerve resulting in pain in the thigh and leg
Seizure Disorders	Disturbance in brain function causing uncontrollable contraction of muscles
Spina Bifida	Birth defect in which the spinal cord is not completely enclosed

COMMON DISEASES AND CONDITIONS OF THE SPECIAL SENSES

Amblyopia	Also known as *lazy eye* Condition in which muscles are weaker in one eye than in the other
Astigmatism	Eyeball is not perfectly round, causing the eye to focus improperly
Blepharoptosis	Drooping of the upper eyelid
Cataract	Lens of the eye becomes cloudy, preventing light from entering and making it difficult to see clearly Commonly associated with aging
Conjunctivitis	Also known as *pink eye* Inflammation of the lining of the eyelids Highly contagious
Glaucoma	Increased intraocular pressure Loss of peripheral vision May cause blindness if left untreated

Hordeolum	Also known as a *sty* Infection of one of the glands in the eyelid
Hyperopia	Also known as *farsightedness* Ability to see faraway objects more clearly than those close by Most commonly occurs after age 40
Impacted Cerumen	Accumulation of hardened cerumen in the external auditory canal, making it difficult to hear clearly
Macular Degeneration	Deterioration of the central portion of the retina Loss of central vision with intact peripheral vision
Ménière's Disease	Condition of the inner ear that may cause vertigo, tinnitus, and nerve loss
Monochromatism	Also known as *color blindness* Inability to distinguish colors
Myopia	Also known as *nearsightedness* Ability to see nearby objects more clearly than those farther away
Otitis Externa	Also known as *swimmer's ear* Infection of the outer ear
Otitis Media	Inflammation of the middle ear Common in young children
Otosclerosis	Hardening of the oval window resulting in fusion of the stapes and hearing loss
Presbycusis	Progressive hearing loss Most common in the aged
Presbyopia	Loss of the ability to adjust near-to-far and far-to-near vision due to age and the loss of elasticity in the lens
Tinnitus	Ringing or buzzing in the ears

DIAGNOSTIC PROCEDURES AND TREATMENTS RELATED TO THE NERVOUS SYSTEM AND SPECIAL SENSES

DIAGNOSTIC PROCEDURES AND TREATMENTS RELATED TO THE NERVOUS SYSTEM

Computerized Axial Tomography	Also known as *CAT* or *CT scan* X-rays of the layers of the brain with the aid of computer guidance to produce cross-sectional views
Electroencephalography	Also known as *EEG* Process of recording the brain waves
Encephalography	X-ray study of the fluid-containing spaces in the brain
Lumbar Puncture	Also known as a *spinal tap* Puncture with a spinal needle between the L3 and L4 or L4 and L5 vertebrae Cerebrospinal fluid is aspirated for examination
Magnetic Resonance Imaging	Also known as *MRI* Pictures of the brain using magnetic and radio waves
Myelography	X-ray study of the spinal cord following injection of a contrast medium
Transcutaneous Electronic Nerve Stimulation	Also known as *TENS* Electronic impulses applied to nerve endings through the skin used to control pain

DIAGNOSTIC PROCEDURES AND TREATMENTS RELATED TO THE SPECIAL SENSES

Tonometry	Measurement of intraocular pressure to check for glaucoma using a tonometer
Refraction	Examination for visual correction or prescription of glasses
Visual Acuity	Evaluation of the eye and its ability to distinguish details and shapes
Ishihara Method	Evaluation of the ability to distinguish differences in colors
Corneal Transplant	Surgical replacement of diseased or scarred cornea
Myringotomy	Incision of the tympanic membrane to create an opening for placement of tympanostomy tubes
Audiometry	Evaluation and measurement of the ability to hear using an audiometer
Tympanocentesis	Surgical puncture of the tympanic membrane using a needle to remove fluid

Pathophysiology of the Urinary System

COMMON DISEASES AND CONDITIONS OF THE URINARY SYSTEM

Acute Renal Failure	Sudden loss of the kidney's ability to remove waste
Chronic Renal Failure	Gradual, progressive loss of the kidney's ability to remove waste
Cystitis	Inflammation of the bladder that occurs when bacteria infect the lower urinary tract Most often caused by *Escherichia coli*
Dysuria	Difficult or painful urination
Epispadias	Congenital abnormality that causes the opening of the male urethra to be located above the penis
Glomerulonephritis	Inflammation of the glomerulus, which affects the ability of the kidney to remove waste and excess fluids
Hypospadias	Congenital abnormality that causes the opening of the male urethra to be located on the underside of the penis
Incontinence	Inability to control flow of urine • *Stress incontinence*: Most common form of incontinence. Urine may leak when the individual sneezes, coughs, or laughs. • *Urge incontinence*: The bladder contracts without warning, which in turn may allow urine to leak. • *Overflow incontinence*: Blockage prevents complete emptying of the bladder, causing the bladder to overflow. • *Enuresis*: Bed wetting
Polycystic Kidney Disease	Inherited disorder that causes clusters of cysts to form on the kidneys
Pyelonephritis	Infection of the kidney and renal pelvis, usually as a result of a bacterial urinary tract infection
Renal Calculus	Also known as *kidney stones* Caused by deposits of mineral salts in the kidney
Urethritis	Inflammation of the urethra

DIAGNOSTIC PROCEDURES AND TREATMENTS RELATED TO THE URINARY SYSTEM

Catheterization	Insertion of a urinary catheter through the urethra and into the urinary bladder in order to withdraw urine and relieve urinary pressure
Cystoscopy	Visual examination of the urinary bladder using a cystoscope
Dialysis	Procedure that removes waste from the blood when the patient's kidneys are no longer functioning
Intravenous Pyelogram	Also known as *IVP* X-ray of the kidneys and ureters after a contrast medium has been injected
KUB	Also known as a *flat plate* of the abdomen X-ray of the kidney, ureters, and bladder
Lithotripsy	Procedure to destroy kidney stones via ultrasound waves that travel through water
Urinalysis	Visual examination of urine

Pathophysiology of the Reproductive System

COMMON DISEASES AND CONDITIONS OF THE MALE REPRODUCTIVE SYSTEM

Anorchism	Congenital defect resulting in the absence of one or both testes
Benign Prostatic Hypertrophy	Also known as *BPH* Enlargement of the prostate that may occur in men over age 50
Carcinoma of the Testes	Cancer of one or both testes
Cryptorchidism	Failure of one or both testicles to descend into the scrotum
Erectile Dysfunction	Also known as *ED* Inability to achieve and maintain an erection
Hydrocele	Excessive fluid in the scrotum
Impotence	Inability to achieve or maintain erection of the penis
Orchitis	Inflammation of the testes
Prostate Cancer	Slow-growing cancer that affects the prostate
Prostatic Hyperplasia	Abnormal cell growth within the prostate
Prostatitis	Inflammation of the prostate gland
Varicocele	Varicose vein of the testicle

COMMON DISEASES AND CONDITIONS OF THE FEMALE REPRODUCTIVE SYSTEM

Amenorrhea	Absence of menstruation
Cervical Cancer	Cancer of the cervix
Cervicitis	Inflammation of the cervix
Dysmenorrhea	Difficult and/or painful menstruation
Endometrial Cancer	Cancer of the inner lining of the uterus (endometrium)
Endometriosis	Endometrial tissue found outside of the uterus, usually within the pelvic area
Fibrocystic Breast Disease	One or several benign cysts within the breast; may become malignant
Hysterectomy	Surgical removal of the uterus

(*continued*)

(Continued)

Mastectomy	Removal of the breast due to cancer
Menopause	Cessation of normal menstrual periods
Menorrhagia	Excessive amount of menstrual blood, with the menstrual period lasting longer than usual
Ovarian Cancer	Cancer of the ovary
Ovarian Cyst	Fluid-filled sac within the ovary
Pelvic Inflammatory Disease	Also known as *PID* Inflammation of the female reproductive organs, usually as a result of a sexually transmitted infection
Premenstrual Syndrome	Also known as *PMS* Irritability, bloating, headache, and anxiety that may occur within two weeks prior to the onset of the menstrual period
Prolapsed Uterus	Falling of the uterus, causing the cervix to protrude through the vaginal opening Usually the result of weakened muscles due to vaginal delivery
Salpingitis	Inflammation of the fallopian tubes
Uterine Fibroids	Also known as *leiomyoma* Benign tumors that grow within the wall of the uterus
Uterine Cancer	Cancer of the uterus Occurs most commonly following menopause
Vaginitis	Inflammation of the vagina caused by yeast, bacteria, or other organisms

SEXUALLY TRANSMITTED INFECTIONS (STIs)

Acquired Immune Deficiency Syndrome	Also known as *AIDS* The final stage of human immunodeficiency virus
Human Immunodeficiency Virus	Also known as *HIV* Affects the immune system Transmitted through semen, amniotic fluid, cerebrospinal fluid, and blood
Syphilis	Highly contagious STI caused by a bacterial organism called a *spirochete* Spread via broken skin or mucous membranes, most often through sexual contact
Gonorrhea	Contagious STI causing inflammation of the mucous membranes
Chlamydial infections	Leading cause of PID Caused by the bacterium *Chlamydia trachomatis* Transmitted via sexual contact
Trichomoniasis	Common STI in men and women; typically, men do not exhibit symptoms Caused by the protozoan *Trichomonas vaginalis*
Genital herpes	Common STI that is highly contagious Most often caused by Herpes Simplex Virus 2 (HSV-2), but can also be caused by Herpes Simplex Virus 1 (HSV-1) No known cure
Human Papilloma Virus	Also known as *HPV* and *genital warts* The most common STI Transferred via genital-to-genital contact Caused by the human papilloma virus

DIAGNOSTIC PROCEDURES AND TREATMENTS RELATED TO THE REPRODUCTIVE SYSTEM

DIAGNOSTIC PROCEDURES AND TREATMENTS RELATED TO THE MALE REPRODUCTIVE SYSTEM

Circumcision	Surgical removal of the foreskin of the penis
Prostatectomy	Surgical removal of all or a portion of the prostate gland
Testicular Self-Examination	Also known as *TSE* Self-examination performed by gently rolling the testicles between the thumb and forefingers of both hands
Vasectomy	Male sterilization procedure Removal of a portion of the vas deferens

DIAGNOSTIC PROCEDURES AND TREATMENTS RELATED TO THE FEMALE REPRODUCTIVE SYSTEM

Amniocentesis	Puncture of the amniotic sac with an ultrasound-guided needle to remove amniotic fluid for study
Breast Self-Examination	Self-examination performed by palpating the breasts in the shower using flat fingertips circling the breasts from the nipple outward
Cauterization	Destruction of abnormal cells or tissue by using either electrical or chemical heat
Cryotherapy	Freezing a section of the cervix Used to destroy abnormal cells of the cervix
Dilation and Curettage	Also known as *D & C* Dilation of the cervix and curettage (scraping) of the inside of the uterus
Mammogram	X-ray of the breasts
Pap Smear	Obtaining microscopic samples of the cervix and surrounding tissue to examine them for the presence of abnormal cells

Pathophysiology of the Endocrine System

COMMON DISEASES AND CONDITIONS OF THE ENDOCRINE SYSTEM

Acromegaly	Chronic disease of middle-aged adults Caused by excess production of growth hormone in adulthood Can result in diabetes mellitus, hypertension, and an increased risk of cardiovascular disease
Cushing's Syndrome	Excess of glucocorticoids causing edema of the face and fatty tissue on the back ("moon face" and "buffalo hump")
Diabetes Mellitus	Metabolic disease due to hyperglycemia and glycosuria as a result of poor insulin secretion and/or action
Dwarfism	Lack of growth hormone, causing the individual to be abnormally small If it occurs during childhood, it is called *cretinism*
Gigantism	Excessive production of growth hormone, causing the individual to be abnormally tall

(*continued*)

(Continued)

Hyperthyroidism	Excess thyroid hormone production, resulting in increased metabolic rate, increased sweating, nervousness, and weight loss Graves' disease • *Exophthalmia*: bulging eyes • *Goiter*: enlarged thyroid due to lack of iodine
Hypothyroidism	Decrease in thyroid hormone production, resulting in decreased metabolic rate, increased fatigue, depression, and sensitivity to cold
Myxedema	Severe life-threatening form of adult hypothyroidism
Tetany	Uncontrolled twitching of the muscles due to hypoparathyroidism

DIAGNOSTIC PROCEDURES AND TREATMENTS RELATED TO THE ENDOCRINE SYSTEM

Thyroidectomy	Surgical removal of the thyroid gland
Thyroid Function Tests	Laboratory test that measures how well the thyroid gland is functioning
Thyroid Scan	Measures the size and shape of the thyroid gland and provides information on its activity
Glucose Tolerance Test	Laboratory test that measures how the patient's body metabolizes glucose; confirmatory test for diabetes Also know as *GTT*

5 APPLICATION

Directions: Select the best answer for each of the following questions. Check your answers in the Answer Key at the end of the book.

1. If a patient was scheduled for a proctoscopy, what will the physician be viewing when he or she performs the procedure?
   a. The patient's stomach
   b. The patient's gallbladder
   c. The patient's rectum
   d. The patient's prostate
   e. The patient's colon

2. A highly contagious skin infection usually caused by streptococcus or staphylococcus, transferred via skin-to-skin contact and handling contaminated objects, is known as which of the following?
   a. Herpes simplex
   b. Impetigo
   c. Measles
   d. Ringworm
   e. Scabies

3. Inflammation of the joints caused by formation of crystals in the joints is known as which of the following?
   a. Arthritis
   b. Gout
   c. Rheumatoid arthritis
   d. Spondylitis
   e. Bursitis

4. Which of the following statements best describes psoriasis?
   a. Hereditary condition
   b. Chronic red, raised areas of the skin
   c. Skin is scaly and itchy
   d. All of the above
   e. None of the above
5. A disease of the lung caused by chronic inhalation of dust is known as which of the following?
   a. Severe acute respiratory syndrome
   b. Pneumoconiosis
   c. Asbestosis
   d. Legionnaire's disease
   e. Pneumothorax
6. Which of the following best describes a Colles fracture?
   a. Part of the bone is crushed
   b. Occurs in the vertebrae
   c. Occurs in the ankle
   d. Occurs when the bone is twisted apart
   e. None of the above
7. Which of the following best describes those conditions common in the aged patient?
   a. Hyperopia, presbyopia, amblyopia, otitis externa
   b. Presbycusis, cataracts, presbyopia, otitis media
   c. Cataracts, presbycusis, presbyopia, hyperopia
   d. Conjunctivitis, otitis externa, presbyopia, amblyopia
   e. Presbyopia, hyperopia, amblyopia, otitis media
8. A severe form of adult hypothyroidism is known as
   a. Myxedema
   b. Tetany
   c. Acromegaly
   d. Cushing's syndrome
   e. Hashimoto's thyroiditis
9. Hives are also known as:
   a. Vitiligo
   b. Urticaria
   c. Eczema
   d. Vulgaris
   e. Varicella
10. When there is decreased oxygen to the myocardium, a spasm of the heart muscle occurs. Which of the following terms best describes this condition?
    a. Congestive heart failure
    b. Myocardial infarction
    c. Coronary artery disease
    d. Angina pectoris
    e. Rheumatic heart disease
11. Which of the following procedures allows visualization of heart activity and measures pressures within the heart's chambers?
    a. Echocardiogram
    b. Cardiac catheterization
    c. Transesophageal echocardiogram
    d. Holter monitor
    e. Arteriogram
12. All of the following are different types of urinary incontinence except
    a. Urge
    b. Nocturia
    c. Stress
    d. Enuresis
    e. Overflow
13. Which of the following best describes a fracture that occurs on an angle?
    a. Comminuted
    b. Compression
    c. Oblique
    d. Open
    e. Pott's
14. The term used to describe a benign tumor that grows within the wall of the uterus is
    a. Pelvic inflammatory disease
    b. Endometriosis
    c. Prolapsed uterus
    d. Uterine fibroids
    e. Uterine cancer
15. Which of the following statements regarding neoplasms is true?
    a. Benign tissue growth
    b. Malignant tissue growth
    c. Abnormal tissue that grows more rapidly than normal
    d. Both B and C
    e. All of the above
16. Which of the following best describes the wasting away of muscles due to lack of use?
    a. Atrophy
    b. Multiple sclerosis
    c. Myasthenia gravis
    d. Amyotrophic lateral sclerosis
    e. Fibromyalgia
17. The excessive production of growth hormone that causes abnormally tall individuals is known as
    a. Tetany
    b. Acromegaly
    c. Gigantism
    d. Cushing's syndrome
    e. Dwarfism

18. Which of the following best describes a muscle sprain?
    a. Overstretching of ligaments that support a joint
    b. Twisting or pulling a muscle or tendon
    c. Tearing of ligaments that support a joint
    d. Both A and B
    e. Both A and C

19. Which of the following best describes intussusception?
    a. Protrusion of an organ through the wall of the cavity that contains it
    b. Telescoping or sliding of one part of the intestine into another
    c. Narrowing of the pyloric sphincter
    d. Dilated, inflamed veins of the rectal mucosa
    e. Chronic liver cell destruction

20. Cellulitis is defined as which of the following?
    a. An acute infection of cells
    b. An acute infection of nerves
    c. An acute infection of connective tissue
    d. Both A and B
    e. Both A and C

21. Which of the following is a diagnosis for an abnormal curvature of the spine?
    a. Scoliosis
    b. Kyphosis
    c. Lordosis
    d. All of the above
    e. None of the above

22. All of the following statements regarding sickle cell anemia are true except:
    a. Red blood cells are abnormally shaped.
    b. Life-threatening form of anemia
    c. May be a carrier without having the disease
    d. Malignancy of red blood cells
    e. Occurs most often in African Americans

23. A record showing the tracing of the heart's electrical activity and rhythm is known as:
    a. Echocardiogram
    b. Electrocardiogram
    c. EKG
    d. Both A and C
    e. Both B and C

24. Which of the following best describes pleurisy?
    a. Type of bacterial pneumonia
    b. Air in the pleural space that causes the lung to collapse
    c. Inflammation of the lining around the lungs
    d. Inflammation of the lungs caused by bacteria
    e. Accumulation of fluid in the lungs

25. If a patient has been diagnosed with hypertension, which of the following best describes his or her blood pressure readings?
    a. 130/80 or greater
    b. 130/90 or greater
    c. 140/80 or greater
    d. 140/90 or greater
    e. 150/90 or greater

26. All of the following statements regarding diphtheria are true except:
    a. Acute infection of the throat
    b. Caused by bacteria
    c. Potentially fatal childhood disease
    d. Thick, dry, sticky mucus clogs organs, mainly the lungs
    e. Acute infection of the respiratory tract

27. Which of the following statements about multiple sclerosis is not correct?
    a. Patient may experience episodic tremors
    b. Autoimmune disorder
    c. Patient may experience mood swings
    d. Causes destruction of neurons
    e. Patient may experience vision changes

28. Poor muscle control and spasticity that may be a result of brain damage that occurred before or during birth is known as which of the following?
    a. Bell's palsy
    b. ALS
    c. Cerebral palsy
    d. Epilepsy
    e. CVA

29. When the muscles in one eye are weaker than the muscles in the other eye, the condition is known as:
    a. Hyperopia
    b. Myopia
    c. Presbyopia
    d. Diplopia
    e. Amblyopia

30. When there is a decrease in the number of alveoli and those left are enlarged and unable to function properly, the condition is best defined as which of the following?
    a. Emphysema
    b. Cystic fibrosis
    c. Asthma
    d. SARS
    e. Pertussis

31. The ability to see faraway objects more clearly than those nearby is known as:
    a. Hyperopia
    b. Myopia

c. Presbyopia
d. Diplopia
e. Amblyopia

32. Which of the following best defines tracheotomy?
   a. Creating an opening and passing a tube within the trachea to enable air passage or removal of secretions
   b. Emergency procedure performed to obtain an airway
   c. Establishing an airway by passing a tube through the nose or mouth into the trachea
   d. Both A and B
   e. Both B and C

33. A patient diagnosed with Ménière's disease may experience which of the following?
   a. Nerve loss
   b. Tinnitus
   c. Vertigo
   d. All of the above
   e. None of the above

34. Tonometry is best defined as which of the following?
   a. Measuring intraocular pressure to check for glaucoma
   b. Evaluation and measurement for visual correction or prescription of glasses
   c. Evaluation and measurement of the ability to hear
   d. Evaluation of the ability to distinguish difference in colors
   e. Measurement of the ability to see tone on tone

35. Which of the following best defines electroencephalography?
   a. Process of recording layers of the brain with the aid of computer guidance
   b. Recording of fluid-containing spaces in the brain
   c. Process of recording brain waves
   d. Study of the spinal cord following an injection of a contrast medium
   e. Electronic impulses applied to nerve endings through the skin used to control pain

36. When a lumbar puncture is made, which of the following best identifies where within the vertebral column the puncture occurs?
   a. Between the L1 and L2 vertebrae
   b. Between the L3 and L4 vertebrae
   c. Between the L4 and L5 vertebrae
   d. Both A and B
   e. Both B and C

37. An inherited disorder that causes clusters of fluid-filled sacs to form on the kidneys is known as
   a. Glomerulonephritis
   b. Renal calculus
   c. Pyelonephritis
   d. Polycystic kidney disease
   e. Cystitis

38. Otosclerosis is defined as hardening of the ____________.
   a. Cochlea
   b. Oval window
   c. Incus
   d. Malleus
   e. Tympanic membrane

39. Destruction or elimination of abnormal tissue through extremely cold applications, usually of liquid nitrogen, is known as which of the following?
   a. I & D
   b. Debridement
   c. Cauterization
   d. Cryosurgery
   e. Excisional biopsy

40. Which of the following is most often caused by *Escherichia coli*?
   a. Renal calculi
   b. Hypospadias
   c. Dysuria
   d. Glomerulonephritis
   e. Cystitis

41. Benign prostatic hypertrophy is best defined as
   a. Abnormal cell growth within the prostate
   b. Enlargement of the prostate
   c. Excessive fluid in the scrotum
   d. Inflammation of the prostate gland
   e. Slow-growing form of cancer that affects the prostate

42. Which of the following best defines dysmenorrhea?
   a. Absence of menstruation
   b. Excessive amount of menstrual blood
   c. Difficult and/or painful menstruation
   d. Cancer of the endometrium
   e. Menstrual period that lasts longer than usual

43. Which of the following terms best describes an inflammation of the female reproductive organs that is usually the result of a sexually transmitted infection?
   a. Salpingitis
   b. PID
   c. Vaginitis
   d. Cervicitis
   e. Endometritis

44. All of the following statements regarding trichomoniasis are true except:
   a. Men typically do not exhibit symptoms
   b. Common STI in women
   c. Leading cause of PID
   d. Caused by a protozoan
   e. Common STI in men

45. Destruction of abnormal cells or tissue by using either electrical or chemical heat is known as which of the following?
    a. Vasectomy
    b. Circumcision
    c. D & C
    d. Cryotherapy
    e. Cauterization

46. Which of the following best describes the procedure in which an X-ray of the kidneys and ureters is performed after a contrast medium has been injected?
    a. KUB
    b. Lithotripsy
    c. IVP
    d. Cystoscopy
    e. Renal X-ray

47. Which of the following best describes petechiae?
    a. Pinpoint hemorrhages found on the skin
    b. Chronic red, raised areas of the skin that are scaly and itchy
    c. Chronic inflammatory disorder that affects the face
    d. Any acute or chronic skin inflammation
    e. Caused by a highly contagious parasite

48. All of the following statements regarding diabetes mellitus are true except:
    a. Metabolic disease due to hyperglycemia
    b. Occurs as the result of poor insulin secretion
    c. Excess of glucocorticoids
    d. Metabolic disease due to glycosuria
    e. Occurs as the result of poor insulin action

49. Pathophysiology is defined as which of the following?
    a. Study of the changes that happen to the structures of the body
    b. Study of the changes that happen to the functions of the body
    c. Changes within the body that lead to disease
    d. All of the above
    e. None of the above

50. Acromegaly may have secondary complications such as:
    a. Diabetes mellitus
    b. Increased risk of cardiovascular disease
    c. Hypertension
    d. All of the above
    e. None of the above

51. Regarding decubitus ulcers, all of the following are true except:
    a. Also known as *bed sores*
    b. Caused by patients lying in the same position for too long
    c. Bacterial infection of the hair follicles
    d. Also known as *pressure ulcers*
    e. Caused by lack of blood flow to a bony prominence

52. When one or both testicles fail to descend into the scrotum, the condition is known as
    a. BPH
    b. Orchitis
    c. Cryptorchidism
    d. Varicocele
    e. Prostatic hyperplasia

53. Which of the following best defines paraplegia?
    a. Paralysis of all four extremities
    b. Paralysis from the waist up
    c. Paralysis of both legs
    d. Paralysis of both legs and the lower part of the body
    e. Paralysis of the lower part of the body

54. All of the following are signs or symptoms of hyperthyroidism except:
    a. Increased sweating
    b. Increased metabolic rate
    c. Weight loss
    d. Nervousness
    e. Fatigue

55. Which of the following fractures is most commonly found in children?
    a. Open
    b. Greenstick
    c. Colles
    d. Comminuted
    e. Transverse

56. Which of the following best describes the medical condition that causes thickening and hardening of the walls of the arteries due to a buildup of fatty plaques in the coronary arteries?
    a. Arteriosclerosis
    b. Atherosclerosis
    c. Angina
    d. Aneurysm
    e. Ischemia

6 Basic Nutrition

CONTENTS

Nutrition and the Major Nutrients

NUTRITION

Nutrition refers to the processes associated with taking in and metabolizing food for growth, repair, and maintenance of the body. In order to benefit the body, food taken in must provide nutrition. Nutritious foods provide energy that allows vital functions to occur, help build and repair tissue, and regulate metabolic processes.

MAJOR NUTRIENTS

Nutrients may be either organic or inorganic, and the body requires more than 50 nutrients to function properly. These nutrients fall into one of six classifications (Figure 6-1):

- Carbohydrates
- Proteins
- Fats
- Vitamins
- Minerals
- Water

NUTRIENT CLASS	BODILY FUNCTIONS	FOOD SOURCES
CARBOHYDRATES	Provides work energy for body activities, and heat energy for maintenance of body temperature.	Cereal grains and their products (bread, breakfast cereals, macaroni products), potatoes, sugar, syrups, fruits, milk, vegetables, nuts.
PROTEINS	Build and renew body tissues; regulate body functions and supply energy. Complete proteins; maintain life and provide growth. Incomplete proteins; maintain life but do not provide for growth.	Complete proteins: Derived from animal foods—meat, milk, eggs, fish, cheese, poultry. Incomplete proteins: Derived from vegetable foods—soybeans, dry beans, peas, some nuts and whole grain products.
FATS	Give work energy for body activities and heat energy for maintenance of body temperature. Carrier of vitamins A and D, provide fatty acids necessary for growth and maintenance of body tissues.	Some foods are chiefly fat, such as lard, vegetable fats and oils, and butter. Many other foods contain smaller proportions of fats—nuts, meats, fish, poultry, cream, whole milk.
MINERALS Calcium	Builds and renews bones, teeth, and other tissues; regulates the activity of the muscles, heart, nerves; and controls the clotting of blood.	Milk and milk products except butter; most dark green vegetables; canned salmon.
PHOSPHORUS	Associated with calcium in some functions needed to build and renew bones and teeth. Influences the oxidation of foods in the body cells; important in nerve tissue.	Widely distributed in foods; especially cheese, oat cereals, whole wheat products, dry beans and peas, meat, fish, poultry, nuts.

FIGURE 6-1 Basic food groups.

There are two types of vitamins: water-soluble and fat-soluble. With the exception of vitamins A, D, and K, vitamins cannot be formed within the body, so they must be taken in through the foods consumed.

Fat-Soluble Vitamins

- Vitamin A
- Vitamin D
- Vitamin E
- Vitamin K

Water-Soluble Vitamins

- Vitamin B_1
- Vitamin B_2
- Vitamin B_{12}
- Vitamin C
- Niacin

NUTRIENT CLASS	BODILY FUNCTIONS	FOOD SOURCES
MINERALS (*continued*) Iron	Builds and renews hemoglobin, the red pigment in blood which carries oxygen from the lungs to the cells.	Eggs, meat, especially liver and kidney; deep-yellow and dark green vegetables; potatoes, dried fruits, whole-grain products; enriched flour, bread, breakfast cereals.
Iodine	Enables the thyroid gland to perform its function of controlling the rate at which foods are oxidized in the cells.	Fish (obtained from the sea), some plant-foods grown in soils containing iodine; table salt fortified with iodine (iodized).
VITAMINS A	Necessary for normal functioning of the eyes, prevents night blindness. Ensures a healthy condition of the skin, hair, and mucous membranes. Maintains a state of resistance to infections of the eyes, mouth, and respiratory tract.	One form of vitamin A is yellow and one form is colorless. Apricots, cantaloupe, milk, cheese, eggs, meat organs, (especially liver and kidney), fortified margarine, butter, fish-liver oils, dark green and deep yellow vegetables.
B Complex B_1 (Thiamine)	Maintains a healthy condition of the nerves. Fosters a good appetite. Helps the body cells use carbohydrates.	Whole grain and enriched grain products; meats (especially pork, liver and kidney). Dry beans and peas.
B_2 (Riboflavin)	Keeps the skin, mouth, and eyes in a healthy condition. Acts with other nutrients to form enzymes and control oxidation in cells.	Milk, cheese, eggs, meat (especially liver and kidney), whole grain and enriched grain products, dark green vegetables.

FIGURE 6-1 ***(continued)***

NUTRIENT CLASS	BODILY FUNCTIONS	FOOD SOURCES
VITAMINS (*continued*) Niacin	Influences the oxidation of carbohydrates and proteins in the body cells.	Liver, meat, fish, poultry, eggs, peanuts; dark green vegetables, whole grain and enriched cereal products.
B_{12}	Regulates specific processes in digestion. Helps maintain normal functions of muscles, nerves, heart, blood—general body metabolism.	Liver, other organ meats, cheese, eggs, milk, leafy green vegetables.
C (Ascorbic Acid)	Acts as a cement between body cells, and helps them work together to carry out their special functions. Maintains a sound condition of bones, teeth, and gums. Not stored in the body.	Fresh, raw citrus fruits and vegetables—oranges, grapefruit, cantaloupe, strawberries, tomatoes, raw onions, cabbage, green and sweet red peppers, dark green vegetables.
D	Enables the growing body to use calcium and phosphorus in a normal way to build bones and teeth.	Provided by vitamin D fortification of certain foods, such as milk and margarine. Also fish-liver oils and eggs. Sunshine is also a source of vitamin D.
WATER	Regulates body processes. Aids in regulating body temperature. Carries nutrients to body cells and carries waste products away from them. Helps to lubricate joints. Water has no food value, although most water contains mineral elements. More immediately necessary to life than food—second only to oxygen.	Drinking water, and other beverages; all foods except those made up of a single nutrient, as sugar and some fats. Milk, milk drinks, soups, vegetables, fruit juices. Ice cream, watermelon, strawberries, lettuce, tomatoes, cereals, other dry products.

FIGURE 6-1 ***(continued)***

Dietary Guidelines

Dietary guidelines are developed by the U.S. Department of Agriculture and the Department of Health and Human Services (Figure 6-2). These guidelines are updated every five years and provide advice on proper eating and nutrition.

Special Needs Diets and Restrictions

Occasionally, the patient's diet must be adjusted to meet his or her specific needs, and the patient may be required to avoid certain foods or to significantly limit the amounts taken in.

CLEAR LIQUID DIET

The clear liquid diet is often prescribed in preparation for certain laboratory tests, examinations, and surgery. It requires avoidance of all solid foods and milk products.

The clear liquid diet consists of the following:

- Clear soup and broth
- Plain gelatin
- Black coffee
- Tea
- Carbonated beverages
- Popsicles

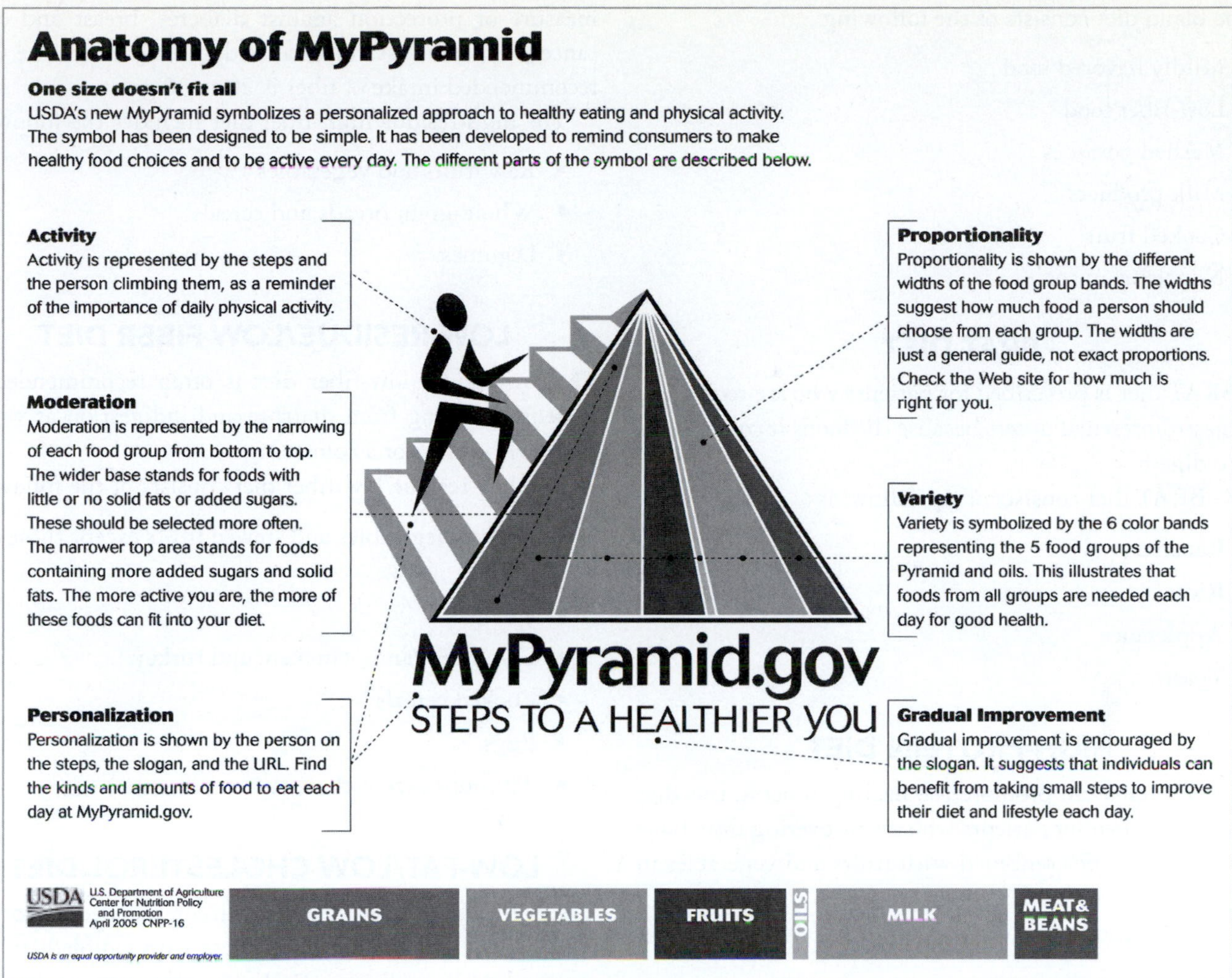

Anatomy of MyPyramid
One size doesn't fit all
USDA's new MyPyramid symbolizes a personalized approach to healthy eating and physical activity. The symbol has been designed to be simple. It has been developed to remind consumers to make healthy food choices and to be active every day. The different parts of the symbol are described below.
Activity
Activity is represented by the steps and the person climbing them, as a reminder of the importance of daily physical activity.
Moderation
Moderation is represented by the narrowing of each food group from bottom to top. The wider base stands for foods with little or no solid fats or added sugars. These should be selected more often. The narrower top area stands for foods containing more added sugars and solid fats. The more active you are, the more of these foods can fit into your diet.
Personalization
Personalization is shown by the person on the steps, the slogan, and the URL. Find the kinds and amounts of food to eat each day at MyPyramid.gov.
Proportionality
Proportionality is shown by the different widths of the food group bands. The widths suggest how much food a person should choose from each group. The widths are just a general guide, not exact proportions. Check the Web site for how much is right for you.
Variety
Variety is symbolized by the 6 color bands representing the 5 food groups of the Pyramid and oils. This illustrates that foods from all groups are needed each day for good health.
MyPyramid.gov
STEPS TO A HEALTHIER YOU
Gradual Improvement
Gradual improvement is encouraged by the slogan. It suggests that individuals can benefit from taking small steps to improve their diet and lifestyle each day.
USDA U.S. Department of Agriculture Center for Nutrition Policy and Promotion April 2005 CNPP-16
USDA is an equal opportunity provider and employer.
GRAINS
VEGETABLES
FRUITS
OILS
MILK
MEAT& BEANS

FIGURE 6-2 The 2005 Food Guide Pyramid.

FULL LIQUID DIET

The full liquid diet is often prescribed for patients who are unable to chew or digest solid food due to gastrointestinal problems or recent surgery.

The full liquid diet consists of the clear liquid diet in addition to the following:

- Milk and milkshakes
- Ice cream
- Custard
- Creamed or strained soup
- Fruit and vegetable juices
- Strained fruit

MECHANICAL SOFT DIET

The mechanical soft diet is often prescribed for patients who are unable to chew due to dental problems, have difficulty swallowing, or are recovering from surgery and the doctor has determined that they are able to tolerate solid food.

The mechanical soft diet consists of the following:

- All soups
- All liquids
- Cooked vegetables
- Canned fruit
- Ground meat and vegetables
- Tender fish and poultry

BLAND DIET

The bland diet is often prescribed for patients with gastrointestinal problems and/or allergies. Food items on this diet contain no seasoning or fiber, as these can irritate the stomach and cause gas.

The bland diet consists of the following:

- Mildly flavored food
- Low-fiber food
- Mashed potatoes
- Milk products
- Cooked fruit
- Noncitrus juices

BRAT DIET

The BRAT diet is prescribed for patients who are recovering from gastrointestinal upsets because the foods it contains are easy to digest.

The BRAT diet consists of the following:

- Bananas
- Rice
- Applesauce
- Toast

HIGH-PROTEIN DIET

Because proteins can promote the healing process, this diet is often prescribed for patients who are recovering from bone injury. It should be combined with fruits and vegetables in order to maintain a balanced diet.

The high-protein diet consists of the following:

- Meat
- Dairy products
- Legumes

DIABETIC DIET

The diabetic diet varies among individuals in order to meet each patient's needs. Most diabetics are encouraged to consume a moderate-carbohydrate diet of 1600–2000 calories daily spread out over several small meals rather than three large meals in order to maintain consistent glucose levels. Several factors are considered when determining each patient's needs. Among them are the following:

- Type of insulin therapy the patient is receiving
- Severity of the diabetes
- Activity and exercise
- Calories required to maintain proper weight

HIGH-RESIDUE/HIGH-FIBER DIET

The high-residue/high-fiber diet is often recommended for patients with existing heart disease and also as a preventive measure or protection against diabetes, breast and colon cancer, hypercholesterolemia, and constipation. The daily recommended intake of fiber is 20 to 30 g.

The high-residue/high-fiber diet includes the following:

- Raw fruits and vegetables
- Whole-grain breads and cereals
- Legumes

LOW-RESIDUE/LOW-FIBER DIET

The low-residue/low-fiber diet is often recommended for patients suffering from diarrhea and indigestion as well as those with colitis or a colostomy.

The low-residue/low-fiber diet consists of the following:

- Cooked vegetables and stewed fruits except those high in fiber
- Bananas
- Lean beef, lamb, chicken, and turkey
- Cooked cereals
- Eggs
- All soups except those that are creamed

LOW-FAT/LOW-CHOLESTEROL DIET

The low-fat/low-cholesterol diet is recommended for patients with hypercholesterolemia and those with gallbladder, pancreatic, and liver disease. Daily fat intake should be 20 to 30 g.

The low-fat/low-cholesterol diet consists of the following:

- Fruits and vegetables
- Fat-free milk
- Whole-grain breads and cereals

LOW-SODIUM (SALT) DIET

The low-sodium (salt) diet is often recommended for patients with congestive heart failure, kidney disease, and hypertension because sodium may cause water retention. The amount of sodium allowed will vary, depending on the patient's condition.

The low-sodium (salt) diet guidelines are as follows:

- Severe salt restriction allows 500 mg of sodium daily.
- Moderate salt restriction allows 1500–2000 mg of sodium daily
- Mild salt restriction allows 3000–5000 mg of sodium daily

FOOD-RELATED DISEASES AND DISORDERS

Anorexia Nervosa	Eating disorder characterized by dangerously low body weight, poor body image, and fear of becoming overweight
Botulism	Rare but serious condition caused by the toxins produced by the *Clostridium botulinum* bacterium. This bacterium can survive in environments with little oxygen, such as in canned food. Symptoms typically begin 12 to 36 hours following ingestion of the bacterium and include vision problems, difficulty swallowing, nausea, and vomiting.
Bulimia	Eating disorder characterized by an obsession over body image The bulimic will eat large amounts of food in a short period of time and then vomit and/or use laxatives.
Binge Eating	Eating disorder that occurs when an individual frequently consumes large amounts of food
Food Allergies	The reaction of the immune system soon after eating food(s) to which the body has developed antibodies, which in turn triggers the release of histamine Symptoms vary from itching and watery eyes to a severe reaction resulting in anaphylaxis
Food Poisoning	Occurs when contaminated food is eaten. Contamination may occur when food is incorrectly handled or cooked or is stored improperly. Most commonly caused by salmonella bacteria, *Escherichia coli (E. coli), Clostridium perfringens,* or *Staphylococcus aureus.*
Obesity	Excessive body fat as a result of consuming more calories than are used via exercise or physical activity
Trichinosis	A type of roundworm infection that may occur when raw or undercooked meat from an infected animal is eaten.

6 APPLICATION

Directions: Select the best answer for each of the following questions. Check your answers in the Answer Key at the end of the book.

1. Which of the following is not one of the six nutrient classifications?
   a. Water
   b. Vitamins
   c. Minerals
   d. Vegetables
   e. Proteins

2. ________________ is not a fat-soluble vitamin:
   a. Vitamin K
   b. Vitamin B_{12}
   c. Vitamin D
   d. Vitamin A
   e. Vitamin E

3. Which of the following choices includes all three of the vitamins that can be formed within the body?
   a. A, D, K
   b. A, B_1, C
   c. B_1, B_2, B_{12}
   d. E, K, C
   e. Niacin, A, D

4. A clear liquid diet consists of the following:
   a. Plain gelatin
   b. Tea
   c. Black coffee
   d. None of the above
   e. A, B and C

5. The special needs diet most often prescribed for patients recovering from bone injury is the:
   a. BRAT diet
   b. High-protein diet
   c. Bland diet
   d. Mechanical soft diet
   e. High-residue/high-fiber diet

6. According to the text, the "B" in the BRAT diet is what food?
   a. Bran
   b. Broccoli
   c. Beans
   d. Bananas
   e. Baby food

7. The correct daily fat intake for a patient on a low-fat/low-cholesterol diet is:
   a. Between 35 and 45 g
   b. No fat should be consumed
   c. Between 20 and 30 g
   d. Between 5 and 15 g
   e. Between 45 and 55 g

8. "Symptoms typically begin 12–36 hours following ingestion of the bacterium and include vision problems, difficulty swallowing , nausea, and vomiting" describes:
   a. Bulimia
   b. Food allergies
   c. Botulism
   d. Trichinosis
   e. B and D

9. "Enables the thyroid gland to perform its function of controlling the rate at which foods are oxidized in the cells" is descriptive of:
   a. Minerals
   b. Iodine
   c. Vitamin B_2
   d. Phosphorus
   e. Riboflavin

10. What vitamin enables the body to use calcium and phosphorus in a normal way to build bones and teeth?
   a. C
   b. B_{12}
   c. B_1
   d. A
   e. D

Section 2

Interoffice Relations and Effective Therapeutic Communications

7 Verbal, Nonverbal, and Written Communications

CONTENTS

Professionalism

Professionalism is exhibited by treating everyone, including patients, co-workers, supervisors, and those from outside the office, in a courteous, conscientious, and businesslike manner. All forms of communication should be delivered with a positive attitude, in a respectful manner, and should be appropriate for the intended receiver. Maintaining professionalism is of the utmost importance whether communicating verbally, nonverbally, or in writing.

Communication

Communication is important in all aspects of business, but especially in healthcare, as the exchange of information and interaction between the patient and the healthcare provider will help shape outcomes and actions.

POSITIVE COMMUNICATION

Positive communication between the patient and the caregiver will help patients feel more comfortable, increasing their well-being and the likelihood that they will follow the physician's instructions. Examples of positive communication are smiling, showing empathy, listening carefully, and being friendly.

NEGATIVE COMMUNICATION

Though typically not intentional, negative communication can have the opposite effect of positive communication.

- ❑ **Content**—Address all areas of interest and fully answer all questions.
- ❑ **Conciseness**—Get to the point; say what needs to be said in as few words as possible.
- ❑ **Clarity**—Choose words that accurately and precisely convey meaning.
- ❑ **Coherence**—Create a logical, easy-to-follow train of thought.
- ❑ **Check**—Ask for feedback or clarification to ensure comprehension.

FIGURE 7-1 Five Cs of better communication.
From *Medical Assisting: Foundations and Practices* by M. S. Frazier, C. Malone, and C. Morgan, Upper Saddle River, NJ: Pearson Education, Inc., 2010, p. 69. Reprinted with permission.

Examples of negative communication are mumbling, showing disrespect, and avoiding eye contact.

Verbal Communication

Verbal communication is based on words, sounds, and tone of voice. Figure 7-1 shows the five Cs of better communication.

COMMUNICATION CYCLE

The communication cycle includes a source, message, channel, and receiver (Figure 7-2).

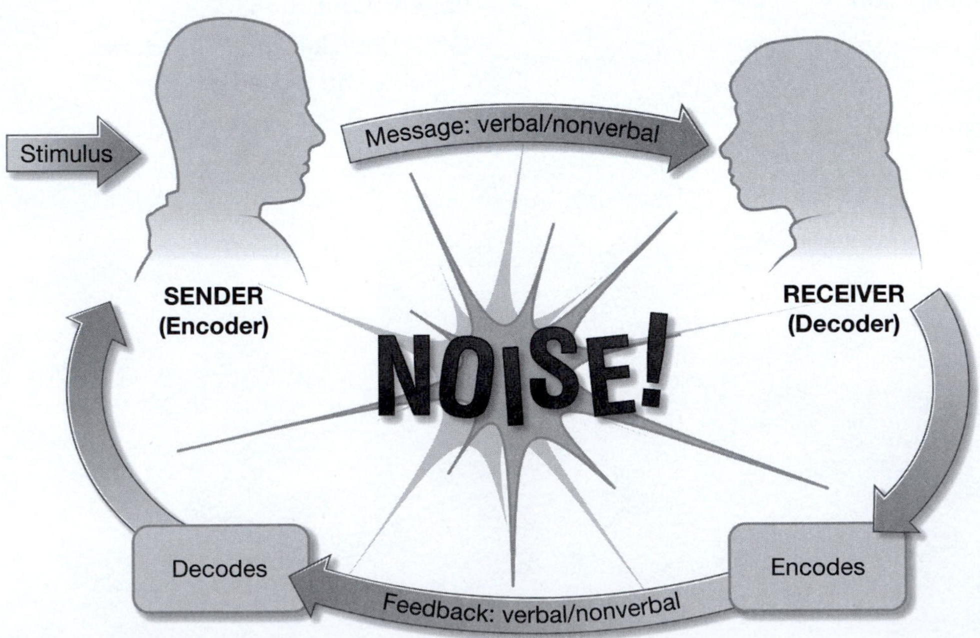

FIGURE 7-2 The communication cycle.

DIRECTIVE COMMUNICATION TECHNIQUES

You can assist the communication process by directing questions to the patient in order to obtain specific information.

Close-Ended Questions

Questions that can be answered with a simple "yes" or "no" are referred to as *close-ended questions*. For example, "Are you in pain?" is a close-ended question.

Open-Ended Questions

Questions that require more than "yes" or "no" are referred to as *open-ended questions*. This type of question is very helpful in gathering information about the patient—for example, "Can you please describe your pain?"

LISTENING SKILLS

Listening is vital to successful communication and involves not only receiving the words being spoken, but also observing nonverbal cues regarding what the patient may be thinking.

DIRECTIVE COMMUNICATION TECHNIQUES

Technique	Description	Example
Open-Ended Statement	Encourage the patient to discuss the problem freely.	"Please describe your pain for me."
Close-Ended Statement	Direct the patient to make a yes/no or simple response.	"Are you having pain?"
Reflecting	Direct the conversation back to the patient by repeating the patient's words.	Patient: "I'm afraid of what the doctor will find." MA: "You're afraid of what the doctor will find?"
Acknowledgment	Indicate understanding.	"I understand what you are saying."
Restating	State what the patient has said but in different terms.	Patient: "I can't sleep." MA: "You say you're having trouble getting to sleep at night?"
Adding to an Implied Statement	Verbalize implied information.	Patient: "I'm usually relaxed." MA: "And today you're not relaxed?"
Seeking Clarification	Request more information to better understand the problem.	Patient: "I don't feel good." MA: "Tell me what your symptoms are."
Silence	Remain silent or make no gesture in response to a statement.	Patient: "I don't know what's wrong, but something is."

THE THREE FORMS OF LISTENING

Active Listening	Listening that is two-way and requires a response *Example*: "What brings you to the office today?" requires a response.
Passive Listening	Listening that is one-way and does not require a response. *Example*: Listening to the news.
Evaluative Listening	Listening that allows the medical assistant to evaluate the information as it is being disseminated and form an immediate response and an opinion It is important to listen carefully to everything the patient says. *Example*: CMA: "What brings you to the office today?" Patient: "I have had a headache, blurred vision, and jaw tightness." While the CMA is listening to and processing what the patient is saying, he or she is determining what other information may be needed, which may prompt a question such as "How long has this been occurring?"

THE DIFFERENCES BETWEEN ASSERTIVE AND AGGRESSIVE BEHAVIOR

Assertive	Maintaining a positive, yet firm perspective based on your values; being the boss without being "bossy"
Aggressive	Imposing your point of view on others (i.e., being "bossy")

ASSERTIVE VERSUS AGGRESSIVE BEHAVIOR

In order to be an effective medical assistant, most circumstances require the cooperation of peers and/or patients. The use of assertive behavior skills will help you get cooperation.

There is a difference between assertive and aggressive behavior. The former behavior is desirable; the latter is not.

COMPARISON OF ASSERTIVE AND AGGRESSIVE BEHAVIOR

Assertive Behavior	Aggressive Behavior
"This medication works best when it is taken on a regular daily basis."	"You know you can't expect this medication to work when you're not taking it every day."
"Let me find someone who can answer that question for you."	"That's not my job."
"Your behavior is inappropriate."	"Why did you do that? It was stupid."
Knocking on an exam room door and then coming in to say, "Excuse me, Dr. Thompson. You are needed on the telephone."	Rushing into an exam room to say, "Doctor, you've got a telephone call."

Nonverbal Communication

Many times the nonverbal message being sent is more accurate than the verbal message. It is important to listen not only with your ears but also with your eyes.

BODY LANGUAGE

Nonverbal communication is most commonly known as *body language*. In most instances, body language will tell the real story of how the patient is feeling versus what he or she tells you verbally. Examples of nonverbal communication are as follows:

- Facial expressions: may or may not reflect judgment.
- Eye contact: depending on whether it is or is not maintained, it may reflect the individual's level of interest, attention, and sensitivity.
- Gestures: may be positive or negative.
- Posture: may or may not reflect interest and a feeling of self-worth.
- Therapeutic touch: may convey empathy and sensitivity, but be aware of the recipient's reaction; not everyone likes to be touched by persons they don't know well.

It is important to remember that patients will pay attention to your body language, just as you are aware of theirs.

PERSONAL SPACE

Depending on the culture they come from, the comfort level of individuals engaged in conversation will vary, depending on the space between them (Box 7-1).

PROFESSIONAL APPEARANCE

Careful grooming, good hygiene, and appropriate dress are important, as these are other forms of nonverbal communication. Your appearance speaks volumes about how you care for yourself and can have an impact on how you communicate with those around you. Excessive makeup, facial piercings,

Box 7-1 Personal Space Measurements Typical in the United States

Intimate Distance	0–18"	Shows affection, provides comfort and protection.
Personal Distance	18"–4'	Most communication takes place at this distance.
Social Distance	4'–12'	Less personal, used in social and business encounters.
Public Distance	greater than 12'	Least personal, observed in lectures, church, and impersonal social encounters.

Source: Medical Assisting: Foundations and Practices by M. S. Frazier, C. Malone, and C. Morgan, Upper Saddle River, NJ: Pearson Education, Inc., 2010, p. 71. Reprinted with permission.

and tattoos will most likely have a negative effect on the way patients, especially children and the elderly, interact with you.

Written Communication

Written communication must be professional, courteous, and businesslike, project a positive tone, and protect the confidentiality of the physician and the patient. This requires some diplomacy.

PROOFREADER'S MARKS

Proofreading, or checking for errors in content and typing when preparing written documents, is critical. The professionalism of the office is judged, in part, by the appearance of its correspondence and documents. Therefore, the importance of proofreading cannot be overemphasized. Even small omissions, such as commas, are noticed by readers. Standard proofreader's marks are shown in Figure 7-3.

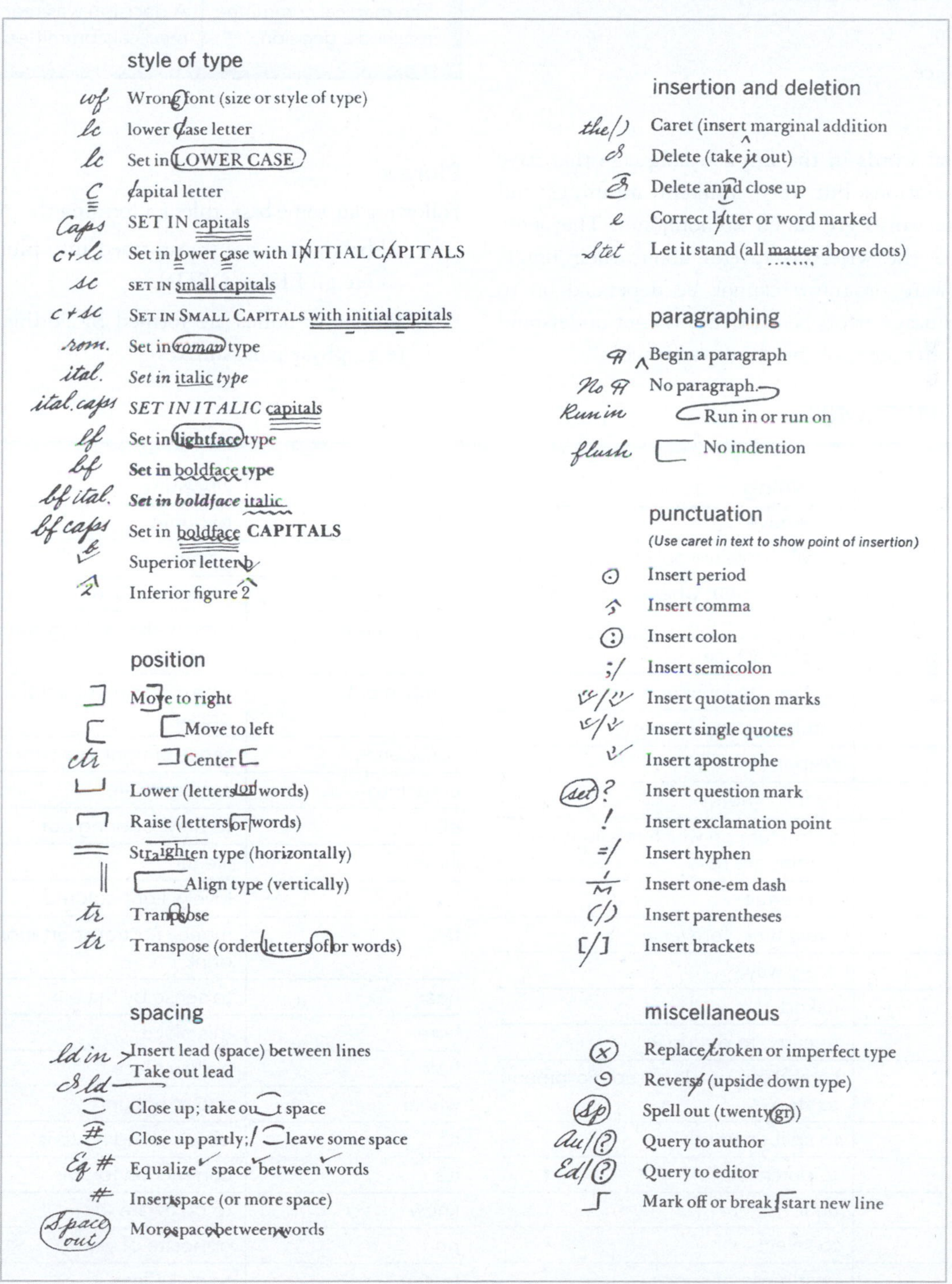

FIGURE 7-3 Proofreader's marks.

FUNDAMENTAL WRITING SKILLS

The use of correct words when preparing office correspondence includes avoiding the use of the following:

- Technical terms
- Gender bias (indicating either male or female by the type of language used)
- Long sentences and paragraphs
- Excessive use of the personal pronoun *I*
- Repetition
- Passive voice

ACTIVE COMPARED TO PASSIVE VOICE

Active Voice	Passive Voice
The medical assistant took the patient's blood pressure measurement.	The patient's blood pressure measurement was taken by the medical assistant.
The surgeon performed an appendectomy on the patient.	An appendectomy was performed on the patient by the surgeon.
The medical committee reached a decision.	A decision was reached by the medical committee.

Spelling

There are several words in the English language that have similar pronunciations but very different meanings and spellings. These words are called homophones. They pose problems unless the writer is careful about their usage. Computer software programs cannot be depended on to correct all word usage errors because they do not understand the data input or content of the correspondence.

Plurals

Following are some basic rules for forming the plurals of words:

- Abbreviations are transformed into plurals by adding an *s* (e.g., EKGs, DRGs).
- Plurals of nouns are formed by adding an *s* or an *es* (e.g., physicians, suffixes).

COMMON HOMOPHONES

Word	Meaning	Word	Meaning
accept	to receive	cite	to quote
except	to take or leave out	sight	vision
advice	opinion about what to do for a problem	site	position, place
advise	to offer advice	complement	what makes a thing complete; to complete
affect	to exert an influence	compliment	an expression of admiration; to praise
effect	result; accomplishment	conscience	sense of right and wrong
all ready	prepared	conscious	awake; aware
already	by this time	elicit	to draw or bring out
altar	a structure on which religious ceremonies are held	illicit	illegal
alter	to change	fair	lovely; light-colored
always	every time; forever	fare	money for transportation, food, or drink
all ways	every way	hear	to sense by the ear
bare	naked	here	this place
bear	to carry; to put up with	hole	hollow place
brake	something used to stop movement; to stop	whole	entire; unhurt
break	to split or smash	its	of or belonging to it
buy	to purchase	it's	contraction for *it is*
by	near	know	to be aware of
choose	to select	no	opposite of *yes*
chose	past tense of *choose*	lessen	to make less

(*Continued*)

Word	Meaning	Word	Meaning
lesson	something learned	then	at that time; next
loose	free; not secured	their	belonging to them
lose	to be deprived of	they're	contraction of *they are*
pair	set of two	there	that place or position
pare	to trim	through	by means of; finished
pear	fruit	threw	past tense of *throw*
patience	calm endurance	thorough	careful; complete
patients	a doctor's clients	to	toward
personal	private; intimate	too	also
personnel	a group of employees	two	one more than one in number
precede	to come before	waist	midsection
proceed	to go forward	waste	to squander
quiet	silent; calm	weak	feeble
quite	very	week	seven days
right	proper or just; correct	weather	state of the atmosphere
rite	a ritual	whether	indicating a choice between alternatives
write	to put words on paper	who's	contraction of *who is*
stationary	standing still	whose	possessive of *who*
stationery	writing paper	your	possessive of *you*
taught	past tense of *teach*	you're	contraction of *you are*
taut	tight		
than	besides		

Numbers

In general, the following rules apply when using numbers in written correspondence:

- Numbers 1 to 10 are spelled out—one to ten.
- For numbers greater than ten, it is acceptable to use the numerical designation, as in 128, 1020, or 32.
- The only exception to this rule is when the number occurs at the beginning of a sentence. Then it should be spelled out.

USE OF NUMBERS IN CORRESPONDENCE

Type	Explanation of When to Use
Decimals	Write numerals without commas (23.04).
Figures	Use only numerals (including 1–10) in tables, statistical data, dates, money, percentages, and time.
Measurements	Use numerals and spell out the unit of measure (e.g., 23 inches).
Percentages	Use numerals and spell out *percent* (.e.g., 20 percent).
Tables	When typing numerals or placing them in columns, align them as follows: • Arabic numerals (1, 2, 3) are aligned on the right. • Numerals with decimals (1.33) are aligned on the decimal point. • Roman numerals (I, II, III) are aligned on the left.
Time	Do not use zeros when writing on-the-hour time. Use A.M. and P.M. with the time designation (e.g., 10 A.M., not 10:00 A.M.).

Grammar

Traditional grammar recognizes eight parts of speech: noun, pronoun, verb, adjective, adverb, preposition, conjunction, and interjection. Many words can function as more than one part of speech. Common grammatical errors are shown below.

Punctuation

The rules of use for common punctuation marks are shown on the following page.

DOCUMENT PROCESSING

EIGHT PARTS OF SPEECH

Part of Speech	Definition
Noun	Names a person, place, or thing *Examples:* medical assistant, office
Pronoun	Substitutes for a noun *Examples:* I, me, you, he, him, she, her, it, we, us, they, them
Verb	Helping verb: comes before the main verb. Main verb: asserts action, being, or state of being *Examples:* operate, write, speak, obtain, is, are, am
Adjective	Modifies a noun or pronoun, usually answering the questions "Which one?" "What kind?" or "How many?" *Example:* responsible medical assistant
Adverb	Modifies a verb, adjective, or adverb, usually answering the questions "When?" "Where?" "Why?" "How?" "Under what conditions?" and "To what degree?" *Examples:* gently, extremely, nicely, quietly
Preposition	Indicates the relationship between the noun and pronoun that follows it and another word in the sentence *Examples:* about, above, after, for, in, on, over, through
Conjunction	Connects words or word groups *Examples:* and, but, nor, or
Interjection	Word used to express strong feeling *Examples:* oh, hooray, hurrah, ouch

COMMON GRAMMATICAL ERRORS

Error	Example
Noun/verb mismatch	"The office feels this is a bad idea." (The office cannot feel, but people can.)
Adjective used as an adverb	"I did good on that exam." (The word *well* should replace *good*.)
Sentence that ends with a preposition	"This is something we need to work on." (A proper rewrite is, "This is something on which we need to work.")
Run-on sentence	"This lab is a dangerous place, patients should not be back here." (A semicolon should replace the comma.)
Misuse of words that sound alike but differ in spellings and meanings	"Their here, just two quiet." (The sentence should read, "They're here, just too quiet.")

Source: Medical Assisting: Foundations and Practices by M. S. Frazier, C. Malone, and C. Morgan, Upper Saddle River, NJ: Pearson Education, Inc., 2010, p. 121. Reprinted with permission.

RULES OF USE FOR COMMON PUNCTUATION MARKS

Mark	Use(s)
Period (.)	Indicates the end of a sentence and separates the part of an abbreviation.
Comma (,)	Separates words, phrases, or two independent clauses and sets off elements that interrupt or add information in a sentence.
Semicolon (;)	Sets apart independent clauses and items in a list that contain commas.
Colon (:)	Follows a salutation in a business letter, precedes a list, separates independent clauses, helps express time.
Apostrophe (')	Indicates a missing letter from a contracted word and the possessive case of nouns.
Diagonal (/)	Separates the numbers in dates (e.g., 6/1/07) and fractions (e.g., $^1/_2$) and sometimes indicates abbreviations (e.g., w/o).
Parentheses ( )	Set off part of a sentence that is not part of the main thought.
Quotation marks (" ")	Indicate a direct quote.
Ellipsis (...)	Shows that a thought trails off or represents missing material (e.g., "I was going to, but . . .").

Source: Medical Assisting: Foundations and Practices by M. S. Frazier, C. Malone, and C. Morgan, Upper Saddle River, NJ: Pearson Education, Inc., 2010, p. 121. Reprinted with permission.

Components of the Business Letter

All business letters contain the same basic components: the heading, date, inside address, salutation, body, closing, and reference initials. In some cases, such as insurance correspondence, there may be special components added for clarification, such as the insurer's identification number.

BASIC COMPONENTS OF THE BUSINESS LETTER

Salutation	Courteous greeting Typed at the left margin Spaced two lines below the inside address Agreement between the name in the salutation and the name in the inside address
Body	Contains the purpose of the letter Begins two spaces below the salutation Single-spaced, with a double space between each paragraph Either blocking or indentation of the paragraphs of the body, depending on the style (format) of the letter
Complimentary Close	Contains courtesy word(s), such as "Sincerely," "Sincerely yours," or "Yours truly" Appears two spaces below the end of the body of the letter
Signature Line	Contains the name and title of the writer Typed four spaces below the complimentary close The signature of the writer placed directly above the typed signature line before the letter is sent
Reference Initials	Indicate who keyboarded the letter Placed at the lower left margin in lowercase
Enclosure	A notation made on the letter indicating that documents included with the letter have been enclosed. This notation is made one line below the name and title of the individual sending the letter.
Copy Notation	Used when a copy of the letter is sent to someone other than the addressee Noted at the bottom left of the letter by typing the initial "c:"

Letter Styles

Letter styles vary, depending on the purpose of the letter. Letter styles include block, modified block (standard), and modified block with indented paragraphs (Figures 7-4A–C). The block and modified block forms are the ones most commonly used in the medical office.

Memos

Interoffice memoranda, also called *memos*, are correspondence sent to people within the office or organization. The memo is a quick, efficient, and inexpensive way to communicate with others in the office setting. It does not require postage, and it is delivered through interoffice mail.

Memos may be used to inform office personnel about the following:

- Meetings
- General changes that affect all employees, such as a change in office hours
- Special projects
- News items

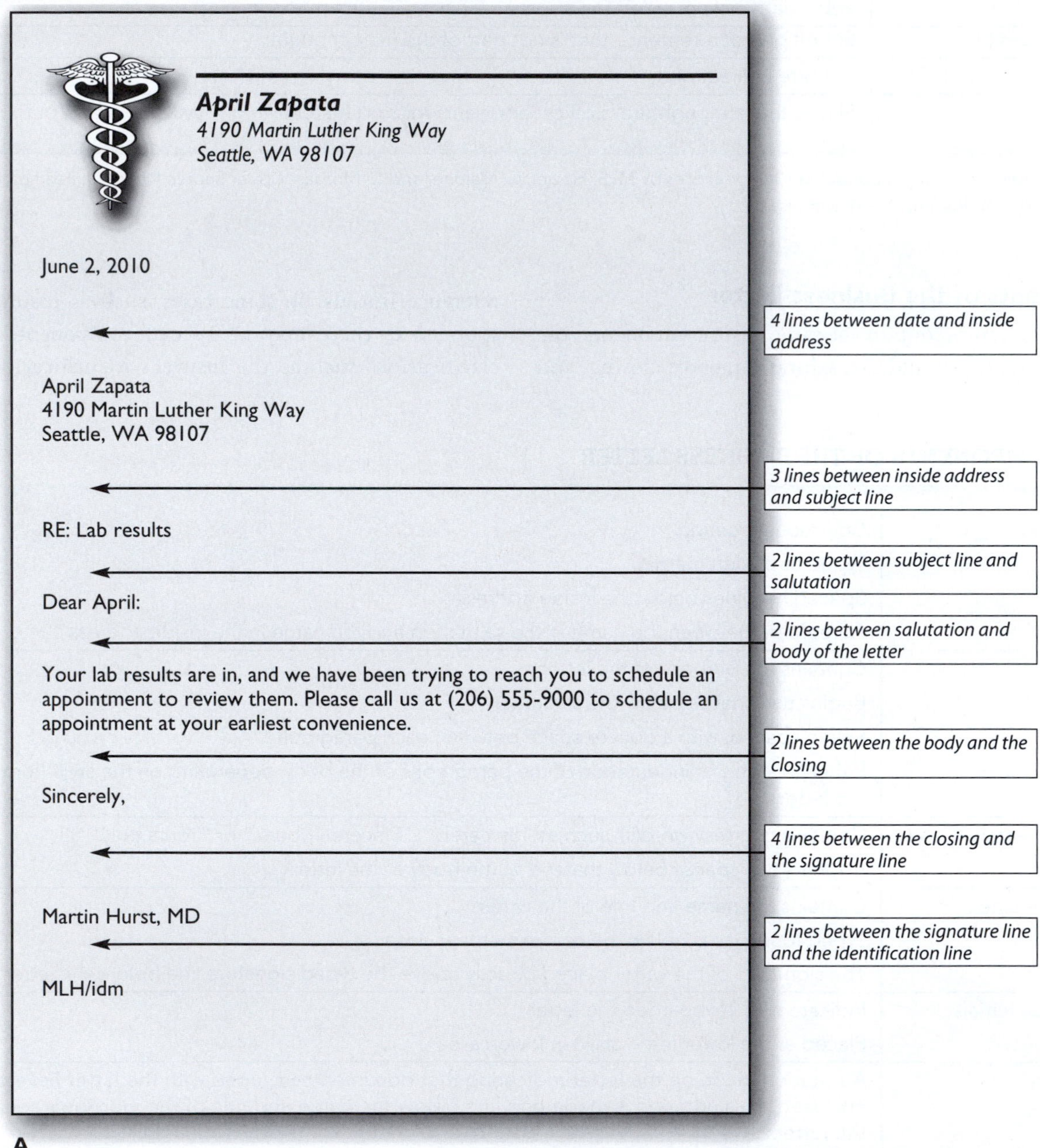

April Zapata
4190 Martin Luther King Way
Seattle, WA 98107

June 2, 2010

April Zapata
4190 Martin Luther King Way
Seattle, WA 98107

RE: Lab results

Dear April:

Your lab results are in, and we have been trying to reach you to schedule an appointment to review them. Please call us at (206) 555-9000 to schedule an appointment at your earliest convenience.

Sincerely,

Martin Hurst, MD

MLH/idm

FIGURE 7-4A Block style.

From *Medical Assisting: Foundations and Practices* by M. S. Frazier, C. Malone, and C. Morgan, Upper Saddle River, NJ: Pearson Education, Inc., 2010, p. 125. Reprinted with permission.

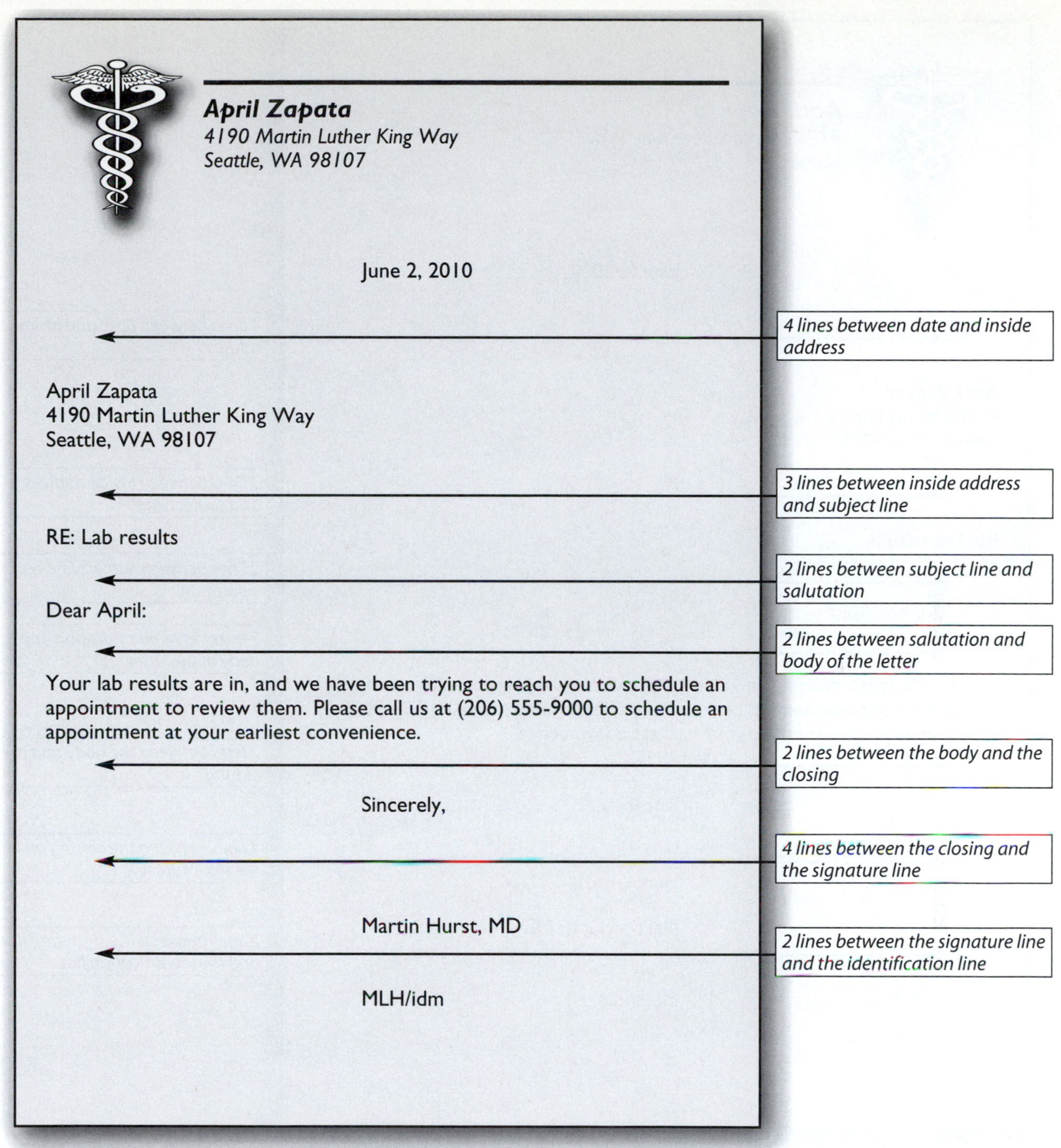

April Zapata
4190 Martin Luther King Way
Seattle, WA 98107

June 2, 2010

April Zapata
4190 Martin Luther King Way
Seattle, WA 98107

RE: Lab results

Dear April:

Your lab results are in, and we have been trying to reach you to schedule an appointment to review them. Please call us at (206) 555-9000 to schedule an appointment at your earliest convenience.

Sincerely,

Martin Hurst, MD

MLH/idm

FIGURE 7-4B Modified block style.

From *Medical Assisting: Foundations and Practices* by M. S. Frazier, C. Malone, and C. Morgan, Upper Saddle River, NJ: Pearson Education, Inc., 2010, p. 126. Reprinted with permission.

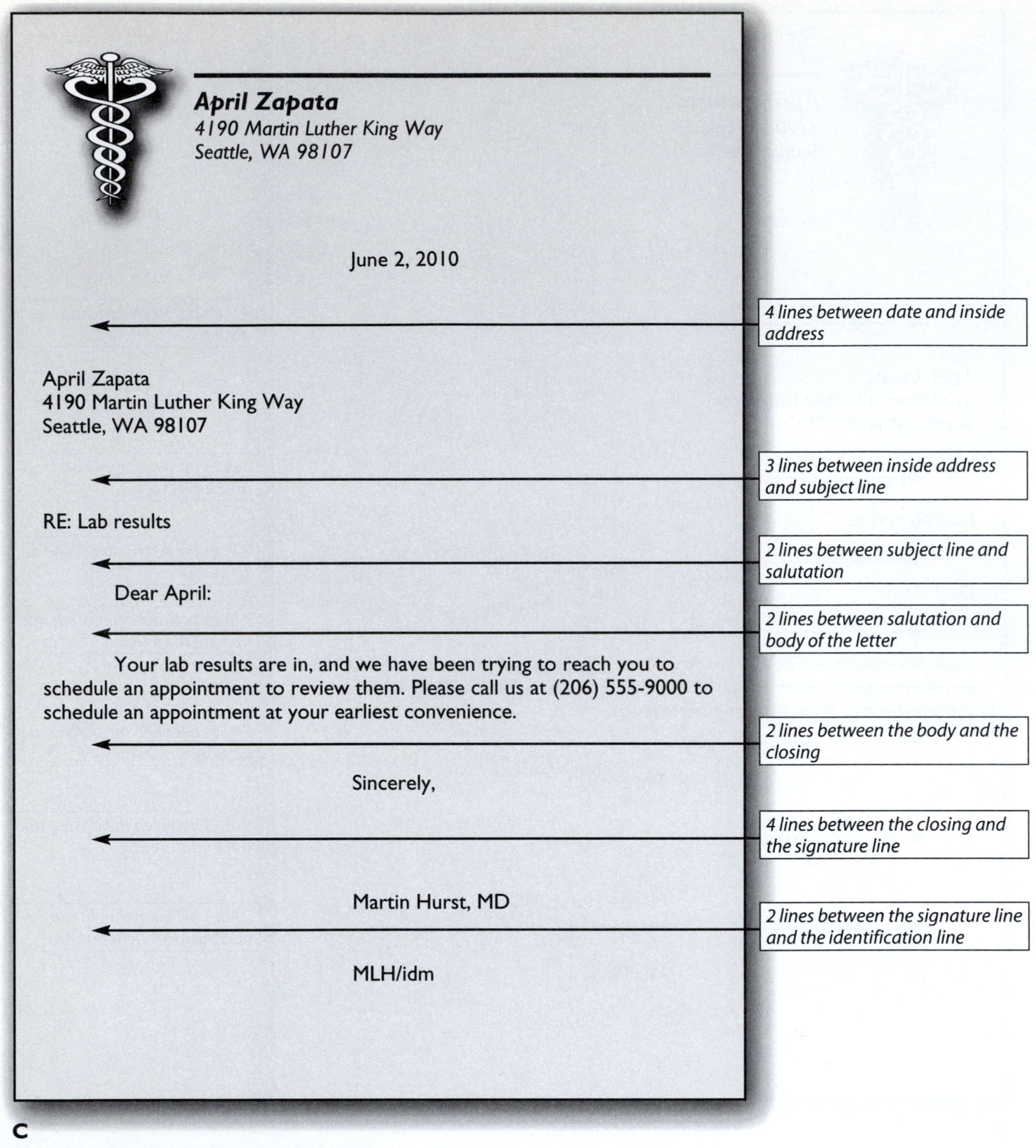
April Zapata
4190 Martin Luther King Way
Seattle, WA 98107

June 2, 2010

April Zapata
4190 Martin Luther King Way
Seattle, WA 98107

RE: Lab results

Dear April:

Your lab results are in, and we have been trying to reach you to schedule an appointment to review them. Please call us at (206) 555-9000 to schedule an appointment at your earliest convenience.

Sincerely,

Martin Hurst, MD

MLH/idm

FIGURE 7-4C Modified block style with indentations.

From *Medical Assisting: Foundations and Practices* by M. S. Frazier, C. Malone, and C. Morgan, Upper Saddle River, NJ: Pearson Education, Inc., 2010, p. 127. Reprinted with permission.

Communicating with Special Needs Patients and Their Families

At times, you will need to communicate with special needs patients and their families. It is important to treat these patients with the same respect, dignity, empathy, and professionalism that you would use with any other patient.

HEARING-IMPAIRED PATIENTS

The degree of hearing loss can vary greatly. It is important to first understand the level of loss, as this will help determine how best to communicate with the patient. The manner in which you communicate will vary, depending on whether or not the patient can lip-read, has a hearing aid, or uses an interpreter. If the patient uses an interpreter, be sure to maintain eye contact and speak directly with the patient. Some general guidelines to follow when working with hearing-impaired patients are as follows:

- Make sure that you are in a quiet, well-lit room.
- Face the patient.
- Speak slowly and clearly.
- Don't have anything in your mouth, such as gum or candy.
- Have paper and pen available so that the patient can communicate in writing if desired.

VISUALLY IMPAIRED PATIENTS

It is important to ask a visually impaired patient if he or she needs assistance in going to and from the exam room. Don't automatically assume that the patient needs your guidance and assistance. If the patient does request assistance, offer your arm and provide guidance, making sure to alert the patient about any steps, slopes, or ramps.

The manner in which you speak will play a significant role in your communication with a visually impaired patient. Some general guidelines to follow when working with visually impaired patients are as follows:

- Speak clearly and pay attention to the speed and volume of your speech.
- Face the patient.
- Explain in detail any procedures the patient may have performed.
- Have large-print patient education materials available.

MENTALLY AND EMOTIONALLY IMPAIRED PATIENTS

When working with mentally and/or emotionally impaired patients, it is important to first determine the patient's level of communication and understanding. Be sure to speak slowly and clearly. Stay calm, and keep your messages short and to the point. If the patient will be undergoing any type of procedure or will require you to touch the patient, be sure to explain to the patient what you will be doing.

NON-ENGLISH-SPEAKING PATIENTS

It is unlikely that an office will have a multilingual staff available to communicate with patients from all ethnic and cultural backgrounds. In the event that nobody within the practice is familiar with the patient's language, you may need to rely on nonverbal communication initially. However, this can be dangerous, as there are many opportunities for misunderstanding or error when neither of the parties is absolutely sure of what is being communicated by the other. If you are working in a culturally diverse area, it is best to have a list of interpreters available to call when needed. Most acute care facilities can arrange to have multilingual interpreters available if enough advance notice is given.

ANGRY PATIENTS

Some of the greatest difficulty in communicating occurs when a patient is angry. It is important to remember that the patient is most likely not angry with you, but rather with the situation. The patient's anger may be based on fear and anxiety or loss of control. You should take care not to become defensive and respond to the angry patient in the same manner in which the patient is responding to you. Remain calm and ask, "What can I do to help you?"

Patient Education

Patient education may occur at any point during the visit, as well as before and afterward. This education can be presented in several forms and often begins when the patient calls for an appointment. It can include information on office hours, policies, insurance form submissions, and after-hours emergency telephone numbers.

In addition to patient education regarding office policy, there may be times when it is necessary to provide clinical patient education regarding preparation for procedures or taking medications properly, information regarding test results, postvisit care, and when to call the office.

Patient education is supported by the use of descriptive informational office practice brochures; literature from established healthcare organizations such as the American Cancer Society, the American Diabetic Association, and the American Heart Association; and bulletin displays on various aspects of health. Some offices provide a brief video presentation about selected procedures or health concerns.

Always ensure that patient education is provided at a level the patient understands. It is best to ask the patient to repeat back what he or she has heard. This offers an opportunity to assess the patient's level of understanding. If it is apparent that the patient didn't quite understand the first communication, restate the information at an appropriate level and ask the patient to repeat it again. If the education being provided seems to confuse the patient or if a great deal of education is occurring, it is best to provide written information for the patient to refer to.

Many offices that use electronic medical records are sending out targeted patient education information via e-mail. Various patient teaching methods are shown on the following page.

PATIENT TEACHING METHODS

Method	Description	Advantages	Disadvantages	Usefulness
Lecture	Formal report or instructions delivered to the patient, with little interaction between teacher and learner	Efficient No limit to the number of the learner	No interaction to handle individual learner's confusion May be boring for the learner	Patients who need general knowledge (e.g., new mothers) Large groups (e.g., for smoking cessation, weight reduction)
Role-Play	Short play in which the learner participates in "playing out" the story	Learner sees how others might do something Learner involvement	Time-consuming Learner must be willing to play the role	Patients with chronic diseases (e.g., hypertension, diabetes) Patients learning new interactions (e.g., how to direct a home health aide) Handling unusual situations that cannot be demonstrated, such as calling 911 in an emergency
Case Problems	Applies information to real situations	Believable Concrete rather than abstract	Significant facts may be missing Effectiveness depends on the teacher	Patients who must apply new knowledge (e.g., a patient with angina or diabetes, a new mother)
Demonstration/ Return Demonstration	Showing patients how to do something and then immediately having them do the same procedure	Presents standards for performance, both visual and oral Allows learner to know that it can be done	May be difficult to see Limited to a small group Learners may be nervous	Patients who need to understand cause and effect Patients who must learn new skills (e.g., colostomy care, diabetic injections, baby care, CPR)
Contracting	Setting up goals with clear behaviors and responsibilities for the patient	Requires learner's involvement Promotes learner's strengths Identifies acceptable goals	Requires learner to make decisions May be threatening to learners Time-consuming	Patients with chronic disease Well patients who wish to change their health habits
Use of a Significant Other	Teaching a close relative or friend the same information the patient receives	Provides learner with support and reinforcement Learning continues at home	Other person must be willing to help Other person may be a negative influence Other person may foster dependence	Elderly patients and those with disabilities Patients whose compliance is in question
Past Experiences	Building learning on what has been learned in the past rather than creating a new set of knowledge	Identifies potential problems Makes the learner more comfortable	Depends on learner's ability to recall Requires insight	Patients who are anxious or overwhelmed Patients who must change their behavior (e.g., take medication, use a proper diet, exercise)

(*Continued*)

Method	Description	Advantages	Disadvantages	Usefulness
Group Teaching	Bringing together patients who have common learning needs	Efficient and economical Participants support each other Participants are actively involved	Group may digress Some cultures discourage open discussion Transportation may be a problem Difficult for all participants to agree on a time	Patients and families with common learning needs (e.g., weight reduction, smoking cessation)
Programmed Instruction	Printed instructions that force the patient to understand one concept before going on to the next Every correct response builds toward the next question Can be computer assisted	Active learner participation Individual pacing Encourages independence Provides immediate feedback	May be impersonal and boring Learner must be literate Lack of personal involvement between learner and teacher Learner must be self-motivated	Self-motivated learners Accommodates patients with lower reading levels
Simulations (Games)	A scenario created for learning purposes	Involves the patient in the learning process Nonthreatening Allows learners to see knowledge previously learned	Some patients dislike competition Some patients do not like games Some patients have difficulty following directions or dealing with abstract ideas	Adults and children with acute problems (e.g., cast care), chronic problems (e.g., asthma), or health promotion issues (e.g., dental care, weight control)
Tests of Knowledge	Short questions related to the patient's knowledge of the subject	Evaluates learner's knowledge at that moment Gives learner a feeling of accomplishment Raises learner's awareness	May make learners anxious Time-consuming May embarrass learners with lack of knowledge	Adults and children who must apply knowledge (e.g., diabetic patient, postsurgical patient with a dressing change)
Printed Handouts	Brochures or instruction sheets printed for the main purpose of imparting knowledge to the patient	Promotes consistency Provides visual reinforcement	Must be accompanied by verbal teaching Difficult to create since clarity and simplicity are required	Well patients (health maintenance literature) Patients who must remember difficult information (e.g., presurgical instructions, medication information)
Diagrams	Picture models of concepts	Offers visual reinforcement Attracts attention of the learner Shows proportions and relationships	Must be accurate May require artistic skill to produce	Preschoolers People with limited reading or vocabulary

(*continued*)

(Continued)

Method	Description	Advantages	Disadvantages	Usefulness
Models	A miniature (usually) representation of an object produced in a substance, such as clay or plaster	Encourages learner's participation Offers direct application of skill	May be expensive	School-age children Adults practicing a skill (e.g., CPR, breast self-exam, bathing a child)
Video	A slide presentation or moving picture	Re-creates real-life situations Effective for patients with limited reading skills	Too fast for the elderly adult May be expensive Takes time to set up and run	Groups of patients Health maintenance material (e.g., nutrition, preventive dentistry) Video player in a waiting room

Office Policies and Procedures

All offices should have a policy manual and a procedures manual listing the policies of the office and describing how to carry out tasks within a particular medical practice. These manuals are sometimes combined into one manual called the *policies and procedures manual*. Detailed descriptions of the standard operating procedure (SOPs) and instructions on how to perform both administrative and clinical tasks are included in this manual.

POLICY AND PROCEDURES MANUALS

The primary functions of policies and procedures manuals are as follows:

- List the tasks to be performed within the office, including equipment needed in order to complete the procedure.
- Standardize the procedure for each task.
- Describe job responsibilities and titles.

The procedures manual, when properly updated, is an excellent reference tool for the new employee since it provides guidelines for performing specific tasks. Temporary or substitute employees also find it valuable.

The personnel policy manual, also known as the *employee handbook*, contains information for the employee about the employer-employee relationship, the work environment, and the expectations of the particular medical facility. This manual contains general information about office policies relating to dress and behavior codes, punctuality, office safety, and the role of the employee in an emergency, such as a fire.

Most offices require the employee to sign an acknowledgment that he or she has received a copy of the personnel manual and understands it. This signed acknowledgment is kept in the employee's personnel file.

Employees should be provided with specific information about the following issues or benefits, which is usually found in the policy manual:

- Compensation and reimbursement for work-related activities, such as attending conventions and taking courses (CEU/degree), and parking fees
- Emergency leave
- Grievance (complaint) process
- Health benefits
- Holidays
- Jury duty
- Overtime policy
- Pension plan
- Performance review and evaluation
- Probationary period
- Sick leave
- Termination of employment
- Vacation
- Work hours, including flex time

PATIENT INFORMATION BOOKLET

Patient information booklets should provide patient information on the following:

- Office hours
- Payment guidelines

- Appointment and cancellation policies
- Telephone answering service
- Information about the physician(s)
- After-hours availability
- Directions to the facility
- Parking information

Patient information booklets can help reduce the number of questions by telephone from patients, enhance the office's image, and reduce the number of patients who fail to remember instructions.

7 APPLICATION

Directions: Select the best answer for each of the following questions. Check your answers in the Answer Key at the end of the book.

1. Verbal communication is very important in dealing with patients, co-workers, and physicians. The five Cs of better communication are key components of verbal communication. They include which of the following?
   a. Coherence
   b. Clarity
   c. Content
   d. Conciseness
   e. All of the above
2. An example of a close-ended question is:
   a. Can you please describe your pain?
   b. Are you in pain?
   c. How long have you had this condition?
   d. A and C
   e. None of the above
3. The three forms of listening skills are:
   a. Active, passive, inquisitive
   b. Active, evaluative, inquisitive
   c. Technical, inquisitive, evaluative
   d. Passive, active, evaluative
   e. Clinical, personal, active
4. Which of the following is not an example of nonverbal communication?
   a. Therapeutic touch
   b. Gestures
   c. Open-ended questions
   d. Eye contact
   e. C and D
5. Maintaining personal space can be essential in making patients feel comfortable. Typical personal space categories in the United States include:
   a. Intimate
   b. Arm's length
   c. Body length
   d. Social distance
   e. A and D
6. Which of these should be avoided in office correspondence?
   a. Gender bias
   b. Long sentences
   c. Repetition
   d. Technical terms
   e. All of the above
7. Words that have similar pronunciations but different meanings and spellings are known as:
   a. Synonyms
   b. Similes
   c. Homophones
   d. Pronouns
   e. Adjectives
8. A correct example of the plural of a noun is:
   a. Drugs
   b. Drug's
   c. Boxes'
   d. Drugs'
   e. Prescriptiones
9. According to the text, which of the following is not one of the eight parts of grammar?
   a. Verb
   b. Conjunction
   c. Adverb
   d. Salutation
   e. Preposition

10. Business letters contain several components. "Dear Mr. Smith" is an example of the component known as the:
   a. Signature line
   b. Complimentary close
   c. Salutation
   d. Enclosure
   e. None of the above

11. When working with a hearing-impaired patient, you should always:
   a. Use sign language
   b. Face the patient
   c. Not speak; write everything down
   d. B and C
   e. All of the above

12. Showing a patient how to do something and immediately having the patient do the same procedure describes the patient teaching method known as:
   a. Demonstration/return demonstration
   b. Role-play
   c. Contracting
   d. Lecture
   e. Case problem

13. The primary functions of a policy manual include:
   a. Description of benefits
   b. Description of job responsibilities and titles
   c. Description of the grievance process
   d. All of the above
   e. A and B only

14. Patient information booklets commonly include:
   a. Office hours
   b. Job responsibilities and titles
   c. Directions to the facility
   d. Payment guidelines
   e. A, C, and D

15. _____________ contains information about standardized tasks.
   a. The policy manual
   b. The corporate mission statement
   c. The procedure manual
   d. Either A or B
   e. The patient information booklet

16. Which of the following proofreader's marks is an indication that brackets should be inserted?
   a. [
   b.]
   c. [/]
   d. (/)
   e. [ ]

17. There are four basic parts to the communication cycle. Which of the following is not part of that cycle?
   a. Receiver
   b. Message
   c. Channel
   d. Stimulus
   e. Source

18. Listening is vital to successful communication and involves receiving messages. Which form of listening requires a response?
   a. Evaluative
   b. Active
   c. Nonverbal
   d. Passive
   e. None of the above

19. In regard to the use of numbers in correspondence, which of the following sentences is correct?
   a. Twenty patients canceled this week.
   b. There were 5 cancellations today.
   c. The total patient count for the day was 35.
   d. A and C
   e. B and C

20. In a business letter, the reference initials are placed:
   a. Directly above the signature line
   b. Two spaces below the body of the letter
   c. At the lower left margin in lowercase
   d. Two lines below the address
   e. Two spaces below the salutation

21. For the following question, choose the best answer. "Why did you do that? It was stupid" is an example of:
   a. Open-ended question
   b. Close-ended question
   c. Aggressive behavior
   d. Assertive behavior
   e. Active questioning

22. For the following question, choose the best answer. "Your behavior is inappropriate" is an example of:
   a. Open-ended question
   b. Close-ended question
   c. Aggressive behavior
   d. Assertive behavior
   e. Active questioning

8 Human Relations

CONTENTS

Stages of the Life Cycle

DEVELOPMENTAL STAGES OF THE LIFE CYCLE

Stage	Characteristics
Prenatal Period	Conception to birth Body structures and organs formed Development influenced by the environment
Infancy	Childbirth to toddler period Motor ability and coordination develop Language and sensory skills develop Basic emotions and feeling expressed Trust develops Attachment to caregivers
Childhood	*Early Childhood* Ages 3 to 5 Linguistic, physical, and cognitive skills develop Concept of self begins to develop *Middle Childhood* Ages 6 to 11 Logical thinking develops Advances in reading and writing occur Moral and psychosocial development occurs rapidly Achievement important
Adolescence	*Early Adolescence* Ages 12 to 14 Operational thinking occurs Sexual maturation occurs Desire for independence begins Friendships important *Late Adolescence* Ages 15 to 19 Positive identity formed Decisions made concerning college, career, and workplace Sexual relationships formed Ability to relate to others increases
Adulthood	*Early Adulthood* Ages 20 to 30s Career choices made Intimacy develops *Middle Adulthood* Ages 40 to 50s Vocational success achieved Personal responsibility realized Emotional and physical changes occur *Late Adulthood* Age 60 to death Physical and mental capacity changes occur Relationships change Satisfaction may be at this stage

Developmental and Behavioral Theories

Several psychologists and psychiatrists have developed explanations and predictions regarding why people behave the way they do.

MASLOW'S HIERARCHY OF NEEDS

Abraham Maslow was a twentieth-century psychologist who developed a hierarchy of human needs. Maslow's hierarchy of needs states that human beings must have their basic physiological and safety needs met before they can move to the next level of development and eventually reach the highest level: self-actualization (Figure 8-1).

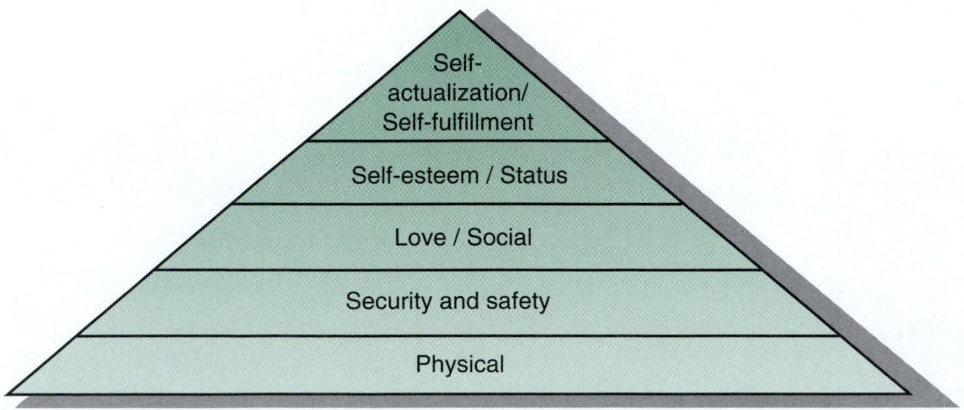

FIGURE 8-1 Maslow's hierarchy of needs.

FREUD'S STAGES OF PSYCHOSEXUAL DEVELOPMENT

Sigmund Freud was an Austrian neurologist of the late nineteenth to mid-twentieth centuries who developed several theories related to psychology and human development. Many of these theories are no longer accepted, but they provide the foundations of modern psychology.

One of Freud's theories concerns the stages of psychosexual development, which focuses on the development of personality in childhood. Freud believed that sexual drive was the result of an instinctual sexual appetite beginning at birth and progressing to adulthood.

STAGES OF PSYCHOSEXUAL DEVELOPMENT

Stage	Age	Characteristic
Oral	Birth to 18 months	The mouth is the center of pleasure.
Anal	18 months to 3 years	Toilet-training: the anus is the center of pleasure.
Phallic	4 to 6 years	The genitals are the center of pleasure.
Latency	7 years to puberty	Sexual concerns are not important; sexual drives are seen as dormant.
Genital	Puberty to adulthood	Genitals are the center of pleasure; this is expressed as adult sexuality.

ERIK ERIKSON'S STAGES OF PSYCHOSOCIAL DEVELOPMENT

Erik Erikson, a twentieth-century psychologist and psychoanalyst, developed a theory about the social development of human beings. Erik Erikson believed that individuals go through eight stages of development as they progess through life. This is in contrast to the five stages identified in Freud's theory of psychosexual development.

Erik Erikson believed that at each stage, a new conflict can occur. When this happens, there will be either a positive or a negative outcome. Erik Erikson believed that the outcome of the conflict will play an important role in the development of the individual's personality

THE STAGES OF PSYCHOSOCIAL DEVELOPMENT

Age and Stage		Conflict	
		Positive	Negative
Birth to 1 year	Infancy	Trust	Mistrust
2 to 3 years	Toddler	Autonomy	Shame and doubt
4 to 6 years	Preschool	Initiative	Guilt
7 to 12 years	Childhood	Industry	Inferiority
13 to 19 years	Adolescence	Identity	Role confusion
20 to 34 years	Early adulthood	Intimacy	Isolation
35 to 65 years	Middle adulthood	Generativity	Stagnation
65 years and older	Late adulthood	Ego integrity	Despair

PIAGET'S THEORY OF COGNITIVE DEVELOPMENT

During the twentieth century, Jean Piaget, a biologist and psychologist, developed a theory dividing child development and learning into four stages that exist as a result of *mapping* understood concepts to physical experiences within the child's environment.

THE THEORY OF COGNITIVE DEVELOPMENT

Age	Stage	Focus
Birth to 2 years	Sensorimotor	Movement and senses
2 to 7 years	Preoperational	Language and symbols
7 to 11 years	Concrete operational	Abstract concepts
11 to 15+ years	Formal operational	Logical and analytical reasoning

JUNG'S THEORIES

Carl Jung, a twentieth-century psychiatrist, developed theories based on the human unconscious and personality types.

JUNG'S THEORIES

Personal Unconscious	Personal memories that were once in the conscious but have been forgotten or repressed because they are threatening to the individual Unique to each individual
Collective Unconscious	Part of the unconscious mind that is inherited and shared by all humans
Extroversion	The tendency of those individuals who seek out excitement and enjoy interaction with others
Introversion	The tendency of those individuals who prefer less interaction with others and tend to be more reserved

PAVLOV'S CLASSICAL CONDITIONING THEORY

Ivan Pavlov was a physician and psychiatrist of the late nineteenth and early twentieth centuries. While conducting a study on the digestion process of dogs, he discovered that malnourished dogs would salivate when his assistants entered the room to feed them. He began to precede the feeding of the dogs with the ringing of a bell. Eventually, the dogs salivated at the sound of the bell alone. This is an example of the simplest form of learning.

SKINNER'S OPERANT CONDITIONING THEORY

B. F. Skinner, a psychologist of the late 1950s through the early 1970s, developed a theory of learning more complex than that of Pavlov. This theory, called *operant conditioning*, is based on voluntary behavior during a previous experience and the idea that a response (positive or negative) occurs as a result of that behavior. An example of operant conditioning is when a patient, on the advice of his or her physician, loses weight and in turn receives praise and encouragement from the physician.

Death

Elizabeth Kübler-Ross was a psychiatrist of the late 1960s and 1970s who developed the model on death and dying that now bears her name. She determined that any time loss occurs, an individual may progress through five stages of grief. It is important to understand that not all individuals

KÜBLER-ROSS'S FIVE STAGES OF GRIEF

Denial	This stage is marked by refusal to believe that dying is taking place. The patient (or family member) may need time to adjust to the reality of approaching death. This stage cannot be hurried.
Anger	At this stage, the patient may be angry at everyone and may direct this intense anger at God, family members, and even healthcare professionals. The patient may focus this anger on the person closest to him or her; usually this is a family member. In reality, the patient is angry about dying.
Bargaining	This stage involves an attempt to gain time by making promises in return. The patient may bargain with God and may also indicate a need to talk.
Depression	This stage is marked by deep sadness over the loss of health, independence, and eventually life. There is the additional sadness of leaving loved ones behind. The grieving patient may become withdrawn.
Acceptance	This stage is characterized by a sense of peace and calm. The patient may make comments such as "I have no regrets. I'm ready to die." It is better to let the patient talk and not make denial statements such as "Don't talk like that. You're not going to die."

go through all five stages, and they may not go through the stages in the order listed on page 122.

Defense Mechanisms

Freud believed that coping skills were formed to help reduce anxiety and maintain the self-image. Defense mechanisms, he stated, are the subconscious reactions human beings may use when trying to manage anxiety by denying, misinterpreting, or distorting reality. Overuse of some of these defense mechanisms may lead to self-destructive behavior, as the mechanisms may prevent the individual from addressing the cause of the anxiety.

DEFENSE MECHANISMS

Defense Mechanism	Example(s)	Use/Purpose
Compensation Covering up weaknesses by emphasizing a more desirable trait or by overachievement in a more comfortable area	A high school student too small to play football becomes the star long-distance runner for the track team.	Allows a person to overcome weakness and achieve success
Denial An attempt to screen out or ignore unacceptable realities by refusing to acknowledge them	A woman, though told that her father has metastatic cancer, continues to plan a family reunion 18 months in advance.	Temporarily isolates a person from the full impact of a traumatic situation
Displacement Transferring emotional reactions from one object or person to another object or person	A husband and wife are fighting, and the husband becomes so angry that he hits a door instead of his wife; a student gets a C on a paper she worked hard on and goes home and yells at her family.	Allows feelings to be expressed through or to less dangerous objects or people
Identification An attempt to manage anxiety by imitating the behavior of someone who is feared or respected	A student nurse imitates the nurturing behavior she observes one of her instructors using with clients.	Helps a person avoid self-devaluation
Intellectualization A mechanism by which an emotional response that normally would accompany an uncomfortable or painful incident is evaded by the use of rational explanations that remove from the incident any personal significance and feelings	The pain over a parent's sudden death is reduced by saying, "He wouldn't have wanted to live disabled."	Protects a person from pain and traumatic events
Introjection A form of identification that allows for the acceptance of others' norms and values, even when they are contrary to one's previous assumptions	A seven-year-old boy tells his little sister, "Don't talk to strangers." He has introjected this value from the instructions of parents and teachers.	Helps a person avoid social retaliation and punishment; particularly important for the child's development of the superego
Minimization Not acknowledging the significance of one's behavior	A person says, "Don't believe everything my wife tells you. I wasn't so drunk that I couldn't drive."	Allows a person to decrease responsibility for behavior
Projection Blaming other persons or the environment for unacceptable desires, thoughts, shortcomings, and mistakes	A mother is told that her child must repeat a grade in school, and she blames this on the teacher's poor instruction; a husband forgets to pay a bill and blames his wife for not giving it to him earlier.	Allows a person to deny the existence of shortcomings and mistakes; protects the self-image

(continued)

(Continued)

Defense Mechanism	Example(s)	Use/Purpose
Rationalization Justification of certain behaviors by faulty logic and ascription of motives that are socially acceptable but did not in fact inspire the behavior	A mother spanks her toddler too hard and says that it was acceptable because he couldn't feel it through the diaper anyway.	Helps a person cope with the inability to meet goals or certain standards
Reaction Formation Acting exactly opposite to the way one feels	An executive resents his bosses for calling in a consulting firm to make recommendations for change in his department but verbalizes complete support of the idea and is exceedingly polite and cooperative.	Aids in reinforcing repression by allowing feelings to be acted out in a more acceptable way
Regression Resorting to an earlier, more comfortable level of functioning that is characteristically less demanding and responsible	An adult throws a temper tantrum when he does not get his own way; a critically ill client allows the nurse to bathe and feed him.	Allows a person to return to a point in development when nurturing and dependency were needed and accepted with comfort
Repression An unconscious mechanism by which threatening thoughts, feelings, and desires are kept from becoming conscious; the repressed material is denied entry into consciousness	A teenager, seeing his best friend killed in a car accident, becomes amnesic about the circumstances surrounding the accident.	Protects a person from a traumatic experience until he or she has the resources to cope
Sublimation Displacement of energy associated with more primitive sexual or aggressive drives into socially acceptable activities	A person with excessive, primitive sexual drives invests psychic energy in a well-defined religious value system.	Protects a person from behaving in irrational, impulsive ways
Substitution Replacement of a highly valued, unacceptable, or unavailable object by a less valuable, less acceptable, or available object	A woman wants to marry a man exactly like her dead father and settles for someone who looks a little bit like him.	Helps a person achieve goals and minimizes frustration and disappointment
Undoing An action or words designed to cancel disapproved thoughts, impulses, or acts in which the person relieves guilt by making reparation	A father spanks his child and the next evening brings home a present for him; a teacher writes an exam that is far too easy and then constructs a grading curve that makes it difficult to earn a high grade.	Allows a person to reduce guilty feelings and atone for mistakes

Mental Disorders

Mental disorders can be divided into three major categories:

- **Neuroses:** mild emotional disturbances that impair judgment.
- **Psychoses:** severe mental disorders that interfere with the individual's perception of reality.
- **Personality disorder:** antisocial reactions, paranoias, and narcissistic behavior.

Patient Advocacy

At some point during their care, patients may need an advocate. Patient advocates are individuals who help patients make sure that their voices are heard and their wishes are carried out. Typically, a family member will serve as the patient advocate; however, there may be times when a member of the medical office may need to serve in this capacity and ensure that the patient is receiving quality care.

MAJOR DIAGNOSTIC CATEGORIES OF MENTAL DISORDERS

Category	Example
Anxiety Disorder	Phobias, panic attacks, compulsive rituals
Cognitive Disorder	Delirium, dementia, amnesia (resulting from brain damage or the effects of toxic substances or drugs), degenerative disorders such as Alzheimer's disease
Disorder Diagnosed in Infancy and Childhood	Mental retardation, attention deficit disorders such as hyperactivity or inability to concentrate, and developmental problems
Disorder with Physical Symptoms and No Organic Cause (Somatoform)	Paralysis, heart palpitations, dizziness; also referred to as *hypochondriasis*
Dissociative Disorder	Dissociative amnesia, in which important events cannot be remembered after a traumatic event, and dissociative identity disorder (multiple personality disorder), in which two or more personalities or identities are present in one person
Eating Disorders	Characterized by abnormal eating patterns, distorted body image, fear, guilt, and depression
Factitious Disorders	Characterized by physical and/or psychological symptoms that are consciously created by the patient, which the patient knows are not real; such as pretending to be sick (or to sicken others) to get attention
Impulse Control Disorder	Inability to resist the impulse to perform some act that is harmful to the individual or others, such as pathological gambling, stealing (kleptomania), setting fires (pyromania), or having violent rages
Mood Disorder	Major depression, bipolar disorder (manic depression), chronic depressive mood
Personality Disorder	Inflexible behavior patterns that cause distress or the inability to function; these include paranoid, narcissistic, and antisocial disorders
Schizophrenia and Other Psychotic Disorders	Characterized by delusions, hallucinations, and severe disturbances in thinking and emotion
Sexual and Gender Identity Disorder	Transsexualism (wanting to be the other gender), impaired sexual performance (lack of orgasm, premature ejaculation, or lack of sexual desire), or unusual or bizarre sexual acts
Substance-Related Disorder	Related to either excessive use of or withdrawal from alcohol, amphetamines, caffeine, cocaine, hallucinogens, nicotine, opiates, and other drugs

When patients are not feeling well, have recently received devastating news, or are depressed or frightened, they may react in a very uncharacteristic way. It is important that the patient advocate and medical personnel listen to them and remain empathetic.

It is also important to understand psychological theories, defense mechanisms, and mental disorders as you work with patients and advocate for their care.

8 APPLICATION

Directions: Select the best answer for each of the following questions. Check your answers in the Answer Key at the end of the book.

1. Which of the following is not one of the developmental stages of the life cycle?
   a. Infancy
   b. Adolescence
   c. Childhood
   d. Prepubescence
   e. Prenatal period

2. Piaget's theory of cognitive development includes which of the following stages?
   a. Generativity
   b. Autonomy
   c. Sensorimotor
   d. Formal operational
   e. C and D

3. In the life cycle, adolescence is characterized by:
   a. Importance of friendships
   b. Development of trust
   c. Beginning of the desire for independence
   d. A and B
   e. A and C

4. Which of the following is the first stage of Freud's stages of psychosexual development?
   a. Genital
   b. Anal
   c. Oral
   d. Phallic
   e. Latency

5. The concept at the top of Maslow's hierarchy of needs is:
   a. Safety
   b. Physiological
   c. Self-actualization
   d. Love/social
   e. Self-esteem/status

6. Which of these examples contain all of the needs in the physiological stage of Maslow's hierarchy?
   a. Food, physical safety, water
   b. Food, water, sense of belonging
   c. Water and physical safety
   d. Food, shelter, water
   e. Sense of belonging and sense of accomplishment

7. Erik Erikson's psychosocial development theory includes how many stages?
   a. Six
   b. Eight
   c. Seven
   d. Five
   e. Four

8. In Erik Erikson's theory, each stage has a major conflict and each conflict can have a positive or negative outcome. The positive outcome of the childhood stage is industry. What is the negative outcome?
   a. Inferiority
   b. Guilt
   c. Role confusion
   d. Isolation
   e. Despair

9. Ivan Pavlov conducted a famous series of experiments involving the feeding of dogs preceded by the ringing of a bell. His theory is known as:
   a. Behavioral conditioning
   b. Classical conditioning
   c. Canine conditioning
   d. Operant conditioning
   e. None of the above

10. The operant conditioning theory was developed and proposed by whom?
    a. B. F. Skinner
    b. Sigmund Freud
    c. Christian Barnard
    d. Erik Erikson
    e. Jean Piaget

11. The final stage in the five stages of grief as proposed by Elizabeth Kübler-Ross is:
    a. Depression
    b. Anger
    c. Denial
    d. Acceptance
    e. Bargaining

12. Which of these is not one of Freud's defense mechanisms?
    a. Identification
    b. Projection
    c. Fight or flight
    d. Denial
    e. Compensation

13. Mental disorders are divided into the following three major categories:
    a. Neuroses, alcohol addiction, psychoses
    b. Psychoses, personality disorder, neuroses
    c. Drug addiction, alcohol addiction, neuroses
    d. Neuroses, psychoses, personality disorder
    e. Depression, repression, psychoses

14. In Piaget's theory of cognitive development, the focus of the preoperational stage is:
    a. Language and symbols
    b. Movement and senses
    c. Movement and abstract concepts
    d. Analytical reasoning
    e. Logical and analytical reasoning

15. A young adult sees his best friend fall through the ice of a frozen pond and drown. He becomes amnesic about the circumstances of the event. This is an example of which defense mechanism?
    a. Minimization
    b. Denial
    c. Compensation
    d. Repression
    e. Undoing

Section 3

Medical Laws, Legal Issues, and Ethical Considerations

9 Medical Law and Ethical Considerations

CONTENTS

Licensure

Licensure in general is defined as granting permission to practice. In order for a physician to practice medicine, he or she is required to have a current license, which is granted by the state in which the physician is practicing. A physician's license informs patients that the physician has met the licensure qualifications by successfully completing his or her medical education and training, including residency, and has demonstrated competency by passing the licensure examination.

MEDICAL PRACTICE ACTS

Each state regulates the practice of medicine within that state. These medical practice acts establish the requirements for licensure, the duties attached to that license, and the basis for revocation or suspension of the license.

Physician licensure is granted by the board of medical examiners in each state. The medical license may be obtained one of three ways: examination, reciprocity, or endorsement.

- **Examination:** The qualifying examination accepted for licensure varies from state to state; however, all states accept the United States Medical Licensing Exam (USMLE), which consists of four separate exams broken down into steps:

  Step 1: Required written exam, commonly referred to as the *boards*, which is typically taken at the end of the second year of medical school and tests the examinee's knowledge and ability to apply important fundamental scientific concepts as they relate to the practice of medicine.

  Step 2 CK: Required written exam that tests the examinee's ability to apply clinical knowledge.

  Step 2 CS: Optional in some states, a series of encounters with hypothetical patients that assesses the examinee's ability to successfully complete a patient history and a physical exam, determine diagnoses, and write progress notes.

  Step 3: Required written exam that covers general topics required to understand and practice general medicine. Steps 1 and 2 CS must be successfully completed prior to applying for Step 3.

Other qualifying examinations are the Federation Licensing Examination (FLEX) and the National Board of Medical Examiners (NBME) exam, among others.

There are two circumstances in which the licensure exam may be waived:

- **Reciprocity:** In some cases, physicians who hold a current license in one state and wish to practice medicine in another state may not be required to take that state's licensure exam because the physician's current license requirements are recognized.
- **Endorsement:** When physicians have successfully completed a nationally recognized examination considered to have high standards, their current license and examination scores may be recognized and they may not have to take the state examination.

REVOCATION OR SUSPENSION OF THE MEDICAL LICENSE

A physician's license may be revoked or suspended for one of the following reasons:

- Unprofessional conduct
- Conviction of a crime
- Inability to perform due to physical or emotional incapacity

REGISTRATION

Once physicians have obtained a medical license, they are required to reregister their license with the state in which they practice either annually or biannually. In addition to submitting the proper forms and fees when reregistering, physicians are expected to submit their required number of completed CMEs (Continuing Medical Education credits). CMEs are required to ensure that physicians are aware of current practices in their field of medicine.

Law

LEGAL TERMINOLOGY

Accessory	An individual who contributes to the commission of a crime
Assumption of Risk	Medical malpractice defense when the physician must prove that the patient was aware of the risks involved in a procedure
Bench Trial	A trial in which a judge serves without a jury
Burden of Proof	Presenting testimony at a trial to prove either guilt or innocence
Contributory Negligence	Plaintiff's actions or failure to act that contributed to the injury

(*Continued*)

Damages	Money awarded to a patient as a result of damage or injury sustained
Defamation of Character	Statement(s) about an individual that can damage his or her reputation • *Slander*: spoken defamation • *Libel*: written defamation
Emancipated Minor	An individual under the age of 18 who is no longer under the care, custody, or supervision of a parent
Expressed Consent	Written or verbal statement by the patient (or legal guardian) that the patient agrees to the prescribed procedure
Guardian ad litem	A court-appointed adult who acts on behalf of a child
Implied Consent	Agreement to a procedure through actions only
Locum tenens	Latin term meaning "placeholder"; a physician who covers for an absent physician is referred to as a "*locum* doctor"
Malfeasance	Performing an incorrect treatment
Misfeasance	Performing the correct treatment with errors
Nonfeasance	Failure to perform a treatment
Non compos mentis	Latin term meaning "not of sound mind"
Proximate Cause	Plaintiff must prove that the defendant's actions or failure to act caused injury
Qui tam	Legal action brought about by an informer also known as a *whistle-blower*
Quid pro quo	Latin term meaning "something for something"
Res ipsa loquitor	Latin term meaning "the thing speaks for itself"
Res judicata	Latin term meaning "the thing has been decided"
Respondeat superior	Latin term literally translated as "let the master answer." The physician is liable for the negligent actions of anyone who works for him or her.
Standard of Care	The requirement that the physician provide the same knowledge, skill, and care that a similarly trained physician would provide
Statute of Limitations	The period of time that a patient has to file a lawsuit
Subpoena	An order to appear in court
Subpoena duces tecum	An order to appear in court with records

ADMINISTRATIVE LAW

Administrative law, also known as *regulatory law*, is passed by the federal government. It addresses public transportation, the environment, and taxation.

CRIMINAL LAW

Criminal law is concerned with the safety and welfare of the public. Violations of criminal law are classified as either a misdemeanor or a felony based on the severity of the crime. Criminal law varies from state to state.

- **Felonies:** Considered serious crimes.
- **Misdemeanors:** Considered less severe than felonies.

FELONY CATEGORIES

Felony Degree	Action of Person Being Charged
First	Committed the crime
Second	Was at the scene of the crime and assisted in the crime
Third	Assisted in the crime before the crime occurred
Fourth	Assisted the person who committed the crime after the fact

Source: Medical Assisting: Foundations and Practices by M. S. Frazier, C. Malone, and C. Morgan, Upper Saddle River, NJ: Pearson Education, Inc., 2010, p. 42. Reprinted with permission.

Box 9-1 The Four Ds of Negligence

- *Duty* refers to the physician-patient relationship. The patient must prove that this relationship has been established. When the patient has made an appointment and been seen by the physician, a relationship has been established. Further office visits and treatment will establish that the physician had a duty or obligation to the patient. (Contract)
- *Dereliction or neglect of duty* refers to a physician's failure to act as any ordinary and prudent physician (a peer) within the same community would act in a similar circumstance when treating a patient. To prove dereliction or neglect of duty, a patient must prove that the physician's performance or treatment did not comply with the acceptable standard of care based on the norm of the ordinary and prudent physician. (Standard of Care)
- *Direct cause* requires the patient to prove that the physician's dereliction or neglect of duty was the direct cause of the injury that resulted.
- *Damages* refers to any injuries received by the patient. The court may award compensatory damages to pay for these injuries.

CIVIL LAW

Civil law is concerned with the relationships between individuals and between individuals and the government. Civil law includes tort law and contract law.

TORT LAW

Tort law is the part of civil law concerned with injuries due to an inappropriate action or failure to act. Torts are categorized as either unintentional or intentional:

- **Unintentional tort:** Occurs when a mistake was made. Most medical malpractice cases involve unintentional torts and occur as a result of negligence. In order for a physician to be found guilty of negligence, all four Ds of negligence must be proven (Box 9-1).
- **Intentional tort:** Occurs when someone intentionally injures another individual.

INTENTIONAL TORTS

Assault	Unauthorized attempt or threat to touch another person. *Example:* Telling a patient her temperature will be taken whether she wants it or not after she refuses to allow it.
Battery	Actual physical touching of another person without the person's consent; includes physical abuse. *Example:* Taking a patient's temperature against the patient's will.
Defamation of Character	Making or publishing false or malicious statements about another person's character or reputation. *Example:* Telling patients they should not see the cardiologist across the street because that cardiologist has a drinking problem.
Duress	Act of coercing someone into an act. *Example:* Telling patients they must have a tetanus vaccine or they will develop a life-threatening infection. The patients feel they have no choice but to comply, even though they do not want the vaccine.
Fraud	Deceitful act made to conceal the truth. *Example:* Falsifying a patient's medical record to conceal a medical mistake.
Invasion of Privacy	Releasing private information about another person without the person's consent. *Example:* Releasing a patient's medical records without the patient's consent or a court order.
Tort of Outrage	Intentionally inflicting emotional distress on another person. *Example:* The physician yells at a patient for failing to follow instructions.
Undue Influence	Intentionally persuading people to do things they do not want to do. *Example:* Convincing single mothers that they should give their children up for adoption when they clearly do not want to.

Source: Medical Assisting: Foundations and Practices by M. S. Frazier, C. Malone, and C. Morgan, Upper Saddle River, NJ: Pearson Education, Inc., 2010, p. 42. Reprinted with permission.

CONTRACT LAW

A contract is a voluntary agreement between two parties resulting in benefit for both of them. There are three parts to a contract:

- **Offer:** The contract is initiated.
- **Acceptance:** Both parties agree to the terms of the contract.
- **Consideration:** Services are provided and a fee is paid.

COMMON TERMS ASSOCIATED WITH CONTRACT LAW

Term	Definition
Abandonment	When a healthcare professional initiates care of a patient and leaves the patient without completing the care or finding an acceptable substitute
Breach of Contract	When either party in a contract fails to comply with the terms of the agreement
Expressed Contract	Either written or verbal agreement to a contract
Implied Contract	Agreement to a contract through actions only
Termination of Contract	Occurs when the physician has finished treating the patient and the patient has paid the associated fees

PUBLIC DUTIES OF THE PHYSICIAN

Physicians have responsibilities to the general public. The reporting requirements may vary from state to state, so the medical assistant should be familiar with the physician's responsibilities in the particular state.

PHYSICIAN-PATIENT RELATIONSHIP

The patient and physician must agree to form a relationship in order for a contract to occur. Once the physician-patient relationship has been established, the patient has certain responsibilities and rights, as does the physician.

In addition to the rights described in the Patients' Bill of Rights, discussed later in the chapter, the patient has the following responsibilities:

- Honesty in communication
- Cooperation with the physician
- Payment of fees

The physician's rights and responsibilities are as follows:

- Right to accurate information from the patient
- Right to choose whom to accept as a patient, but without discrimination based on race, religion, or another classification that applies to an entire group of people
- Right to decide what types of medicine to practice
- Right to establish the location of the office and the office hours
- Right to take a vacation, with the responsibility of providing a qualified substitute who is available to continue to care for the patient. If the physician fails to provide a qualified substitute, it is considered abandonment.
- Most responsibilities of the physician are determined by the licensing board, but the physician's primary responsibility is to intentionally do no harm.

Terminating the Physician-Patient Relationship

The patient may decide to terminate the physician-patient relationship at any time without providing formal notice. If the patient does provide the reason for terminating the relationship, that information must be documented in the patient's chart.

If a physician determines that it is best to terminate the physician-patient relationship, the physician is required to follow legal protocol in order to do so. Typical reasons for physician termination are the patient's failure to pay, failure to comply with the suggested treatment, and failure to keep appointments.

The legal protocol for terminating the relationship with a patient requires the physician to notify the patient in writing and provide the following information:

- The physician's intent to terminate the relationship and the reason
- A statement that the patient's medical records will be available for transfer to another physician
- An offer to refer the patient to another physician
- A statement that the physician will continue to provide care until a set date (typically 30 days from the time the letter is received)

PUBLIC DUTIES OF THE PHYSICIAN

Duty	Description
Births	Issuing a legal certificate, which will be maintained during a person's life as proof of age. Many benefits and documents, including Social Security, a passport, and a driver's license, depend on having a valid birth certificate.
Deaths	Physician signs a certificate indicating the cause of a natural death. Check with your state's public health department to determine the specific requirements. For example, in the case of a stillbirth before the 20th week of gestation, the medical assistant will have to determine if both a birth certificate and a death certificate are required. A coroner or health official will have to sign a certificate in the following cases: • No physician present at the time of death • Violent or unlawful death • Death as a result of criminal action • Death from an undetermined cause
Reportable Communicable Diseases	Physicians must report all diseases that can be transmitted from one person to another and are considered a general threat to the public. The list of reportable diseases differs from state to state. The report can be sent either by mail or phone. The following childhood vaccines and toxoids are required by law (National Childhood Vaccine Injury Act of 1986): • Diphtheria, tetanus toxoids, pertussis vaccine (DTP) • Pertussis vaccine (whooping cough) • Measles, mumps, rubella (MMR) • Poliovirus vaccine, live • Poliovirus vaccine, inactivated • Hepatitis B vaccine • Tuberculosis test
Reportable Injuries	Certain injuries are reportable according to state requirements. These injuries include gunshot and knife wounds, rape and battered persons injuries, and spousal, child, and elder abuse.
Child Abuse	Questionable injuries of children, including bruises, fractured bones, and burns, must be reported. Signs of neglect, such as malnutrition, poor growth, and lack of hygiene, are reportable in some states.
Elder Abuse	Physical abuse, neglect, and abandonment of older adults is reportable in most states. The reporting agency varies by state but generally includes social service agencies.
Drug Abuse	Abuse of prescription drugs is reportable according to the law. Such abuse can be difficult to determine since the abuser may seek prescriptions for the same drug from several different physicians. A physician will want to see a patient before prescribing a medication.

A copy of the letter should be placed in the patient's chart. The letter should be mailed via U.S. Postal Service certified mail, return receipt requested.

Legislation

PATIENT SELF-DETERMINATION ACT

The Patient Self-Determination Act provides protection for the patient and the physician and also provides guidance for the patient's caregiver to make decisions based on the wishes of the patient.

Living Will

A living will is a document that allows patients of sound mind to make decisions regarding the use (or nonuse) of life support and nutritional support prior to the time when death is imminent and such support would be implemented.

Durable Power of Attorney

This document allows an appointed individual to act on behalf of the patient and make decisions for that patient regarding his or her health care.

Uniform Anatomical Gift Act

Individuals 18 years of age and older and of sound mind can determine which of their organs (if any) are to be used for transplantation or medical research at the time of death. The Uniform Anatomical Gift Act includes the following:

- The intent to donate must be stated in writing.
- The donor may determine which organs or tissues are to be used for transplant.
- The donor's valid statement takes precedence over other individuals' wishes, except when autopsy is required.
- Survivors (in specific order of priority) may act on the donor's behalf if the donor has not acted during his or her lifetime.
- The physician performing the transplant operation cannot determine death or the time of death of the donor.
- For the purpose of organ donation, money cannot be exchanged.

PATIENTS' BILL OF RIGHTS

Figure 9-1 shows the Patients' Bill of Rights.

GOOD SAMARITAN ACT

The Good Samaritan Act protects healthcare workers from liability when they provide first aid in emergency situations.

CONTROLLED SUBSTANCES ACT OF 1970

The Controlled Substances Act of 1970 requires that physicians handle highly addictive medications in a certain manner.

I. **Information Disclosure** You have the right to receive accurate and easily understood information about your health plan, health care professionals, and health care facilities. If you speak another language, have a physical or mental disability, or just do not understand something, assistance will be provided so you can make informed health care decisions.

II. **Choice of Providers and Plans** You have the right to a choice of health care providers that is sufficient to provide you with access to appropriate high-quality health care.

III. **Access to Emergency Services** If you have severe pain, an injury, or a sudden illness that convinces you that your health is in serious jeopardy, you have the right to receive screening and stabilization emergency services whenever and wherever needed, without prior authorization or financial penalty.

IV. **Participation in Treatment Decisions** You have the right to know all your treatment options and to participate in decisions about your care. Parents, guardians, family members, or other individuals that you designate can represent you if you cannot make your own decisions.

V. **Respect and Nondiscrimination** You have a right to considerate, respectful, and nondiscriminatory care from your doctors, health plan representatives, and other health care providers.

VI. **Confidentiality of Health Information** You have the right to talk in confidence with health care providers and to have your health care information protected. You also have the right to review and copy your own medical record and request that your physician amend your record if it is not accurate, relevant, or complete.

VII. **Complaints and Appeals** You have the right to a fair, fast, and objective review of any complaint you have against your health plan, doctors, hospitals, or other health care personnel. This includes complaints about waiting times, operating hours, the conduct of health care personnel, and the adequacy of health care facilities.

FIGURE 9-1 The Patients' Bill of Rights.
From *Medical Assisting: Foundations and Practices* by M. S. Frazier, C. Malone, and C. Morgan, Upper Saddle River, NJ: Pearson Education, Inc., 2010, p. 63. Reprinted with permission.

All physicians must be registered with the Drug Enforcement Administration (DEA) and be issued a specific DEA number.

HEALTH INSURANCE PORTABILITY AND ACCOUNTABILITY ACT OF 1996 (HIPAA)

HIPAA was enacted to help lower healthcare administration costs, ensure patient privacy, and prevent fraud and abuse. See Chapter 10.

OCCUPATIONAL SAFETY AND HEALTH ACT (OSHA)

OSHA includes regulations that protect healthcare workers and patients from health hazards and addresses the following:

- Requires employers to classify jobs that involve exposure to blood
- Mandates universal precautions and requires employers to provide personal protective equipment (PPE) for their employees
- Requires a written plan or schedule for cleaning and decontaminating, as well as the method of disposal for regulated biohazardous material
- Requires a written exposure plan
- Requires employees' medical records to be kept confidential during their employment plus 30 years

CLINICAL LABORATORY IMPROVEMENT ACT (CLIA)

CLIA consists of regulations of the Centers for Medicare and Medicaid Services (CMS) concerning laboratory testing on humans. The regulations are based on the complexity of the test(s) being performed.

Ethics

Ethics are moral guidelines that help determine what is considered to be appropriate behavior. Medical ethics focus on the rights, welfare, and concerns of patients and are guidelines for appropriate conduct and behavior. Medical organizations such as the American Medical Association (AMA), the American Association of Medical Assistants (AAMA), and the American Medical Technologists (AMT) each have their own set of guidelines (Boxes 9-2, 9-3, and 9-4).

It is important to understand that unethical behavior is not always unlawful; however, unlawful behavior is always unethical.

Box 9-2 AMA Principles of Medical Ethics

Preamble

The medical profession has long subscribed to a body of ethical statements developed primarily for the benefit of the patient. As a member of this profession, a physician must recognize responsibility not only to patients, but also to society, to other health professionals, and to self. The following principles adopted by the American Medical Association are not law, but standards of conduct which define the essentials of honorable behavior for the physician.

Human Dignity

I. A physician shall be dedicated to providing competent medical service with compassion and respect for human dignity.

Honesty

II. A physician shall deal honestly with patients and colleagues, and strive to expose those physicians deficient in character or competence, or who engage in fraud or deception.

Responsibility to Society

III. A physician shall respect the law and recognize a responsibility to seek changes in those requirements which are contrary to the best interests of the patient.

Confidentiality

IV. A physician shall respect the rights of patients, of colleagues, and of other health professionals, and shall safeguard patient confidence within the constraints of the law.

Continued Study

V. A physician shall continue to study, apply and advance scientific knowledge, make relevant information available to patients, colleagues, and the public, obtain consultation, and use the talents of other health professionals where needed.

Freedom of Choice

VI. A physician shall, in the provision of appropriate patient care, except in emergencies, be free to choose whom to serve, with whom to associate, and the environment in which to provide service.

Responsibility to Improved Community

VII. A physician shall recognize a responsibility to participate in activities contributing to an improved community.

Box 9-3 AMT Standards of Practice

1. While engaged in the Arts and Sciences, which constitute the practice of their profession, AMT professionals shall be dedicated to the provision of competent service.
2. The AMT professional shall place the welfare of the patient above all else.
3. The AMT professional understands the importance of thoroughness in the performance of duty, compassion with patients, and the importance of the tasks which may be performed.
4. The AMT professional shall always seek to respect the rights of patients and of health care providers, and shall safeguard patient confidences.
5. The AMT professional will strive to increase his/her technical knowledge, shall continue to study, and apply scientific advances in his/her specialty.
6. The AMT professional shall respect the law and will pledge to avoid dishonest, unethical or illegal practices.
7. The AMT professional understands that he/she is not to make or offer a diagnosis or interpretation unless he/she is a duly licensed physician/dentist or unless asked by the attending physician/dentist.
8. The AMT professional shall protect and value the judgment of the attending physician or dentist, providing this does not conflict with the behavior necessary to carry out Standard Number 2 above.
9. The AMT professional recognizes that any personal wrongdoing is his/her responsibility. It is also the professional health care provider's obligation to report to the proper authorities any knowledge of professional abuse.
10. The AMT professional pledges personal honor and integrity to cooperate in the advancement and expansion, by every lawful means, of American Medical Technologists.

Box 9-4 Code of Ethics of the American Association of Medical Assistants

Preamble

The Code of Ethics of AAMA shall set forth principles of ethical and moral conduct as they relate to the medical profession and the particular practice of medical assisting.

Members of the AAMA dedicated to the conscientious pursuit of their profession, and thus desiring to merit the high regard of the entire medical profession and the respect of the general public which they serve, do hereby pledge themselves to strive always to:

Human Dignity

I. Render service with full respect for the dignity of humanity;

Confidentiality

II. Respect confidential information obtained through employment unless legally authorized or required by responsible performance of duty to divulge such information;

Honor

III. Uphold the honor and high principles of the profession and accept its disciplines;

Continued Study

IV. Seek to continually improve the knowledge and skills of medical assistants for the benefit of patients and professional colleagues;

Responsibility for Improved Community

V. Participate in additional service activities aimed toward improving the health and well-being of the community.

Laws can be enforced by government authorities via penalties and prison sentences; however, ethical standards are much more difficult to enforce, and failure to adhere to them rarely results in a penalty. Unethical behavior may cause the professional to be shunned by the organization with which he or she is associated.

BIOETHICS

Ethical decisions pertaining to life issues are referred to as *bioethics*. Examples of current bioethical issues are shown on the following page.

EXAMPLES OF CURRENT BIOETHICAL ISSUES

Abortion	Planned interrruption of pregancy by either mechanical or chemical means
Artificial Insemination	Injection of sperm (either spousal or donor) into the vagina by means other than intercourse
Euthanasia	Also known as *physician-assisted suicide* by lethal injection or overdose of chemicals
In Vitro Fertilization	Placement of sperm and ova in a petri dish with the hope that an embryo will develop, followed by implantation in the uterus or freezing for later use

GENETICS

Genetics is the study of heredity, or how traits are passed from one generation to the next.

Genetic engineeing involves altering an individual's genes in order to alter genetic traits and cure or eliminate genetic diseases such as sickle cell anemia.

EXAMPLES OF CURRENT BIOETHICAL ISSUES RELATED TO GENETIC ENGINEERING

Cloning	Copying one cell to create a genetically identical organism
Genetic Testing	Tests using blood, saliva, or tissue to determine whether a person is predisposed to develop or carry certain genetic characteristics or disesases
Gene Therapy	Altering or eliminating harmful genes or inserting normal genes into defective cells
Stem Cell Research—Adult	Adult stem cells are found within organs and not specialized, but typically surrounded by those cells that are. Adult stem cells maintain and repair tissue and can be used to treat a variety of conditions and diseases. Research is conducted to determine the viability of the cells as well as the stem cell's ability to divide and regenerate into a limited number of cell types.
Stem Cell Research—Embryonic	Embryonic stem cells are not specialized yet and can be manipulated to become any type of specialized body cell. Research is conducted to determine the viability of the cells as well as the stem cell's ability to divide and regenerate into all cell types found within the body.

TRANSPLANTS

In addition to organ and tissue transplants that take place once someone has died, there are also transplants that can occur while the individual is still alive. These transplants fall into one of three categories:

CATEGORIES OF LIVE TRANSPLANTS

Autograft	Transplanting tissue within the self *Example*: Transplanting skin from the thigh to the torso
Homograft	Transplanting tissue between *members of* the same species *Example*: Blood tranfusion
Heterograft	Transplanting tissue from one species to another *Example*: Transplanting a pig's heart valve into a human heart

9 APPLICATION

Directions: Select the best answer for each of the following questions. Check your answers in the Answer Key at the end of the book.

1. The practice of medicine within each state is regulated by:
   a. The surgeon general of the United States
   b. The state itself
   c. The American Medical Association
   d. The U.S. attorney general
   e. A and C

2. What are the three ways medical licensure may be obtained?
   a. Reciprocity, registration, examination
   b. Registration, endorsement, examination
   c. Endorsement, examination, reciprocity
   d. Clinical demonstration, registration, examination
   e. Clinical demonstration, reciprocity, examination

3. Performing the correct treatment with errors is the definition of:
   a. Malfeasance
   b. Misfeasance
   c. Nonfeasance
   d. Proximate cause
   e. None of the above

4. The physician is liable for the negligent actions of anyone who works for him or her. This is the definition of what legal term?
   a. Proximate cause
   b. Standard of care
   c. *Quid pro quo*
   d. *Res judicata*
   e. *Respondeat superior*

5. What are the three parts of a contract?
   a. Offer, acceptance, renegotiation
   b. Offer, counteroffer, acceptance
   c. Offer, acceptance, consideration
   d. Offer, refusal, consideration
   e. Offer, renegotiation, acceptance

6. What legislative act protects healthcare workers from liability when they provide first aid in an emergency situation?
   a. Good Samaritan Act
   b. Patients' Bill of Rights
   c. Occupational Safety and Health Act
   d. Red Cross Act
   e. None of the above

7. Which of these is not an intentional tort?
   a. Fraud
   b. Duress
   c. Battery
   d. Assault
   e. Shoplifting

8. Physical touching of another person without the person's consent is the definition of:
   a. Battery
   b. Assault
   c. Duress
   d. Undue influence
   e. Tort of outrage

9. Which of these is not one of the four Ds of negligence?
   a. Duty
   b. Direct cause
   c. Duplicity
   d. Damages
   e. Dereliction of duty

10. A physician's license may be revoked or suspended for the following reasons:
    a. Conviction of a crime
    b. Refusal to accept new patients
    c. Unprofessional conduct
    d. A and B
    e. A and C

11. The following are included in the Patients' Bill of Rights:
    a. Complaints and appeals
    b. Information disclosure
    c. Confidentiality of health information
    d. A and B but not C
    e. A, B, and C

12. There are four degrees of felonies. Which is the most serious?
    a. First
    b. Second
    c. Third
    d. Fourth
    e. They are all equal

13. Civil law is concerned with:
   a. Felonies and contracts
   b. Felonies and misdemeanors
   c. Contracts and misdemeanors
   d. Torts and contracts
   e. Torts and misdemeanors

14. A healthcare professional initiates care of a patient without completing the care or finding an acceptable substitute. This is known as:
   a. Breach of contract
   b. Abandonment
   c. Termination of contract
   d. Assumption of risk
   e. Contributory negligence

15. Intentionally persuading people to do things they do not want to do is known as:
   a. Duress
   b. Undue influence
   c. Fraud
   d. Breach of contract
   e. Misrepresentation

16. ___________ are ethical decisions that pertain to certain life issues.
   a. Biogenetics
   b. Bioethics
   c. Medi-ethics
   d. Genetic ethics
   e. None of the above

17. Genetic engineering–related bioethical issues include:
   a. Artificial insemination
   b. Gene therapy
   c. In vitro fertilization
   d. Stem cell research
   e. B and D

18. Copying one cell to create a genetically identical organism is known as:
   a. In vitro fertilization
   b. Gene therapy
   c. Stem cell research—adult
   d. Cloning
   e. Stem cell research—embryonic

19. A physician who decides to terminate the physician-patient relationship must notify the patient in writing and address the following items:
   a. The date when care will no longer be provided
   b. The intent to terminate the relationship and why
   c. An offer to refer the patient to another physician
   d. All of the above
   e. A physician may not terminate the physician-patient relationship

20. Altering or eliminating harmful genes or inserting normal genes into defective cells is known as:
   a. Gene therapy
   b. Gene manipulation
   c. Stem cell research
   d. Cloning
   e. Genetic testing

21. All but one of the following are principles of both the AMA and the AAMA Code of Ethics:
   a. Freedom of choice
   b. Responsibility to improve the community
   c. Confidentiality
   d. Continued study
   e. Human dignity

22. Which of the following statements is not correct?
   a. Ethics are difficult to enforce.
   b. Unlawful behavior is always unethical.
   c. Unethical behavior rarely results in a penalty.
   d. Unethical behavior may cause the professional to be shunned by his or her associated organization.
   e. Unethical behavior is always unlawful.

10 HIPAA

CONTENTS

Health Insurance Portability and Accountability Act of 1996 (HIPAA)

The U.S. Congress passed HIPAA after many complaints by patients that they were not allowed to continue paying insurance premiums to the same company when they moved from one place of employment to another. In addition to having portability problems, patients feared that information about their health might prevent them from obtaining insurance coverage. Congress determined that patient privacy must be maintained for the patient's protected health information (PHI). PHI is any information that would identify a patient:

- Name
- Address
- Telephone number
- Date of birth
- Social Security number
- E-mail address
- Medical record number
- Insurance information, including ID and group number
- Driver's license number
- Photos

The intention of HIPAA was to do the following:

- Improve portability and continuity within group and individual insurance
- Combat waste, fraud, and abuse in health insurance and within the healthcare delivery system
- Promote the use of medical savings accounts (MSAs)
- Improve access to long-term care services and coverage
- Simplify health insurance information
- Provide a way to pay for reform and related initiatives

TITLE I

Title I of HIPAA addresses portability of insurance coverage when employees change or lose their jobs. It accomplishes the following:

- Increases the chance that a new employee will be able to obtain health insurance when beginning a new job.
- Provides for continuous coverage when an employee changes jobs.
- Helps reduce the likelihood that an employee will lose his or her health insurance.
- Helps employees who lose their jobs to access insurance coverage that they may purchase on their own.

TITLE II

Title II of HIPAA is concerned mostly with healthcare providers. It addresses the prevention of fraud and abuse, administrative simplification, and medical liability reform.

- It is commonly known as the *privacy rule*.
- It requires insurance providers to notify patients in writing about how their medical information is handled and under what circumstances their PHI may be released.
- Patients have more control over their health information and who may have access to it.
- It safeguards patient information and establishes rules by which healthcare providers must abide.
- It prevents fraud and abuse.
- It sets standards and requirements regarding electronic transmission of health information.
- It requires the use of Employer Identification Numbers (EINs).

Business Associate Agreements

HIPAA states that only those who need to know should have access to patient information.

On being hired, employees must complete HIPAA training, and those records must be maintained. The business associate agreement applies to individuals such as the cleaning staff and consultants who work in the office, as well as to any medical staff not employed by the office but who are shadowing or externing. These are individuals who do not need access to patient information but who may come in contact with it while completing their duties.

Privacy Officer

Every office should have one person designated as the HIPAA privacy officer. This person is responsible for making sure that the office is HIPAA compliant. The privacy officer should be an effective communicator with the ability to answer questions regarding suspected HIPAA violations and complaints. Box 10-1 shows the penalties for HIPAA violations.

Box 10-1 Penalties for HIPAA Violations

General penalty for the failure to comply with requirements and standards:

- Not more than $100 for each violation up to $25,000 for all violations of an identical requirement during a calendar year.

Wrongful disclosure of protected health information:

- A person who knowingly and in violation of HIPAA regulations:
  - Uses or causes to be used a unique health identifier
  - Obtains private health information relating to an individual
  - Discloses individually identifiable health information to another person

Shall be punished by:

- A fine of not more than $50,000, imprisoned for not more than 1 year, or both
- If the offense is committed under false pretenses, be fined not more that $100,000, imprisoned for not more than 5 years, or both
- If the offense is done with the intent to sell, transfer, or use private health information for commercial purposes or to cause harm, be fined not more than $250,000, imprisoned not more than 10 years, or both

Source: Medical Assisting: Foundations and Practices by M. S. Frazier, C. Malone, and C. Morgan, Upper Saddle River, NJ: Pearson Education, Inc., 2010, p, 60. Reprinted with permission.

Confidentiality

Patient information should never be released without a patient's signed consent or a court order.

Medical information about a patient should be shared only when the patient agrees to let the designated individuals have access to it. Occasionally, patient medical information is used for health research and may be disclosed to public health agencies such as the Centers for Disease Control. Specific names are usually not given to researchers. Their use of patient information is covered by HIPAA.

Federal law protects patient records dealing with substance abuse treatment.

Some state laws specially protect human immunodeficiency virus/acquired immune deficiency syndrome (HIV/AIDS) information and mental health records. In order to obtain a copy of these records or have them forwarded, the patient may need to sign a form that outlines the release of specific information.

Chart Ownership

The physician or the facility where the physician works owns the medical records, but the patient has the legal right of *privileged communication* and access to his or her records. Therefore, the patient must authorize release of these records in writing. The patient may also request a copy of the records.

Releasing Patient Information

Generally, only a patient can authorize the release of his or her own medical records. However, there are some exceptions to the rule; generally, the following persons can sign a release:

- Parents of minor children
- Legal guardian
- Agent (someone the patient selects to act on his or her behalf in a healthcare power of attorney)

Under some circumstances, a minor, rather than the parent, must sign the release. Patients with questions about who can authorize release of their medical records should check with their healthcare provider.

Disclosure without Consent

Although medical records are confidential, there are times when they can be released without a patient's consent. In special cases, records may be released to:

- Healthcare workers who need the records to care for a patient, such as when a patient is referred.
- Qualified people or organizations that perform services for the physician, practice, or hospital, such as data processing, transcription, converting records to

disks, EHR support, administrative functions, or other such related services

- Certain government authorities, as permitted or required by law, to assist in public health activities such as tracking diseases or medical devices as well as investigating or regulating health-related issues such communicable diseases, and use of prescription drugs
- Appropriate authorities to protect victims of abuse or neglect
- Law enforcement officials or judicial orders in response to a subpoena or another process that may involve a lawsuit if a patient's medical condition is an issue in the suit

Computers and HIPAA

The same legal standards of confidentiality and HIPAA compliance apply to all patient records, whether on paper or on the computer. It is important to reassure patients that their information will be used appropriately within the medical office. It is absolutely essential that other patients should not be able to see computerized records any more easily than paper records.

All persons who have access to patient records are required to have a unique password. Medical management programs often have several tiers of security, allowing one system administrator (the person in charge of the computer program) to limit access to different areas of the patient record. Not everyone needs the clinical information portion of the patient's record, so that portion may be limited to those who need to know.

HIPAA compliance mandates that computer systems must be located in a secured and private space. This can be accomplished by placing the computer in an area of the office where there is limited public walk-through traffic. The computer screen should be set to a *screen saver* after a few short minutes, and the use of a *privacy screen* should be mandatory. Passwords should also be changed frequently and should not be written down anywhere near the computer.

HIPAA requires healthcare organizations to protect the privacy and security of confidential health information and calls for standard formats of electronic transactions. These standardized national requirements apply to the electronic transmission of patient history and health records such as health insurance enrollment details and claims. The need to maintain confidentiality and privacy of medical information, as well as rules for medical document security, including standards related to electronic signatures, are also outlined in HIPAA.

Data must be backed up (copied to disks or CD-ROMs) at regular intervals, and those backup files must be stored in a secure location outside the office. Again, confidentiality is of the utmost importance, and access to backup files should be carefully guarded.

Fax Machines and HIPAA

In order to maintain patient confidentiality, fax machines must be kept in areas of the office that are not accessible to patients.

HIPAA states that fax machines should be used only when no other, more secure mode of transmission is available. Any faxed documents must have an accompanying HIPAA-compliant fax cover sheet containing the disclaimer that faxed information cannot be shared with any other party without the patient's written consent.

10 APPLICATION

Directions: Select the best answer for each of the following questions. Check your answers in the Answer Key at the end of the book.

1. Which of the following items are included as protected health information (PHI)?
   a. E-mail address
   b. Date of birth
   c. Name(s) of children
   d. A and C
   e. A and B

2. Which of the following is not true concerning Title II of HIPAA?
   a. Helps reduce the likelihood that employees will lose their health insurance
   b. Commonly known as the *privacy rule*
   c. Prevents fraud and abuse
   d. Safeguards patient information
   e. Sets standards and requirements regarding electronic transmission of health information
3. The patient medical record is owned by:
   a. The patient's insurance company
   b. The patient
   c. The physician or facility where the physician works
   d. The state in which the patient resides
   e. A and B
4. In special cases, medical records may be released to certain parties. Which of the following is not included for special consideration?
   a. Qualified people or organizations for approved research
   b. Parents
   c. Healthcare workers who need the records to care for a patient
   d. Lawyers and parties in a lawsuit if a patient's medical condition is an issue in the suit
   e. None of the above
5. Any faxed patient documents must include:
   a. A patient insurance form
   b. A release signed by the physician
   c. A HIPAA-compliant fax cover sheet
   d. A release signed by the patient
   e. B and D
6. Title I of HIPAA addresses:
   a. Fraud and abuse by the physician
   b. Privacy violation
   c. Portability of insurance coverage when an employee changes or loses his or her job
   d. All of the above
   e. A and C
7. Patient information should never be released without:
   a. A court order or an insurance release
   b. A court order or a patient's signed consent
   c. An insurance release or a patient's signed consent
   d. The physician's signature
   e. An insurance release and the physician's signature
8. Which of the following are true?
   a. All persons who have access to patient records must have a password.
   b. HIPAA compliance mandates that computer systems must be kept in a secured and private place.
   c. HIPAA requires the privacy and security of confidential health information to be protected by healthcare organizations.
   d. B and C
   e. A, B, and C
9. The general penalty for HIPAA violations ranges from:
   a. $1000 to $2500
   b. $80 to $8000
   c. $100 to $25,000
   d. Six months' imprisonment
   e. A and D
10. PHI includes the patient's
   a. Name and address
   b. Driver's license number and name
   c. Social Security number and date of birth
   d. Name and insurance information
   e. All of the above

Section 4 Administrative Competencies and Skills

11 Administrative Functions

CONTENTS

Reception

Patient reception requires a multiskilled individual who is able to multitask and whose manner, physical appearance, and tone of voice project a professional, confident, and caring attitude.

The receptionist greets and assists incoming patients and performs many important duties that make the office run smoothly and efficiently. Some of these duties are quiet and behind the scenes; others require constant interaction with patients.

RECEPTION ROOM

One of the most forgotten duties of the medical assistant is taking care of the reception area. Many office staff still refer to this area as the *waiting room*; however, many others now call it the *reception area* to avoid the negative term *waiting*. This area must be kept clean and free from any hazards that may injure the patient. It is often the reception area where the patient develops his or her first impression of the office.

The receptionist needs to monitor the cleanliness of the room. If the room begins to get messy, the receptionist may need to take the time to straighten it out. Magazines, brochures, patient education documents, and children's toys should be arranged neatly.

DUTIES OF THE RECEPTIONIST

Box 11-1 lists the duties of the receptionist.

Personal Characteristics and Appearance of the Receptionist

The receptionist is the first person a patient will see on entering the office. Projecting a positive public image is important, since the receptionist's appearance reflects on the entire staff.

Receptionists need to be mindful of the following:

- Careful grooming
- Appropriate dress
- Good hygiene, including daily bathing
- Use of a deodorant without a strong scent
- Good oral care
- Clean, well-pressed clothing
- Professionalism of makeup, hairstyles, and jewelry worn by male and female receptionists
- Accessories that are conservative and minimal—generally limited to one finger ring, a watch with a second hand, a name tag, and a professional association pin
- Long hair worn tied back and off the shoulders
- Nails that are well trimmed, with only clear polish
- Name pins/tags that are visible at all times

OPENING THE OFFICE

The individual responsible for opening the office should arrive 15–30 minutes prior to the start of office hours and should do the following:

- Check the security alarm and disengage it.
- Turn on all lights and check the general status of the reception room.
- Check to make sure that all paper charts are pulled and prepared for that day's patients.
- Have charge slips printed in advance for the day, with any balances due highlighted.
- Make sure that all office machines are turned on and ready for use.
- Add paper to the copier, fax machine, and any printers in the office.

Box 11-1 Duties of a Medical Receptionist

- Opening the office
- Pulling charts for the next day's appointments
- Collating patient records
- Checking in patients
- Greeting patients as they arrive
- Updating patient demographics
- Helping new patients fill out paperwork
- Collecting insurance co-payments and patient balances due
- Keeping the reception area clean and safe
- Managing reception area disturbances
- Handling reception area emergencies
- Handling incoming calls
- Scheduling appointments
- Escorting patients to exam rooms
- Respecting patients' time
- Documenting patient no-shows
- Closing the office

Telephone Techniques

The manner in which the receptionist answers the telephone frequently determines how the conversation will flow. It also provides the first impression that callers, including potential new patients, receive of the office. Following are some important techniques that will assist the receptionist in answering the medical office's telephone in the most professional manner.

TELEPHONE TIPS

Smiling	Always answer the telephone with a smile. Callers will be able to "hear" the warmth or indifference in your voice.
Greeting	It is important to answer the telephone quickly, usually by the third ring, and with a friendly, professional greeting.
Using Clear Speech	It is important to speak clearly on the telephone. Four words are used in reference to the speaking voice: • *Clarity:* quality or state of being understandable • *Enunciation:* clear articulation and pronunciation of words • *Inflection:* pitch and tone of voice and the way the person utters words and phrases • *Pitch:* the sound of the voice as it ranges from high to low
Using the Correct Volume	Be sure to speak loud enough for the patient to hear you, yet not so loud that patients in the reception area can hear.
Speaking at a Normal Rate	Speak at a normal rate, not too slow or too fast.
Identifying the Caller	Take steps to protect patient information. Ask the caller for identifying information such as his or her first and last names, Social Security number, and/or date of birth.

TELEPHONE TRIAGE

Triage is a process used to determine the order in which patients should be treated. The severity of the patient's illness or injury determines the order of treatment. Telephone triage is the process of determining the order in which to take patients' calls; this is an issue for the telephone screening process.

Emergency Calls

Every office should have a written protocol for handling emergency calls. It can be difficult to determine a true emergency by talking to someone on the telephone. It is critical to get the caller's name and telephone number immediately in case the caller is disconnected. The receptionist will then ask the patient specific questions (Box 11-2).

Box 11-2 Questions to Ask When Handling a Telephone Emergency

- What is your name?
- What is your telephone number?
- Where are you?
- What is your relationship to the caller? (if a parent, spouse, friend, or passerby is calling)
- What is the emergency?
- When did the emergency occur?
- How severe is the emergency?
- What are the patient's symptoms? (problem breathing, bleeding, extreme pain, other symptoms)
- What has been done for the patient?
- Has anyone called an ambulance?
- Who is the patient's primary physician?

Note: Some specialists, such as obstetricians and cardiologists, may have additional questions they wish to have the receptionist ask the caller.

Following are some of the types of emergency calls that come into the medical office:

- Allergic reactions (anaphylactic shock)
- Asthma
- Broken bone
- Drug overdose
- Eye injury or foreign body in the eye
- Gunshot or stab wound
- Heart attack
- Inability to breathe (or difficulty breathing)
- Loss of consciousness
- Premature labor
- Profuse bleeding
- Severe pain, including chest pain
- Severe vomiting and/or diarrhea
- Suicide attempt or suicide threats
- High temperature

PLACING CALLERS ON HOLD

One of the most sensitive issues relating to telephone courtesy is the use of the hold function. The *hold function* refers to the ability to keep more than one caller on the line at a time. Holding the call is permissible when you are speaking with a caller on one line and another call comes in (Procedure 11-1).

procedure 11-1

ANSWERING THE TELEPHONE AND PLACING CALLS ON HOLD

Objective: Ensure that the telephone is answered in a professional manner and, if necessary, that patients are placed on hold appropriately

EQUIPMENT AND SUPPLIES

- telephone
- message pad
- pen, notepad

METHOD

1. Answer the telephone by at least the third ring, with the mouthpiece 1 to 2 inches from your mouth.
2. Smile and speak clearly, using inflection, a pleasant tone, and a moderate rate of speech.
3. Answer using the greeting your office prefers (e.g., "Thank you for calling Dr. Smith's office. This is Carlos. How may I help you?").
4. At this point, callers will typically identify themselves. If not, ask them to do so and then verify the information against the patient's medical record.
5. Listen to the caller closely to verify the reason for the call, which may include, but is not limited to, the following:
   - A patient calling to schedule an appointment
   - A patient calling to request a prescription refill
   - Another physician's office calling about a mutual patient
   - An insurance company calling about a patient's claim
6. Once you have determined the reason for the call, act accordingly while providing excellent customer service. The most common actions you will take during a telephone call are scheduling an appointment, taking a message, transferring the caller to a co-worker, or requesting a prescription refill.
7. In busy offices, you may need to answer more than one incoming telephone line. When this occurs, you will combine the procedure just described with the following steps.
8. While speaking with one caller, another incoming line may ring. When this occurs, you must notify the current caller that another line is ringing and ask if the current caller can hold. Wait for the caller's response, then place the first call on hold.
9. Answer the second call following the procedures described, ask the second caller if he or she can hold, wait for a response, and then place the second call on hold. (If the second call is an emergency, you would not ask the person to hold and would assist the caller immediately.)
10. Return to the first call, thank the caller for holding, and continue assisting the person. When you return to that caller, do not ask "Who are you waiting for?" because this gives the impression that you have forgotten about that person.
11. Once the first call is completed, return to the second call, thank the person for holding, and continue assisting that caller.
12. If the caller asks to speak with another employee who is not readily available and it is necessary to place the call on hold, be sure to check back with the caller about every 30 seconds. This lets the caller know that you are actively working on his or her behalf, and it provides an opportunity for the caller to leave a message instead of continuing to hold.

TELEPHONE MESSAGES

Receptionists often take messages from patients, other physicians, healthcare facilities, and businesses. When taking a telephone message, it is important to obtain the following information:

- First and last names of the caller (with spelling verified)
- Telephone number, including the area code, at which he or she can be reached for a callback
- The reason for the call
- The name of the person the caller is trying to reach. If the caller is a patient requesting a medication refill, it is important to also document the name of the patient's pharmacy as well as the pharmacy's telephone number and fax number.

All telephone messages regarding a patient should be placed in the patient's chart as documentation of an interaction that occurred between the office and the patient.

TELEPHONE FEATURES

Voice Messaging System	Allows messages (voice mail) to be left or recorded when the intended recipient is unavailable to answer the telephone.
Call Forwarding	Allows a telephone user to forward calls to another telephone. This feature is often used if the office uses an answering service for after-hours calls.
Caller ID	Allows telephone owners to know who is calling each time the telephone rings.
Privacy Manager	Allows patients to block access to their home telephones. You will be asked to state the location from which you are calling. Once you have given this information, unless you are cleared, you will be directed to a voice mail system, where you will leave a message.
Speakerphone	Allows the receptionist to hear and speak without having to pick up the handset of the telephone.
Headsets	Allows the receptionist to have a hands-free receiver, which helps to prevent neck and shoulder injury and allows both hands to be used while documenting calls.

Incoming and Outgoing Mail

PROCESSING INCOMING MAIL

To facilitate time management within the medical office, all mail should be handled only once. Following are suggestions to help the handling of incoming mail:

- Sort the mail before opening it into first class, personal/confidential, second, third, and fourth class.
- Discard or recycle all unwanted third-class mail.
- Place a current date and time of arrival on each piece of mail.
- Do not open mail marked "personal" or "confidential." Place it in the physician's box unopened unless otherwise instructed.
- Attach all enclosures in each envelope with a paper clip.
- Annotate the mail as soon as possible after it is opened.
- Route the mail immediately after opening it.

PREPARING OUTGOING MAIL

Letter and Envelope Sizes

Letterhead stationery, which contains the name and address of the sender, comes in three commonly used sizes:

- Standard
- Monarch or executive
- Baronial

Common letter sizes, their matching envelope sizes, and the typical use for each size follow.

COMMON LETTER AND ENVELOPE SIZES

Stationery	Stationery Dimensions	Corresponding Envelope	Envelope Dimensions	Commonly Used For
Standard	8½″ × 11″	No. 10	9½″ × 4 1/8″	Most office correspondence
Monarch or Executive	7¼″ × 10½″	No. 7	7½″ × 3 7/8″	May be used by physicians for social correspondence
Baronial	5½″ × 8½″	No. 6¾	6½″ × 3 5/8″	Brief letters and memoranda

Folding Letters

Following are the recommended methods for folding and inserting letters into envelopes so that the contents can remain confidential and be easily removed:

Number 10 Envelope (standard business envelope)

- Bring up the bottom third of the letter and fold it with a crease.
- Fold the top of the letter down to 3/8 inch from the first creased edge.
- Make a second crease at the fold and place this edge into the envelope first.

Number 6 3/4 Envelope

- Bring the bottom edge up to 3/8 inch from the top edge.
- Make a crease at the fold.
- Fold the right edge one-third of the width of the paper and press a crease at this fold.
- Fold the left edge to 3/8 inch from the previous crease and insert this edge into the envelope first.

Envelope Formats

The U.S. Postal Service (USPS) has recommended guidelines when typing envelopes. They are meant to improve the handling and delivery of mail. Optical character recognition (OCR) equipment used by the USPS scans, reads, and sorts the envelopes. For optimal efficiency of OCR scanning, the address must be typed on the envelope, using single spacing and all capital letters with no punctuation.

The last line of the address must include the city, state two-letter code (Figure 11-1), and ZIP code. It cannot exceed 27 characters in length.

TWO-LETTER ABBREVIATIONS

UNITED STATES and TERRITORIES

Alabama	AL	Montana	MT
Alaska	AK	Nebraska	NE
Arizona	AZ	Nevada	NV
Arkansas	AR	New Hampshire	NH
California	CA	New Jersey	NJ
Canal Zone	CZ	New Mexico	NM
Colorado	CO	New York	NY
Connecticut	CT	North Carolina	NC
Delaware	DE	North Dakota	ND
District of Columbia	DC	Ohio	OH
Florida	FL	Oklahoma	OK
Georgia	GA	Oregon	OR
Guam	GU	Pennsylvania	PA
Hawaii	HI	Puerto Rico	PR
Idaho	ID	Rhode Island	RI
Illinois	IL	South Carolina	SC
Indiana	IN	South Dakota	SD
Iowa	IA	Tennessee	TN
Kansas	KS	Texas	TX
Kentucky	KY	Utah	UT
Louisiana	LA	Vermont	VT
Maine	ME	Virgin Islands	VI
Maryland	MD	Virginia	VA
Massachusetts	MA	Washington	WA
Michigan	MI	West Virginia	WV
Minnesota	MN	Wisconsin	WI
Mississippi	MS	Wyoming	WY
Missouri	MO		

FIGURE 11-1 Two-letter abbreviations for U.S. states.

ZIP Codes

The five-digit ZIP code has increased the post office's efficiency in handling mail. ZIP codes begin on the East Coast with the number 0, eventually increasing to the number 9 on the West Coast and Hawaii. The first three numbers of the ZIP code identify the city, and all five digits combine to identify the individual post office and zone within the city. Four more digits have been added to the ZIP code by the USPS.

CLASSIFICATIONS OF MAIL

Type	Description
First Class	Letters, postcards, business reply cards; letters weighing less than 11 ounces; sealed and unsealed, handwritten or typed material
Priority	First-class mail weighing more than 11 ounces; maximum weight of 70 pounds; postage calculated based on weight and destination
Second Class	Newspapers and periodicals that have received second-class mail authorization; not allowed for newspapers and periodicals mailed by the general public
Third Class	Catalogs, booklets, photographs, flyers, and other printed materials; must be marked "Third Class"; must be sealed; no size limitation; includes bulk mail
Fourth Class	Books, computer media, and merchandise not included in first and second class; must weigh between 16 ounces and 70 pounds; size limitations apply
Express Mail/ Next-Day Service	Available seven days a week; up to 70 pounds in weight and 108 inches around; expected delivery by noon; shipping containers supplied; pickup service in some areas

CLASSIFICATIONS OF MAIL

The classifications of mail vary according to weight, type, and destination. Mail is weighed in ounces and pounds. The most common types of mail are first class, priority, second class, third class, fourth class, and express mail.

SPECIAL POSTAL SERVICES

Certified Mail	Mail that is not valuable but would be difficult to replace if lost should be sent as certified mail. Examples of the types of documents that should be sent certified mail are as follows: • Contracts • Mortgages • Birth certificates • Deeds • Checks Sent at the first-class rate, with a special fee added for certified mail Assists in tracking and collecting this mail A receipt verifying delivery can be requested for a fee. Records of certified mail maintained at the post office for two years
Registered Mail	Safest way to send first-class or priority mail Fee is paid, and a signed record is kept for each piece of registered mail Tracked as it moves throughout the mail system Insured for the value declared at the time of registration For an additional fee, the sender can request a return receipt indicating the time, place of delivery, and the receiver's signature.
Certificate of Mailing	A document that demonstrates proof that mail was posted Useful for mailing items such as tax returns, which need to be received by a certain date
Special Delivery	Can be requested from the postal service when fast delivery of an item is required Items will be delivered outside of regular delivery service hours (e.g., on Sundays and holidays). There is a fee for this service.
Special Handling	Can be requested for third- and fourth-class items Fee based on weight
Insurance	Can be purchased for third-class, fourth-class, and priority mail If mail is lost or damaged, sender will be reimbursed for the content. Sender receives a receipt from the post office at the time the insurance is purchased.
Postal Money Orders	Purchased at the post office Is replaceable if lost or stolen Can be mailed instead of cash Available in several denominations
Forwarding Mail	First-class mail can be forwarded to another address without paying an additional fee. The post office will forward mail for up to six months.
Returned Mail	If mail is returned and marked "undeliverable," it cannot be remailed until new postage is added.

SIZE REQUIREMENTS FOR MAIL

The USPS has standardized envelope sizes in order to machine sort mail.

Minimum Mail Size	Must be at least 0.0007 inch thick Mail ¼ inch or less in thickness must be 3½ inches in height and at least 5 inches long.
Maximum Mail Size	Maximum size for mail is no more than 108 inches in length and girth combined. Maximum weight for anything mailed is 70 pounds. Postage is generally based on a package's weight; however, items that are bulky and lightweight are charged a 15-pound balloon rate surcharge.

ELECTRONIC MAIL

Letters, reports, and pictures may all be transmitted electronically and are referred to as *electronic mail* (*e-mail*). E-mail may be sent over telephone lines, cables, computers, and satellites and allows the recipient to edit, correct, and transmit documents very quickly to another location. E-mail cannot be used if the original signature on the document needs to be sent.

E-mail correspondence related to the patient is considered part of the patient's record, and confidentiality guidelines apply.

Office Equipment

In order for a medical office to maintain effective flow of documents, certain office machines and equipment are most beneficial.

IMPORTANT OFFICE EQUIPMENT

Copier	Copies, reduces, enlarges, and collates documents in the medical office Available in several sizes
Color Laser Printer	Used in conjunction with a computer for letter-quality printing Creates images with a laser beam and then transfers the color image to paper with pressure and heat
Scanner	"Reads" text and graphic files and transforms them into a usable document
Fax Machine	Sends and receives printed documents via telephone lines
Postage Meter	Used by offices with large mailings to stamp envelopes and packages
Telephone System	Many types of business telephone systems available Most medical offices use a multiline telephone. • Some offices separate the lines; a particular line's button must be pressed to answer it. • Other offices use a system that feeds calls to the appropriate individual or area via a queue or waiting line.
Transcription Machine	Tape recorder–type devices that allow a transcriptionist to listen to a physician's dictation and transfer the information to a printed form

Medical Records

The medical record contains all the written documentation related to the patient's healthcare. Each patient's medical record contains essentially the same categories of material, but the information is unique to each patient.

It is important to keep in mind that the medical record is a legal document, a permanent record, and a tool used to communicate between staff members not only in your office, but also between offices, regarding the services delivered to the patient.

SIX Cs OF CHARTING

When making entries into the patient's chart, the following should be kept in mind:

- Client's words
- Clarity
- Completeness
- Conciseness
- Chronological order
- Confidentiality

MEDICAL RECORD COMPONENTS

Patient Registration	Includes the following: • Patient's full name • Address • Contact information, including home phone, work phone, and cell phone • E-mail address if applicable • Date of the visit • Patient's age • Date of birth (DOB) • Social Security number • Driver's license number (if applicable) • Medical insurance information • Person responsible for payment

(*Continued*)

Family and Medical History	Includes the following: • Patient's current medical problem, with details of the present illness • Chief complaint (CC) • Family medical history • Patient's past medical history and surgeries • Allergies • Current prescriptions, medications, and over-the-counter medications
Physical Examination Results	Results of the examination include the following: • Patient's general appearance • Nutrition • Blood pressure (B/P) • Head—eyes, ears, nose, and throat examination (EENT); mouth, and scalp • Results of neck and thyroid examinations • Results of thorax and breast exams • Lymphadenopathy • Examinations of the heart and lungs, abdomen, pelvic, genital and rectal areas, and skin • Overall impression • Treatment plan
Results of All Tests	All results of tests performed on patients should be tracked and filed in patients' records.
Records from Referred Physicians or Hospital Visits	Records from past office visits to other physicians should be placed in the patient record.
Informed Consent Forms	Documents stating that a patient understands and consents to a treatment offered and knows the potential outcome and side effects of that treatment, including the expected outcome if the treatment is not performed
Diagnosis and Treatment Plan	Includes the physician's diagnosis, treatment plan, and options presented to the patient, as well as any instructions given to the patient
Patient Correspondence and Follow-up Care	Any patient correspondence sent to the medical office, including procedures, follow-up visits, medical office care, and any notations involving the patient, should be included in the patient's medical record.
Consultation Report	A physician may ask another physician to provide a second opinion on a patient's case. The consultation report will include: • Patient's name and medical record number • Date of consultation • Medical transcriptionist's name • Referring physician • Reason for the consultation • Physical and laboratory evaluations • Consulting physician's impression and recommendations
Operative Note	Describes a surgical procedure
Pathology Report	Generated by the pathologist after examining tissue and organs removed during a surgical procedure (such as a biopsy) or at an autopsy
Radiology Report	Completed by the radiologist Documents results of diagnostic procedures, such as X-rays, CT scans, MRI scans, nuclear medicine procedures (bone and thyroid scans), and other fluoroscopic examinations
Discharge Summary	Completed on every hospitalized patient and summarizes the hospitalization

TYPES OF MEDICAL RECORDS

Chronological Record	Follows the patient over a period of time, with each visit consisting of a new entry by date, rather than by symptoms or diagnosis Most recent visit/diagnosis is found on top of the records of previous visits. One of the most common types of medical records
Problem-Oriented Medical Record (POMR)	The patient problem list found at the front of the chart As new problems and diagnoses are identified, they are noted on the problem list. Helps the healthcare provider identify trends in the patient's medical history or emerging diagnoses Assists healthcare providers and physicians not familiar with a particular patient to obtain a "snapshot" regarding previous visits and problems at a glance The four parts of the POMR: • *Database*: the physical examination, patient history, and results of baseline laboratory or diagnostic procedures • *Problem list*: list of patient problems kept in the front of the chart, much like a table of contents; each problem is titled and numbered • *Plan*: a written plan for each numbered problem identified on the problem list • *Progress notes*: consists of several sections, with the first initial spelling out the word SOAP; also known as *SOAP notes*
Source-Oriented Medical Record	Patient information found in reverse chronological order and organized in different sections The sections commonly used include the history and physical, examinations, insurance, progress notes, medications, laboratory test results, and consultations. Most recent information is seen first in each section of the medical record. Commonly used in medical clinics

SOAP CHARTING FOR 1/24/XX

S	Subjective symptoms provided by the patient and/or family; actual patient's words are recorded	"I'm thirsty and eating all the time, but I'm not gaining any weight. I feel tired all the time."
O	Objective findings from vital signs, physical examination, and laboratory and diagnostic tests	B/P: 158/96; T: 98°F; P: 76; R: 16 Skin turgor (resiliency) poor. Wt. 10# less than 6 weeks ago Urine 4+ sugar, FBS positive
A	Assessment, including the physician's diagnosis	Uncontrolled diabetes
P	Plan, including recommended treatments, further tests, medications, consultation, surgery, and physical therapy	Dx: Lab tests for diabetes Tx: Begin diabetic diet and insulin Instruct on diet and exercise follow-up

COMPONENTS OF THE MEDICAL RECORD

A standard medical record is one of the most important items in an office setting. It is imperative to be familiar with all of its components.

FILING/STORING OF MEDICAL RECORDS

Choosing the type of file system for medical forms and reports, including the file folder coding system used in the office, is an important decision since all files must be maintained within that system.

CATEGORIES OF FILES

Active Records	Patients who have been seen within the past three years and are currently being treated
Inactive Records	Patients who have not been seen within the past three years or another time period determined by office policy
Closed Records	Patients who have actively terminated their contact with the physician

FILE STORAGE

Vertical	Two to four stacked pullout drawers holding up to 100 files per drawer Heavy and space-consuming
Lateral	Set up with shelves allowing for easy access to files Often uses a color-coded method for visual recognition of files
Movable	Electrically powered or manually controlled file units that move on tracks in the floor Save space because the file units can be moved close together when they are not needed

Rules for Filing

Three commonly used systems for filing are alphabetic, numeric, and subject filing. Because the numeric system provides the most privacy, it is the one most commonly used in the office.

FILING SYSTEMS

Alphabetic System (See page 160.)	Divides names and titles into units The unit is the portion of the name that is used for filing or indexing purposes. • Unit 1 Jergens (last name) • Unit 2 Jacob (first name) • Unit 3 James (middle name)
Numeric System	A number is assigned to each patient's medical record. The number assigned is usually a six-digit number divided into three sections of two digits each (e.g., 05-72-21). Also known as the *patient identification system* Used in hospitals and many larger clinics There are several types of numerical filing: • *Straight numerical filing*: each record filed sequentially based on its assigned number • *Terminal digit filing*: based on the last six digits of the ID number • *Middle digit filing*: uses the same six-digit numbering system as the terminal digit system; however, it places the middle digits as the primary numbers • *Unit numbering*: assigns a number to a patient the first time he or she is seen; all subsequent visits use the same number • *Serial numbering:* patient receives a different medical record number for each hospital visit
Subject Matter	Used for general files, such as invoices, correspondence, resumes, and personnel records

CORRECTIONS TO MEDICAL RECORD

There are three types of corrections to medical records:

- **Corrections to handwritten entries:** Do not erase or totally obliterate the original error with commercial products like correcting fluid. Simply draw a single line through the error so that the original entry can still be seen, initial above the line, date it, and write "error." Once this is done, write in the correction.
- **Corrections to typewritten entries:** If an error is made while keyboarding, it should be corrected the same way any other errors are corrected. However, if the error is noted later, draw a line through it, enter your initials and the date, and write in the correction.
- **Corrections in electronic entries:** If you are using an electronic medical record (EMR), errors may be corrected by deleting them as you would with any other type of computer program prior to saving the entry. However, if an error is discovered after the entry is saved, an additional entry called an *addendum* will be required. An addendum is an addition to the original document. In this case, the addendum should be titled "correction." When an EMR is used, the entry will be automatically dated and signed electronically when it is saved.

RULES FOR ALPHABETIC FILING

Rules	Example
Names are filed: last name, first name, middle name (or middle initial). Each letter in the name is a separate unit.	Krause, Marvin K. is placed before Krause, Marvin L.
Initials come before a full name.	Brown, H. is placed before Brown, Henry.
Hyphenated names are treated as one unit. This applies to the names of individuals and businesses.	Amy Freeman-Smith is indexed under F for Freeman. It is considered Freemansmith for indexing purposes.
Titles (and initials) are disregarded for filing but placed in parentheses after the name.	Dr. Beth Ann Williams is indexed as Williams, Beth Ann (Dr).
Married women are indexed using their legal name. The husband's name can be used for cross-referencing.	Mrs. Mary Jane Smith is indexed as Smith, Mary Jane (Mrs. John).
Seniority units, such as Jr. and Sr., are filed in chronological (age) order from first to last.	Jacob James Jurgens, Sr. comes before Jacob James Jurgens, Jr.
Numeric seniority terms are filed before alphabetic terms.	Jurgens, Jacob James III is indexed before Jurgens, Jacob James, Jr.
Mac and Mc can be filed either alphabetically as they occur or grouped together, depending on the preference of the office.	
Foreign language names are indexed as one unit.	Mary St. Claire is indexed as Stclaire, Mary. Carol van Damm is indexed as Vandamm, Carol.
If company names are identical, the address—by state, then city, then street—may be used in the index. The ZIP code is not used to index files.	ABC Drugs, 123 Michigan Blvd., Chicago, IL is indexed before ABC Drugs, 1450 N. Ash, Kalispell, MT.
If individuals' names are identical, use the birth date or mother's maiden name. Avoid using an address since that can change.	Mark Richard Jones is indexed as Jones, Mark Richard (5/12/65) and Jones, Mark Richard (2/12/89).
Disregard apostrophes.	Megan O'Connor is indexed as OConnor, Megan.
Business organizations are indexed as they are written.	Lincoln Memorial Hospital is correct.
Disregard short words, such as *a, and, the*, and *of*.	The Whitefish Drug Store is indexed as Whitefish Drug Store (The).
Numeric characters are indexed before alpha characters.	23rd Avenue Clinic is indexed before Nineteenth Street Medical Center. A separate file is set up for all numeric files.
Names with religious titles, such as Sister Mary Murphy, would be filed with the last name first and then with the religious title.	Murphy, Sister Mary.
Compound words are filed as they are written.	South West Physician Service is filed before Southwest Physician Service.

RETENTION OF MEDICAL RECORDS

The following are general guidelines for how long medical records should be kept:

- The American Medical Association recommends keeping medical records for 10 years.
- Patients' immunization records should be kept indefinitely in case patients need them in the future.
- Each state varies on the legal time limits (statute of limitations) for keeping records and documents. In many cases, the statute of limitations is two years, and it begins to run at the point of discovery of damage and the connection between that damage and the treatment. In some circumstances, this could be many years later. Special rules apply when treating a child or an incompetent patient, and the time period is longer.
- Most states require that all patient records be retained for 2 to 7 years after the last treatment or 7 years after the patient reaches the age of majority (age 18 or 21 in most states), whichever comes later.

Establishing and Maintaining the Appointment Schedule

Office hours are usually determined by the physician or group of physicians in a practice. The scheduling system used in each office is dependent on a variety of factors, including the physician's preference, type and size of the practice, equipment availability, staff availability, amount of flexibility required by the physician(s), insurance coverage issues, and patient needs.

The appointment book is considered a legal document and should be treated as such. Old appointment books should be kept for at least three years.

The two basic types of appointment scheduling systems are open office hours and scheduled appointments. When patients arrive without an appointment and are generally seen in the order of arrival (unless a patient with an emergent condition arrives), the system is known as *open* office hours scheduling. Scheduled appointments are just that.

TYPES OF SCHEDULING SYSTEMS

Specified Time Scheduling	Each patient is given a specific time slot. The time allocated to each patient will depend on the reason for the office visit or the type of examination or testing that is to be done.
Wave Scheduling	Each hour is divided into equal segments of time, depending on how many patients can be seen within an hour. All patients scheduled for that hour are told to come in at the beginning of the hour. These patients are then seen in the order in which they arrive. The purpose of wave scheduling is to begin and end each hour on time. It provides built-in flexibility to accommodate unforeseen situations.
Modified Wave Scheduling	This method uses the hour as the base of each block of time. There are many variations of this type of scheduling. Three patients may be scheduled at intervals during the first half hour, with none scheduled for the second half hour. Alternatively, three patients arrive on the hour and are seen within the first half of the hour in the order of their arrival. During the second half of the hour one patient would be scheduled, with another patient scheduled on the three-quarter hour.
Scheduling by Grouping Procedures	Similar procedures and examinations are scheduled during a particular block of time.
Double Booking Patients	Two patients are scheduled to be seen during the same time slot without allowing for any additional time in the schedule.
Open Office Hours System	Patients may arrive at any time during the posted office hours. Patients are seen in the order of their arrival.

See page 162 for a comparison of scheduling methods.

SCHEDULING PROCESS

The appointment schedule should show the periods of time blocked out on the daily schedule when appointments are unavailable due to physicians' meetings, surgery time, vacations, and hospital rounds. The periods of time the physician is unavailable is known as the *matrix.* The appointment matrix should be completed several weeks, if not months, in advance.

COMPARISON OF SCHEDULING METHODS

Specified Time	Wave	Modified Wave
1:00 Ed Trombley—ear irrigation	1:00 Ed Trombley Jerry Richard Janet Orlando	1:00 Ed Trombley
1:20 Jerry Richard—well-baby checkup with vaccines		1:10 Jerry Richard
1:40 Janet Orlando—Pap smear		1:20 Janet Orlando
2:00 Lena Mezza—well-baby checkup with vaccines	2:00 Lena Mezza David Ingiolo Christina Soave	1:30
2:20 David Ingiolo—B/P check		1:40
2:40 Christina Soave—skin rash (poss. contagious)		2:00 Lena Mezza
3:00	3:00	2:10 David Ingiolo
3:20		2:20 Christina Soave
3:40		2:30
4:00	4:00	2:40

11 APPLICATION

Directions: Select the best answer for each of the following questions. Check your answers in the Answer Key at the end of the book.

1. Speech is an important communication technique; one of the elements of speech is enunciation. Enunciation is defined as:
   a. The sound of your voice as it ranges from high to low
   b. The pitch and tone of your voice
   c. The quality of being understandable
   d. Clear articulation and pronunciation of words
   e. B and C
2. Which of the following is not considered a classification of mail?
   a. Priority
   b. Express mail
   c. UPS next day
   d. Second class
   e. Fourth class
3. It is important to obtain the following information when taking a telephone message:
   a. The reason for the call
   b. The name of the person the caller is trying to reach
   c. The callback number, including the area code
   d. All of the above
   e. A and B
4. The dimensions of standard-size stationery are:
   a. 3" × 5"
   b. 5" × 7"
   c. 7¼" × 10½"
   d. 5½" × 8½"
   e. 8½" × 11"

5. The corresponding envelope for standard size-stationery is:
   a. No. 10
   b. No. 9
   c. No. 7 1/8
   d. No. 6¾
   e. No. 8½

6. When addressing envelopes, the abbreviation for the state name contains how many letters?
   a. Three
   b. Two
   c. Four
   d. Both A and B are acceptable.
   e. State names are not abbreviated when addressing envelopes.

7. The safest way to send first-class or priority mail is:
   a. Registered mail
   b. Certified mail
   c. Bulk mail
   d. Second-class mail
   e. Both B and D

8. Items that should be sent certified mail include:
   a. Contracts and deeds
   b. Mortgages and contracts
   c. Deeds and birth certificates
   d. All of the above
   e. None of the above

9. A certificate of mailing is:
   a. A document proving that mail was posted
   b. Another term for certified mail
   c. A fee for special delivery
   d. A receipt from the post office for registered mail
   e. A certificate that must be earned in order to deliver mail

10. The maximum size for mail in length and girth combined is no more than:
   a. 64 inches
   b. 32 inches
   c. 108 inches
   d. 164 inches
   e. 132 inches

11. ____________ contains all the written documentation related to a patient's healthcare.
   a. Consultation report
   b. Pathology report
   c. Consent forms
   d. Medical record
   e. Medical history

12. Which of the following is not one of the four parts of the problem-oriented medical record?
   a. Problem list
   b. Plan
   c. Progress notes
   d. Insurance plan
   e. Database

13. The American Medical Association recommends that medical records be kept for how many years?
   a. Six
   b. 10
   c. Seven
   d. Five
   e. Three

14. How long should a patient's immunization record be kept?
   a. Two years
   b. Four years
   c. Seven years
   d. 10 years
   e. Indefinitely

15. Types of scheduling systems include:
   a. Block scheduling
   b. Wave scheduling
   c. Open office hours
   d. B and C
   e. None of the above

16. The postal abbreviation for the state of Michigan is:
   a. MN
   b. MA
   c. MC
   d. MI
   e. MIC

17. The following is/are true about alphabetic filing rules:
   a. Initials come before a full name.
   b. Alpha characters are indexed before numeric characters.
   c. Names are filed: Last name, first name, middle name.
   d. Names are filed: First name, middle initial, last name.
   e. A and C

18. When using SOAP to chart, the "S," or subjective information, is:
   a. Gathered from the patient
   b. The same as the chief complaint
   c. Data gathered during the visit
   d. Both A and B
   e. Both B and C

19. A record that is considered active indicates:
    a. Patients who have been seen within the past three years
    b. Patients who have actively terminated their contact with the physician
    c. Patients who are currently being treated
    d. Both A and B
    e. Both A and C

20. The numerical filing system that is based on the last six digits of the ID number is known as:
    a. Straight numerical filing
    b. Terminal digit filing
    c. Unit numbering
    d. Serial numbering
    e. None of the above

21. The appointment book is considered a legal document and should be kept for a minimum of how many years?
    a. Three
    b. Five
    c. Seven
    d. 10
    e. None of the above

22. The appointment matrix should reflect which of the following?
    a. Times the physician is available to see patients
    b. Physician surgery time
    c. Physician meetings
    d. Physician vacation
    e. All of the above

23. Which of the following is not required when answering the telephone?
    a. Smiling
    b. Speech
    c. Speed
    d. All are required
    e. None of the above

24. Which of the following statements regarding emergency telephone calls is not true?
    a. It is easy to determine a true emergency when talking with someone on the telephone.
    b. Ask the patient specific questions.
    c. Premature labor is an example of an emergency telephone call.
    d. It is okay to ask who the patient's primary physician is during an emergency telephone call.
    e. Get as much information from the patient as possible while talking on the telephone.

25. Which of the telephone features allows patients to block access to their home telephone?
    a. Caller ID
    b. Call waiting
    c. Privacy manager
    d. Call forwarding
    e. Voice messaging system

12 Electronic Technology

CONTENTS

Computers

A computer is a programmable machine, or system of hardware, that responds to a specific set of instructions and performs a list of instructions in programmed language called *software*. Most physicians' offices use computers to maintain patient records. The same legal standards of confidentiality and compliance with HIPAA apply to all patient records, whether on paper or on the computer. See Chapter 10 for more information on HIPAA.

Generally, computers require the following components to function (Figure 12-1):

- *Memory* makes it possible for a computer to temporarily store data and programs.
- A *mass storage device* enables computers to permanently retain large amounts of data, including times when the computer is turned off. Common mass storage devices include disk drives and zip drives.
- *Input devices*, such as the keyboard and scanners, feed data and instructions into a computer.
- *Output devices*, such as a display screen, a printer, and other devices, allow the user to see what the computer has accomplished.
- *The central processing unit* (CPU) is the brain of the computer and executes a specific set of instructions.

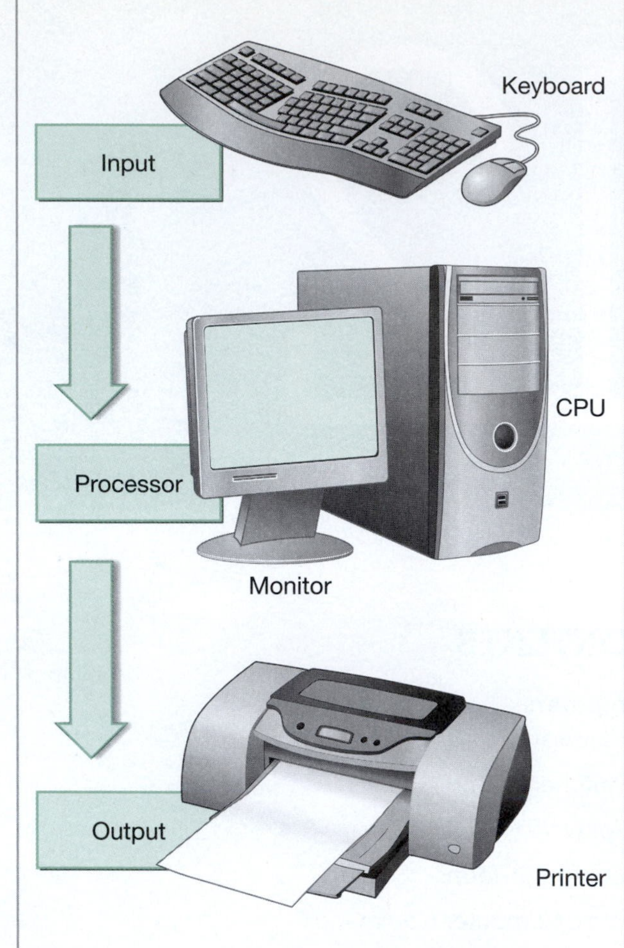

FIGURE 12-1 Components of a computer system.

HARDWARE

Central Processing Unit (CPU)	Directs the computer's activities and sends electronic signals to the right place at the right time
Monitor	Display screen that allows the user to observe that the computer is doing what it has been directed to do Monitors are categorized as monochrome, gray scale, or color.
CD-ROM (Compact Disc Read-Only Memory)	Data storage system that allows data to be stored on a compact disc Capable of holding or storing large amounts of data
Universal Serial Bus Drive (USB)	Small, portable storage device that can hold up to 64 gigabytes (GB) or more of data Also known as a *jump drive, thumb drive*, or *flash drive*
Memory	Measured and stored in kilobytes (kb or k) Each kilobyte is 1000 bytes (or characters) of information. This memory is further divided into RAM and ROM. • RAM, or random-access memory, is the internal storage area in the computer that can be accessed randomly. It is available only when the computer is on. • *ROM*, or read-only memory, is an internal storage area in the computer where data have been recorded. Once data are recorded, they cannot be removed, only read.
Drives	Computers are based on hard-disk drive technology. The hard-disk drive is usually called the *C drive*.

HARDWARE (*Continued*)

Keyboard	Set of keys utilized to input data with function keys, alphanumeric keys, punctuation keys, arrow keys, and conjunction keys
Mouse	Device that gives the user control of the computer
Printers	Transfer information from the computer to paper • *Ink-jet printer:* forms dots when ink is blown onto the paper • *Laser printer:* ink burned onto the paper by a laser

PERIPHERALS Peripherals are the extras that can be attached to hardware to expand the computer's capability.

Scanner	Converts paper records to an electronic format that the computer can read
Digital Camera	Takes pictures without film and stores the images electronically in the camera until they are downloaded

SOFTWARE

Computer software, also known as a *computer program*, is a set of instructions that works with the operating system and allows the computer to perform its functions. The most common program used in the medical office is Microsoft Office. Other medical software programs can perform appointment scheduling, charting, bookkeeping, and insurance billing.

Electronic Medical Records

Electronic medical records (EMRs), sometimes called *electronic health records* (EHRs), are the portions of patients' medical records that are kept on a computer's hard drive or a medical office's computer network rather than on paper. The software within the EMR contains a section for adding information, such as telephone calls or conversations with patients and their families that occur in the office and are related to the patient's medical care.

The EMR is very helpful for gathering and sorting patient data that must be reported out for national measures of conditions such as diabetes and stroke. Of course, all patient identifiers are removed before those reports are forwarded to the organizations that require the data.

Spreadsheets

Spreadsheet software allows the user to create worksheets and perform calculations. Spreadsheets may be used for accounting and bookkeeping as well as for tracking accounts payable.

Graphics

Several graphics programs are available, and some have been developed specifically for use in healthcare. This software is especially helpful for developing patient and staff education material as well as for preparing presentations.

COMPUTER TERMS

Frequently used computer terms and their definitions follow.

FREQUENTLY USED COMPUTER TERMS

Term	Definition
Backup	A copy of work or software batch data stored for processing at periodic intervals
Batch	Data stored for processing at periodic intervals
Boot	To start up the computer
Catalog	List of all files stored on a storage device
Characters per Second	Speed measurement for printers
Cursor	Flashing bar, arrow, or symbol that indicates where the next character will be placed
Daisy-Wheel Printer	An impact printer that "strikes" characters onto a page, much like a typewriter; unable to produce graphic images but does produce letter-quality output

(continued)

(*Continued*)

Term	Definition
Database	Computer application that contains records or files
Data Debugging	Process of eliminating errors from input data
Disk Drive	A container that holds a read/write head, an access arm, and a magnetic disk for storage
DOS	Disk operating system
Downtime	Time a computer cannot be used because of maintenance or mechanical failure
Electronic Mail (E-Mail)	Use of appropriate hardware and software (modem, computer, telephone, etc.) to allow transmission of data electronically from computer to computer
File	A collection of related records
File Maintenance	Data entry operations including additions, deletions, and modifications
Format	Methods for setting margins, tabs, line spacing, and other layout features
GIGO	"Garbage in, garbage out," which means that if incorrect information is input, the result is incorrect output
Hard Copy	A printed copy of data in a file
Hardware	The physical equipment that is used by a computer to process data
Input	To enter data into the computer system; data entered into the system
Interface	Technology that allows two or more unconnected computers to exchange programs and data; also referred to as a *network*
Keyboard	An input device similar to a typewriter keyboard
Menu	A list of options available to the software user
Modem	Hardware device that converts digital signals to analog signals for transfer over communication lines or links
Output	To process data into final form; data produced by the computer system
Peripheral	Device required for the input, output, processing, and storage of data; includes the mouse, disk drives, keyboards, printers, and joysticks
Scrolling	Feature that allows the computer operator to control the location of the cursor within a document
Security Code	A group of characters that allows an authorized computer operator access to certain programs or features; a password
Write-Protect	Feature of storage devices that allows the data to be seen but not changed

BASIC COMPUTER COMMANDS

Depending on personal preference, you can execute certain functions on the computer either by using the keyboard commands below or by using the mouse and clicking with either a right click or left click, single or double.

KEYBOARD COMMANDS FOR WINDOWS

Copy	Ctrl + C	Undo	Ctrl + Z
Paste	Ctrl + V	Redo	Ctrl + Y
Cut	Ctrl + X	Bold	Ctrl + B
Save	Ctrl + S	Underline	Ctrl + U
Print	Ctrl + P	Restart the System	Ctrl + Alt + Delete

THE INTERNET

The Internet is a computer network made up of thousands of interfacing networks worldwide. Access is obtained through a commercial Internet service provider (ISP). The World Wide Web (WWW), or the Web, is a system of Internet servers.

Electronic Signatures

Traditional signatures found on paper documents can now be converted into a mathematical process (or a set of numbers) to create an electronic signature. This set of numbers is recorded temporarily in a computer's working memory or permanently on a storage medium such as a disk.

COMPUTERS AND ERGONOMICS

To safely incorporate computer use in your daily routine and to work effectively, you should be aware of some ergonomic tips, such as to appropriately position your computer equipment.

ERGONOMIC TIPS

Chair	• Hips should be as far back as they can go in the chair. • Feet should be flat on the floor. • Knees should be at the same level as hips or lower. • The back of the chair should be at a 100–110 degree reclined angle.
Keyboard	• An articulating keyboard tray allows adjustment of the angle and height of the keyboard. • Pull up close to your keyboard and position it directly in front of your body. • Adjust the height of the keyboard so that your shoulders are relaxed, the elbows are in a slightly open position, and the wrists and hands are straight.
Monitor	• The monitor should be centered directly in front of you above the keyboard. • The top of the monitor should be approximately 2 to 3 inches above your seated eye level. • Adjust the monitor and source documents so that your neck is in a neutral, relaxed position.
Body	• Shift your position as much as possible. • Take 1- to 2-minute stretch breaks every 20 to 30 minutes.

12 APPLICATION

Directions: Select the best answer for each of the following questions. Check your answers in the Answer Key at the end of the book.

1. ________ makes it possible for a computer to temporarily store data and programs.
   a. Mouse
   b. Monitor
   c. Memory
   d. A and C
   e. A and B
2. The following are considered common computer input devices:
   a. Printer, monitor, and keyboard
   b. Keyboard and monitor
   c. Printer and keyboard
   d. Scanner and keyboard
   e. Scanner and monitor
3. A small, portable device that can hold up to 64 GB or more of data is:
   a. The USB
   b. The CPU
   c. The flash drive
   d. A and C
   e. None of the above
4. The hard disk drive of the computer is usually called the:
   a. C drive
   b. Z drive
   c. USB drive
   d. RAM drive
   e. S drive
5. Certain commands for Microsoft Windows can be executed using two or more keys on the keyboard instead of the mouse. The keyboard command for "paste" is:
   a. Ctrl + P
   b. Ctrl + V
   c. Ctrl + P + S
   d. Ctrl + Alt + Delete
   e. There is no keyboard command for "paste."

6. In Internet terminology, WWW is the:
   a. World Web Wide
   b. World Wide Web
   c. A system of Internet servers
   d. Both A and C
   e. Both B and C

7. *Security code* in computer terminology is commonly known as:
   a. The database
   b. The interface
   c. The password
   d. The menu
   e. The cursor

8. The computer hardware container that holds a read/write head, an access arm, and a magnetic disk for storage is the:
   a. Modem
   b. Cursor
   c. Monitor
   d. Menu
   e. Disk drive

9. Which best describes the central processing unit (CPU)?
   a. Also known as the *thumb drive*
   b. Directs the computer's activities and sends electronic signals to the right place at the right time
   c. The display screen
   d. Is divided into RAM and ROM
   e. Gives the user control of the computer

10. Computer input devices:
   a. Feed data and instructions into the computer
   b. Allow the user to see what the computer has accomplished
   c. Store information
   d. All of the above
   e. None of the above

13 Best Practice Finances

CONTENTS

Payment Methods

Most patients make payments via cash, credit card, or check; most insurance companies make electronic funds transfers.

CASH

Cash can be accepted as a form of payment; however, most patients pay either by check or with a credit card. Receipts must be given for all cash payments. Having large amounts of cash in an office poses a security risk and creates the potential for embezzlement of funds.

DEBIT OR CREDIT CARD

Most offices accept credit and debit cards for the convenience for their patients even though most banks charge the practice a fee of 1 to 3% of the collected charges. One of the benefits of accepting debit and/or credit cards is that the funds are automatically transferred from the patient's bank account and posted to the practice account within 24 hours.

CHECKS

A check is a written order to a bank to pay or transfer money to an individual, a business, or an entity. A check, which is payable on demand, is considered a negotiable instrument. A negotiable instrument permits the transfer of money to another person. In order to be a negotiable instrument, the check must:

- Be written and signed by an authorized payer of the check
- State the sum of money to be paid
- Be payable on demand or at a fixed date in the future
- Be payable to the holder (payee) of the check

TYPES OF CHECKS

Cashier's Checks	• Written using the bank's own check or form • Issued by the bank • Guarantees that the money is available • Usually a charge for this service
Certified Checks	• Written on the payer's own check form • Guarantees that the money is available • Bank teller verifies the check by placing an official stamp directly on it • Bank withdraws the money from the payer's account when it certifies the check
Limited Checks	• Used for payroll checks and insurance payments • Issued on a special check form that contains a preprinted maximum dollar amount for which the check can be written • May also be a time limit during which the check is valid or must be cashed
Bank Drafts	• Checks that are drawn up by a bank against money that is in an account at another bank
Money Orders	• Purchased with cash for the cash value typed on the check • Can be purchased from banks, the USPS, and other authorized agents • There is a charge for this service. • Frequently used by individuals who do not have bank accounts
Traveler's Checks	• Checks preprinted in certain dollar amounts ($10, $20, $50, $100, $500 and $1000) and prepaid • Considered a safe means of carrying money when traveling • Contains a space for two signatures of the payer: one at the time of purchase and the other when the check is cashed

Voucher Checks	• Frequently used for payroll checks since additional information can be supplied to the payee
	• *Three detachable sections:*
	  • Upper portion contains the actual check
	  • Lower portion provides details about the transaction, such as payroll deductions
	  • Third portion is a carbon copy that remains with the payer as a record of the transaction

Third-Party Checks	• A check written by a party unknown to the recipient
Stale Check	• A check that has not been presented for payment within the time frame suggested on the check—typically six months from the time the check was written

PARTS OF A CHECK

American Bankers Association Number	Also known as the *ABA number* • Located in the upper right corner of a printed check • Printed as a fraction on a business check or as a straight series of numbers (1–109/210) on a personal check • Identifies the bank and the state where the bank issuing the check is located
Magnetic Ink Character Recognition	Also known as *MICR* • A combination of characters and numbers located at the bottom left side of checks and deposit slips • A form of identification for the bank and the account • First series of numbers identifies the bank and its location • Second series of numbers identifies the individual account

ELECTRONIC FUNDS TRANSFER (EFT)

Most payments by insurance companies are made via EFT, which is a method of transferring money between bank accounts by computer. Using EFT eliminates the need to write and mail paper checks.

Banking

The basic banking functions are depositing funds, writing checks, transferring funds between bank accounts, withdrawing funds, reconciling statements, and using banking services. Bank records are subject to government examination since the federal government regulates banking practices. In addition, accurate records are needed for preparation of federal tax returns.

BANKING TERMS

Bank Statement (Figure 13-1)	• A statement from the bank used to confirm the amount of funds that are in each account • Includes all debits and credits that have been processed Includes the following information: • Account number • Average collected balance • Minimum balance • Tax ID number (usually the Social Security number of the physician) • Beginning balance • Deposit history, including credit card transaction deposits • Interest and credits • Checks and debits • Service charges • Ending balance
Cash Disbursement	• Payments made to creditors
Credit	• Additions to an account (different than bookkeeping credit)
Debit	• Charges against an account (different than bookkeeping debit)
Deposit	• Money (cash, checks, and money orders) placed into a checking or savings bank account
Interest	• Money earned and paid to the depositor by the financial institution for allowing the use of the depositor's money (interest-earning savings or checking account) OR • Money paid to the financial institution for allowing the borrower to use the financial institution's money (loan)

(continued)

(Continued)

Nonsufficient Funds	Also known as *NSF* • Occurs when there is not enough money in the payer's account to cover the amount of the check or when a stop-payment order was issued by the payer • Many banks charge the account a fee if a deposited check has nonsufficient funds
Payee	• Person to whom a check is made out
Payer	• Person who signs the check to release the money
Reconciliation	• Comparison of the figures on the bank statements with the banking records maintained in the medical office and adjustment of the banking records so that both are in agreement
Returned Check	• May be returned by the bank due to a missing signature or missing endorsement • NSF checks will also be returned.
Stop-Payment Order	• Issued by the payer • The bank will not allow the funds indicated on the check to be disbursed.
Uncollected Funds Hold	Also known as *UCF* or *UFH* • A bank may place a "hold" on a checking account. • May occur when a deposit needs to "clear" so that the bank can make sure that the funds (money) are present before allowing anyone to write a check on that account • Typically occurs with checks written for large sums

STATEMENT OF ACCOUNT

FIRST NORTH
BANK OF CHIGAGO
123 East Pearson, Chicago, IL 60611
(312) 321-1000

Pearson Physicians Group
Shania McWalter, D.O.
123 Michigan Avenue,
Parker Heights, IL 60610

144808
PAGE 1 OF 1
STATEMENT PERIOD
FROM 08/01/11
THRU 08/31/11
CUST # 300-30-3000

--- ADVANTAGE CHECKING ACCOUNT ---

ACCOUNT NBR DD	12345	BEGINNING BALANCE	$2,646.63
AVG COLL BAL	$4,732.52	DEPOSITS/CREDITS	$8,000.00
MINIMUM BAL	$2,502.88	INTEREST PAID	$.00
TAX ID NUMBER	300-30-3000	CHECKS/DEBITS	$7,871.32 -
		SERVICE CHARGES	$5.00 -
		ENDING BALANCE	$2,770.31
		# DEPOSITS/CREDITS	1
		#CHECKS/DEBITS	11

DATE	DESCRIPTION		AMOUNT	BALANCE
08/01	BEGINNING BALANCE			$2,646.63
08/01	CK#	872	24.95-	2,621.68
08/06	CK#	879	3.00-	2,618.68
08/08	CK#	883	75.00-	2,543.68
08/14	CK#	885	15.80-	2,527.88
08/15	CK#	886	25.00-	2,502.88
08/19	DEPOSIT		8,000.00	10,502.88
08/26	CK#	887	32.00-	10,470.88
08/26	CK#	888	2,500.00-	7,970.88
08/28	CK#	890	70.00-	7,900.88
08/28	CK#	889	125.57-	7,775.31
08/28	CK#	884	5,000.00-	2,775.31
08/31	MONTHLY MAINTENANCE FEE		5.00-	2,770.31
08/31	ENDING BALANCE			$2,770.31

CHECK REGISTER

CHECK#	DATE	AMOUNT	CHECK#	DATE	AMOUNT
872	08/01	24.95	886	08/15	25.00
879*	08/06	3.00	887	08/26	32.00
883*	08/08	75.00	888	08/26	2,500.00
884	08/28	5,000.00	889	08/28	125.57
885	08/14	15.80	890	08/28	70.00

* INDICATES NON-CONSECUTIVE CHECK NUMBER(S)

FIGURE 13-1 A sample bank statement.

DEPOSITS

A deposit slip is completed every time a deposit is made into a bank account (Figure 13-2).

- The slip indicates the total dollar amounts of cash and checks being deposited.
- Entries on the slip should be printed in black ink.
- Currency (coins and bills) is totaled separately from checks.
- Each check must be entered on a different line, noting either the payer's name, the check number, or the ABA number, depending on the bank's preferred method.
- If there are more checks than lines provided, the excessive checks can be entered on the back of the deposit slip.
- The currency and coin totals and check totals are added together. Then this amount, the total for the deposit, is entered on the bottom line of the deposit slip.

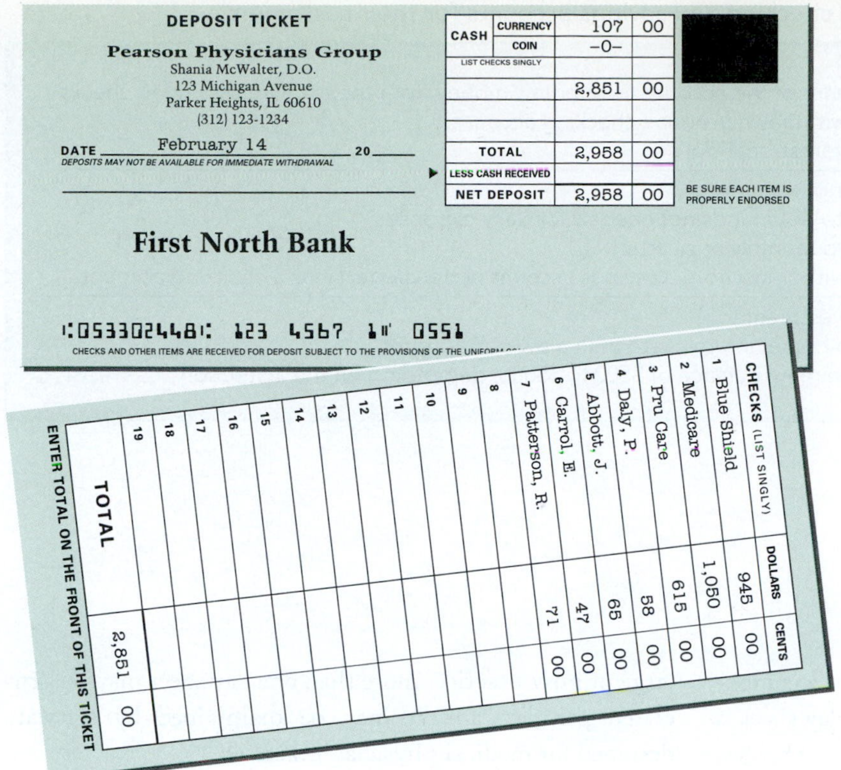

DEPOSIT TICKET

Pearson Physicians Group
Shania McWalter, D.O.
123 Michigan Avenue
Parker Heights, IL 60610
(312) 123-1234

DATE February 14 20
DEPOSITS MAY NOT BE AVAILABLE FOR IMMEDIATE WITHDRAWAL

CASH	CURRENCY	107	00
	COIN	-0-	
LIST CHECKS SINGLY		2,851	00
TOTAL		2,958	00
LESS CASH RECEIVED			
NET DEPOSIT		2,958	00

BE SURE EACH ITEM IS PROPERLY ENDORSED

First North Bank

⑆053302448⑆ 123 4567 1⑈ 0551

CHECKS AND OTHER ITEMS ARE RECEIVED FOR DEPOSIT SUBJECT TO THE PROVISIONS OF THE UNIFORM

CHECKS (LIST SINGLY)	DOLLARS	CENTS
1 Blue Shield	945	00
2 Medicare	1,050	00
3 Pru Care	615	00
4 Daly, P.	58	00
5 Abbott, J.	65	00
6 Carrol, E.	47	00
7 Patterson, R.	71	00
8		
9		
10		
11		
12		
13		
14		
15		
16		
17		
18		
19		
TOTAL	2,851	00

ENTER TOTAL ON THE FRONT OF THIS TICKET

FIGURE 13-2 A sample deposit ticket.

When making deposits, the following procedures are usually followed:

- Prepare and make deposits daily.
- Maintain all records of daily receipts (for checks, cash, money orders, and credit card transactions) together in a safe location.
- Compare the total on the deposit slip against the total on the day sheet.
- Keep a duplicate copy of all deposits on file in the office. Photocopy the deposit slip before submitting it to the bank. Some offices copy checks for later reference.
- Keep bank receipts of all deposits on file in the office.
- Immediately note all deposits in the checkbook.

ENDORSEMENTS

In order to transfer money from one person to another, the check must be endorsed. Federal banking regulations require an endorsement on the back of the check within the top $1^1/_2$ inches on the left side of the check as it is turned over. This upper left-hand corner is referred to as the *trailing edge* of a check. An endorsement can either be a payee's written signature or rubber-stamped.

TYPES OF ENDORSEMENTS

Endorsement	Description	Example
Blank	Carries the signature of the payee Can be cashed by anyone Not used in the business office	Shania McWalter
Full	Indicates the payer's name, company, account number, and bank name and the payee's name	Pay to the order of First Town Bank Shania McWalter, D.O. 123-123456
Restrictive	Specifies to whom money should be paid and the money's purpose, such as "For Deposit Only" The physician's signature can be rubber-stamped. Considered the safest endorsement	Pay to the order of First Town Bank For Deposit Only Shania McWalter, D.O. 123-123456

TYPES OF ACCOUNTS Banks maintain both checking and savings accounts for their customers.

Checking Account	• Allows the owner of the account to withdraw money from the account by writing checks • Cash can be withdrawn from the checking account • Usually not interest-bearing
Savings Account	• Interest-bearing account • Can be used to hold funds not needed for daily expenses • Interest earned monthly or quarterly • Cash can be withdrawn from a savings account or transferred into a checking account.
Money Market Savings Account	• Used as an investment tool • Usually pays a higher interest rate than a savings account • Requires a minimum balance of $500 to $5000, depending on the institution

Day Sheet

The day sheet, which contains five basic sections, is a component of the pegboard system (Figure 13-3). The day sheet is used to list or post each day's financial transactions: charges, payments, adjustments, and credits. The day sheet, one for each day of the month, must be balanced at the end of each day. The balance from the previous day is carried over to the present day's day sheet as part of the balancing process. In a large or busy practice, more than one day sheet may be generated per day, and it may be maintained by software designed for medical physician practices.

To make sure that the accounts and entries are correct, the day sheet(s) need to be balanced at the end of the day. Use a calculator to balance day sheets and always double-check each total.

DAY SHEET SECTIONS

Section	Description
Section 1	The individual transactions, such as patient charges, are posted in this column. The ledger card, charge slip, and receipt forms are used when posting in this row and column. Included in this section are: • Patient's name • Description of the transaction • Charges and credits • Previous and current balances
Section 2	This is the deposit portion of the day sheet. Some forms include a detachable slip that can be used as a deposit slip for making a deposit in a bank account. A payment made by the patient would also be listed in the appropriate right-hand column (cash, check, insurance).
Section 3	This is an optional column and depends on the needs of the practice. For example, it can be used to specify the type of service that was provided (office visit, office surgery, hospital visit).
Section 4	This is the totals column/row. Each column feeding into the bottom section is totaled at the end of each day.
Section 5	This section is critical in checking that the accounts balance. It also keeps track of the cumulative accounts receivable amounts owed by all of the patients. This column is useful in determining, by looking at just one number, how much money is still owed to the physician.

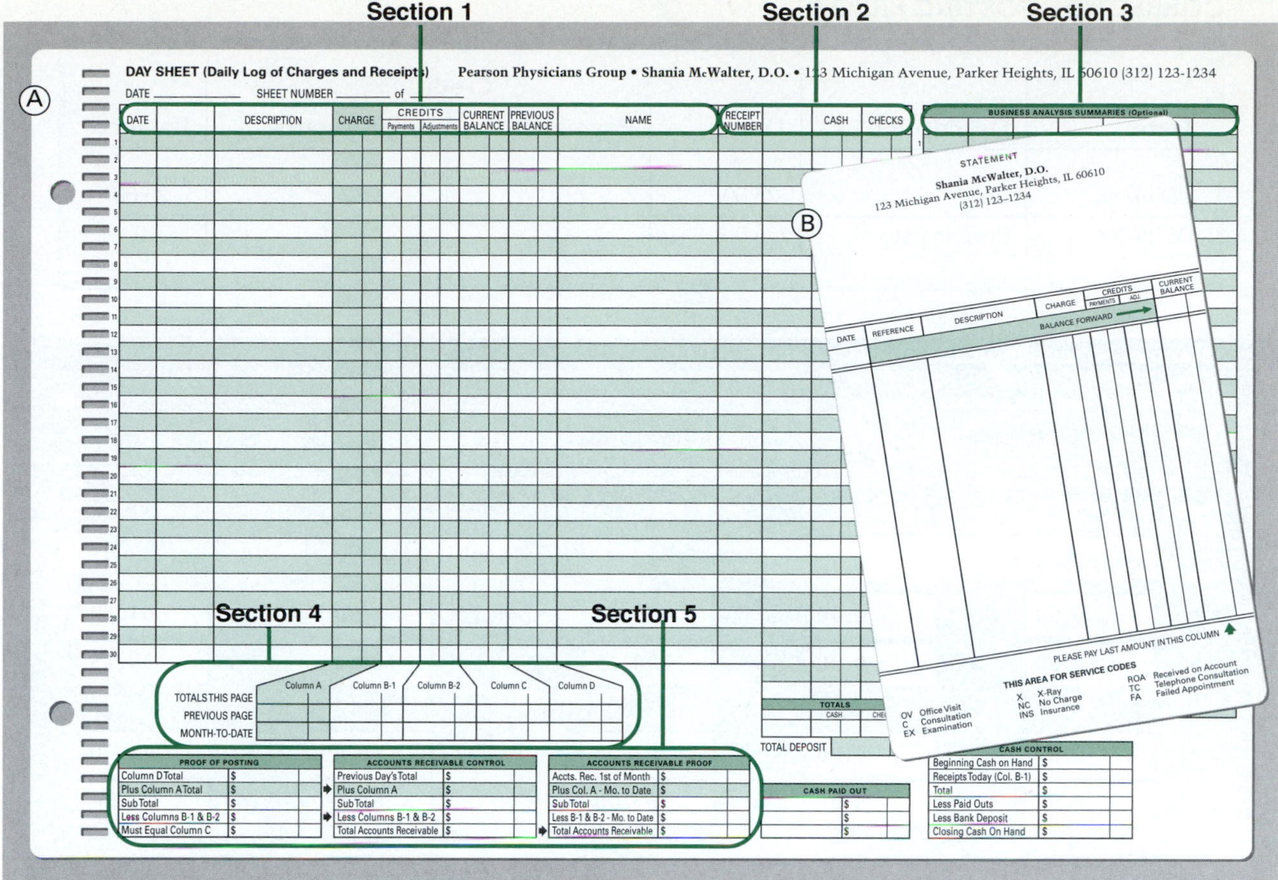

FIGURE 13-3 Example of a pegboard system.

BALANCING THE DAY SHEET

1. Total columns A, B1, B2, C, and D and place the total for each column in the boxes marked "Totals This Page." These column totals then must be added to the numbers brought forward and entered into the "Previous Page" column. This will provide the "Month to Date" total. "Month to Date" totals are important since they indicate all the credits, charges, and transactions that have occurred from the first day of the month to the present day.
2. The "Proof of Posting" box is used to ensure that all entries and the totals columns are correct. The numbers used to calculate this figure are taken from the "Totals This Page" column box.
   a. Enter the amount from today's column D total, which is the sum of the previous balances, in the appropriate box.
   b. Place the total for column A, which represents all the charges for this day, in the appropriate box ("Plus Column A Total"), and create a subtotal by adding the column D and column A totals.
   c. Add columns B1 and B2, which are both credit columns (payments and adjustments); then enter this amount in the box "Less Columns B1 and B2." This amount will then be subtracted (minus) from the subtotal of column D and column A.
   d. If the calculations have been correct, this new subtotal obtained after subtracting columns B1 and B2 should be equal to column C, which is the current balance.

   Note: When doing a proof of posting, column D is added to column A minus the sum of columns B1 and B2, and this must equal column C. Therefore, a proof of posting formula is:

   $$D + A - (B1 + B2) = C$$

   This means that the previous balance (D) plus the charge (A) minus the sum of the payments and adjustments (B1 and B2) is equal to the current balance (C).

CORRECTING POSTING ERRORS

Date	Description	Debit	Credit: Payments	Credit: Adjustments	Balance
06/19/XX	OV	25.00			25.00
06/19/XX	Error in pstg	(25.00)			0

Columbus Scheduling/Columbus Corporation 0.00

File Edit Patient Billing Service Codes Clinic Daily Reports Forms Utilities Window Help

Ledger Card

Name: Mary A. Jones | Bill Type: 1 | Acct.: 100 | Doctor: 10 | Selected Ledger: Z

Curr	0.00	+60.	0.00	+120.	100.25	Surplus	0.00	Ins.	61.10
+30..	0.00	+90.	0.00	Total	100.25	End Bal	100.25	Pat.	39.15

Current Ledger

Curr	0.00	+60.	0.00	+120.	63.00	Surplus	0.00	Ins.	61.10
+30..	0.00	+90.	0.00	Total	63.00	End Bal	63.00	Pat.	1.90

Eff Date	#	Doc	CPT	Description	Bill	%	Ins. Bal.	Pat. Bal.	Amount	Total
01/30/20XX	2	1	67891	Balance Forward	P		000.00	000.00	000.00	375.00
01/30/20XX	3	1		Payment Check 00					66.00	309.00
01/30/20XX	1	1		Payment Check 01					198.00	111.00
01/30/20XX	2	1		Office Visit					50.00	161.00
02/07/20XX	1	1	45678	Cash Received	P		000.00	000.00	000.00	98.00
		***		END			***			63.00

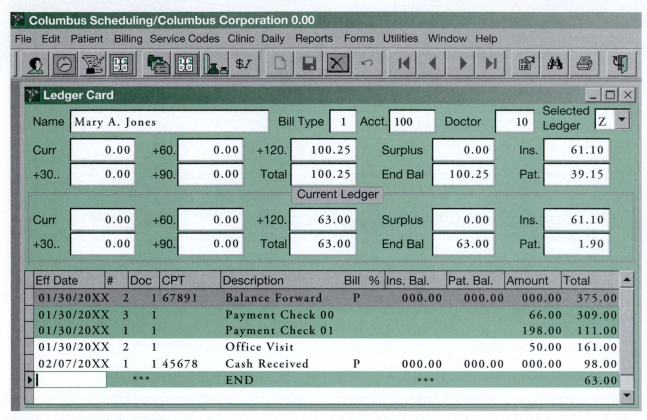

FIGURE 13-4 Electronic ledger card.

Ledger Cards

Ledger cards are used to record the charges, adjustments, and payments for the patient. In most offices, the ledger cards are maintained by a software program designed for medical physician practices and may be used to generate the monthly statements. An electronic ledger card is shown in Figure 13-4, and paper ledger cards are shown in Figure 13-5.

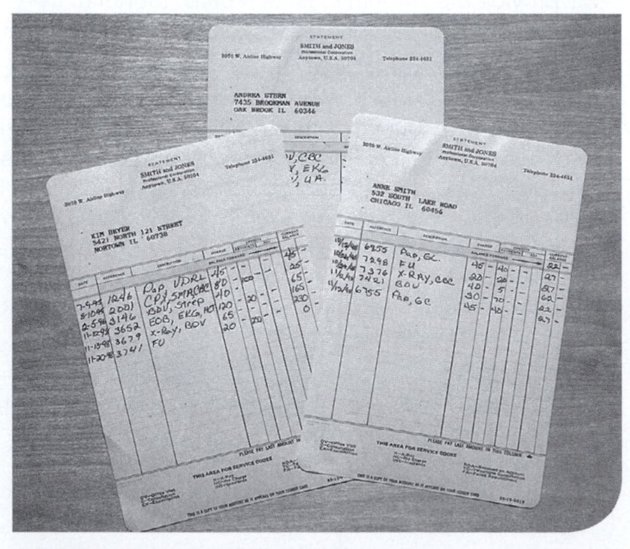

FIGURE 13-5 Paper ledger cards.

Billing and Collections

The process of setting up a fee schedule, extending credit, billing, and collection is an important part of the medical practice. Payment for medical services can be achieved in one of three ways.

PAYMENT METHODS

Payment at the Time of Service	• The preferred method • Significantly reduces the cost of billing, including the generation of bills, postage fees, and the use of human resources
Billing the Patient for Services and Extending Credit	• If credit is extended and the patient will make set payments to the physician in four or more installments, the patient must sign a Truth in Lending form. • The form must clearly state the amount financed, the finance charge, and the total of the payments
Collection Agency	• Used as a last resort • Most collection agencies will keep up to 50% or more of the amount collected.

BILLING AND COLLECTIONS TERMINOLOGY

Accounting	• System of reporting the financial results of a business • The basis of accounting is the ability to make an analysis, a statement, or a summary of financial matters.
Accounting Formula	• Assets = Liabilities + Net Worth
Accounts Payable	Also known as *AP* • Money the physician owes to others for supplies, equipment, and services that have not yet been paid
Accounts Receivable	Also known as *AR* • Money owed to the practice by insurance companies and patients that have not yet paid
Accounts Receivable (AR) Ratio	• Provides a measurement of how quickly the outstanding accounts are being paid • Referred to as "Days in AR" • AR Ratio equals the Current Accounts Receivable Balance divided by the Average Gross Monthly Charges
Adjustment	• Entering a change into the account record such as a discount, a write-off, or an amount not allowed by an insurance company (disallowance) • A discount is entered as a credit since this amount will be subtracted from the total amount owed.
Age Analysis	• Process of determining how long an account has been past due and instituting the necessary collection procedures
Assets	• Everything owned by the medical practice, such as cash, bank accounts, money owed to the physician, equipment, and real estate
Assignment of Benefits Form	• Used by the office so that insurance payments are made directly to the physician
Balance	• Difference between the debit (money owed) and the credit (money paid)
Bookkeeping	• Process of managing the accounts for a business • Continual process that should be done on a daily basis
Co-payment	• Predetermined amount of money set by the insurance company that the patient must pay for medical services at every visit
Credit	• Indicates that a payment has been received on an account • To credit an account means to subtract the payment from the account.
Credit Balance	• Overpayment has occurred. • This may happen when either the patient or the insurance company pays more than is due. • Noted on the patient's account either in red or by enclosing the amount in parentheses
Debit	• Indicates that a charge has been entered and added to the account balance

(continued)

(Continued)

Ledger Card	• Used to record the charges, adjustments, and payments for the patient • May be used to generate the monthly statement
Liabilities	• Money the medical practice owes to its creditors, such as money owed for medical supplies to a vendor (supplier)
Professional Courtesy	Also known as *PC* • The physician's decision not to charge other physicians, staff, family members, or clergy • May be granted only by the physician • Not looked on kindly by the government • Must meet insurance requirements and must be recorded in the patient's record
Statute of Limitations	• The time period within which a legal collection suit may be brought against a debtor
Superbill Encounter Form or Charge Slip (Figure 13-6)	• Document generated by the medical office and used as a statement and an insurance reporting form • Provides a comprehensive list of patient services, with respective diagnostic and procedural codes and fees • Can be used to input computer information for billing • Provides the patient with a record of the account's activity (charges, payments, adjustments) and can be used as a receipt • Provides a record that can be used for insurance purposes
Third-Party Payer(s)	• A party or person other than the patient, such as an insurance company, who assumes responsibility for paying the patient's bill
Usual, Customary, and Reasonable	Also known as *UCR* • *Usual:* what a physician usually charges for a procedure or service • *Customary:* fee charged for the same procedure by the majority of physicians with the same or similar training to perform that procedure • *Reasonable:* fee a physician charges for a modified procedure or service that is more difficult and requires more time and effort

Laws related to collections are outlined in the following table. Every medical office should have a collection policy in place, as it is not advantageous to have a haphazard method for collecting overdue accounts. The collection process for most practices includes noting the account status in the patient's record. This is especially helpful if the patient calls

LAWS GOVERNING COLLECTION

Law	Description
Notice on "Use of Telephone for Debt Collection" from the Federal Communications Commission	Provides guidelines for the specific times that credit collection phone calls can be made. It prohibits use of the telephone for harassment and threats. Telephone calls for the purpose of collections must be made between 8 A.M. and 9 P.M.
Fair Debt Collection Practices Act of 1978	Provides a guide for determining what are considered the fair collections practices for creditors
Equal Credit Opportunity Act of 1975	Prohibits discrimination in granting credit. This law mandates that women and minorities must be issued credit if they qualify for it, based on the premise that if credit is given to one patient, it should be given to all qualified patients who request it.
Fair Credit Reporting Act of 1971	Provides guidelines for collecting an individual's credit information. Individuals are able to learn what credit information is available about them. Consumers can correct and update this information.
Truth in Lending Act of 1969	Requires full written disclosure concerning the payment of any fee that will be collected in more than four installments. Also referred to as Regulation Z of the Consumer Protection Act.

Pearson Physicians Group 312-123-1234

Patient Number	Ticket Number	Service Date	Pat Prior Balance
Patient Name		Gender	Ins
Address		Phone	Other
SSN	Referring Dr.		Total
Primary Insurance Co.	Policy/Group ID		Paymt
Secondary Insurance Co.	Policy/Group ID		Bal Due

Location

☐ ______
☐ ______
☐ ______
☐ ______
☐ ______
☐ ______
☐ ______
☐ ______
☐ ______
☐ ______
☐ ______
☐ ______

Cardiologist

☐ ______
☐ ______
☐ ______
☐ ______
☐ ______
☐ ______
☐ ______
☐ ______
☐ ______
☐ ______
☐ Other:

X	Code	Service
		New Patient
	99203	Limited/Simple (30m)
	99204	Comprehensive (45m)
	99205	Complex (60m)
		New Patient Consult
		(Need Referring MD)
	99243	Brief (40m)
	99244	Full Consult (60m)
	99245	Very Complex (80m)
		Established Patient
	99211	Nurse Visit
	99212	Very Brief FU (10m)
	99213	Limited/Simple FU (15m)
	99214	Comprehensive FU (25m)
	99215	Complex FU (40m)
		New Cons. 2nd Opin.
	99274	Moderate 2nd Opinion
	99275	Complex 2nd Opinion
		Home Health
	99375	Home Health 30 days
		Drugs:
	J3420	B-12 Injection
	J1940	Lasix
	90724	Flu (Dx V-04.8)
	G0008	MC Flu Admin Fee
		Misc Rx ______
	90782	IM Injections
	90784	IV Injections
	A4615	O2 Cannula

X	Code	Service
		Office Procedures
	93000	EKG w/ Interp
	93015	Stress Tread w/ Interp
	93040	Rhythm strip w/ Interp
	93307	2D Echo Compl.
	93320	Doppler Compl.
	93325	Color Flow Compl.
	93308	2D Echo F/U
	93321	Doppler F/U
	ES	Stress Echo
	BUB	Echo/Bubble/Doppler
		Event Monitor
	93268	Loop- Non MC
	G0005	Loop - Hookup - MC
	G0007	Loop - Interp - MC
	93012	Chest Plate Tech - Non MC
	93014	Chest Pl - Interp Non MC
	G0016	Chest Pl - Interp MC
		Holter Monitor
	93224	Holter w/ Interp Global
		Other
	92960	Cardioversion
	93734	Pacer Eval - Single
	93735	Pacer Eval - Sngl w/ Prg
	93731	Pacer Eval - Dual
	93732	Pacer Eval - Dual w/ Prg
	99499	Review outside records
	99080	Special Reports

X	Code	Service
		Diagnostic w/o Interp
		(Technical only)
	93005	EKG
	93017	Stress Tread
	93225	Holter Hookup
	93226	Holter Scan
	93307-TC	2D Echo
	93320-TC	Doppler Compl.
	93325-TC	Color Flow
	93308-TC	2D Echo F/U
	93321-TC	Doppler F/U
	93880-TC	Carotid Doppler
	Phys	**Interpretation**-Supervision,
		Interpretation & Report Only
	93010	EKG Interp & Reortt only
	TR	Regular Stress Test--S, I & R
	NU	Nuclear Stress Test--S, I & R
	ES-26	Stress Echocardiogram--S, I & R
	307	Echocardiogram 2-D
	320-26	Doppler Echocardiogram
	325-26	Color Flow
	308	Echocardiogram 2-D F/U
	321-26	Doppler F/U
	227	Holter Monitor - I & R only
	71250-26	UltraFast CT
	XXXXX	**LAB ORDERED**
		(see attached sheet)
	36415	VeniPuncture (non MC)
	99000	Specimen Collection (Lab)

Next Appointment:
Return in: ___ (Wks) (Mo) (Yr)

Bl:

Before next appointment:
☐ Ekg ☐ Echo ☐ Doppler ☐ CXR ☐ Event Monitor
☐ TM ☐ Stress Echo ☐ CFD ☐ Holter ☐ Lab ______

Hospital Admission:

☐ Admit Cath
☐ Admit to ______ unit at:

☐ BAP ☐ WMC ☐ CMC ☐ SHMC
☐ Other: ______

Notes:

Cardiac Diagnoses

FIGURE 13-6 Superbill.

to schedule an appointment or inquire about medication refills. Generally, once a patient's account is in the hands of a collection agency, most offices will terminate the physician-patient relationship using the proper notification procedure as described in the office manual.

Collection agencies charge for their services, either a flat fee per account or a percentage of the amount collected. Be certain not to include the patient's diagnosis when turning over an account for collection. This is a violation of the patient's privacy and the HIPAA guidelines.

Once the patient is told that his or her account is going to a collection agency, it must, by law, be turned over for collection; otherwise, it could be considered an idle threat. After the account has been turned over, no further collection attempts can be made by the physician's office. If the patient contacts the office after the account has been turned over for collection, the patient should be referred to the collection agency.

Petty Cash

Petty cash is available for incidentals such as reimbursements, postage due, or other miscellaneous expenses within the medical office. Petty cash must be tracked and recorded in a daily financial log. Usually a designated amount of cash is placed in a drawer or box at the beginning of each month for this purpose. This amount will vary from office to office, depending on the needs of the office, and usually ranges from $50 to $100.

Accounts Payable

Accounts payable (AP) are the amounts the physician owes to others for supplies, equipment, and services that have not yet been paid. Examples of AP expenditures in a medical office include the following:

- Office supplies, such as paper goods, day sheets, appointment cards, and scheduling books
- Medical supplies and equipment
- Equipment repair and maintenance, including housekeeping
- Utilities such as telephones and electricity
- Taxes
- Payroll
- Rent

PAYROLL

Typically, the largest AP account in the medical office is for payroll.

PAYROLL SCHEDULES

Weekly	• 52 pay periods a year • Employees paid every week on the same day of the week
Biweekly	• 26 pay periods a year • Employees paid every two weeks
Semimonthly	• 24 pay periods a year • Employees paid on predetermined dates during the month, for example, on the 15th and 30th of every month
Monthly	• 12 pay periods a year • Employees paid on the same date every month.

PAYROLL TERMINOLOGY

Deductions	• Money withheld from the employee's paycheck, depending upon the taxes, health and life insurance premiums, and any other deductions
Federal Insurance Contributions Act	Also known as *FICA* • Includes monies contributed by the employer and monies withheld from the employee's gross wage to cover Social Security and Medicare taxes • Deposits must be made monthly.
Federal Unemployment Tax	Also known as *FUTA* • Employers required to pay this tax, as mandated by the Federal Unemployment Tax Act • Solely the responsibility of the employer; the employee does not contribute • Calculated quarterly
Gross Annual Wage	• Annual wage before taxes and any withholdings are deducted • For hourly employees, use the following formula: (Hourly wage × Number of hours worked per week) × 52 Weeks in a year = Gross pay (or Hourly wage × 2080 Full-time hours in a year = Annual pay)

Income Tax Withholding (Figure 13-7)	• Deductions that must be paid by both the employee and the employer
Salary	• A predetermined amount of money every pay period that does not depend on the number of hours working within that period
W-2 Form (Figure 13-8)	• Must be completed at the end of each year and provided to each employee • By law, employers must mail or hand deliver W-2 forms by January 31 of the year immediately following upcoming tax reporting season.
W-4 Form (Figure 13-9)	• Each employee must complete a W-4 form when hired. The W-4 form must include the following: • Employee's name and current address • Social Security number • Marital status • Number of exemptions to be claimed

MARRIED Persons—**WEEKLY** Payroll Period
(For Wages Paid Through December 2009)

If the wages are–		And the number of withholding allowances claimed is—										
At least	But less than	0	1	2	3	4	5	6	7	8	9	10
		The amount of income tax to be withheld is—										
$0	$310	$0	$0	$0	$0	$0	$0	$0	$0	$0	$0	$0
310	320	1	0	0	0	0	0	0	0	0	0	0
320	330	2	0	0	0	0	0	0	0	0	0	0
330	340	3	0	0	0	0	0	0	0	0	0	0
340	350	4	0	0	0	0	0	0	0	0	0	0
350	360	5	0	0	0	0	0	0	0	0	0	0
360	370	6	0	0	0	0	0	0	0	0	0	0
370	380	7	0	0	0	0	0	0	0	0	0	0
380	390	8	1	0	0	0	0	0	0	0	0	0
390	400	9	2	0	0	0	0	0	0	0	0	0
400	410	10	3	0	0	0	0	0	0	0	0	0
410	420	11	4	0	0	0	0	0	0	0	0	0
420	430	12	5	0	0	0	0	0	0	0	0	0
430	440	13	6	0	0	0	0	0	0	0	0	0
440	450	14	7	0	0	0	0	0	0	0	0	0
450	460	15	8	1	0	0	0	0	0	0	0	0
460	470	16	9	2	0	0	0	0	0	0	0	0
470	480	17	10	3	0	0	0	0	0	0	0	0
480	490	19	11	4	0	0	0	0	0	0	0	0
490	500	20	12	5	0	0	0	0	0	0	0	0
500	510	22	13	6	0	0	0	0	0	0	0	0
510	520	23	14	7	0	0	0	0	0	0	0	0
520	530	25	15	8	1	0	0	0	0	0	0	0
530	540	26	16	9	2	0	0	0	0	0	0	0
540	550	28	17	10	3	0	0	0	0	0	0	0
550	560	29	19	11	4	0	0	0	0	0	0	0
560	570	31	20	12	5	0	0	0	0	0	0	0
570	580	32	22	13	6	0	0	0	0	0	0	0
580	590	34	23	14	7	0	0	0	0	0	0	0
590	600	35	25	15	8	1	0	0	0	0	0	0
600	610	37	26	16	9	2	0	0	0	0	0	0
610	620	38	28	17	10	3	0	0	0	0	0	0
620	630	40	29	19	11	4	0	0	0	0	0	0
630	640	41	31	20	12	5	0	0	0	0	0	0
640	650	43	32	22	13	6	0	0	0	0	0	0
650	660	44	34	23	14	7	0	0	0	0	0	0
660	670	46	35	25	15	8	1	0	0	0	0	0
670	680	47	37	26	16	9	2	0	0	0	0	0
680	690	49	38	28	17	10	3	0	0	0	0	0
690	700	50	40	29	19	11	4	0	0	0	0	0
700	710	52	41	31	20	12	5	0	0	0	0	0
710	720	53	43	32	22	13	6	0	0	0	0	0
720	730	55	44	34	23	14	7	0	0	0	0	0
730	740	56	46	35	25	15	8	1	0	0	0	0
740	750	58	47	37	26	16	9	2	0	0	0	0
750	760	59	49	38	28	17	10	3	0	0	0	0
760	770	61	50	40	29	19	11	4	0	0	0	0
770	780	62	52	41	31	20	12	5	0	0	0	0
780	790	64	53	43	32	22	13	6	0	0	0	0
790	800	65	55	44	34	23	14	7	0	0	0	0
800	810	67	56	46	35	25	15	8	1	0	0	0
810	820	68	58	47	37	26	16	9	2	0	0	0
820	830	70	59	49	38	28	17	10	3	0	0	0
830	840	71	61	50	40	29	19	11	4	0	0	0
840	850	73	62	52	41	31	20	12	5	0	0	0
850	860	74	64	53	43	32	22	13	6	0	0	0
860	870	76	65	55	44	34	23	14	7	0	0	0
870	880	77	67	56	46	35	25	15	8	1	0	0
880	890	79	68	58	47	37	26	16	9	2	0	0
890	900	80	70	59	49	38	28	17	10	3	0	0
900	910	82	71	61	50	40	29	19	11	4	0	0
910	920	83	73	62	52	41	31	20	12	5	0	0
920	930	85	74	64	53	43	32	22	13	6	0	0
930	940	86	76	65	55	44	34	23	14	7	0	0
940	950	88	77	67	56	46	35	25	15	8	1	0
950	960	89	79	68	58	47	37	26	16	9	2	0
960	970	91	80	70	59	49	38	28	17	10	3	0
970	980	92	82	71	61	50	40	29	19	11	4	0
980	990	94	83	73	62	52	41	31	20	12	5	0
990	1,000	95	85	74	64	53	43	32	22	13	6	0

FIGURE 13-7 Federal Tax Withholding Table.

Control number: B1-049097-0	Company # 007252	ERU 000	State Form		
Employer's name, address, and ZIP code **Pearson Physicians Group** **123 Machigan Avenue** **Parker Heights, IL 60610**			1 Wages, tips, other compensation 32094.40 3 Social Security wages 32094.40 5 Medicare wages and tips 32094.40	2 Federal income tax withheld 5559.06 4 Social Security tax withheld 1989.85 6 Medicare tax withheld 465.37	
Employer's identification number			7 Social Security tips	8 Allocated tips	
Employee's social security number			9 Advance EIC payment	10 Dependent care benefits	
Employee's name, address, and ZIP code			11 Nonqualified plans	12 Benefits included in Box 1	
			13 See instr. for Box 13	14 Other	
			15 Statutory emp. / Deceased / Pension plan X / Legal rep.	942 emp. / Deferred comp. / Void	
18 State and Employer's state ID number	17 State wages, tips, etc. 32094.40	18 State income tax 1305.46	19 Locality Name CASDI	20 Local wages, tips, etc.	21 Local income tax 412.97

1995 Wage and Tax Statement
For Employee's Records
Department of the Treasury - Internal Revenue Service
FORM W2
COPY C

FIGURE 13-8 A sample W-2 form.

Government regulations require that records be maintained for each employee relating to the following payroll items:

- Amount of gross pay
- Social Security number of the employee
- Number of exemptions of each employee (taken from the W-4 form completed by the employee at the time of hire)
- Deductions for Social Security, as well as for federal, state, and local taxes
- State disability insurance and unemployment tax, where applicable
- Any pretax deductions such as 401K contributions

Supplies

Maintaining an adequate level of supplies within the office is required in order to have the office run smoothly and efficiently. When ordering supplies, the person with this responsibility should attempt to have an ample amount of supplies on hand without having too much or too little.

- Too much inventory not only costs money from the paid goods perspective, but also reduces the available space.
- Many offices use a card system; on the card, specific information regarding the product is recorded. The card may note the item name, the name and address of the vendor, the unit price, the quantity typically ordered, date the order was placed, the date the order was received, and any other information of note.
- Whenever an item is removed from the supply cabinet, it should be marked on the inventory sheet. A staff member is assigned the responsibility of reordering all supplies when the number of items reaches the levels determined to be low and appropriate for reordering. The minimum number for a particular item will be determined by the frequency with which that item is used within that office. For example, a gynecologists's office may require a minimum of 10 boxes of drapes to be kept in inventory at all times because drapes are a frequently used item. However, in a pediatrician's office, the minimum required number of boxes of drapes to keep on hand may be three because they are used less often.
- Supplies should be rotated on the shelves so that the newer supplies are at the back and the older ones are used first.

TYPES OF SUPPLIES AND EQUIPMENT

Administrative Supplies	Keep the office running *Examples*: copy paper, toner, postage, pens
Capital Equipment	Major expenditures *Examples*: exam tables and computers
Clinical Supplies	Keep the office running *Examples*: surgical instruments, table paper, bandages
Durable Equipment	Used indefinitely
Incidental Supplies	Not essential to smooth running of the office *Examples*: binder clips, paper clips and staples

Form W-4 (20XX)

Purpose. Complete Form W-4 so that your employer can withhold the correct federal income tax from your pay. Because your tax situation may change, you may want to refigure your withholding each year.

Exemption from withholding. If you are exempt, complete only lines 1, 2, 3, 4, and 7 and sign the form to validate it. Your exemption for 20XX expires February 16, 20XX. See Pub. 505, Tax Withholding and Estimated Tax.

Note. You cannot claim exemption from withholding if (a) your income exceeds $800 and includes more than $250 of unearned income (for example, interest and dividends) and (b) another person can claim you as a dependent on their tax return.

Basic instructions. If you are not exempt, complete the **Personal Allowances Worksheet** below. The worksheets on page 2 adjust your withholding allowances based on itemized deductions, certain credits, adjustments to income, or two-earner/two-job situations. Complete all worksheets that apply. However, you may claim fewer (or zero) allowances.

Head of household. Generally, you may claim head of household filing status on your tax return only if you are unmarried and pay more than 50% of the costs of keeping up a home for yourself and your dependent(s) or other qualifying individuals. See line **E** below.

Tax credits. You can take projected tax credits into account in figuring your allowable number of withholding allowances. Credits for child or dependent care expenses and the child tax credit may be claimed using the **Personal Allowances Worksheet** below. See Pub. 919, How Do I Adjust My Tax Withholding? for information on converting your other credits into withholding allowances.

Nonwage income. If you have a large amount of nonwage income, such as interest or dividends, consider making estimated tax payments using Form 1040-ES, Estimated Tax for Individuals. Otherwise, you may owe additional tax.

Two earners/two jobs. If you have a working spouse or more than one job, figure the total number of allowances you are entitled to claim on all jobs using worksheets from only one Form W-4. Your withholding usually will be most accurate when all allowances are claimed on the Form W-4 for the highest paying job and zero allowances are claimed on the others.

Nonresident alien. If you are a nonresident alien, see the Instructions for Form 8233 before completing this Form W-4.

Check your withholding. After your Form W-4 takes effect, use Pub. 919 to see how the dollar amount you are having withheld compares to your projected total tax for 20XX. See Pub. 919, especially if your earnings exceed $125,000 (Single) or $175,000 (Married).

Recent name change? If your name on line 1 differs from that shown on your social security card, call 1-800-772-1213 to initiate a name change and obtain a social security card showing your correct name.

Personal Allowances Worksheet (Keep for your records.)

A Enter "1" for **yourself** if no one else can claim you as a dependent . . . . **A** ______

B Enter "1" if:
- You are single and have only one job; or
- You are married, have only one job, and your spouse does not work; or
- Your wages from a second job or your spouse's wages (or the total of both) are $1,000 or less.

. . **B** ______

C Enter "1" for your **spouse.** But, you may choose to enter "-0-" if you are married and have either a working spouse or more than one job. (Entering "-0-" may help you avoid having too little tax withheld.) . . . . **C** ______

D Enter number of **dependents** (other than your spouse or yourself) you will claim on your tax return . . . . **D** ______

E Enter "1" if you will file as **head of household** on your tax return (see conditions under **Head of household** above) . **E** ______

F Enter "1" if you have at least $1,500 of **child or dependent care expenses** for which you plan to claim a credit . . **F** ______
(**Note.** Do **not** include child support payments. See **Pub. 503,** Child and Dependent Care Expenses, for details.)

G **Child Tax Credit** (including additional child tax credit):
- If your total income will be less than $54,000 ($79,000 if married), enter "2" for each eligible child.
- If your total income will be between $54,000 and $84,000 ($79,000 and $119,000 if married), enter "1" for each eligible child plus "1" **additional** if you have four or more eligible children. **G** ______

H Add lines A through G and enter total here. (**Note.** This may be different from the number of exemptions you claim on your tax return.) ▶ **H** ______

For accuracy, complete all worksheets that apply.
- If you plan to **itemize or claim adjustments to income** and want to reduce your withholding, see the **Deductions and Adjustments Worksheet** on page 2.
- If you have **more than one job** or are **married and you and your spouse both work** and the combined earnings from all jobs exceed $35,000 ($25,000 if married) see the **Two-Earner/Two-Job Worksheet** on page 2 to avoid having too little tax withheld.
- If **neither** of the above situations applies, **stop here** and enter the number from line H on line 5 of Form W-4 below.

Cut here and give Form W-4 to your employer. Keep the top part for your records.

Form **W-4**
Department of the Treasury
Internal Revenue Service

Employee's Withholding Allowance Certificate

▶ **Whether you are entitled to claim a certain number of allowances or exemption from withholding is subject to review by the IRS. Your employer may be required to send a copy of this form to the IRS.**

OMB No. 1545-0010
20XX

1 Type or print your first name and middle initial	Last name	2 Your social security number
Home address (number and street or rural route)	3 ☐ Single ☐ Married ☐ Married, but withhold at higher Single rate. **Note.** If married, but legally separated, or spouse is a nonresident alien, check the "Single" box.	
City or town, state, and ZIP code	4 **If your last name differs from that shown on your social security card, check here. You must call 1-800-772-1213 for a new card.** ▶ ☐	

5 Total number of allowances you are claiming (from line **H** above **or** from the applicable worksheet on page 2) | 5 |

6 Additional amount, if any, you want withheld from each paycheck . . . . | 6 | $

7 I claim exemption from withholding for 20XX, and I certify that I meet **both** of the following conditions for exemption.
- Last year I had a right to a refund of **all** federal income tax withheld because I had **no** tax liability **and**
- This year I expect a refund of **all** federal income tax withheld because I expect to have **no** tax liability.

If you meet both conditions, write "Exempt" here . . . . ▶ | 7 |

Under penalties of perjury, I declare that I have examined this certificate and to the best of my knowledge and belief, it is true, correct, and complete.

Employee's signature
(Form is not valid unless you sign it.) ▶ **Date** ▶

8 Employer's name and address (Employer: Complete lines 8 and 10 only if sending to the IRS.)	9 Office code (optional)	10 Employer identification number (EIN)

For Privacy Act and Paperwork Reduction Act Notice, see page 2. Cat. No. 10220Q Form **W-4** (20XX)

FIGURE 13-9 A sample W-4 form.

TERMS ASSOCIATED WITH PURCHASING, RECEIVING, AND PAYING FOR SUPPLIES

Billing Statement	Summary of the month's invoices from a particular vendor
Invoice	Describes the purchased quantity and dollar amount of supplies ordered Should be verified with the original order and packing slip
Packing Slip	Lists the quantities ordered, shipped, and back-ordered
Purchase Order	Also known as a *PO* A preapproved order with a reference number that is provided to the vendor as a means of tracking the order
Terms of Payment	Found on the invoice from the vendor and notifies when payment in full is due; varies by vendor Some vendors offer a set percentage discount if the entire bill is paid within a short period of time.

13 APPLICATION

Directions: Select the best answer for each of the following questions. Check your answers in the Answer Key at the end of the book.

1. "Written using the bank's own check or form" and "issued by the bank" describe which type of check?
   a. Limited check
   b. Cashier's check
   c. Certified check
   d. Traveler's check
   e. Voucher check
2. Money earned and paid to the depositor by a financial institution for allowing the use of the depositor's money is:
   a. A deposit
   b. An electronic funds transfer (EFT)
   c. Interest
   d. A cash disbursement
   e. None of the above
3. Which of the following is/are true about deposit slips?
   a. Currency is totaled separately from checks.
   b. Entries should be printed in blue ink.
   c. Each check must be entered on a separate line.
   d. A and B
   e. A and C
4. __________ is a component of the pegboard system and is used to list or post each day's financial transaction.
   a. The day sheet
   b. The ledger card
   c. The general ledger
   d. The balance sheet
   e. The AR aging report
5. "Assets equal liabilities and net worth" is commonly known as the:
   a. Age analysis
   b. Credit balance
   c. Bookkeeping formula
   d. Accounting formula
   e. Income statement
6. Money the medical practice owes to a supplier is a:
   a. Liability
   b. Debit
   c. Credit
   d. Receivable
   e. None of the above
7. ___________ must be completed at the end of each year and provided to each employee.
   a. W-4 form
   b. Annual deduction analysis
   c. W-2 form
   d. A and C
   e. A and B

8. The government requires payroll records to be maintained for each employee; these records must include the:
   a. Employee's Social Security number
   b. Pretax deductions
   c. Withholding tax deductions
   d. Gross pay amount
   e. All of the above

9. The W-2 form includes the following items:
   a. Gross wages
   b. Health insurance contributions
   c. Federal income tax withheld
   d. A and C
   e. None of the above

10. ____________requires full written disclosure concerning the payment of any fee that will be collected in more than four installments:
    a. Fair Debt Collection Practices Act of 1978
    b. Fair Credit Reporting Act of 1971
    c. Truth in Lending Act of 1969
    d. Equal Credit Opportunity Act of 1975
    e. Federal Communication Act of 1963

11. Examples of accounts payable (AP) expenditures in a medical office are:
    a. Taxes and patient co-pays
    b. Office supplies and rent
    c. Patient co-pays and payroll
    d. Utilities and patient co-pays
    e. B and D

12. ____________describes the fee charged for a procedure by the majority of physicians with the same or similar training to perform that procedure.
    a. Usual
    b. Customary
    c. Typical
    d. Reasonable
    e. Average

13. In accounting terms, money owed to the practice that has not yet been paid is known as:
    a. Accounts receivable
    b. Accounts payable
    c. Balance
    d. Credit balance
    e. Liability

14. The bank's statement of account includes:
    a. Withdrawals and deposits
    b. Deposits and cleared (processed) checks
    c. The mid-month balance
    d. A and C
    e. A and B

15. The process of comparing the bank statement to the office's banking records and the adjustment of those records so that both are in agreement is known as:
    a. Income statement adjustment
    b. Balance sheet adjustment
    c. Readjustment
    d. Reconciliation
    e. Age analysis

16. Regarding ABA, which of the following statements is not true?
    a. Located in the bottom left corner of a printed check
    b. Printed as a fraction on a business check
    c. Identifies the bank issuing the check
    d. Identifies the area issuing the check
    e. ABA stands for American Bankers Association Number

17. Which of the following is the preferred method for payment of medical services?
    a. Collection agency
    b. Billing the patient
    c. Extending credit
    d. Payment at time of service
    e. None of the above

18. Regarding adjustments, which of the following is not true?
    a. It is entered as a debit on the day sheet because it is a discount.
    b. It can be recorded as a write-off.
    c. An insurance disallowance is considered an adjustment.
    d. Discounts are recorded as an adjustment.
    e. Subtract this from the amount owed.

19. Which of the following is not true about petty cash?
    a. Must be tracked daily
    b. Must be recorded in the daily financial log
    c. Used for incidentals
    d. Designated amount is usually $100 to $200
    e. All of the above statements are true.

20. Which of the following check endorsements is considered the safest?
    a. Open
    b. Blank
    c. Full
    d. Limited
    e. Restrictive

14 Managed Care and Insurance

CONTENTS

Health insurance was originally designed to help patients with catastrophic medical expenses that occurred as a result of an unexpected illness or injury. Health benefits existed as a contract between the subscriber (insured) and the carrier (insurance company or third-party payer). The first medical or health insurance plans were not intended to cover all costs associated with health care. Over the years, insurance plans for medical and health care have expanded. As the cost of medical care has escalated, new and different types of health care plans and many regulations have also come into being.

TERMINOLOGY

Term	Definition
Acceptance of Assignment	An agreement between the physician and the insurance company stating that the physician will accept the amount provided by the insurance company as payment in full
Allowed Charge	The highest amount that third-party payers will pay for services
Assignment of Benefits	Patient's written authorization giving the insurance company the right to pay the physician directly for billed charges
Beneficiary	Person receiving benefits
Benefits	Payments made by the insurance company to the physician/facility on behalf of the patient
Benefit Period	Period of time for which payments for insurance are available
Birthday Rule	Used by insurance claims administrators to determine which parent's benefit plan will be the primary insurance plan of a dependent child who is covered by the employer-sponsored insurance plans of both parents The plan of the parent whose birthday falls earlier in the year (not the older parent) will be the primary plan. *Example:* If one parent's birthday is March 30 and the other parent's birthday is September 24, the parent with the March birthday would cover the child on his or her insurance plan, while the other parent's plan would be considered secondary insurance for the dependent child. If both parents have the same birth date, the parent who has had the coverage longer is considered to have the primary plan. This rule applies only to parents who are legally married.
Capitation Rate	Also known as *prospective payment* The provider is paid a predetermined amount every month, regardless of the number of times the patient is seen within the month.
Claim	Written and documented request for reimbursement of an eligible expense under an insurance plan
CMS	Centers for Medicare and Medicaid Services Formerly known as the Health Care Financing Administration (HCFA)
Coinsurance	A specific percentage of the total cost that must be paid by the insured to the provider when services are rendered
Coordination of Benefits	Also known as *COB* Procedures to prevent duplication of payment by more than one insurance carrier
Copayment	A predetermined amount of money the patient is responsible for paying for various services
Closed-Panel HMO	HMO that requires subscribers to go only to providers on a panel
Crossover Claim	A patient claim that is eligible for both Medicare and Medicaid. It is also called Medi/Medi.
Deductible	Amount of eligible charges each patient must pay each calendar year before the plan begins to pay benefits
Dependents	Spouse, children, and occasionally others who are covered by the insured's health plan
Disability Insurance	Insurance that usually begins paying the patient (not the doctor or the hospital) after the insured has been disabled (unable to work) for a specific period of time
Exclusions	Services that are not covered under the insured's health plan
Exclusive Provider Organization	Also known as *EPO* Combination of PPO and HMO concepts. It allows the patient to select from an exclusive panel of providers, but the patient must pay higher deductibles if a PPO is selected.

(continued)

TERMINOLOGY (*Continued*)

Explanation of Benefits	Also known as *EOB* Document provided by the insurance carrier to the beneficiary describing the benefits provided (Figure 14-1)
Fee Schedule	Schedule of the amount paid by a specific insurance company for each procedure or service. Amounts are determined by a claims administrator and applied to claims subject to the fee schedule of a provider's managed care contract.
Fee-for-Service	An established set of fees for services by a healthcare provider and paid for by the patient
Formulary	Specific to each insurance carrier, a list of medications that will be covered under that insurance plan
Gatekeeper	A PCP who refers patients to other providers for services he or she cannot perform
Group Policy	An insurance policy covering a group of employees under one master contract. The coverage is the same for all employees and dependents covered under that policy.
Guarantor	Individual responsible for paying the medical bill
Health Maintenance Organization	Also known as *HMO* A managed care agency that provides healthcare services for a group at fixed prepaid payments
Indemnity Plan	Traditional health insurance plan that allows the patient to choose the physician and the facility where he or she will receive healthcare services. This type of plan pays for all or most covered services.
Individual Policy	Insurance purchased directly from an insurance company without going through a group plan
Integrated Delivery System	Also known as *IDS* One in which provider sites have contracts with an insurance company
Managed Care Plan	General term used to describe health insurance plans in which insurance is received for a monthly premium and limitations of the insurance are defined based upon the type of plan chosen There are three basic types of managed care plans: • Health maintenance organization (HMO) • Preferred provider organization (PPO) • Point-of-service plan (POS)
Major Medical	Health insurance policy designed to offset major medical expenses as a result of catastrophic illnesses or injury
Medical Foundation	A charitable organization that provides medical care for free or at low cost
Medical Savings Account	Healthcare plan that pays the provider a predetermined amount on a monthly basis; in turn, the provider is responsible for providing quality, cost-effective care.
Medical Necessity	Medical services and/or procedures supported by the patient's symptoms/diagnosis
Nonparticipating Provider	Also known as *non*PAR A provider who decides not to accept an allowable charge as the full fee for care
Open-Panel HMO	HMO that allows subscribers to go to providers who are not on a panel There are three models under this category: • *Direct contract model:* individual physicians in the community provide contracted healthcare services to subscribers. • *Individual practice association (IPA) model:* similar to the direct contract model in that the providers are not employees of the HMO. • *Network model:* contracted services are provided by more than one provider group.
Participating Provider	Also known as *PAR* One who accepts assignment of benefits and is paid directly by the plan
Point-of-Service Plan	Also known as *POS* One in which a patient may choose an HMO or a non-HMO provider but must pay a deductible for using a non-HMO provider
Policyholder	The person whose name is on the insurance policy and is responsible for paying the premium

(*Continued*)

Preauthorization	A requirement to obtain prior approval for surgery and other procedures in order to receive reimbursement.
Preferred Provider Organization	Also known as *PPO* One in which the patient must use a provider under contract to the insurance company and the insurance company reimburses the provider at a discounted rate
Premium	Amount paid to obtain and maintain insurance
Prepaid Plan	A group of physicians or other healthcare providers who have a contractual agreement to provide services to subscribers on a negotiated fee-for-service or capitated basis (also called a *managed care plan*)
Primary Care Provider	Also known as *PCP* Gatekeeper provider who refers patients to other providers for services he or she cannot perform
Primary Insurance	Medical insurance coverage provided through the patient's employer
Referral	Sending the patient to another provider for a specific plan of care
Resource-Based Relative Value System	Also known as *RBRVS* Standardized fee schedule designed by Medicare and based on the costs of providing care in different geographic regions
Rider	Supplemental policies added to basic insurance coverage for additional fees *Examples:* Vision and dental insurance
Self-Insured	Organizations that are large enough to fund their own insurance programs OR Individuals who purchase insurance directly through the insurance company without going through a group plan
Self-Referral	A patient's decision to see another provider for a specific plan of care
Secondary Insurance	Occurs when the patient's spouse has medical insurance through his or her provider and the patient also has medical insurance through his or her own employer. The spouse's insurance is considered secondary.
Subscriber	Person who holds a health benefit plan/contract/policy. This plan, contract, or policy may include other family members.
Third-Party Payer	Insurance carrier that intervenes and pays the physician on behalf of the patient
Utilization Review	Review of healthcare services to determine if the services are a necessary, appropriate, and efficient use of resources

Health Maintenance Organization (HMO)

An HMO is a type of managed care plan in which a range of healthcare services provided by a limited group of providers (such as physicians and hospitals) are made available to plan members for a predetermined fee called the *capitation rate*. The HMO concept was developed to control the explosion of healthcare costs as a result of overutilization of services.

An HMO has two important components:

- All medical services are provided based on a predetermined (per capita) fee rather than a fee-for-service basis. If the actual cost of services exceeds the predetermined (or capitation) amount, then the provider must absorb the excess costs. This provides an incentive for the provider to control costs.
- A member patient must use the providers and hospitals identified by the HMO. The HMO will pay for any covered services that are provided by designated providers, hospitals, durable medical equipment, and pharmacies. Therefore, preapproval must be granted through the primary care provider (PCP) when and if a patient has to seek consultation or medical services outside of the network. The exception to this rule is recognized emergency services.

Uniform
Medical Plan
Your Health, Your Plan Your Choice

Explanation of Benefits

This is not a bill.
06/08/2007

Your UMP ID Number: W125370058
Subscriber Name: CHRIS R LONEMA
Patient Name CHRIS R LONEMA
Claim Number: K100925-0038

If you have questions, contact us:

By Mail:
Uniform Medical Plan
PO Box 84578 98124-1578
Seattle, WA

By Phone/E-mail:
Local: 425-555-3000
Toll Free: 1-800-555-6004
E-mail: www.ump.hca.wa.gov

CHRIS R LONEMA
3160 GRAND AVE 12345
EVERETT WA

Provider Information

CATHERINE N DORTON ARNP
7620 44TH ST NE 12345
MARYSVILLE WA

Provider Name:	Date(s) of Service	Service(s) Provided	Amount Charged	UMP Allowed	PPO Savings	Non-Cov'd Amount	Deductible	Copay	Co-Ins. %	UMP Paid	Patient's Responsibility	See Notes Section
CATHERINE N DORTON ARNP	05/07/07 - 05/07/07	87621 90 PATHOLOGY-PHYS CHGS	125.00	66.94	58.06			6.69	90	60.25	6.69	PPU
CATHERINE N DORTON ARNP	05/07/07 - 05/07/07	88142 90 PATHOLOGY-PHYS CHGS	72.00	28.31	43.69			2.83	90	25.48	2.83	PPU
		TOTALS	197.00	95.25	101.75	0.00	0.00	9.52		85.73	9.52	

Other Insurance Paid Amount	0.00	
(*) See Notes Adjustment	0.00	
UMP Final Paid Amount/Check	85.73	# 43984431

Total Payment to Provider: *******85.73 **Total Payment to Enrollee:** ********0.00

NOTES:

THANK YOU FOR USING A UNIFORM MEDICAL PLAN PARTICIPATING PROVIDER

PPU THIS IS YOUR PLANS PARTICIPATING PROVIDERS CONTRACTUAL ALLOWANCE FOR THIS SERVICE. PROVIDER AGREES TO REDUCE THE FEE TO THE AMOUNT ALLOWED.

DEDUCTIBLE
YOU HAVE MET 200.00 OF YOUR 200.00 DEDUCTIBLE FOR 01/01/2007 - 12/31/2007

200706113300 ENV 8241 3 OF 3 F L1561026164

FIGURE 14-1 Explanation of benefits (EOB).

VARIOUS TYPES OF MANAGED CARE ORGANIZATIONS (MCOs) AND THEIR CHARACTERISTICS

HMO	PPO	POS	EPO
• State licensed • Most stringent guidelines • Limited network of providers • Members assigned to PCPs • Members must use network except in emergencies or pay a penalty • Usually there is a financial reward to providers for managing the cost of care	• Limited network of providers but larger than HMO • Members may be assigned to PCPs but restrictions on accessing other physicians not as tight as in HMO • Financial penalty for accessing non-network providers less severe than in an HMO • Usually there is no reward to providers for managing the cost of care	• Hybrid of HMO and PPO networks • Members may choose from a primary or secondary network • Primary network is HMO-like • Secondary network is often a PPO network • Out-of-pocket expenses are lower within the primary network and higher when using the secondary network • Members have more choices with less expense than with a PPO	• Doesn't have an HMO license • Members are eligible for benefits only when they use network providers • Financial penalties for members leaving the network are similar to those of HMO • Priced lower than a PPO but higher than an HMO
IPA Model HMO	**Staff Model HMO**	**Network Model HMO**	**Group Model HMO**
• An association formed by physicians with separately owned practices (solo or small group) • HMO may contract with physicians separately or through the IPA	• HMO hires the physicians and pays them salaries • HMO owns the network • HMO owns the clinic sites and health centers	• HMO uses two or more group practices or a group practice plus a combination of staff physicians and contracted independent physicians to form a network of providers • Allow members to choose their providers	• HMO contracts with multi-specialty groups • May be open-panel or closed-panel

Source: Comprehensive Health Insurance: Billing, Coding, and Reimbursement by D. Vines, A Braceland, E. Rollins, and S. Miller, Upper Saddle River, NJ: Pearson Education, Inc., 2008, p. 272. Reprinted with permission.

A patient who joins an HMO may either choose a personal provider from a list or be assigned a PCP, who is generally an internist, a family practitioner, an obstetrician/gynecologist, or a pediatrician. The PCP must provide all primary care services since the HMO will not pay for the costs of a nonmember provider except in an emergency.

Preferred Provider Organization (PPO)

A PPO requires the patient to use a medical provider or hospital that is under contract with the insurer for an agreed-on-fee. The PPO is similar to an HMO but differs in four main areas:

- A PPO is a fee-for-service program; it is not based on prepayment.
- PPO physicians and hospitals are reimbursed for each medical service they provide.
- PPO members or enrollees are not restricted to certain designated providers or hospitals.
- PPO members may receive care from a non-PPO provider; however, they will generally have to pay more out-of-pocket expenses when they do this.

PPOs manage cost containment in the following ways:

- They negotiate fees with providers that are less than the current market fees.
- They provide financial incentives for PPO members to use a PPO provider.
- They carefully monitor the quality and type of services offered by PPO providers.

Point-of-Service Plan (POS)

To allow for more flexibility, some HMOs and PPOs have created a POS. Within this plan, patients may choose to use either the panel of providers within the HMO network or non-HMO providers.

If the enrollee chooses to use a provider within the network:

- The enrollee is responsible only for the regular co-payment.
- Deductible amounts do not apply.
- The same benefits apply if the patient is referred by a provider to a specialist outside the network (with authorization from the HMO).

If an enrollee chooses to see an out-of-network provider without authorization, this is known as *self-referral*. The enrollee may be responsible for greater out-of-pocket expenses, including larger deductible and co-insurance charges.

Blue Cross/Blue Shield (BCBS)

BCBS is a commercial insurance carrier and covers nearly one-third of the people in the United States.

- Blue Cross (BC) covers hospitalization.
- Blue Shield (BS) covers physician benefits.

Most patients have BCBS, which covers both hospitalization and physician benefits; however, there is the option of carrying only BC or BS.

BCBS may be fee-for-service, managed care, a federal employee program (FEP), Medicare supplemental, or BC anywhere. The type of coverage is noted on the patient's insurance card.

Worker's Compensation

Worker's compensation is government-mandated insurance for injuries directly related to work.

- Payment of premiums is the employer's responsibility; the employee pays nothing.
- Providers must enroll with their state's worker's compensation plan before they can agree to accept cases.
- In worker's compensation cases, the provider of services must complete a report called a Doctor's First Report and must submit further reports at predetermined intervals.
- A patient's records related to a worker's compensation case must be kept in a separate file from the patient's regular records kept by the physician.

Medicare

Medicare is health insurance for the elderly that is provided by the U.S. government. It has the following characteristics:

- It is operated by the Social Security Administration.
- It is paid for largely through Social Security funds.
- It is designed for persons 65 years of age and older and for the severely disabled.
- It covers approximately 32 million elderly citizens as well as 2 million permanently disabled persons.
- Eligible patients are issued a Medicare card after applying for services.

ADVANCE BENEFICIARY NOTICE (ABN)

All patients covered by Medicare must sign an ABN prior to receiving covered services that may be denied by Medicare (Figure 14-2). When patients sign an ABN, they acknowledge that they are financially responsible for any noncovered services.

Medicare is a multipart health care benefit system.

MEDICARE PART A

- Covers inpatient hospital expenses, inpatient care in a skilled nursing facility, and hospice and home health care
- Covers all expenses for the first 60 days of hospitalization, except for an initial amount, or deductible, which is paid by the patient
- Also pays for a portion of inpatient hospital costs for an additional 30 days
- Does not cover extended nursing-home care or the costs of lengthy or chronic illnesses
- Most individuals are covered automatically when the insured becomes eligible for Social Security benefits.
- Patient must apply to receive Medicare benefits from the Social Security Administration.

MEDICARE PART B

- Covers medical expenses for doctors, medical services, outpatient hospital care, durable medical equipment, and some medical services not covered by Part A
- In order to qualify for Part B Medicare coverage, the insured must pay a monthly premium.
- Coverage is not automatic, nor does it pay for all services.
- The patient pays a yearly deductible.
- After the deductible is met, Medicare will pay for 80% of the approved amount of covered services and the insured is liable for the 20% co-insurance.

(A) **Notifier(s):**
(B) **Patient Name:** *(C)* **Identification Number:**

ADVANCE BENEFICIARY NOTICE OF NONCOVERAGE (ABN)

NOTE: If Medicare doesn't pay for ***(D)***_____________ below, you may have to pay.

Medicare does not pay for everything, even some care that you or your health care provider have good reason to think you need. We expect Medicare may not pay for the ***(D)***_____________ below.

*(D)*_______________	***(E)* Reason Medicare May Not Pay:**	***(F)* Estimated Cost:**

WHAT YOU NEED TO DO NOW:

- Read this notice, so you can make an informed decision about your care.
- Ask us any questions that you may have after you finish reading.
- Choose an option below about whether to receive the ***(D)***_____________listed above.

Note: If you choose Option 1 or 2, we may help you to use any other insurance that you might have, but Medicare cannot require us to do this.

***(G)* OPTIONS:** **Check only one box. We cannot choose a box for you.**

☐ **OPTION 1.** I want the ***(D)***__________ listed above. You may ask to be paid now, but I also want Medicare billed for an official decision on payment, which is sent to me on a Medicare Summary Notice (MSN). I understand that if Medicare doesn't pay, I am responsible for payment, but **I can appeal to Medicare** by following the directions on the MSN. If Medicare does pay, you will refund any payments I made to you, less co-pays or deductibles.

☐ **OPTION 2.** I want the ***(D)***__________ listed above, but do not bill Medicare. You may ask to be paid now as I am responsible for payment. **I cannot appeal if Medicare is not billed.**

☐ **OPTION 3.** I don't want the ***(D)***__________listed above. I understand with this choice I am **not** responsible for payment, and **I cannot appeal to see if Medicare would pay.**

***(H)* Additional Information:**

This notice gives our opinion, not an official Medicare decision. If you have other questions on this notice or Medicare billing, call **1-800-MEDICARE** (1-800-633-4227/**TTY**: 1-877-486-2048).
Signing below means that you have received and understand this notice. You also receive a copy.

***(I)* Signature:**	***(J)* Date:**

According to the Paperwork Reduction Act of 1995, no persons are required to respond to a collection of information unless it displays a valid OMB control number. The valid OMB control number for this information collection is 0938-0566. The time required to complete this information collection is estimated to average 7 minutes per response, including the time to review instructions, search existing data resources, gather the data needed, and complete and review the information collection. If you have comments concerning the accuracy of the time estimate or suggestions for improving this form, please write to: CMS, 7500 Security Boulevard, Attn: PRA Reports Clearance Officer, Baltimore, Maryland 21244-1850.

Form CMS-R-131 (03/08) Form Approved OMB No. 0938-0566

FIGURE 14-2 Advance beneficiary notice (ABN).

MEDICARE PART C

- It is also known as a *Medicare advantage plan.*
- It was formerly known as Medicare + Choice.
- It is offered by private insurance companies.
- It replaces Medicare parts A, B, and D.
- There is limited choice regarding which physicians the patient may see.

MEDICARE PART D

- Participation is voluntary.
- Prescription drugs are covered under a separate medical policy.
- It was implemented in 2006.
- It is offered as a supplemental plan for Medicare recipients to purchase.
- It covers a predetermined list of prescription drugs at participating pharmacies.
- For Medicare recipients who opt to participate in Medicare Part D, there are annual deductibles, applicable co-payments, or co-insurance and maximum benefits that apply.

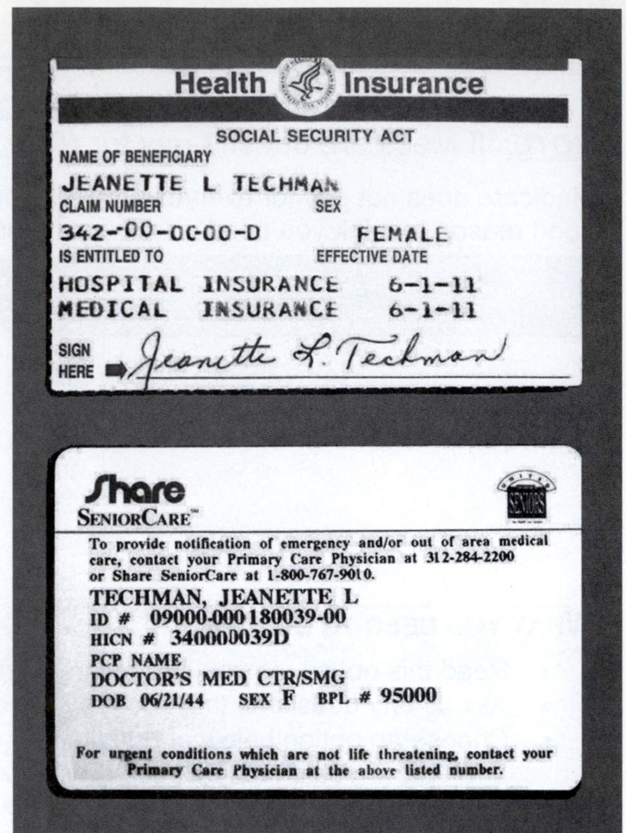

FIGURE 14-3 Medicare and supplemental private insurance cards.

NATIONAL PROVIDER IDENTIFIER (NPI)

Effective May 2007, HIPAA requires all healthcare providers to include their NPI when submitting claim forms to Medicare. The NPI is a unique 10-digit number assigned by the CMS and replaces the unique provider identification number (UPIN).

MEDIGAP PLANS

Patients with Medicare may purchase supplemental insurance plans known as *Medigap plans* (Figure 14-3). These plans may cover deductibles, co-insurance, and services not otherwise covered by Medicare. Medicare is considered the primary insurance; the supplemental plan is secondary.

DIAGNOSIS-RELATED GROUPS (DRGs)

DRGs were developed in the late 1960s with the intention of providing a means of monitoring the quality of care and the utilization of services in a hospital setting. Payment rates based on DRGs have now been established as the basis for a hospital's Medicare reimbursements. While DRGs have an effect on hospital reimbursements, they are not used to calculate payments made to outpatient providers.

Medicaid

Medicaid was designed for the medically indigent or persons without funds. Even though it is not a direct federal program, it qualifies as government insurance.

- Funding for each state's Medicaid program comes from state funds, with some federal money to offset costs.
- The program is administered by individual states, and the rules for eligibility and payment vary from state to state.
- The patient must qualify for benefits on a monthly basis.

MEDI/MEDI

Eligibility for Medicare does not automatically confer Medicaid eligibility. In some cases, a person is eligible for both Medicare and Medicaid. This is referred to as Medi/Medi.

TRICARE and CHAMPVA

TRICARE is the U.S. Department of Defense's worldwide healthcare program for active duty and retired uniformed services members and their families (Box 14-1).

Box 14-1 TRICARE Coverage

- **TRICARE Prime**—a managed care option similar to a civilian HMO
- **TRICARE Extra**—a PPO option in which beneficiaries choose a doctor, hospital, or other medical provider within the TRICARE provider network
- **TRICARE Standard**—a fee-for-service option
- **TRICARE for Life**—an option available to Medicare-eligible beneficiaries age 65 and over

Source: http://www.tricare.mil.

CHAMPVA (Civilian Health and Medical Program of the Veterans Administration) is available for the spouse, widow, widower, and/or children of veterans with total or permanent service-connected disabilities, as well as for the surviving spouse or dependents of veterans who have died as a result of service-connected disabilities.

Claims Processing

The health insurance claim form provides communication between the insurance company and the physician for the services the patient has received. There are three main points to this communication process that are critical in order to receive proper reimbursement from the insurance carrier:

- The correct claim form must be used.
- Information provided in the health insurance claim form must be accurate. One minor mistake can cause the claim to be rejected.
- The claim form must be submitted to the correct insurance carrier.

TYPES OF CLAIM FORMS

The CMS-1500 (previously known as the HCFA 1500) is the most common health insurance claim form and is used to file claims for physicians' services (Figure 14-4). Basic guidelines for completing the CMS-1500 are as follows:

- Use original approved forms.
- Use all capital letters.
- Avoid punctuation.
- Do not use titles (e.g., Mr., Mrs.).
- Use eight-digit dates.
- Erasures, overtyping, or whiteout are not allowed.
- No highlighters or pen marks are allowed.
- No tape or staples can be used.

The CMS-1450, also known as the UB-04, is used to file claims for institutional providers such as those who practice in hospitals, skilled nursing facilities, and home health agencies (Figure 14-5).

Most insurance carriers now require claims to be submitted electronically unless documentation is required to help support the claim.

Three types of health insurance claim forms are used to submit claims to TRICARE and CHAMPVA:

- DD Form 2642, Patient's Request for Medical Payment, is completed and sent by the patient or a family member after medical services have been provided. Payment is sent directly to the patient or family member as reimbursement.
- CMS-1500 is completed and sent by the physician's office. Payment will be sent to the physician's office to cover services already provided to the patient.
- UB-04 is completed and sent by the hospital for services provided to the patient in a hospital setting. Payment will be sent directly to the hospital.

PAPER CLAIMS

Only small providers (institutional organizations with fewer than 25 full-time employees and physicians with fewer than 10 full-time employees) may file paper claims. Paper claims are completed manually and are more likely to have errors than those prepared electronically.

ELECTRONIC CLAIMS

HIPAA, which took effect October 16, 2003, requires claims to be transmitted electronically in the HIPAA format by providers who are not considered small. For more information on HIPAA, see Chapter 10.

Electronic claims are sent to an insurance carrier or clearinghouse via dial-up modem, direct data entry, or over the Internet rather than on paper.

CMS-1500 CLAIM FORM

1500

HEALTH INSURANCE CLAIM FORM

APPROVED BY NATIONAL UNIFORM CLAIM COMMITTEE 08/05

PICA | PICA | CARRIER

1. MEDICARE (Medicare #) MEDICAID (Medicaid #) TRICARE CHAMPUS (Sponsor's SSN) CHAMPVA (Member ID#) GROUP HEALTH PLAN (SSN or ID) FECA BLK LUNG (SSN) OTHER (ID)

1a. INSURED'S I.D. NUMBER (For Program in Item 1)

2. PATIENT'S NAME (Last Name, First Name, Middle Initial)

3. PATIENT'S BIRTH DATE MM DD YY SEX M F

4. INSURED'S NAME (Last Name, First Name, Middle Initial)

5. PATIENT'S ADDRESS (No, Street)

6. PATIENT RELATIONSHIP TO INSURED Self Spouse Child Other

7. INSURED'S ADDRESS (No, Street)

CITY STATE

8. PATIENT STATUS Single Married Other

CITY STATE

ZIP CODE TELEPHONE (Include Area Code) ( )

Employed Full-Time Student Part-Time Student

ZIP CODE TELEPHONE (Include Area Code) ( )

9. OTHER INSURED'S NAME (Last Name, First Name, Middle Initial)

10. IS PATIENT'S CONDITION RELATED TO:

11. INSURED'S POLICY GROUP OR FECA NUMBER

a. OTHER INSURED'S POLICY OR GROUP NUMBER

a. EMPLOYMENT? (Current or Previous) YES NO

a. INSURED'S DATE OF BIRTH MM DD YY SEX M F

b. OTHER INSURED'S DATE OF BIRTH MM DD YY SEX M F

b. AUTO ACCIDENT? YES NO PLACE (State)

b. EMPLOYER'S NAME OR SCHOOL NAME

c. EMPLOYER'S NAME OR SCHOOL NAME

c. OTHER ACCIDENT? YES NO

c. INSURANCE PLAN NAME OR PROGRAM NAME

d. INSURANCE PLAN NAME OR PROGRAM NAME

10d. RESERVED FOR LOCAL USE

d. IS THERE ANOTHER HEALTH BENEFIT PLAN? YES NO *If yes,* return to and complete item 9 a-d

SECOND FOLD

PATIENT AND INSURED INFORMATION

READ BACK OF FORM BEFORE COMPLETING & SIGNING THIS FORM.

12. PATIENT'S OR AUTHORIZED PERSON'S SIGNATURE I authorize the release of any medical or other information necessary to process this claim. I also request payment of government benefits either to myself or to the party who accepts assignment below.

SIGNED DATE

13. INSURED'S OR AUTHORIZED PERSON'S SIGNATURE I authorize payment of medical benefits to the undersigned physician or supplier for services described below.

SIGNED

WHCF-10-ENV / WHCF-10-ENV-SS

14. DATE OF CURRENT MM DD YY ILLNESS (First symptom) OR INJURY (Accident) OR PREGNANCY (LMP)

15. IF PATIENT HAS HAD SAME OR SIMILAR ILLNESS, GIVE FIRST DATE MM DD YY

16. DATES PATIENT UNABLE TO WORK IN CURRENT OCCUPATION FROM MM DD YY TO MM DD YY

17. NAME OF REFERRING PHYSICIAN OR OTHER SOURCE

17a.

17b. NPI

18. HOSPITALIZATION DATES RELATED TO CURRENT SERVICES FROM MM DD YY TO MM DD YY

19. RESERVED FOR LOCAL USE

20. OUTSIDE LAB? YES NO $ CHARGES

21. DIAGNOSIS OR NATURE OF ILLNESS OR INJURY (Relate Items 1,2,3 or 4 to Item 24E by Line)

1. 3.

2. 4.

22. MEDICAID RESUBMISSION CODE ORIGINAL REF. NO.

23. PRIOR AUTHORIZATION NUMBER

FIRST FOLD

24. A. DATE(S) OF SERVICE From MM DD YY To MM DD YY	B. PLACE OF SERVICE	C. EMG	D. PROCEDURES, SERVICES, OR SUPPLIES (Explain Unusual Circumstances) CPT/HCPCS MODIFIER	E. DIAGNOSIS POINTER	F. $ CHARGES	G. DAYS OR UNITS	H. EPSDT Family Plan	I. ID. QUAL.	J. RENDERING PROVIDER ID. #
1								NPI	
2								NPI	
3								NPI	
4								NPI	
5								NPI	
6								NPI	

25. FEDERAL TAX ID NUMBER SSN EIN

26. PATIENT'S ACCOUNT NO.

27. ACCEPT ASSIGNMENT? (For govt. claims, see back) YES NO

28. TOTAL CHARGE $

29. AMOUNT PAID $

30. BALANCE DUE $

31. SIGNATURE OF PHYSICIAN OR SUPPLIER INCLUDING DEGREES OR CREDENTIALS (I certify that the statements on the reverse apply to this bill and are made a part thereof)

SIGNED DATE

32. SERVICE FACILITY LOCATION INFORMATION

a. b.

33. BILLING PROVIDER INFO & PH. # ( )

a. b.

PHYSICIAN OR SUPPLIER INFORMATION

NUCC Instruction Manual available at: www.nucc.org

WCMS-1500CS

APPROVED OMB 0938-0999 FORM CMS-1500 (08/05)

FIGURE 14-4 CMS-1500 claim form.

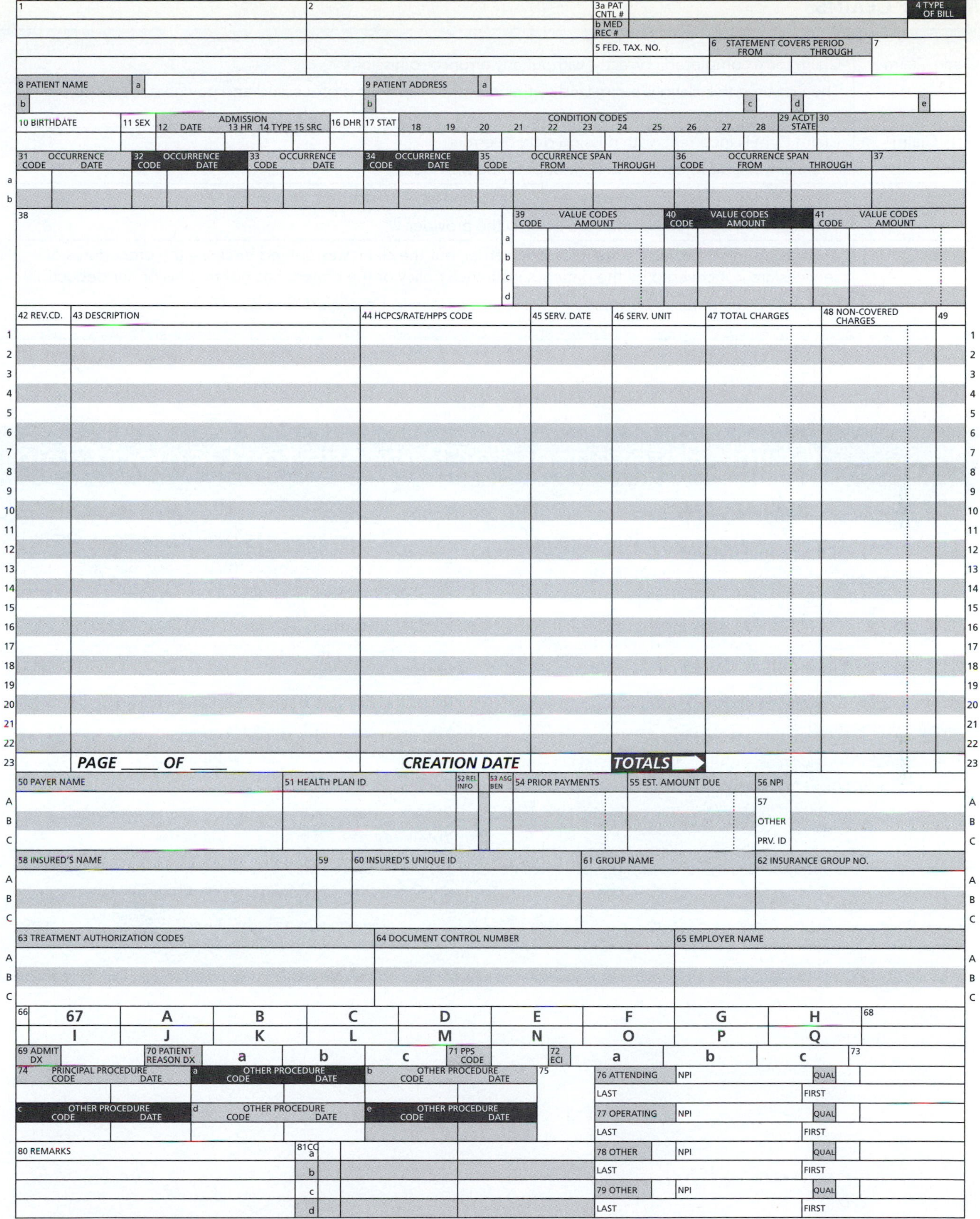

1 | 2 | 3a PAT CNTL # | b MED REC # | 4 TYPE OF BILL
5 FED. TAX. NO. | 6 STATEMENT COVERS PERIOD FROM THROUGH | 7
8 PATIENT NAME a | b
9 PATIENT ADDRESS a | b | c | d | e
10 BIRTHDATE | 11 SEX | ADMISSION 12 DATE 13 HR 14 TYPE 15 SRC | 16 DHR | 17 STAT | CONDITION CODES 18 19 20 21 22 23 24 25 26 27 28 | 29 ACDT STATE | 30
31 OCCURRENCE CODE DATE | 32 OCCURRENCE CODE DATE | 33 OCCURRENCE CODE DATE | 34 OCCURRENCE CODE DATE | 35 OCCURRENCE SPAN CODE FROM THROUGH | 36 OCCURRENCE SPAN CODE FROM THROUGH | 37
a
b
38 | 39 VALUE CODES CODE AMOUNT | 40 VALUE CODES CODE AMOUNT | 41 VALUE CODES CODE AMOUNT
a b c d

42 REV.CD.	43 DESCRIPTION	44 HCPCS/RATE/HPPS CODE	45 SERV. DATE	46 SERV. UNIT	47 TOTAL CHARGES	48 NON-COVERED CHARGES	49
1							
2							
3							
4							
5							
6							
7							
8							
9							
10							
11							
12							
13							
14							
15							
16							
17							
18							
19							
20							
21							
22							
23	PAGE ____ OF ____	CREATION DATE		TOTALS			

50 PAYER NAME | 51 HEALTH PLAN ID | 52 REL INFO | 53 ASG BEN | 54 PRIOR PAYMENTS | 55 EST. AMOUNT DUE | 56 NPI | 57 OTHER PRV. ID
A B C
58 INSURED'S NAME | 59 | 60 INSURED'S UNIQUE ID | 61 GROUP NAME | 62 INSURANCE GROUP NO.
A B C
63 TREATMENT AUTHORIZATION CODES | 64 DOCUMENT CONTROL NUMBER | 65 EMPLOYER NAME
A B C
66 | 67 | A | B | C | D | E | F | G | H | 68
I | J | K | L | M | N | O | P | Q
69 ADMIT DX | 70 PATIENT REASON DX a b c | 71 PPS CODE | 72 ECI a b c | 73
74 PRINCIPAL PROCEDURE CODE DATE | a OTHER PROCEDURE CODE DATE | b OTHER PROCEDURE CODE DATE | 75
c OTHER PROCEDURE CODE DATE | d OTHER PROCEDURE CODE DATE | e OTHER PROCEDURE CODE DATE
76 ATTENDING NPI QUAL LAST FIRST
77 OPERATING NPI QUAL LAST FIRST
80 REMARKS | 81CC a b c d
78 OTHER NPI QUAL LAST FIRST
79 OTHER NPI QUAL LAST FIRST

FIGURE 14-5 CMS-1450 (UB-04) claim form.

STATUS OF CLAIMS

Clean Claim	Claim form completed correctly, without any errors or omissions The first time this claim is submitted to the insurance carrier, it is processed and payment is sent to the provider.
Dirty Claim	Claim form is incorrect, with missing data or errors The claim will be rejected and sent back to the provider.
Invalid Claim	Claim form that has been completed but has some type of incorrect information The claim will be rejected and sent back to the provider.
Denied Claim	Claim form was received by the insurance carrier, but the claim was denied because the procedures or services are not covered by the patient's insurance policy or the patient has not met his or her deductible. Ineligible procedures or services can also cause a claim to be denied. See Box 14-2.

Box 14-2 Quick References for Reasons for Denied Claims

Reason claim was denied: Need supporting documentation

Tip for avoiding this denial: When calling for preauthorization of any procedure, ask the insurance company customer service representative if supporting documentation will be required. If so, copy the chart notes, operative report, laboratory report, or other documentation and send it in with the CMS-1500 billing form.

Reason claim was denied: Diagnosis code does not match procedure performed

Tip for avoiding this denial: Before sending the claim, look at the diagnosis codes the physician assigns to the patient in the *ICD-9* coding book to verify that the code matches the procedure.

Reason claim was denied: Patient is no longer eligible for coverage

Tip for avoiding this denial: Before scheduling any procedure, call to verify coverage with the insurance carrier.

Reason claim was denied: Missing information on the CMS-1500 claim form

Tip for avoiding this denial: Quickly scan all CMS-1500 claim forms prior to sending to determine any missing information or blank boxes.

Reason claim was denied: Past timely filing limits

Tip for avoiding this denial: Submit all insurance claim forms in a timely manner, usually within 30 days of the date of the procedure.

Reason claim was denied: Preauthorization was not obtained before performing the service

Tip for avoiding this denial: Before scheduling any procedure, call to verify coverage with the insurance carrier.

Source: Medical Assisting: Foundations and Practices by M. S. Frazier, C. Malone, and C. Morgan, Upper Saddle River, NJ: Pearson Education, Inc., 2010, p. 307. Reprinted with permission.

14 APPLICATION

Directions: Select the best answer for each of the following questions. Check your answers in the Answer Key at the end of the book.

1. The highest amount that third-party payers will pay for services is called:
   a. Acceptance of assignment
   b. Assignment of benefits
   c. Allowed charge
   d. Co-payment
   e. None of the above

2. A patient claim that is eligible for both Medicare and Medicaid is called a/an:
   a. Indemnity plan
   b. Crossover claim
   c. Open-panel HMO claim
   d. Primary care provider (PCP)
   e. Formulary claim

3. A person who holds a health benefit plan/contract/policy is:
   a. A third-party payer
   b. A gatekeeper
   c. A dependent
   d. A subscriber
   e. A and C

4. Medicare is:
   a. Operated by the Social Security Administration
   b. Provided by a charitable organization
   c. The same as an HMO
   d. Designed for persons 65 years of age and older
   e. A and D

5. Medicare is divided into four parts: A, B, C, and D. The following choices is/are true of Medicare Part D:
   a. It is also known as a *Medicare advantage plan*.
   b. Prescription drugs are covered under a separate medical policy.
   c. It is offered as a supplemental plan for Medicare recipients to purchase.
   d. A and C
   e. B and C

6. TRICARE is the:
   a. Newest PPO plan
   b. Medical care plan for retired persons
   c. U.S. Department of Defense's healthcare program for active duty military personnel
   d. U.S. Department of Defense's healthcare program for active duty and retired uniformed services members and their families
   e. Plan designed for civilians to use when they are drawing unemployment benefits

7. Frequently a patient is sent to another provider for a specific plan of care. This is known as a:
   a. Referral
   b. Subscriber
   c. Rider
   d. Managed care patient
   e. B and D

8. The definition of *self-insured* is:
   a. An individual's purchase of a plan directly from the insurance company without going through a group plan
   b. Medical insurance coverage provided by the patient's employer
   c. An insurance carrier's intervention and payment of the physician on behalf of the patient
   d. Organizations large enough to fund their own insurance plan
   e. A and D

9. A group of physicians or other healthcare providers who have a contractual agreement to provide services to subscribers on a negotiated fee-for-service basis constitute (a):
   a. Primary insurance
   b. Major medical
   c. Medical savings account
   d. Point-of-service plan
   e. Prepaid plan

10. ________________ is the most common health insurance claim form.
   a. CHAMPVA
   b. CMS-1500
   c. MEDICARE
   d. UB-40
   e. CMS-1450

11. The following is/are true of worker's compensation:
   a. Payment of premiums is the employer's responsibility.
   b. It is a form of government-mandated insurance for injuries directly related to work.
   c. The provider of services must complete a report called the Doctor's First Report
   d. All of the above
   e. B and C only

12. ____________ is defined as an arrangement whereby the provider is paid a predetermined amount every month, regardless of the number of times the patient is seen within the month.
   a. Retrospective payment
   b. Fee schedule
   c. Capitation rate
   d. Preauthorization
   e. POS

13. A written and documented request for reimbursement of an eligible expense under an insurance plan is:
   a. A claim
   b. An indemnity plan
   c. An integrated delivery system
   d. A self-referral
   e. None of the above

14. Two important components of an HMO are:
   a. It is a government-mandated program.
   b. Medical services are provided based on a predetermined (per capita) fee.
   c. A member must use the providers and hospitals identified by the HMO.
   d. B and C
   e. A and C

15. How does a PPO differ from an HMO?
   a. PPO members are not restricted to certain designated providers or hospitals.
   b. Deductible amounts do not apply.
   c. PPOs are paid through Social Security funds.
   d. Funding comes from state funds.
   e. None of the above

15 Diagnostic and Procedural Coding

CONTENTS

The process of insurance billing includes the accurate identification of the diagnostic, procedure, and service codes on the medical insurance claim form. Diagnostic codes are located in the *International Classification of Disease, Ninth Revision Clinical Modifications* (ICD-9-CM) listing. The procedure and service codes are located in the *Current Procedural Terminology* (CPT) listing. HIPAA requires correct coding of services and may sanction providers who do not comply with the rules. The medical assistant must understand how to code and bill with accuracy. For more information on HIPAA, see Chapter 10.

Diagnostic Coding

Based on the physician's evaluation, each patient will be diagnosed in medical terms. These medical terms are converted into numeric and alphanumeric diagnosis codes. The diagnosis codes are systematically classified in the ICD, which is published by a specialized agency of the United Nations known as the World Health Organization (WHO).

ICD-9

The ICD-9 contains more than 17,000 diagnosis codes and contains three volumes of information.

ICD-9 VOLUMES

Volume I	Also known as the Tabular List Contains 17 chapters of disease and injury codes Supplementary classifications for V and E codes Has five appendices Codes arranged in numerical order
Volume II	Also known as the Alphabetic Index Lists the same diseases and injuries found in Volume I in alphabetical order Contains an index of poisoning and adverse effects of chemicals and drugs and an index of injuries caused by external effects, such as accidents
Volume III	Deals with inpatient diagnosis and treatment Used to code inpatient hospital-billed procedures Not used in most ambulatory care settings, such as physicians' offices

Steps in Coding

Diagnoses are given a three-digit main code. The fourth and fifth digits are required for certain conditions that define the code to a higher level of specificity. The coding procedure is as follows:

1. Locate the diagnosis (or diagnoses) in the patient's medical chart.
2. Begin with Volume II, the Alphabetic Index, where diagnoses and conditions are listed alphabetically by condition, not body system. Once the diagnosis or condition is found, be sure to read all cross references and any additional information provided to help in determining the correct code. Once the code is found, note the three- to five-digit code associated with the diagnosis or condition.
3. Next, turn to the numeric index (Volume I, Tabular List) and find the code number noted in Volume II. After reading the description, determine whether the code noted is the correct one.
4. The diagnosis may need greater specification that requires an additional fourth or fifth digit. The additional digits provide more specificity. Be sure to read all of the information associated with that particular diagnosis to ensure that the correct diagnosis has been chosen.

   Special notes and symbols used in ICD-9-CM coding, such as "not otherwise specified (NOS)," are listed as reference material in the code books and should be used only when a higher level of specificity is not available.
5. Record the diagnostic code on the insurance claim form.

Primary Diagnosis

The primary diagnosis represents the patient's major health problem for that particular visit. Asking "why was the patient seen today?" will help determine the primary diagnosis for that particular visit.

Determining the primary diagnosis is important when you file an insurance claim for a patient who has more than one diagnosis. A patient may have hypertension and is seen for an acute problem such as otitis media. The otitis media would be the primary diagnosis.

V Codes

The ICD-9 coding system allows for visits (V codes) not directly related to the patient's illness or injury. V codes may be used in the following ways:

- They may add supportive information to the patient or family history.
- They may be used as a primary code to describe a person who may not have a current illness but who is seeing the physician for well-baby care, birth control advice, pregnancy test, or immunizations.
- They are used as supportive information when some circumstance or problem is present, such as an allergy to penicillin.

E Codes

The ICD-9 coding system also allows the use of E codes to describe external causes of injury and poisoning or adverse effects (Figure 15-1). Examples include falls, fire, motor vehicle accidents, and poisioning.

The following guidelines must be followed when using E codes:

- They should not be used as primary or principal diagnoses (they do not stand alone).
- They are used as additional information to help support a particular diagnosis and further define the cause of a poisoning or adverse effect, such as therapeutic use, attempted suicide, or accident.
- E codes (E930–E949) are mandatory when coding the use of drugs.

ABBREVIATIONS AND SYMBOLS Instructional notes such as abbreviations and symbols are included in the listings to guide the user on how to code accurately and precisely.

NEC	Not elsewhere classifiable
NOS	Not otherwise specified
[ ]	Brackets enclose synonyms, alternative terminology, or explanatory phrases.
( )	Parentheses enclose supplementary words (nonessential modifiers) that may be present in the narrative description of a disease without affecting the code assignment.
}	The brace encloses a series of terms, each of which is modified by the statement appearing to the right of the brace.
•	The bullet indicates a new code.
♦	Indicates a revision in the Tabular List and a code change in the Alphabetic Index
➤ ➤	Indicates revised text
Boldface type	Used for all codes and titles in the Tabular List
Italic type	Used for all exclusion notes and to identify codes that should not be used for describing the primary diagnosis

ICD-10

The U.S. Department of Health and Human Services has established a deadline of October 1, 2013, when diagnostic coding will be completed using the *International Classification of Diseases, Tenth Revision* (ICD-10).

The diagnosis codes in the ICD-10 have increased specificity and include recently discovered or diagnosed diseases. The ICD-10 has more than 140,000 codes as well as organizational and content modifications and new features. One significant change will be the identification of left versus right. Currently, with the ICD-9, there is no differentiation between the two.

Adoption of the ICD-10 code sets is expected to:

- Support value-based purchasing and Medicare's antifraud and abuse activities by accurately defining services and providing specific diagnosis and treatment information;
- Support comprehensive reporting of quality data;
- Ensure more accurate payments for new procedures, fewer rejected claims, improved disease management, and harmonization of disease monitoring and reporting worldwide; and
- Allow the United States to compare its data with international data to track the incidence and spread of disease and treatment outcomes because the United States is one of the few developed countries not using ICD-10.

E CODES

SUPPLEMENTARY CLASSIFICATION OF EXTERNAL CAUSES OF INJURY AND POISONING (E000-E999)

This section is provided to permit the classification of environmental events, circumstances, and conditions as the cause of injury, poisoning, and other adverse effects. Where a code from this section is applicable, it is intended that it shall be used in addition to a code from one of the main chapters of *ICD-9-CM*, indicating the nature of the condition. Certain other conditions which may be stated to be due to external causes are classified in Chapters 1 to 16 of *ICD-9-CM*. For these, the "E" code classification should be used for more detailed analysis.

Machinery accidents [other than those connected with transport] are classifiable to category E919, in which the fourth-digit allows a broad classification of the type of machinery involved.

Categories for "late effects" of accidents and other external causes are to be found at E929, E959, E969, E977, E989, and E999.

EXTERNAL CAUSE STATUS (E000)

Note: A code from category E000 should be used in conjunction with the external cause code(s) assigned to a record to indicate the status of the person at the time the event occurred. A single code from category E000 should be assigned for an encounter.

● E000 **External cause status**

● **E000.0 Civilian activity done for income or pay**
Civilian activity done for financial or other compensation
Excludes: *military activity (E000.1)*

● **E000.1 Military activity**
Excludes: *activity of off duty military personnel (E000.8)*

● E000.8 **Other external cause status**
Activity NEC
Hobby not done for income
Leisure activity
Off-duty activity of military personnel
Recreation or sport not for income or while a student
Student activity
Volunteer activity
Excludes: *civilian activity done for income or compensation (E000.0)*
military activity (E000.1)

● E000.9 **Unspecified external cause status**

ACTIVITY (E001-E030)

Note: Categories E001 to E030 are provided for use to indicate the activity of the person seeking healthcare for an injury or health condition, such as a heart attack while shoveling snow, which resulted from, or was contributed to, by the activity. These codes are appropriate for use for both acute injuries, such as those from chapter 17, and conditions that are due to the long-term, cumulative effects of an activity, such as those from chapter 13. They are also appropriate for use with external cause codes for cause and intent if identifying the activity provides additional information on the event.

These codes should be used in conjunction with other external cause codes for external cause status (E000) and place of occurrence (E849).

This section contains the following broad activity categories:
E001 Activities involving walking and running
E002 Activities involving water and water craft
E003 Activities involving ice and snow
E004 Activities involving climbing, rappelling, and jumping off
E005 Activities involving dancing and other rhythmic movement
E006 Activities involving other sports and athletics played individually
E007 Activities involving other sports and athletics played as a team or group
E008 Activities involving other specified sports and athletics
E009 Activity involving other cardiorespiratory exercise
E010 Activity involving other muscle strengthening exercises
E011 Activities involving computer technology and electronic devices
E012 Activities involving arts and handcrafts
E013 Activities involving personal hygiene and household maintenance
E014 Activities involving person providing caregiving
E015 Activities involving food preparation, cooking and grilling

707

Add 4th or 5th digit | Nonspecific code | Unspecified code | Manifestation code

FIGURE 15-1 An E-code section of the ICD-9-CM 2010.

Procedural Coding

Reimbursement from insurance companies is based on codes submitted for services rendered. The process of transforming a narrative description of procedures into numbers is referred to as *procedural coding*. The CPT manual provides a comprehensive list of procedure and service codes that is used to convert the narrative descriptions into a numerical code.

CPT CODING

CPT codes are reviewed and updated yearly by the American Medical Association. Utilizing codes from the most current edition of the CPT manual is essential for maximum reimbursement and clean claims.

The CPT manual is organized numerically or alphanumerically in sections according to classified types of service. The most commonly used codes are evaluation and management (E/M) services (office visits, consultations, the physician's component for emergency services and inpatient hospital care, etc.) and are located in the front of the book. Codes for anesthesia, surgery, radiology, pathology and laboratory, and miscellaneous medical services follow. Several appendices follow the numeric and alphabetical listings, including a complete list of all modifiers used in procedural coding along with descriptions, as well as a quick reference summary of codes that have been added, deleted, or revised.

Steps in Procedural Coding

Procedures are assigned a five-digit code.

1. To the highest level of certainty, begin by identifying what service was provided or what procedure was performed. You will find this information documented in the patient's chart.
2. Once you know what service was provided or what procedure was performed, look for the appropriate level of service or procedural term in the Alphabetic Index. Codes within this index are listed alphabetically by main term and modifying terms. Note the code associated with the narrative description of the procedure performed.
3. Look through the list of modifers to determine if one is needed.
4. Using the code noted from the Alphabetic Index, verify that it is correct by looking in the Tabular List.
5. Record the procedure code on the insurance claim form.

CPT MANUAL: EXAMPLES OF SECTIONS AND CODES

CPT Section	CPT Code
Evaluation and Management	99201–99499
Anesthesia	00100–01999
	99100–99140
Surgery	10021–69999
Radiology	70010–79999
Pathology and Laboratory	80048–89356
Medicine	90281–99199
	99500–99602

Evaluation and Management (E/M)

E/M is based on the following criteria:

- History of the patient
- Complexity of the examination
- Degree of difficulty in medical decision making

Of these three factors, medical decision making can be the most complex.

There are four levels of decision making with E/M:

- Straightforward
- Low complex
- Moderate complex
- High complex

The E/M codes are service oriented and designed to link the procedure or diagnosis with the amount of time it takes the physician to diagnose and treat the patient. It is important

COMMONLY USED CATEGORIES OF E/M CODES

Office (and Other Outpatient) Services	99201–99215
Hospital Observation Services	99217–99220
Hospital (Inpatient) Services	99221–99239
Consultations (Office)	99241–99245
Consultations (Inpatient)	99251–99255
Emergency Department Services	99281–99288
Pediatric Critical Care Patient Transport	99289, +99290
Critical Care Services	99291, +99292
Inpatient Pediatric and Neonatal Critical Care	99293–99300
Nursing Facility Services	99304–99318
Rest Home, Custodial Care, Domiciliary	99324–99337
Oversight Services for Domiciliary, Rest Home or Home	99339–99340
Home Services	99341–99350

Source: CPT 2008, Copyright 2008 American Medical Association. All rights reserved.

to understand that simply because a physician spent more time with the patient, this will not automatically cause the decision-making component to go to the next level.

For coding purposes, all patients are either established patients or new patients.

NEW AND ESTABLISHED PATIENTS

New Patient	Patient who has never been seen by anyone in the practice OR Has not been seen by anyone in the practice for more than three years
Established Patient	Patient who has been seen within the past three years by anyone in the practice

Modifiers

Modifiers are codes that report changes from the usual use of the code (e.g., a procedure that was done on both arms instead of only one). See Figure 15-2.

HCPCS CODING

To report services and procedures for Medicaid and Medicare patients, the Healthcare Common Procedure Coding System (HCPCS) is used. This system includes two coding levels: Level I and Level II.

HCPCS LEVELS

Level I	Provides the same codes as the CPT manual
Level II	Has codes that are not available in the CPT manual Twenty-two sections Five-digit alphanumeric codes Used for items that Medicare covers, such as durable medical equipment (DME), materials, supplies, and injections Level II codes begin with a letter, followed by four numbers (Figure 15-3) HCPCS modifiers consist of two letters and can be used in addition to CPT modifiers

Insurance Fraud

Fraud is an intentional representation that an individual knows to be false or does not believe to be true and makes, knowing that the representation could result in some unauthorized benefit to him- or herself or some other person. Insurance fraud is often committed within the Medicare system.

The most frequent kind of fraud arises from false statements or misrepresentations that claim to provide proof to entitlement or payment under the Medicare program. The violator may be a physician or another practitioner, a hospital or another institutional provider, a clinical laboratory or another supplier, an employee of any provider, a billing service, a beneficiary, a Medicare carrier employee, or any person in a position to file a claim for Medicare benefits.

Medicare uses a computerized system known as the Correct Coding Initiative (CCI) to help prevent overpayment for procedures.

Under the broad definition of fraud are other violations, including the offering or acceptance of kickbacks, upcoding, and unbundling.

OTHER VIOLATIONS

Kickback	Receiving or paying money in order to influence the referral of a Medicare or Medicaid patient
Upcoding	Using a higher-level code than the level of service provided in order to receive increased reimbursement
Unbundling	Billing separately for multiple services that would normally be covered under one code and one charge

Compliance

Every medical office should have a compliance plan. Offices without this plan may be at risk for liability issues. The compliance plan also demonstrates to the physician, fraud investigators, or insurance carriers that the medical office is attempting to locate and correct errors.

The following are basic components of an effective compliance plan:

- Conducting periodic audits of billing and coding practices
- Developing written standards and procedures for compliance
- Training and educating staff members on procedures
- Investigating violations and disclosing incidents to appropriate government agencies
- Discussing in staff meetings how to avoid erroneous or fraudulent conduct

Symbols

- ▲ Revised code
- • New code
- ▶◀ New or revised text
- ➲ Reference to *CPT Assistant, Clinical Examples in Radiology*, and *CPT Changes*
- ✚ Add-on code
- ⊘ Exemptions to modifier 51
- ⊙ Moderate sedation
- ⁄⁄ Product pending FDA approval
- ○ Reinstated or recycled code
- # Out-of-numerical sequence code

Modifiers (See Appendix A for Definitions)

22 Increased procedural services
23 Unusual anesthesia
24 Unrelated evaluation and management service by the same physician during a postoperative period
25 Significant, separately identifiable evaluation and management service by the same physician on the same day of the procedure or other service
26 Professional component
32 Mandated services
47 Anesthesia by surgeon
50 Bilateral procedure
51 Multiple procedures
52 Reduced services
53 Discontinued procedure
54 Surgical care only
55 Postoperative management only
56 Preoperative management only
57 Decision for surgery
58 Staged or related procedure or service by the same physician during the postoperative period
59 Distinct procedural service
62 Two surgeons
63 Procedure performed on infants less than 4 kgs
66 Surgical team
76 Repeat procedure or service by same physician
77 Repeat procedure or service by another physician
78 Unplanned return to the operating/procedure room by the same physician following initial procedure for a related procedure during the postoperative period
79 Unrelated procedure or service by the same physician during the postoperative period
80 Assistant surgeon
81 Minimum assistant surgeon
82 Assistant surgeon (when qualified resident surgeon not available)
90 Reference (outside) laboratory
91 Repeat clinical diagnostic laboratory test
92 Alternative laboratory platform testing
99 Multiple modifiers

Anesthesia Physical Status Modifiers

P1 A normal healthy patient
P2 A patient with mild systemic disease
P3 A patient with severe systemic disease
P4 A patient with severe systemic disease that is a constant threat to life
P5 A moribund patient who is not expected to survive without the operation
P6 A declared brain-dead patient whose organs are being removed for donor purposes

Modifiers Approved for Hospital Outpatient Use Level I (CPT)

25 Significant, separately identifiable evaluation and management service by the same physician on the same day of the procedure or other service
27 Multiple outpatient hospital E/M encounters on the same date
50 Bilateral procedure
52 Reduced services
58 Staged or related procedure or service by the same physician during the postoperative period
59 Distinct procedural service
73 Discontinued outpatient hospital/ambulatory surgical center (ASC) procedure prior to the administration of anesthesia
74 Discontinued outpatient hospital/ambulatory surgical center (ASC) procedure after the administration of anesthesia
76 Repeat procedure or service by same physician
77 Repeat procedure by another physician
78 Unplanned return to the operating/procedure room for a related procedure during the postoperative period
79 Unrelated procedure or service by the same physician during the postoperative period
91 Repeat clinical diagnostic laboratory test

Level II (HCPCS/National)

LT Left side (used to identify procedures performed on the left side of the body)
RT Right side (used to identify procedures performed on the right side of the body)
BL Special acquisition of blood and blood products
CA Procedure payable only in the inpatient setting when performed emergently on an outpatient who expires prior to admission
CR Catastrophe/disaster related
E1 Upper left, eyelid
E2 Lower left, eyelid
E3 Upper right, eyelid
E4 Lower right, eyelid
FA Left hand, thumb
F1 Left hand, second digit
F2 Left hand, third digit
F3 Left hand, fourth digit
F4 Left hand, fifth digit
F5 Right hand, thumb
F6 Right hand, second digit
F7 Right hand, third digit
F8 Right hand, fourth digit
F9 Right hand, fifth digit
FB Item provided without cost to provider, supplier or practitioner, or full credit received for replaced device (examples, but not limited to covered under warranty, replaced due to defect, free samples)
FC Partial credit received for replaced device
GA Waiver of liability statement on file
GG Performance and payment of a screening mammogram and diagnostic mammogram on the same patient, same day
GH Diagnostic mammogram converted from screening mammogram on same day
LC Left circumflex, coronary artery
LD Left anterior descending coronary artery
RC Right coronary artery
Q0 Investigational clinical service provided in a clinical research study that is in an approved clinical research study
Q1 Routine clinical service provided in a clinical research study that is in an approved clinical research study
QM Ambulance service provided under arrangement by a provider of services
QN Ambulance service furnished directly by a provider of services
TA Left foot, great toe
T1 Left foot, second digit
T2 Left foot, third digit
T3 Left foot, fourth digit
T4 Left foot, fifth digit
T5 Right foot, great toe
T6 Right foot, second digit
T7 Right foot, third digit
T8 Right foot, fourth digit
T9 Right foot, fifth digit

FIGURE 15-2 Modifier page from the CPT.

MEDICAL AND SURGICAL SUPPLIES

A4212 Non-coring needle or stylet with or without catheter

A4213 Syringe, sterile, 20cc or greater, each

A4215 Needle, sterile, any size, each

A4216 Sterile water, saline and/or dextrose (diluent/flush), 10 ml
MCM: 2049

A4217 Sterile water/saline, 500 ml
MCM: 2049

A4218 Sterile saline or water, metered dose dispenser, 10 ml

A4220 Refill kit for implantable infusion pump
CIM: 60-14

A4221 Supplies for maintenance of drug infusion catheter, per week (list drug separately)

A4222 Infusion supplies for external drug infusion pump, per cassette or bag (list drugs separately)

A4223 Infusion supplies not used with external infusion pump, per cassette or bag (list drugs separately)

A4230 Infusion set for external insulin pump, non needle cannula type
CIM: 60-14

A4231 Infusion set for external insulin pump, needle type
CIM: 60-14

A4232 Syringe with needle for external insulin pump, sterile, 3cc
CIM: 60-14

A4233 Replacement battery, alkaline (other than j cell), for use with medically necessary home blood glucose monitor owned by patient, each

A4234 Replacement battery, alkaline, j cell, for use with medically necessary home blood glucose monitor owned by patient, each

A4235 Replacement battery, lithium, for use with medically necessary home blood glucose monitor owned by patient, each

Not valid for Medicare | Non-covered by Medicare | Special coverage instructions | Carrier discretion

19

FIGURE 15-3 HCPCS Level II page.

The Health and Human Services Office of Inspector General (OIG) provides compliance guidance for fraud prevention and detection.

CODE LINKAGE

When completing the health insurance claim form, it is critical for the diagnosis to be related to the procedure. An example of code linkage would be a diagnosis of diabetes mellitus and a glucose tolerance test. However, a diagnosis of hypertension and a procedure to remove five skin tags cannot be linked in a health insurance claim form because there is no connection between the patient's diagnosis and the procedure the physician performed. Coding inaccuracies such as this can result in minor to severe penalties.

15 APPLICATION

Directions: Select the best answer for each of the following questions. Check your answers in the Answer Key at the end of the book.

1. The ninth revision of the *International Classification of Disease* (ICD-9) contains ____ volumes of information.
   a. three
   b. nine
   c. two
   d. five
   e. six

2. An index of poisoning and adverse effects of chemicals and drugs is found in ______________of the ICD-9.
   a. Volume II
   b. Volume III
   c. Volume V
   d. Volume VI
   e. Volume IX

3. The first step in diagnostic coding is:
   a. Record the diagnostic code on the insurance claim form.
   b. Note the three- to five-digit code associated with the diagnosis found in the ICD-9.
   c. Locate the diagnosis in the patient's medical chart.
   d. Phone the patient's insurance provider.
   e. None of the above.

4. The following is/are true of V codes:
   a. Used as additional information to help support a particular diagnosis
   b. Add supportive information to the patient or family history
   c. Are interchangeable with E codes
   d. Used as supportive information when a drug allergy is present
   e. A and D

5. Which family of diagnostic codes is mandatory when coding the use of drugs?
   a. V codes
   b. E codes
   c. M codes
   d. E and M codes
   e. It depends on the facility in which the patient is seen.

6. ICD-10 has an establishment deadline of October 1, 2013. The ICD-10 code sets are expected to:
   a. Support Medicare's antifraud and abuse activities
   b. Allow the United States to compare its data with international data to track the incidence and spread of disease
   c. Support comprehensive reporting of quality data
   d. All of the above
   e. B and C only

7. The ______ manual provides a comprehensive list of procedure and service codes used to convert the narrative descriptions of procedures into a numerical code.
   a. ICD-9
   b. ICD-10
   c. V code
   d. CPT
   e. E code

8. Which of the following is an example of an E/M code?
   a. 99213
   b. 992.13
   c. V76.2
   d. 235.6
   e. 10021

9. E/M is based on what criteria?
   a. The patient's insurance plan and medical history
   b. The complexity of the examination and the insurance plan
   c. The complexity of the examination and the history of the patient
   d. Whether the patient is covered by a PPO or an HMO
   e. C and D

10. Basic components of a medical office effective compliance plan include:
   a. Conducting periodic audits of billing and coding practices
   b. Billing separately for multiple services normally covered under one code
   c. Training and educating staff members on procedures
   d. All of the above
   e. A and C

11. Which of the following symbols indicates a new code in the ICD-9?
   a. { }
   b. ( )
   c. •
   d. ▸◂
   e. ◆

12. Which of the following is not one of the four levels of decision making with E/M?
   a. Straighforward
   b. Low complex
   c. Moderate complex
   d. High complex
   e. Extremely complex

13. The HCPCS is used to report services and procedures for which of the following groups of patients?
   a. Medicare
   b. HMO
   c. Medicaid
   d. A and B
   e. A and C

14. Which of the following is not true about the HCPCS Level II codes?
   a. The codes available are the same as those in the CPT manual
   b. Used for DME
   c. Begin with a letter followed by four numbers
   d. Modifiers consist of two letters
   e. None of the above

15. Which of the following is the correct definition for unbundling?
   a. Using a higher-level code than the level of service provided
   b. Billing separately for multiple services that would normally be covered with one code
   c. Receiving money to influence a Medicare referral
   d. Failure of the diagnosis to support the procedure
   e. Coding at a lower level than documented in order to avoid accusation of fraud

Section 5 Clinical Competencies and Skills

16 Blood-Borne Pathogens and Infection Control

CONTENTS

Pathogens are disease-causing organisms that are transmitted in a variety of ways, including skin-to-skin contact, airborne droplet nuclei, body fluids, and blood (Figure 16-1). It is important that the medical assistant has a clear understanding of how easily all pathogens can be spread from one person to another and the actions that must be taken in order to minimize those transmissions.

Microorganisms

Microorganisms are tiny living substances that can be seen only with the aid of a microscope and are found on the skin and in the urinary, gastrointestinal, and respiratory tracts. These microorganisms, known as *normal flora*, do not cause disease as long as they are not transferred to other areas of the body. For example, when *Escherichia coli* normally found in the gastrointestinal tract enters the urinary tract, it results in a urinary tract infection.

Microbiology is the study of microorganisms.

MICROBIOLOGY STUDY AREAS

Bacteriology	Study of bacteria
Mycology	Study of fungi
Protozoology	Study of protozoa
Virology	Study of viruses

GROWTH

In order for microorganisms to grow, they must have all of the following:

- Food
- Moisture
- Suitable temperature
- Darkness

Some types of microorganisms require oxygen in order to grow and are known as *aerobes*; others do not need oxygen in order to grow and are know as *anaerobes*.

TRANSMISSION

In order to prevent the spread of infection, asepsis must be adhered to. This is true within the medical office, but it is especially true within the hospital setting in order to prevent the spread of *nosocomial infections*, defined as those infections that are acquired while in a medical facility that were not present when the patient entered the facility.

In order for infection to occur, several factors known as the chain of infection must be present. See the table on the next page.

If the preceding chain is broken at any point in the process, an infection will not occur. However, if the chain is not broken and the new host is susceptible, the process begins again, only the new host has now become the reservoir host. See the table that describes the stages of the infection process on the next page. Box 16-1 describes how microorganisms are transmitted.

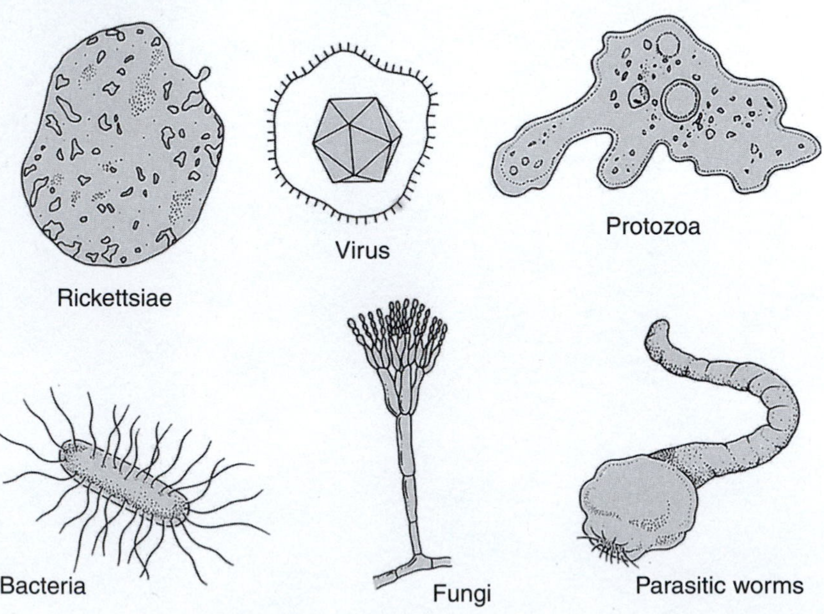

FIGURE 16-1 Pathogens.

CONDITIONS REQUIRED FOR BACTERIAL GROWTH

Condition	Explanation
Moisture	Bacteria grow best in moist areas: skin, mucous membranes, wet dressings, wounds, dirty instruments.
Temperature	Bacteria thrive at body temperature (98.6°F). Low temperatures (32°F and below) retard, but do not kill, bacterial growth. A temperature of 107°F and higher will kill most bacteria.
Oxygen	Aerobic bacteria require an oxygen supply to live. Anaerobic bacteria can survive without oxygen.
Light	Darkness favors the growth of most bacteria. Some bacteria will die if exposed to direct sunlight or light.

THE CHAIN OF INFECTION

1. Infected Reservoir Host	An individual is infected with a pathogen. The individual provides nourishment for the pathogen, allowing it to grow. *Example:* someone infected with the influenza virus
2. Portal of Exit	The infected reservoir host must have a portal of exit, i.e., a means of allowing the pathogen to escape. Portals of exit may be the respiratory, gastrointestinal, urinary, and reproductive tracts, blood, mucous membranes, or an open wound.
3. Means of Transmission	In order for the pathogen to travel from the reservoir host to the new host, the pathogen must have a means of getting from one individual to another through either direct or indirect contact. *Example of indirect contact:* The influenza-infected reservoir host sneezes on a bus. *Example of direct contact:* The influenza-infected reservoir host kisses the new host.
4. Portal of Entry Into New Host	The new host must have a portal of entry by which the pathogen can enter. In the above examples, this would occur either by inhaling the droplet nuclei excreted via the sneeze OR through the mouth via the kiss. The portals of entry are the same as those listed above as portals of exit.
5. Susceptible New Host	In order for the new host to be susceptible, he or she must be unable to fight off the infection. Susceptibility may be caused by poor nutrition, hygiene, or health. Stress may also be a factor.

STAGES OF THE INFECTION PROCESS

Stage	Description
Invasion	The pathogen enters the body through the portal of entry: respiratory, digestive, reproductive, or urinary tracts and skin.
Multiplication	The pathogen reproduces.
Incubation Period	This may vary from several days to months or years, during which time the disease is developing but no symptoms appear.
Prodromal Period	First mild signs and symptoms appear; this is a highly contagious period.
Acute Period	Signs and symptoms are evident and most severe.
Recovery Period	Signs and symptoms begin to subside.

Box 16-1 The Transmission of Microorganisms

- Vector transmission: Parasitic insects carry disease via animals. An example is Lyme disease, which is carried by a tick commonly found on deer.
- Airborne transmission: Microorganisms are moved through the air on dust particles. Examples include rubeola and varicella viruses and *Myco-bacterium tuberculosis*.
- Droplet transmission: The moist droplets from sneezing, coughing, and talking transfer pathogenic microorganisms. Respiratory infections such as the common cold and influenza are spread by droplet transmission.
- Indirect contact, also known as common vehicle transmission: Microorganisms are transferred to a susceptible host by physical contact or by touching a contaminated object such as a food tray, faucets, or equipment. HIV (human immunodeficiency virus) may be transferred from a contaminated needle to the puncture site.
- Direct contact: There is direct contact between an infected area and another skin surface or mucous membrane. Medical personnel are required to wash their hands between patients to avoid skin-to-skin transmission of microorganisms such as *Staphylococcus aureus*.

Source: Medical Assisting: Foundations and Practices by M. S. Frazier, C. Malone, and C. Morgan, Upper Saddle River, NJ: Pearson Education, Inc., 2010, p. 462. Reprinted with permission.

INFLAMMATORY PROCESS

When the body is invaded by a pathogen, there may be an inflammatory response. The four cardinal signs of inflammation and the body's response are found in the adjacent table.

ACUTE INFLAMMATORY PROCESS

Cardinal Sign	The Body's Response
Redness	Leukocytosis
Heat	Fever
Swelling/Edema	Increased pulse rate
Pain	Increased respiration rate
Stiffness	—

BLOOD-BORNE PATHOGENS

Blood-borne pathogens are disease-causing microorganisms that are spread from one individual to another via contact with the infected individual's blood.

MOST COMMON BLOOD-BORNE DISEASES

Acquired immunodeficiency syndrome	Also known as *AIDS* Fatal form of opportunistic illnesses and infections linked to HIV
AIDS-related complex	Also known as *ARC* Syndrome that occurs with HIV-positive individuals, but lacks opportunistic infections and cancers
Hepatitis	Inflammation and infection of the liver, most commonly caused by a virus Symptoms may include fever, loss of appetite, jaundice, nausea, vomiting, malaise, and dark urine
Hepatitis A	Also known as *acute infective hepatitis* Inflammation of the liver caused by the hepatitis A virus (HAV) Transmitted via fecal-oral contamination
Hepatitis B	Inflammation of the liver caused by the hepatitis B virus (HBV) Transmitted via contact with blood and/or body fluids Vaccine available

(*Continued*)

Hepatitis C	Chronic disease of the liver caused by the hepatitis C virus (HCV) Previously known as *non-A and non-B hepatitis* Transmitted primarily through transfusion or sharing of needles Most common form of new hepatitis cases annually
Hepatitis D	Also known as *delta hepatitis* Inflammation of the liver caused by the hepatitis D virus (HDV) Symptoms can be more severe than those of other forms of hepatitis
Hepatitis E	Acute infection of the liver Found mostly in developing countries with poor sanitary conditions Transmitted via food contaminated with human feces
Hepatitis G	Inflammation of the liver Transmitted via needlesticks or contaminated blood
Human immunodeficiency virus	Also known as *HIV* Virus that causes AIDS Enters the body by one of the following methods: • Vaginal, anal, or oral intercourse with an infected individual • Sharing needles • Transfusion of blood from an infected donor • Organ transplant from an infected donor • Transferred from an infected mother to the unborn child • Transferred from an infected mother to the infant via breast milk

MULTIDRUG-RESISTANT ORGANISMS

Bacteria and other pathogens that have developed resistance to antimicrobial drugs are known as *multidrug-resistant organisms* (MRDOs).

COMMON MRDOs

Methicillin-resistant *Staphylococcus aureus*	Also known as *MRSA* Organism highly resistant to antibiotics A form of staphylococcus that has evolved over time as a result of overuse of antibiotics Can either be hospital acquired or community acquired
Vancomycin-Resistant Enterococci	Also known as *VRE* Form of enterococci (bacteria) normally found in the gastrointestinal tract and the female genital tract that is resistant to vancomycin Enterococci infections are one of the most common nosocomial infections.
Multidrug-Resistant Tuberculosis	Also known as *MDR TB* Form of tuberculosis that is resistant to the medications normally used to treat TB

Immunity

The body has a built-in defense mechanism against disease known as *immunity* that can either be acquired or genetic. Acquired immunity involves antibodies that are either acquired passively or actively. Genetic immunity does not involve antibodies, is passed on genetically, and protects against diseases found in other species.

ACQUIRED IMMUNITY

Type of Immunity	Description
Active Acquired Natural	Acquired by having the disease, which results in production of antibodies and "memory cells" that respond when the antigen reappears
Active Acquired Artificial	Acquired by administration of a vaccine that stimulates production of antibodies and memory cells to prevent the disease from occurring
Passive Acquired Natural	Acquired from someone else's antibodies, such as via passage from the mother to the fetus through either the placenta or breast milk
Passive Acquired Artificial	Temporary protection acquired from gamma globulin *Examples:* tetanus immune globulin, rabies antiserum

Infection Control

Figure 16-2 outlines the Centers for Disease Control (CDC)–recommended Standard Precautions for infection control.

ASEPSIS

Asepsis is defined as maintaining an environment that is free from germs, infection, and any form of microbial life. There are two forms of asepsis: medical and surgical. Medical asepsis is primarily concerned with keeping things clean but not necessarily sterile. By contrast, surgical asepsis requires sterile technique.

Proper handwashing is one of the first lines of defense and one of the most important ways to prevent transmission of disease (see Procedures 16-1 and 16-2). Hands should be washed before and after the following:

- Physical contact with patients
- Donning gloves
- Performing procedures
- Handling specimens or other contaminated surfaces
- Blowing your nose
- Sneezing
- Coughing
- Taking breaks
- Eating

SANITIZATION

Sanitization keeps bacteria from growing but does not destroy microorganisms. Sanitization involves careful scrubbing of equipment and instruments with a brush and detergent, rinsing in hot water, and then air drying. This method would be used for cleaning the exam rooms.

Ultrasound can also be used to sanitize instruments, as the sound waves loosen contaminants. The instruments are then rinsed with water and left to air dry.

COMPARISON OF MEDICAL AND SURGICAL ASEPSIS

Medical Asepsis	Surgical Asepsis
Reduces or controls the numbers of microorganisms	Removes all microorganisms from an object or surface
Follows clean technique—using clean equipment and supplies	Follows sterile technique—using sterile equipment and supplies
Hands are washed or clean gloves worn before supplies and equipment are handled	Surgical scrub performed and sterile gloves donned before supplies and equipment are handled
Equipment and supplies placed on clean field	Equipment and supplies placed on sterile field
Used for noninvasive procedures such as taking vital signs	Used for invasive procedures such as suturing and endoscopic procedures

Source: Medical Assisting: Foundations and Practices by M. S. Frazier, C. Malone, and C. Morgan, Upper Saddle River, NJ: Pearson Education, Inc., 2010, p. 479. Reprinted with permission.

Hand Washing

- ☒ Wash hands after touching blood, body fluids, secretions, excretions, and contaminated items, whether or not gloves are worn.
- ☒ Wash hands immediately after gloves are removed, between patient contacts, and when otherwise indicated to avoid transfer of microorganisms to other patients or environments. It may be necessary to wash hands between tasks and procedures on the same patient to prevent cross-contamination of different body sites.
- ☒ Use a plain soap for routine hand washing.
- ☒ Use an antimicrobial agent for specific circumstances, as defined by the infection-control program.

Gloves

- ☒ Wear gloves when touching blood, body fluids, secretions, excretions, and contaminated items.
- ☒ Put on clean gloves just before touching mucous membranes and nonintact skin.
- ☒ Change gloves between tasks and procedures on the same patient after contact with material that may contain a high concentration of microorganisms.
- ☒ Remove gloves promptly after use, before touching noncontaminated items and environmental surfaces, and before treating another patient.

Mask, Eye Protection, Face Shield

- ☒ Wear a mask and eye protection or a face shield to protect mucous membranes of the eyes, nose, and mouth during procedures and patient-care activities that are likely to generate splashes or sprays of blood, body fluids, secretions, and excretions.

Gown

- ☒ Wear a gown to protect skin and to prevent soiling of clothing during procedures and patient care activities that are likely to generate splashes or sprays of blood, body fluids, secretions, or excretions.
- ☒ Remove a soiled gown as promptly as possible.

Patient-Care Equipment

- ☒ Handle used patient care equipment soiled with blood, body fluids, secretions, and excretions in a manner that prevents skin and mucous membrane exposures, contamination of clothing, and transfer of microorganisms to other patients and environments.
- ☒ Ensure that reusable equipment is not used for the care of another patient until it has been cleaned and reprocessed appropriately.
- ☒ Ensure that single-use items are discarded properly.

Environmental Control

- ☒ Ensure that the facility has adequate procedures for the routine care, cleaning, and disinfection of environmental surfaces, beds, bedrails, bedside equipment, and other frequently touched surfaces.

Linen

- ☒ Handle, transport, and process used linen soiled with blood, body fluids, secretions, and excretions in a manner that prevents skin and mucous membrane exposures and contamination of clothing.

Occupational Health and Bloodborne Pathogens

- ☒ Take care to prevent injuries when using needles, scalpels, and other sharp instruments or devices; when handling sharp instruments after procedures; when cleaning used instruments; and when disposing of used needles.
- ☒ Never recap used needles, or otherwise manipulate them using both hands or use any other technique that involves directing the point of a needle toward any part of the body.
- ☒ Do not remove used needles from disposable syringes by hand, and do not bend, break, or otherwise manipulate used needles by hand.
- ☒ Place used disposable syringes and needles, scalpel blades, and other sharp items in appropriate puncture-resistant containers.
- ☒ Use mouthpieces, resuscitation bags, or other ventilation devices as alternatives to mouth-to-mouth resuscitation methods in areas where the need for resuscitation is predictable.

Patient Placement

- ☒ Place a patient who contaminates the environment or who does not or cannot be expected to assist in maintaining appropriate hygiene or environmental control in a private room.

FIGURE 16-2 CDC-recommended Standard Precautions.

procedure 16-1

PROCEDURE FOR CORRECT HANDWASHING

Objective: With the necessary materials you will be able to wash your hands following medically aseptic technique.

EQUIPMENT AND SUPPLIES

- soap (bar or pump)
- paper towels
- waste container
- nail brush or cuticle stick

METHOD

1. Remove and secure most jewelry. Wedding bands and professional watches are allowed. Push the watch higher than your wrist. Avoid touching the contaminated sink front with your uniform.
2. With a paper towel, turn on the water and adjust to a warm temperature. The water should run continuously until you have finished the procedure. Discard the paper towel.
3. With your hands and fingers lower than your elbows, wet your wrists and hands.
4. Apply soap and scrub lather over the hands and fingers, between the fingers, under and around the nails, and rinse. Apply soap and lather to the wrists and forearms. The purpose of this washing order is to wash the dirtiest areas first. A circular motion and friction rubbing will loosen dirt and microorganisms. If you are using bar soap, rinse it before returning it to the soap dish.
5. Use the cuticle stick or nail brush to clean your nails. If you are wearing a wedding band, scrub around it with the nail brush.
6. Rinse off the lather, keeping your hands in a downward position. Avoid splashing and touching the sink or faucets.
7. Dry your hands with a paper towel and discard it.
8. Turn off the faucet with another paper towel and discard it. Using a new paper towel prevents the contamination of clean hands.

CHARTING EXAMPLE

01/22/xx 0900 Discussed with patient that hand washing would reduce germs that she could give to family members while she is recovering from pneumonia. Patient performed return demonstration and stated that she didn't want other family members to get sick. · · · · · · Alexis Smith, CMA (AAMA)

Source: Medical Assisting: Foundations and Practices by M. S. Frazier, C. Malone, and C. Morgan, Upper Saddle River, NJ: Pearson Education, Inc., 2010, p. 470. Reprinted with permission.

procedure 16-2

DEMONSTRATE A STERILE SCRUB (SURGICAL HAND WASHING)

Objective: With the necessary supplies, you will be able to perform surgical hand washing using sterile technique correctly.

EQUIPMENT AND SUPPLIES

- Germicidal liquid soap in dispenser
- Large wall clock
- Sink with hand, knee, or foot on/off controls
- Sterile towel packet
- Sterile scrub sponge
- Orangewood stick or nail file

METHOD

1. Without touching the inside, open the sterile towel packet some distance from potential water spray.

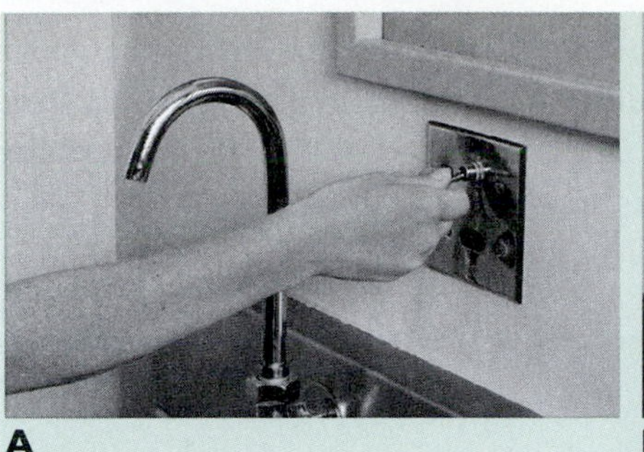
A

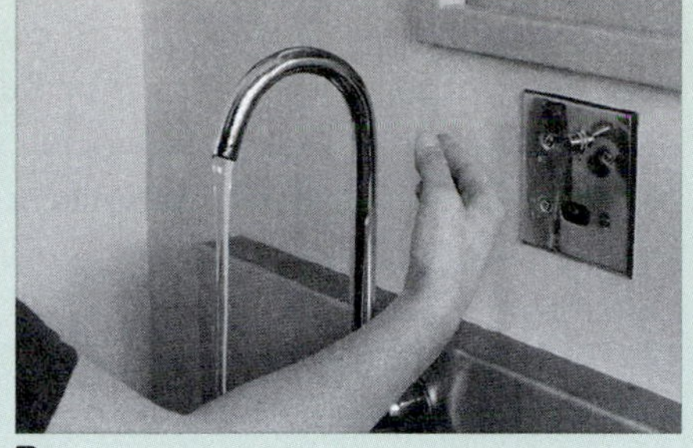
B

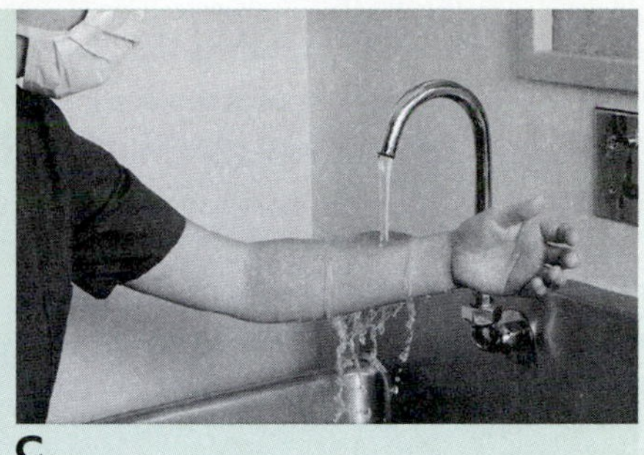
C

FIGURE 16-3 (A) Turn on the water with the hand, knee, or foot controls. (B) Adjust the temperature. (C) Wet your arms from the fingertips to the elbows.

2. Remove all jewelry from your hands and wrists. Use an orangewood stick or nail file to remove dirt from under your fingernails.
3. Turn on the water with hand, knee, or foot controls and adjust the temperature. Wet your arm from the fingertips to the elbows (Figure 16-3).
4. Apply liquid soap to your hands and lower arms. For 5 minutes, use a circular motion to create lather, starting from the fingertips and working toward and including the elbows (Figure 16-4). Be sure to wash between the fingers and under the fingernails.
5. Rinse the lather from your arms, beginning at the fingertips and proceeding to the elbows. Keep your hands above your elbows.
6. Repeat the process, applying liquid soap to your hands and lower arms. Scrub from the fingertips to the elbows with the sponge for 3 minutes (Figure 16-5).
7. Rinse thoroughly and leave the water running. Use a sterile towel to dry your hands (Figure 16-6).
8. Use the towel to turn off a hand-controlled faucet or, if necessary, use your elbow. Otherwise release the foot pedal or move the knee control to turn off the water.

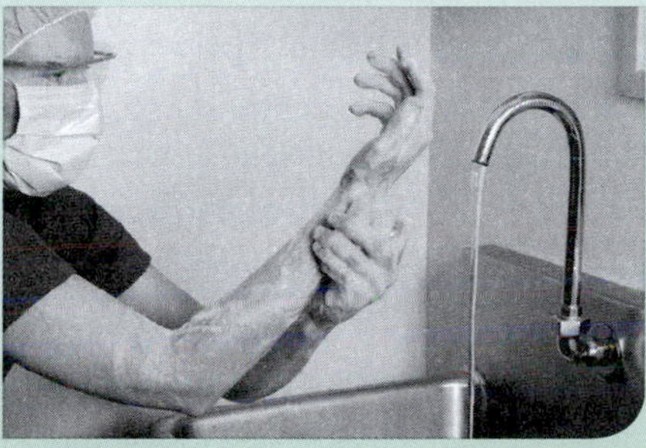

FIGURE 16-5 Scrub from the fingertips to the elbows with the sponge for 3 minutes.

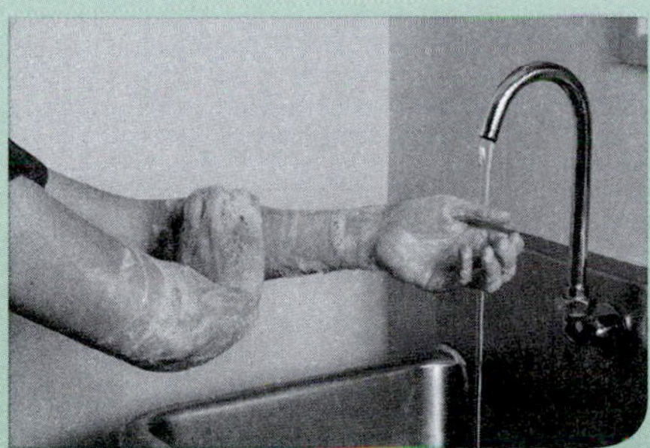

FIGURE 16-4 Use a circular motion to create lather, starting from the fingertips and working toward and including the elbows.

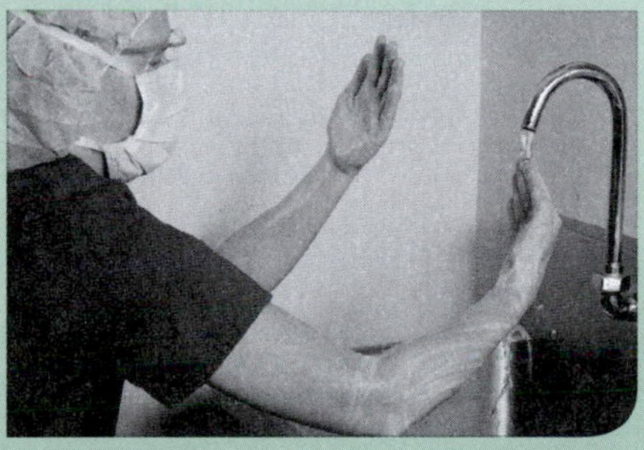

FIGURE 16-6 Rinse thoroughly and leave water running.

Source: Medical Assisting: Foundations and Practices by M. S. Frazier, C. Malone, and C. Morgan, Upper Saddle River, NJ: Pearson Education, Inc., 2010, p. 493. Reprinted with permission.

DISINFECTION

Disinfection destroys or inhibits the growth of pathogens; however, it does not kill spores and some viruses. Information regarding the different types of disinfectant methods that may be used and disinfection methods are shown below.

STERILIZATION

Sterilization is defined as being free of all microorganisms. Items must be sanitized and/or disinfected prior to sterilizing. Sterilization methods are shown below, and sterilization time requirements are shown on the next page.

THREE LEVELS OF DISINFECTION

Low-Level Disinfection	Kills most bacteria and viruses Used on exam tables, countertops, and walls
Intermediate-Level Disinfection	Kills mycobacteria and most viruses and bacteria Used on items that come in contact with skin, but not mucous membranes, such as stethoscopes and blood pressure cuffs
High-Level Disinfection	Kills all microorganisms except bacterial spores Used on items that may come in contact with mucous membranes, such as sigmoidoscopes and glass thermometers

DISINFECTION METHODS

Method	Description and Use
Alcohol (70% Isopropyl)	Used for skin surfaces, equipment such as stethoscopes and thermometers, and table surfaces Causes damage to rubber products, lenses, and plastic Flammable
Chlorine (Sodium Hypochlorite or Bleach)	Use in a dilution of 1:10 (1 part bleach to 10 parts water) Used to eliminate a broad spectrum of microorganisms Has a corrosive effect on instruments, rubber, and plastic products Can cause skin irritation Inexpensive
Formaldehyde	Used to disinfect and sterilize Dangerous product that is regulated by OSHA; must have clearly marked labels
Hydrogen Peroxide	Effective disinfectant for use only on nonhuman surfaces and products May damage rubber, plastics, and metals
Glutaraldehyde	Effective against viruses, bacteria, fungi, and some spores Regulated by OSHA; must have clearly marked labels and be used only in a well-ventilated area Gloves and masks must be worn when using it.

METHODS THAT CAN BE USED TO ACHIEVE STERILIZATION

Steam and Pressure Sterilization	Also known as *autoclaving* Use of steam and pressure to destroy microorganisms on items within the autoclave Most common in the medical office and used to sterilize metal instruments and dressings
Dry Heat Sterilization	Use of dry heat to sterilize items that may be harmed or destroyed by steam, such as needles and other sharps
Chemical Sterilization	Used when steam/pressure sterilization or dry heat sterilization are not appropriate options

STERILIZATION TIME REQUIREMENTS

Time	Article
15 Minutes	Glassware Metal instruments—open tray or individual wrapping with hinges open Syringes (unassembled) Needles
20 Minutes	Instruments—partial metal in double-thickness wrapper or covered tray Rubber products: gloves, tubing, wrapped or unwrapped catheters Solutions in a flask (50–100 mL)
30 Minutes	Dressings—small packs in paper or muslin Solutions in a flask (500–1000 mL) Syringes—unassembled, individually wrapped in gauze Syringes—unassembled, individually wrapped in glass tubes Needles—individually packaged in paper or glass tubes Sutures—wrapped in paper or muslin Instrument and treatment trays—wrapped in paper or muslin Gauze—loosely packed
60 Minutes	Petroleum jelly—in dry heat

OSHA BLOOD-BORNE PATHOGENS STANDARDS AND STANDARD PRECAUTIONS

Medical offices must follow the OSHA regulations for handling contaminated materials. These regulations are available from the U.S. Department of Labor in Washington, D.C. OSHA rules and regulations govern all free-standing healthcare facilities and ensure protection from contracting a contagious disease from any body fluids that may be handled by healthcare workers.

OSHA requires that each medical office have a written Exposure Control Plan to assist in minimizing employee exposure to infectious materials. This plan must be reviewed by all office staff and updated annually.

MANDATORY COMPONENTS OF AN EXPOSURE CONTROL PLAN

Exposure Determination	Listing of job classifications within the office to determine at-risk employees (those with potential exposure to infectious materials)
Method of Compliance	Specific measures to reduce the risk of exposure
Postexposure	Evaluation and follow-up, which specify the steps to follow when an exposure incident occurs

PENALTIES FOR FAILURE TO COMPLY WITH THE OSHA BLOOD-BORNE PATHOGEN STANDARDS

Type of Violation	Violation Defined	Penalty for Violation
Other Than Serious	Directly related to health and safety and on the job, but would not likely cause death or serious harm/injury	Up to $7000 per violation
Serious	Substantial likelihood that death or serious physical harm will occur, and the employer knew or should have known about the hazard	Mandatory $7000 per violation
Willful	Committed intentionally and knowingly	Up to $70,000 per violation, with a minimum penalty of $5000 per violation. If the employee dies, additional penalties may apply and may include six months' imprisonment.
Repeat	Upon reinspection, similar violations discovered	Up to $7000 per violation
Failure to Correct	Initial violation not corrected	Up to $7000 per day following the determined date for correction

PERSONAL PROTECTIVE EQUIPMENT (PPE)

The best ways to prevent exposure to blood-borne pathogens are to wear PPE such as gloves, face shields, and nonabsorbent lab coats when applicable and to maintain strict compliance with the hand hygiene protocol. All PPE must be provided by the employer and be readily available for use.

According the CDC's 2007 Guidelines, Standard Precautions apply in all healthcare settings. The Standard Precautions are designed to prevent transmission of blood-borne pathogens and state that all blood, body fluids, and secretions should be treated as if they were contaminated. PPE that may be used to fulfill the recommendations includes gloves, protective eyewear, masks, and fluid-resistant lab coats.

PPE AND CLOTHING

Clothing and Equipment	When Used
Gloves	Anticipate contact with blood, infectious material, open wounds, or broken skin on hands *Examples:* venipuncture, capillary stick, wound care, injections, minor surgery, cleaning contaminated equipment such as contaminated surfaces of thermometers
Mask	Anticipate spray with blood or infectious materials; often used with eye shields.
Eye/Face Shield	Anticipate spray with infectious materials, droplets of blood, or other infectious matter *Example:* performing a blood smear
Gowns, Lab Coats	Anticipate gross contamination of clothing during a procedure *Examples:* minor surgery, laboratory procedures

16 APPLICATION

Directions: Select the best answer for each of the following questions. Check your answers in the Answer Key at the end of the book.

1. __________ are disease-causing organisms that are transmitted in a variety of ways, including skin-to-skin contact, airborne droplet nuclei, body fluids, and blood.
   a. Inflammatories
   b. Pathogens
   c. Hosts
   d. Infections
   e. B and C

2. The following must be present for microorganisms to grow:
   a. Darkness and food
   b. Food and moisture
   c. Suitable temperature and food
   d. All of the above
   e. A and C only

3. Which of the following is the correct order of occurrence of events in the chain of infection?
   a. Means of transmission, portal of exit, portal of entry into a new host, susceptible new host, infected reservoir host
   b. Infected reservoir host, means of transmission, portal of exit, portal of entry into a new host, susceptible new host
   c. Susceptible new host, portal of entry into a new host, means of transmission, portal of exit, infected reservoir host
   d. Infected reservoir host, portal of exit, means of transmission, portal of entry into a new host, susceptible new host
   e. Portal of entry into a new host, susceptible new host, portal of exit, means of transmission, infected reservoir host

4. Active acquired natural immunity can be defined as immunity that is:
   a. Acquired by administration of a vaccine
   b. Acquired from someone else's antibodies, such as from mother to fetus
   c. Acquired by having the disease
   d. Temporary protection from gamma globulin
   e. A and C

5. ___________________are among the most common blood-borne pathogens.
   a. Typhoid and cholera
   b. AIDS and dysentery
   c. Hepatitis and AIDS
   d. AIDS and tuberculosis
   e. Pneumonia and tuberculosis

6. Hepatitis attacks what organ?
   a. Kidneys
   b. Liver
   c. Pancreas
   d. Spleen
   e. Lungs

7. This level of disinfection kills all bacteria except bacterial spores:
   a. Mega-level disinfection
   b. High-level disinfection
   c. Low-level disinfection
   d. Intermediate-level disinfection
   e. None of the above

8. Use of which of the following chemicals is considered to be an acceptable disinfection method for certain surfaces?
   a. Bromine
   b. Ultraviolet light
   c. 70% isopropyl alcohol
   d. Chlorine bleach
   e. C and D

9. The minimum sterilization time for glassware is:
   a. five minutes
   b. 15 minutes
   c. 20 minutes
   d. 30 minutes
   e. 60 minutes

10. ___________ is defined as being free of all microorganisms.
   a. Disinfected
   b. Sterilization
   c. Aseptic
   d. A and B
   e. B and C

11. Which of the following is not one of the cardinal signs of infection?
   a. Redness
   b. Pain
   c. Fever
   d. Swelling
   e Heat

12. Which of the following statements regarding conditions required for bacterial growth is not correct?
   a. Bacteria grow best in mucous membranes.
   b. Bacteria thrive at body temperature.
   c. Some bacteria can survive without oxygen.
   d. Low temperatures kill bacterial growth.
   e. A temperature of 107°F will kill most bacteria.

13. During the prodromal period of the infection process, which of the following occurs?
   a. Pathogens enter the body.
   b. Pathogens reproduce.
   c. First mild signs and symptoms appear; this is a highly contagious period.
   d. Signs and symptoms are most severe.
   e. Signs and symptoms begin to subside.

14. When parasites carry disease via animals, this is known as:
   a. Direct contact
   b. Droplet transmission
   c. Indirect contact
   d. Vector transmission
   e. None of the above

15. When assisting the physician with a procedure, if you anticipate that you may be sprayed with blood and the likelihood of gross contamination is high, which of the following best describes the PPE that you should don prior to the procedure?
   a. Gloves
   b. Gloves and mask
   c. Gloves, mask, and eye/face shield
   d. Gloves, mask, eye/face shield, and lab coat
   e. Gloves, mask, eye/face shield, lab coat, and gown

17 Patient Preparation and Education

CONTENTS

Patient Interview

In many offices, the medical assistant is responsible for gathering the patient's personal history. This is also known as *interviewing* the patient. It is important that the medical assistant begins the interview by introducing himself or herself and remains professional and organized throughout the interview and visit.

In order to gather accurate data, the medical assistant may need to use varying styles of communication. The style used will depend on the patient and the situation. See Box 17-1 for examples of questions you may ask in order to obtain personal history information from the patient.

COMMUNICATION STYLES

Open-Ended Questions	Require more than a "yes" or "no" answer *Example*: "Mr. Thompson, how would you describe your pain?"
Close-Ended Questions	Allow for a simple "yes" or "no" answer *Example*: "Ms. Ritchie, did you take your medication this morning?"
Reflecting	Repeating the patient's statement so that the patient knows that you understood what he or she said *Example*: "Mrs. Roseberry, you said you have had pain and burning with urination for the past two weeks. Is that correct?"
Examples	Helps the medical assistant understand more clearly what the patient is saying, feeling, and thinking *Example*: "Mr. Ray, with a "1" being no pain and a "10" being unbearable pain, can you please tell me how you would rate the pain level right now?"
Silence	Allows patients to gather their thoughts and/or think of answers to the questions being asked
Indirect Questions	Helpful when interviewing patients you are not familiar with *Examples*: "Do you know . . . ?" "I was wondering . . ." "Can you tell me . . . ?" "Do you happen to know . . . ?" "I'd like to know . . ." "Have you any idea . . . ?"

Box 17-1 Personal History Questions

1. What was the last grade you attended in school?
2. What is your occupation?
3. How long have you done that type of work?
4. Have you been exposed to any toxic or harmful substances such as dust, chemicals, cleaning fluids or fumes, smoke, radiation, pesticides, or paint at work? At home?
5. What do you usually eat for breakfast?
6. Have you gained or lost 10 or more pounds during the past year? Is there a reason?
7. Do you follow a low-fat diet? A low-salt diet?
8. What do you do for exercise? How often?
9. How much alcohol do you drink a day? A month? What is your preferred drink?
10. Do you smoke cigarettes? If yes, how many packs a day? Filtered?
11. Do you smoke a pipe or cigars or chew tobacco? If yes, how much?
12. How many cups of coffee do you drink a day? Tea? Soft drinks with caffeine?
13. Have you ever used heroin, cocaine, or LSD? Over-the-counter drugs? Laxatives? How often?
14. Do you have unusual stress at home or work?
15. What are your hobbies?

PATIENT HISTORY: CHIEF COMPLAINT, PRESENT ILLNESS, PAST MEDICAL HISTORY, FAMILY MEDICAL HISTORY AND SOCIAL HISTORY

Chief Complaint	Also known as *CC* The reason for the office visit consists of: • *Subjective symptoms:* felt by the patient but not able to be seen or measured by the clinician. *Example:* headache • *Objective signs:* felt by the patient and visible/measurable by the clinician. *Example:* fever Important to ask the following questions: • What? • When? • Where? Should be stated in the patient's own words, using quotation marks
Present Illness	Also known as *PI* More detailed description of the CC History of the present illness (HPI) will provide information regarding: • Onset • Duration • Intensity
Past History	Includes all diseases and medical problems the patient has experienced in the past Past history should include the following: • Dates of major illnesses, surgeries, hospitalizations • Medications: prescription and over-the-counter (OTC) • Childhood diseases • Allergies • Immunizations • Last examination
Family History	Includes health problems of blood relatives Family history should include the following information on blood relatives: • Current health • Major health problems • Cause and age of death
Social History	Includes lifestyle patterns that might affect the patient's health Social history should include the following information: • Smoking • Drinking • Recreational drug use • Occupation • Marital status • Sexual preference • Lifestyle, including diet, exercise, sleep habits

REVIEW OF SYSTEMS

The review of systems (ROS) consists of a head-to-toe exam and is part of most physical exams. The sequence most physicians use allows them to begin at the head and work their way down. Depending on the purpose of the exam and the physician's specialty, the physician may examine the entire body or may focus on specific areas.

DOCUMENTATION GUIDELINES

For every encounter with a patient, there should be timely documentation of the interaction and exchange of information that occurs (Box 17-2).

REVIEW OF SYSTEMS (ROS)

Head	Headaches, sinus pain, masses, alopecia (unusual hair loss), dizziness, injury, or trauma
Eyes	Visual acuity, blurred vision, burning, halo effect, tearing, photophobia (sensitivity to light), discharge, redness, jaundice (yellowing of skin and sclera), known eye diseases, date of last eye exam, prescription glasses, contact lenses
Ears	Tinnitus (ringing in the ears), dizziness, hearing loss, discharge, ear infections, exposure to loud noise on a regular basis
Nose	Allergies, obstruction, sense of smell, pain, discharge
Mouth	Dental work, dentures, gums, sense of taste, teeth, salivation (producing saliva), dryness of mouth, tongue, leukoplakia (white patches, possibly cancerous), gingivitis
Throat	Hoarseness, laryngitis (loss of voice), redness, speech defect, masses, pain
Neck	Tenderness, pain, swelling, difficulty swallowing, enlarged nodes
Respiratory	Dyspnea (labored breathing), cough, asthma, wheezing, allergies, hemoptysis (coughing up blood), chest pain, night sweats, orthopnea (difficulty breathing while lying down), shortness of breath (SOB)
Cardiovascular (CV)	Chest pain, hypertension, peripheral edema, cyanosis, fainting, dizziness, heart murmurs, palpitations, arrhythmias
Gastrointestinal (GI)	Nausea, vomiting, anorexia (loss of appetite), bulimia (eating disorder—binge eating followed by purging), indigestion, diarrhea, constipation, hemorrhoids, presence of blood in stool, number of bowel movements daily, hematemesis (vomiting blood)
Genitourinary (GU)	History of urinary tract infection, frequency, hesitation, oliguria (reduced urine), hematuria (blood in urine), dysuria (difficult or painful urination), renal colic (kidney pain), stones, discharge, nocturia (urination during the night)
Female Reproductive	Menstrual history, obstetric history, leukorrhea (white discharge), itching, pain, discharge, date of last Pap smear, breast self-exam history, sexual habits, menopause symptoms, last mammogram (breast exam)
Male Reproductive	Prostate problems, testicular self-exam, discharge, sexual habits, frequency of urination, decreased stream, nocturia, impotence
Endocrine	Growth and development, goiter, excessive thirst, intolerance to temperature change, hormone therapy, diabetes symptoms, irregular menses, symptoms of thyroid disorders
Skin	Rash, urticaria (hives), texture, moles, infection, redness, jaundice, cyanosis, allergies, dryness/oiliness, acne
Musculoskeletal (MS)	Joint pain, swelling, weakness, stiffness, numbness, muscle pain, fractures, discoloration, edema
Neurologic	Fainting, loss of consciousness, headaches, tremor, nervousness, paralysis, pain, memory loss
Psychiatric	Mental health history, emotional stability, depression, stress
General	Weight gain or loss, sleep habits, fatigue, eating habits, smoking, work environment

Box 17-2 The Six Cs of Charting

To better recall the guidelines for charting, remember the six Cs:

1. *Client's* own words must be used exactly and in quotation marks.
2. *Clarity* must be achieved when recording information, using proper spelling and medical terminology and abbreviations.
3. *Completeness* is essential for all information recorded in the medical record.
4. *Conciseness* of the entry saves writing and reading time and chart space.
5. *Chronological* order of information is imperative.
6. *Confidentiality* of patient information is mandatory in every aspect of patient care.

The following are guidelines for proper documentation:

- Provide the date/time of every entry.
- Ensure that your handwriting is legible.
- Use permanent black ink.
- Use proper terminology, correct spelling, and correct grammar.
- Document in sequence as the visit occurs.
- Be concise.
- Correct errors by drawing a single line through the incorrect entry and initialing it. Then record the correct entry.
- Sign every entry.

Because medical assistants are not licensed to practice medicine and diagnose, documentation must not reflect diagnostic terms when recording the chief complaint.

Correct documentation: 05/10/11, Pt c/o excessive pain and burning with urination × 5 days. S. White, RMA (AMT)

Incorrect documentation: 05/10/11 Pt c/o excessive pain and burning with urination × 5 days consistent with UTI. S. White, RMA (AMT)

Vital Signs

A healthy human body will work to maintain homeostasis, and vital signs are an indicator of the body's ability to regulate itself.

It is important that vital signs are recorded for each patient visit, as this will provide information for the physician and allow the physician to compare the current visit's vital signs with those at the previous visit and determine if there are any significant changes with which the physician should be concerned. To see how vital signs are recorded, read the procedure for each vital sign listed.

Temperature (T), pulse (P), respiration (R), and blood pressure (BP) measurements are considered vital signs because they measure some of the body's most vital functions and may provide important information about the body's overall state of health. Many physicians refer to temperature, pulse and respirations as *TPR*.

PERFORMING VITAL SIGNS

Temperature (T)

See Procedure 17-1 for guidelines on the appropriate steps required to measure temperature accurately.

NORMAL BODY TEMPERATURE FOR ADULTS

Method	Fahrenheit	Celsius
Oral	98.6	37
Rectal	99.6	37.6
Axillary	97.6	36.4
Aural	98.6	37
Temporal Artery	98.6	37

SELECTING A METHOD FOR MEASURING BODY TEMPERATURE

Method	Advisable	Inadvisable
Oral	Most adults and children who are able to follow instructions	Patients who have had oral surgery, mouth sores, dyspnea; uncooperative patients; patients on oxygen; infants and small children; patients with facial paralysis or nasal obstruction
Rectal	Infants and small children; patients who have had oral surgery; mouth-breathing patients; unconscious patients	Active children; fragile newborns
Axillary	Small children	Patients who cannot form an airtight seal around the thermometer
Tympanic (Aural)	Small children	Patient with in-the-ear hearing aids or ear infections
Temporal Artery	Infants and small children; patients who have had oral surgery; mouth-breathing patients; unconscious patients	Active children; fragile newborns

procedure 17-1

MEASURING ORAL TEMPERATURE USING AN ELECTRONIC OR DIGITAL THERMOMETER

Objective: Accurately perform all steps of the procedure and provide an accurate temperature reading.

EQUIPMENT AND SUPPLIES

- electronic or digital thermometer (rechargeable)
- probe cover
- waste container
- pen
- patient's chart

METHOD

1. Perform hand hygiene.
2. Assemble equipment.
3. Identify the patient and explain the procedure.
4. Remove the thermometer unit from the base and attach the probe (blue for oral temperature).
5. Remove the thermometer probe from the holder.
6. Insert the thermometer probe into the disposable tip box to secure the tip (Figure 17-1A).
7. Insert the thermometer into the patient's mouth on either side of the frenulum linguae and instruct the patient to close the mouth.
8. When the temperature signal is seen or heard, remove the thermometer from the patient's mouth and read the result in the LED window.
9. Dispose of the thermometer tip in a waste container (Figure 17-1B).
10. Return the thermometer probe to the storage place (Figure 17-1C).
11. Replace the unit on the rechargeable base.
12. Perform hand hygiene.
13. Document the results.

CHARTING EXAMPLE

07/25/XX 4 P.M. T 99.6R · · · · · · · · · · · · E. Leonard, RMA (AMT)

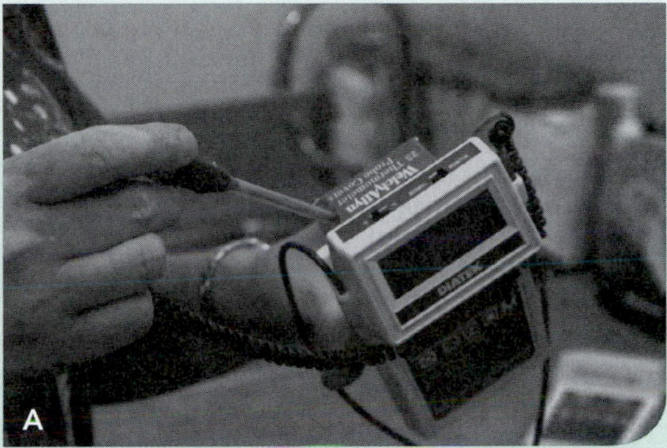

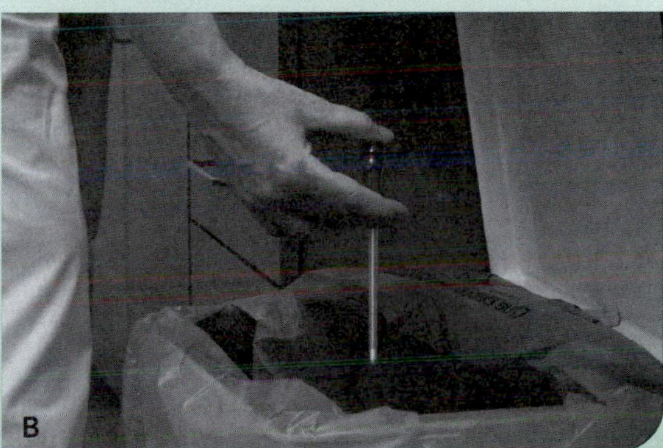

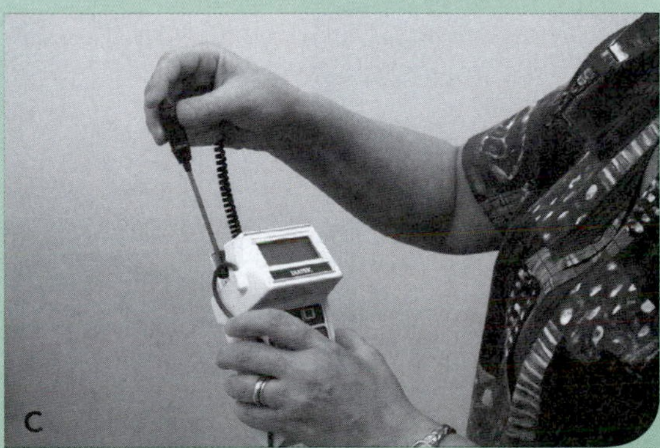

FIGURE 17-1 (A) Insert the thermometer probe into the disposable tip box to secure a tip. (B) After measuring the temperature, press to eject the probe cover. (C) Replace the probe in the holder.

Pulse (P)

Pulse rate is a measurement of the number of times the heart beats per minute (bpm). Each pulse beat represents one heartbeat. The pulse rate in a normal, healthy adult is approximately 70 bpm. A pulse rate above 100 bpm is considered tachycardia; a pulse rate below 60 bpm is considered bradycardia. See the accompanying tables, Figure 17-2, and Procedure 17-2 for more information.

AVERAGE PULSE RATES BY AGE

Less than 1 year	120–160 bpm
2–6 years	80–120 bpm
6–10 years	80–100 bpm
11–16 years	70–90 bpm
Adult	60–80 bpm
Older adult	50–65 bpm

LOCATION OF COMMON PULSE SITES

Site	Location
Radial	Thumb side of the wrist about 1 inch below the base of the thumb (most frequently used site)
Brachial	Inner (antecubital fossa/space) aspect of the elbow (pulse heard when taking BP)
Carotid	At the side of the neck between the larynx and the sternocleidomastoid muscle (pulse used in CPR; pressing both carotids at the same time can cause a reflex drop in BP and pulse)
Temporal	At the side of the head just above the ear
Femoral	In the groin where the femoral artery passes to the leg
Popliteal	Behind the knee; pulse located deeply behind the knee and felt when knee is slightly bent
Posterior Tibial	On the medial surface of the ankle near the ankle bone
Dorsalis Pedis	On the top of the foot slightly lateral to midline; helps assess adequate circulation to foot
Apical	At the apex of the heart to the left of sternum, fourth or fifth intercostal space below the nipple

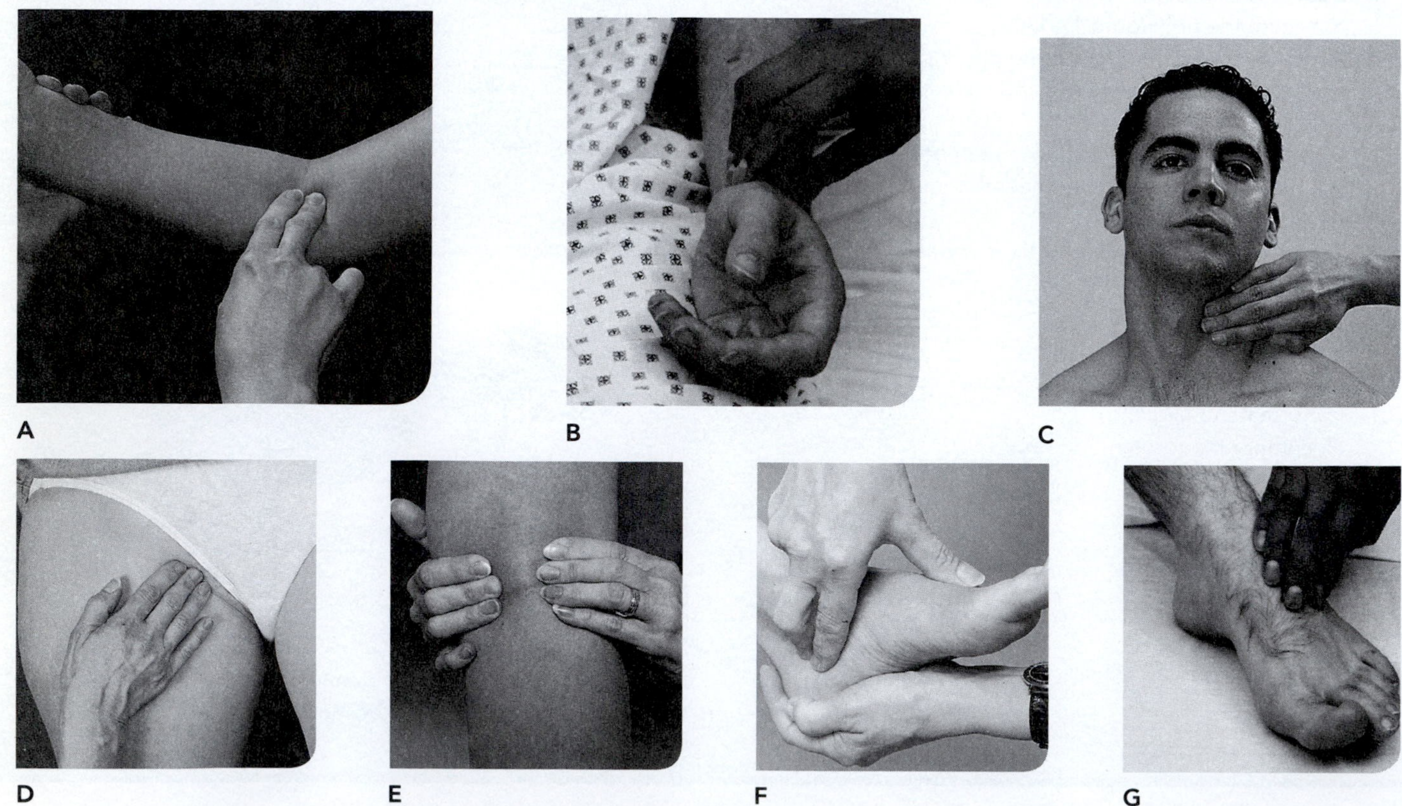

FIGURE 17-2 **(A) Brachial pulse. (B) Radial pulse. (C) Carotid pulse. (D) Femoral pulse. (E) Popliteal pulse. (F) Posterior tibial pulse. (G) Dorsalis pedis pulse.**

procedure

17-2

MEASURING THE RADIAL PULSE

Objective: Accurately perform all steps of the procedure and provide an accurate radial pulse reading.

EQUIPMENT AND SUPPLIES

- paper and pen/pencil
- patient's record
- watch with second hand

METHOD

1. Perform hand hygiene.
2. Identify the patient.
3. Explain the procedure.
4. Ask the patient about any recent physical activity or smoking.
5. Ask the patient to sit down and place the arm in a comfortable, supported position. The hand should be at chest level with the palm down.
6. Place your fingertips on the radial artery on the thumb side of the wrist (Figure 17-3).
7. Check the quality of the pulse.
8. Start counting pulse beats when the second hand on the watch is at 3, 6, 9, or 12.
9. Count the pulse for 1 full minute. The number will always be an even number.
10. Immediately write the pulse beats per minute on a piece of paper.
11. Perform hand hygiene.
12. Record the pulse beats per minute in the patient's record, describing any abnormalities in the pulse rate.

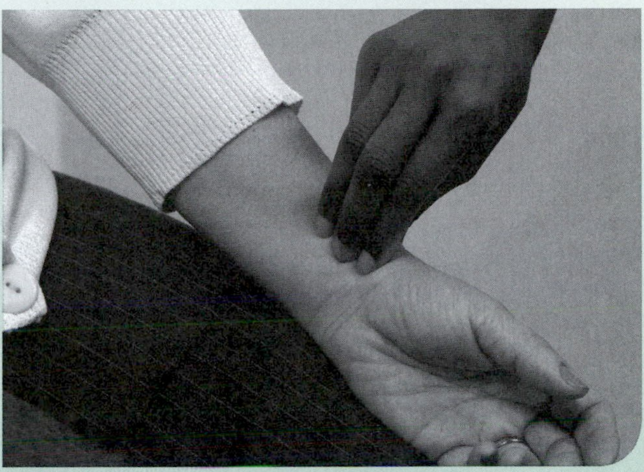

FIGURE 17-3 Measuring a patient's radial pulse.

CHARTING EXAMPLE

2/14/XX 4:00 P.M. Pulse 72 (R) Regular and strong
.... M. King, CMA (AAMA)

CHARACTERISTICS OF PULSE RATE

Rate	Number of pulse beats per minute
Volume	Refers to the strength of the pulse • *Bounding pulse*=strong, forceful pulse • *Thready pulse*=small, fine pulse
Rhythm	Refers to the regularity of the heartbeat • *Arrhythmia*=irregluar rhythm

Respirations (R)

Respirations are the measurement for the act of breathing when the exchange of oxygen and carbon dioxide occurs. Respiratory rates indicate how well oxygen is being delivered throughout the body. One respiratory cycle includes one exhalation and one inhalation. See Procedure 17-3 for guidelines on the appropriate steps required to measure respirations accurately.

procedure
17-3

MEASURING RESPIRATIONS

Objective: Accurately perform all steps of the procedure and provide an accurate respiration measurement.

EQUIPMENT AND SUPPLIES

- watch with a sweep second hand

METHOD

1. Perform hand hygiene.
2. Identify the patient.
3. Assist the patient into a comfortable position.
4. Place your hand on the patient's wrist in a position to take the pulse or place your hand on the patient's chest (Figure 17-4).
5. Count each breathing cycle by observing and/or feeling the rise and fall of the chest or upper abdomen.
6. Count for one full minute using a watch with a sweep second hand. If the rate is atypical or unusual in any way, take it for another minute.
7. Record the respiratory rate in the patient's record, noting the date, time, any abnormality in rate, rhythm, and depth, and your signature.

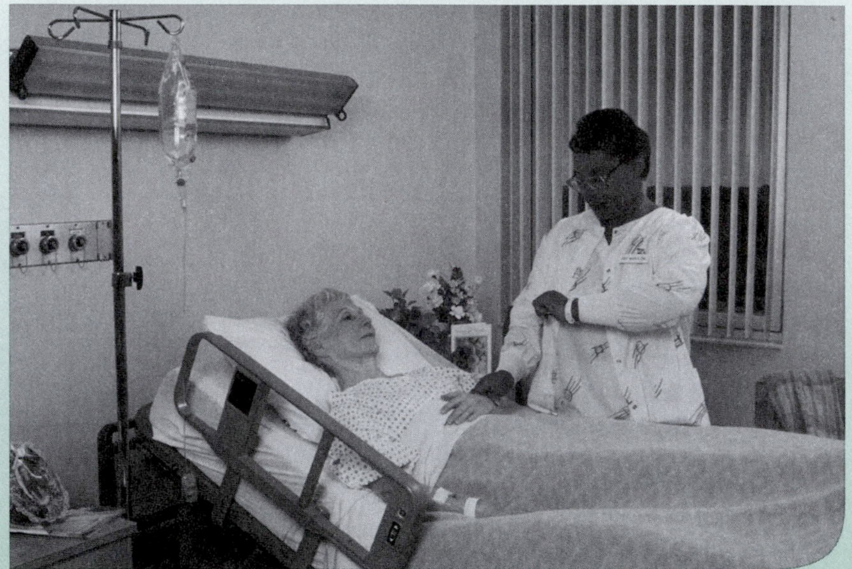

FIGURE 17-4 Place a hand on the chest when respirations are difficult to count. The patient must be unaware that you are counting respirations.

CHARTING EXAMPLE

2/14/XX 4:00 P.M. Resp. 20 and regular ....
.... M. King, CMA (AAMA)

CHARACTERISTICS OF RESPIRATION

Respiratory Rate	Refers to the number of respirations per minute • *Normal:* 16 to 20 per minute (eupnea) • *Rapid:* >40 per minute (tachypnea) • *Slow:* <12 per minute (bradypnea)	**Breath Sounds**	Normal respirations have no noticeable sound Descriptions of breath sounds: • *Stridor*: shrill, harsh sound • *Stertorous*: noisy breathing; sounds like snoring • *Crackles/rales*: crackling sounds simliar to those made when crushing tissue paper • *Rhonchi* (*gurgles*): rattling, whistling made in the throat • *Wheezes*: high-pitched whistling sounds • *Cheyne-Stokes*: irregular breathing that may be slow and shallow at first, then becomes faster and deeper and may stop for a few seconds • *Bubbling breathing sounds*: gurgling
Rhythm	Breathing pattern that occurs at either regular or irregular spacing of breaths		
Depth	Refers to the volume of air with each inhalation and exhalation • *Hypoventilation:* shallow respirations • *Hyperventilation:* deep, rapid respirations		
Respiratory Quality	Refers to breathing patterns that differ from normal effortless breathing		

RESPIRATORY RATE RANGES OF VARIOUS AGE GROUPS

Newborn	30–50
1 year old	20–40
2–10 years old	20–30
11–18 years old	18–24
Adult	14–20

Blood Pressure (BP)

Measurement of blood pressure is an important vital sign and assists in diagnosis and treatment. Many medical conditions and diseases can be indicated by the rise or fall of a patient's blood pressure.

HYPOTENSION AND HYPERTENSION

Hypotension	Low blood pressure, which may be due to: • Shock • Trauma • CNS disorders
Hypertension	Also known as *HTN* High blood pressure Often asymptomatic

It is important that the appropriate size cuff is used when measuring the patient's blood pressure. Using the wrong size cuff can significantly affect the blood pressure reading. See Figure 17-5 and Procedure 17-4.

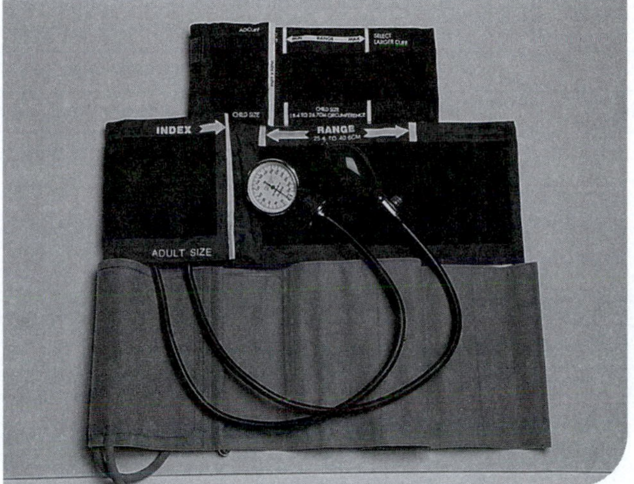

FIGURE 17-5 Three standard sizes of cuffs: a small size for a child or frail adult; a normal adult size; and a large size for measuring blood pressure on the leg (thigh) or on the arm of an obese adult.

BLOOD PRESSURE GUIDELINES

New Classification (2003)		Previous Classification
140/90 or above	Hypertension	High blood pressure >140/90
120/80 to 139/89	Prehypertension	Borderline 130–139/85–89
119/79 or below	Normal	Normal 129/84 or below
		Optimal 120/80 or below

SYSTOLIC AND DIASTOLIC BLOOD PRESSURE DEFINED

Systolic Blood Pressure	Highest pressure that occurs as the left ventricle of the heart is contracting In the BP reading **118**/76, the systolic blood pressure is 118.
Diastolic Blood Pressure	Lowest pressure that occurs when the heart is at rest In the BP reading 118/**76**, the diastolic blood pressure is 76.

AVERAGE NORMAL BLOOD PRESSURE READINGS

Newborn	75/55
6–9 years of age	90/55
10–15 years of age	100/65
16 years to adulthood	118/76
Adult	120/80

TERMS RELATED TO ABNORMAL BLOOD PRESSURE READINGS

Benign	Slow-onset elevated blood pressure without symptoms
Essential	Primary hypertension of unknown cause; may be genetically determined
Hypertension	A condition in which the patient's blood pressure is consistently above the norm for his or her age group; also called *high blood pressure*; below 120/80 is the baseline
Hypotension	Condition of abnormally low blood pressure that may be caused by shock, hemorrhage, and central nervous system (CNS) disorders
Malignant	Rapidly developing elevated blood pressure that may become fatal if not treated immediately
Orthostatic	A temporary fall in blood pressure that occurs when a patient moves rapidly from a lying to a standing position. Dizziness and blurred vision can also be present.
Postural	A temporary fall in blood pressure from standing motionless for extended periods of time
Renal	Elevated blood pressure as a result of kidney disease
Secondary	Elevated blood pressure associated with other conditions, such as renal disease, pregnancy, arteriosclerosis, and obesity

procedure 17-4

MEASURING BLOOD PRESSURE

Objective: Obtain an accurate systolic and diastolic reading.

EQUIPMENT AND SUPPLIES

- sphygmomanometer
- stethoscope
- 70% isopropyl alcohol
- alcohol sponges or cotton balls
- paper and pen/pencil
- patient's record

METHOD

1. Perform hand hygiene.
2. Assemble the equipment. Thoroughly cleanse the earpieces, bell, and diaphragm pieces of the stethoscope. Use an alcohol sponge or cotton ball with 70% isopropyl alcohol. Allow the alcohol to dry.
3. Identify the patient verbally and explain the procedure.
4. Assist the patient into a comfortable position. BP may be taken with the patient in a sitting or lying position. The patient's arm should be at heart level. If the patient's arm is below heart level, the BP reading will be higher than normal; if the arm is above heart level, the BP reading will be lower than normal. Patients should be reminded not to cross their legs or talk during the procedure.
5. Place the sphygmomanometer on a solid surface with the gauge within 3 feet for easy viewing.
6. Uncover the patient's arm by asking the patient to roll back his or her sleeve 5 inches above the elbow. If the sleeve becomes constricting when rolled back, ask the patient to slip the arm out of the sleeve. Never take a BP reading through clothing.
7. Have the patient straighten the arm with the palm up. Apply the proper size cuff of the sphygmomanometer over the brachial artery 1 to 2 inches above the antecubital space (bend in the elbow). Many cuffs are marked with arrows or circles to be placed over the artery. Hold the edge of the cuff in place as you wrap the remainder of the cuff tightly around the arm. If the cuff has a Velcro closure, press it into place at the end of the cuff (Figure 17-6A).
8. Palpate with your fingertips to locate the brachial artery in the antecubital space (Figure 17-6B).
9. Pump air into the cuff quickly and evenly until the level of mercury is 20 to 30 mmHg above the point at which the radial pulse is no longer palpable. Note the level, and rapidly deflate the cuff and wait 60 seconds. The manometer should be at eye level for a more accurate reading.
10. Place the earpieces in your ears and the diaphragm (or bell) of the stethoscope over the area where you feel the brachial artery pulsing. Hold the diaphragm in place with one hand on the chest piece without placing your thumb

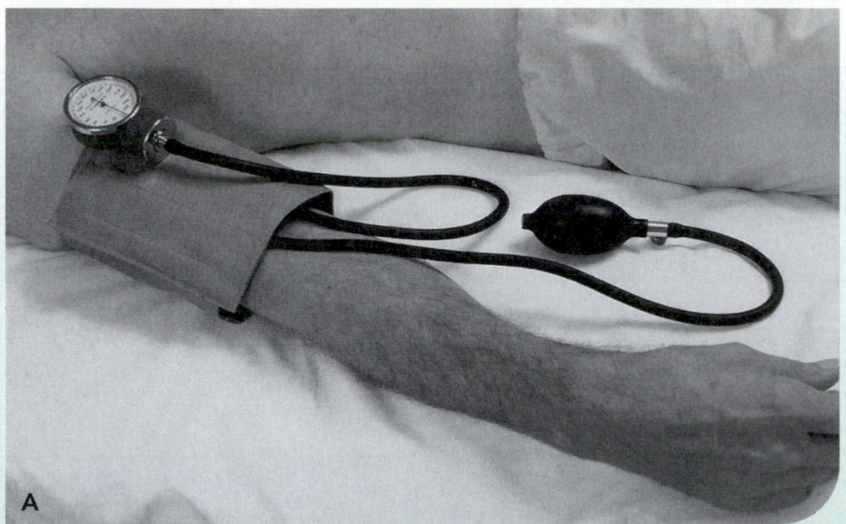

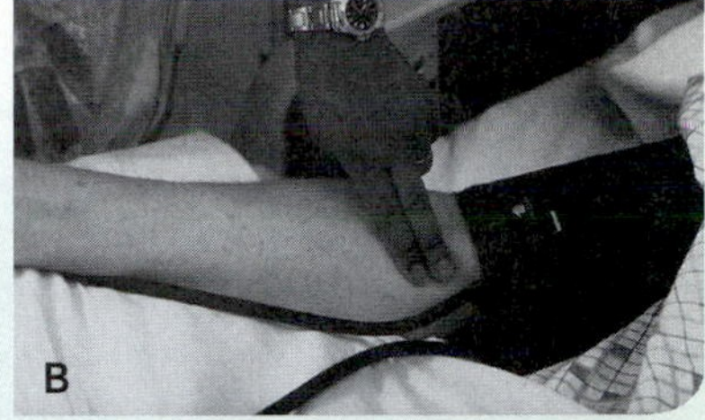

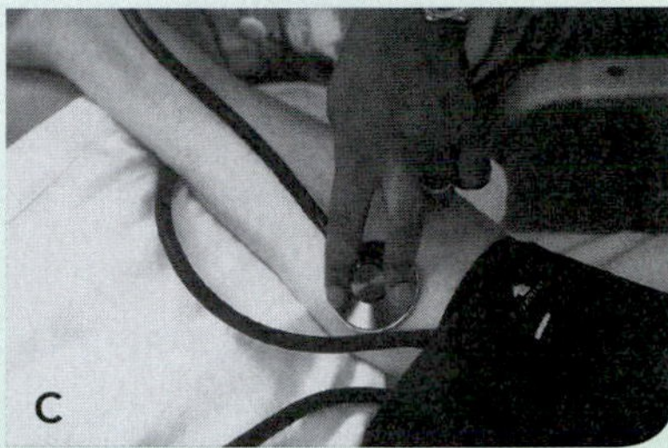

over the diaphragm (Figure 17-6C). The stethoscope tubing should hang freely and not touch any object or the patient during the reading.

11. Close the thumbscrew on the hand bulb by turning clockwise with your dominant hand. Close the thumbscrew just enough so that no air can leak out. Do not close it so tightly that you will have difficulty reopening it with one hand.
12. Slowly turn the thumbscrew counterclockwise with your dominant hand. Allow the pressure reading to fall only 2 to 3 mmHg at a time.
13. Listen for the point at which the first clear sound is heard (phase I of the Korotkoff sounds). Note where this occurred on the manometer. This is the systolic pressure.
14. Slowly continue to allow the cuff to deflate. The sounds will change from loud to a murmur and then fade away (phases I, II, III, and IV of the Korotkoff sounds). Read the mercury column (or spring gauge scale) at the point where the sound is no longer heard. This is the diastolic pressure (phase V of the Korotkoff sounds).
15. Many physicians want both phase IV and phase V reported for the diastolic reading (Figure 17-6D).
16. Quickly open the thumbscrew all the way to release the air and deflate the cuff completely.
17. If you are unsure about the BP reading, wait at least a minute or two before taking a second reading. Never take more than two readings in one arm since blood stasis may have occurred, resulting in an inaccurate reading.
18. Immediately write the BP as a fraction on paper. You may inform the patient of the reading if this is the policy in your office.
19. Remove the cuff.
20. Clean the earpieces of the stethoscope with an alcohol sponge.
21. Perform hand hygiene.
22. Chart the results, including the date, time, BP reading, and your name.

CHARTING EXAMPLE

2/14/XX 9:00 A.M. B/P 134/88 left arm, sitting . . . . M. King, CMA (AAMA)

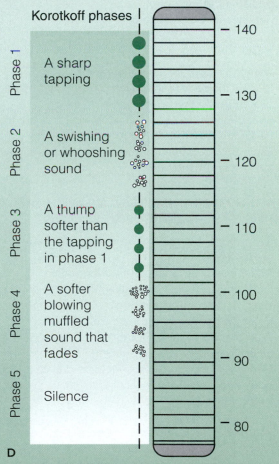

Korotkoff phases

Phase 1 — A sharp tapping

Phase 2 — A swishing or whooshing sound

Phase 3 — A thump softer than the tapping in phase 1

Phase 4 — A softer blowing muffled sound that fades

Phase 5 — Silence

140 — 130 — 120 — 110 — 100 — 90 — 80

D

FIGURE 17-6 (A) Wrap a blood pressure cuff snugly around the upper arm. (B) Palpate the brachial artery on the medial antecubital fossa. (C) Place a stethoscope on the medial antecubital fossa. (D) Korotkoff sounds can be differentiated into five phases. In the illustration, the blood pressure is 138/90 or 138/102/90.

procedure 17-5

MEASURING PEDIATRIC VITAL SIGNS

Objective: Perform all steps of the procedures and provide readings with accuracy according to the instructor's guidelines.

EQUIPMENT AND SUPPLIES

- gloves
- tympanic thermometer
- glass thermometer
- electronic thermometer
- watch with a second hand
- pediatric stethoscope
- pediatric blood pressure cuff

METHOD

1. Gather the appropriate equipment.
2. Identify the patient, introduce yourself, and explain the procedures to the parent.
3. Speak reassuringly to the child to win his or her trust.
4. Perform hand hygiene.
5. Explain to the parent how he or she can assist you in holding the infant.

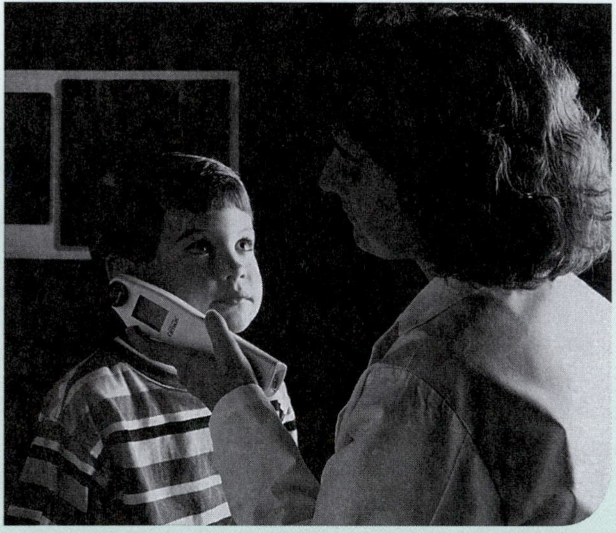

FIGURE 17-7 **Tympanic thermometers are particularly helpful for measuring the temperature of a child.**

OBTAIN TEMPERATURE READING WITH THE TYMPANIC THERMOMETER AS FOLLOWS

1. Remove the thermometer from the base and note that it reads "Ready."
2. Attach the disposable probe cover to the earpiece.
3. Gently pull in a downward direction on the outer ear to straighten the child's ear canal.
4. Insert the probe into the ear canal.
5. Press the scan button (Figure 17-7).
6. Observe the temperature reading.
7. Gently withdraw the thermometer and eject the probe cover into a biohazard waste container.
8. Record the temperature reading using "T" to denote the tympanic reading.
9. Return the thermometer to the base.

OBTAIN TEMPERATURE READING USING THE AXILLARY METHOD AS FOLLOWS

1. Take a nonmercury thermometer out of the container and rinse it with cool water; inspect it for defects.
2. Shake down the thermometer to 95°F/35°C.
3. Place the thermometer in the infant's armpit and hold the infant's arm across the chest for the required 10 minutes.
4. Read the thermometer, then record by designating the reading with "AX" to indicate the method used.
5. Clean and disinfect the thermometer when you are finished with the patient.

OBTAIN TEMPERATURE READING RECTALLY BY USING A DIGITAL THERMOMETER WITH A RED PROBE (RECTAL USE) AS FOLLOWS

1. Put on gloves.
2. Attach the disposable tip to the top of the probe.
3. Lubricate the thermometer to provide easy insertion.
4. Place the child on the bed in a supine or prone position.
5. Insert the thermometer ½ inch into the rectum and it hold in place with your hand to prevent it from being expelled (Figure 17-8).
6. Hold the child securely to restrict movement.
7. Leave the thermometer in place for the required time until it beeps.

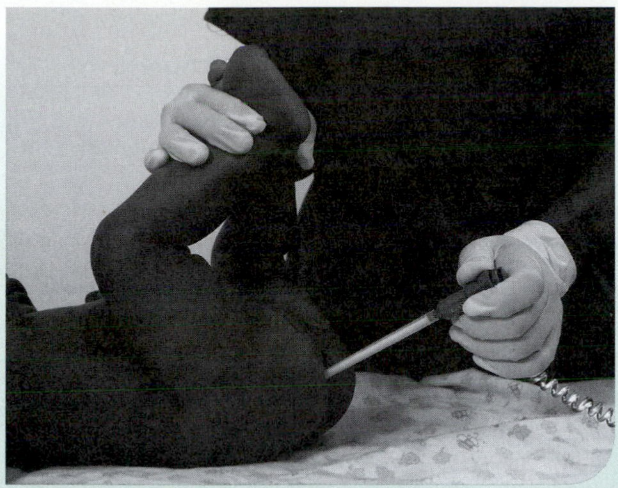

FIGURE 17-8 Obtaining a temperature reading rectally.

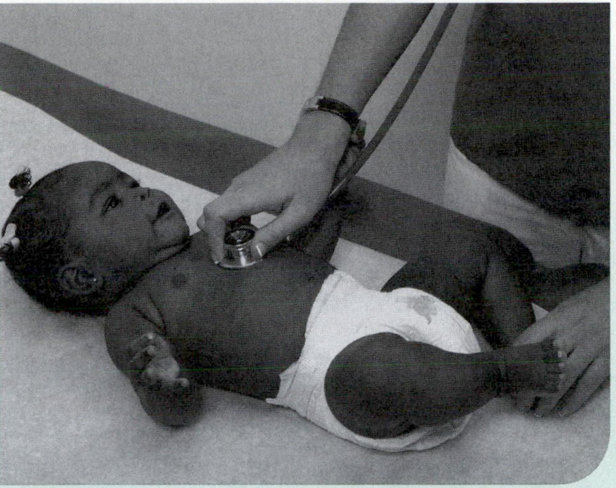

FIGURE 17-9 Measuring the apical pulse of an infant.

8. Remove thermometer, wipe off the lubricant, and take the reading.
9. Record the reading using "R" to indicate the method used.

MEASURE HEART RATE/PULSE BY APICAL MEASUREMENT AS FOLLOWS

1. Place the stethoscope on the child's chest at the midpoint between the sternum and the left nipple (Figure 17-9). Distract the child if necessary to obtain the apical pulse.
2. Listen for the apical beat.
3. Count the apical beat for one full minute.
4. Record the apical pulse using "Ap" before the pulse to indicate the apical reading.

MEASURE INFANT RESPIRATIONS FOR ONE FULL MINUTE AS FOLLOWS

1. Place your hand on the child's chest and count the rise and fall of the chest as 1 respiration.
2. Record the results.

MEASURE THE INFANT'S BLOOD PRESSURE USING A PEDIATRIC CUFF AND STETHOSCOPE AS FOLLOWS

1. Wrap the cuff securely around the upper arm (Figure 17-10).
2. Feel for the brachial pulse.

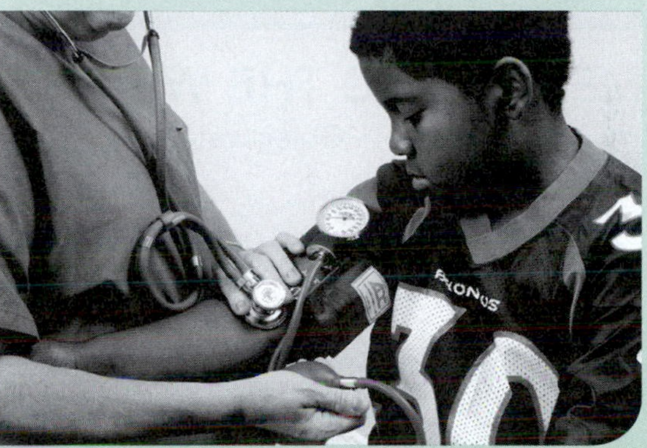

FIGURE 17-10 Taking the child's blood pressure.

3. Place the stethoscope earpieces in the ears and place the diaphragm near the pulse.
4. Pump up the cuff until the pulse is no longer heard.
5. Release the valve slowly, listening for systolic and diastolic sounds.
6. Record the results.

CHARTING EXAMPLE

4/10/XX T 99°F (T), AP 90, R 20, BP 136/78 .... M. King, CMA (AAMA)

NORMAL BODY TEMPERATURE FOR CHILDREN FROM BIRTH TO ADOLESCENCE

Method	Fahrenheit	Celsius
Oral	98.6	37
Aural	98.6	37
Axillary	97.6	36.4
Rectal	99.6	37.6

BASELINE PULSE, RESPIRATION, AND BP VALUES FROM BIRTH TO ADOLESCENCE

Age	Respirations	Pulse	Systolic BP MmHg	Diastolic BP MmHg
Infants	30–60	120–160	74–100	50–70
Toddlers	24–40	90–140	80–112	50–80
Preschoolers	22–34	80–110	82–110	50–78
School Age	18–30	75–100	84–120	54–80
Adolescents	12–16	60–90	100+ age	30–40 less than age

procedure 17-6

MEASURING THE WEIGHT AND HEIGHT OF AN INFANT

Objective: Obtain the weight and height of an infant.

EQUIPMENT AND SUPPLIES

- baby scale
- patient record
- pen
- small towel or protector for scale
- tape measure

METHOD

1. Introduce yourself and identify the infant by stating the infant's name to the parent or caregiver. Have the infant remain with the parent or caregiver while you prepare the equipment. Explain the procedure.
2. Perform hand hygiene.
3. Place a towel or paper protector on the baby scale.
4. Balance the scale by placing all the weights to the far left side. Turn the bolt at the right edge of the scale until the balance bar pointer is at the middle of the balance bar.
5. Undress the infant (or ask the parent or caregiver to undress the infant). A clean diaper may be kept in place. Gently lay the infant on the scale. Always keep one hand on the infant until the weights are adjusted. Do not leave the infant unattended at any time.
6. Keeping one hand over the infant's body as a safety precaution, move the large pound weight into the groove closest to the weight estimated for the baby. Move the smaller ounce weight by tapping it gently until it reaches a point at which the pointer floats in the center of the frame. See Figure 17-11A–B for examples of balance and electronic baby scales.

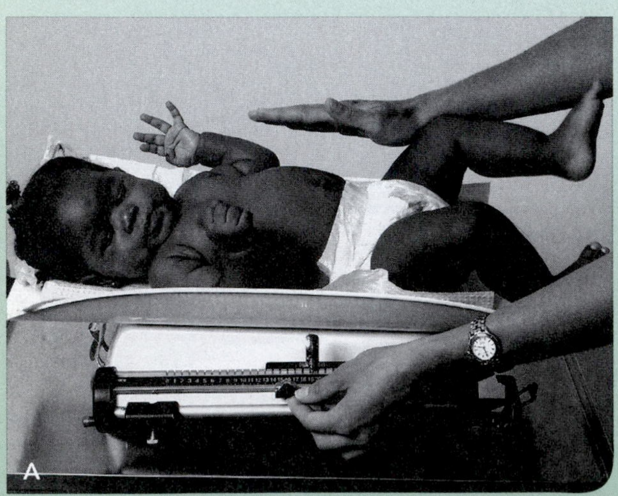

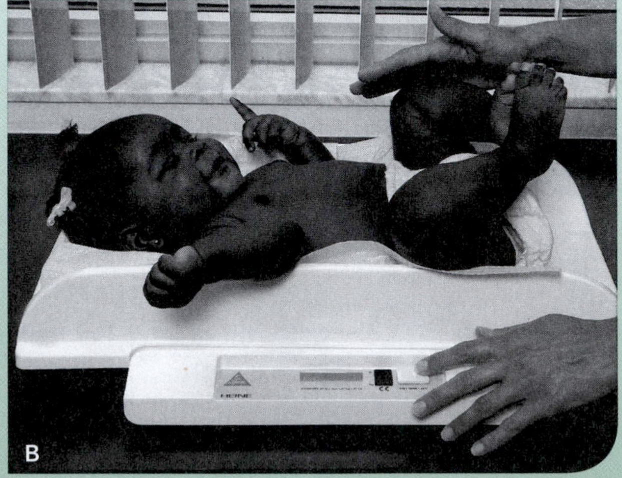

FIGURE 17-11 **(A) Balance baby scale. (B) Electronic baby scale.**

7. Keep the weights in place while the infant is moved to the examination table for height measurement under the parent's or caregiver's care while you record the weight.

CONTINUE WITH MEASURING HEIGHT

8. Holding the tape measure with one hand, place the tape at the top of the side of the infant's head. Stretch the infant out full length as you pull the tape measure down to the bottom of the feet (Figure 17-12). If you are using a table with a measure bar, place the infant's head at one end of the table with the soles of his or her feet touching the footboard so that the toes are pointing toward the ceiling.

Note: It is best, and preferred, to have two people measure the length of an infant. The parent or caregiver can assist by holding the infant's head still. To measure an active child, make pencil marks on the examination table paper at the top of the child's head and at the bottom of the feet at the heels. When the child is removed, measure the area between the marks.

9. Note the height in inches and fractions of an inch, and write it on the paper covering the exam table.
10. Ask the parent or caregiver to hold the infant while the height and weight are charted in the infant's record.

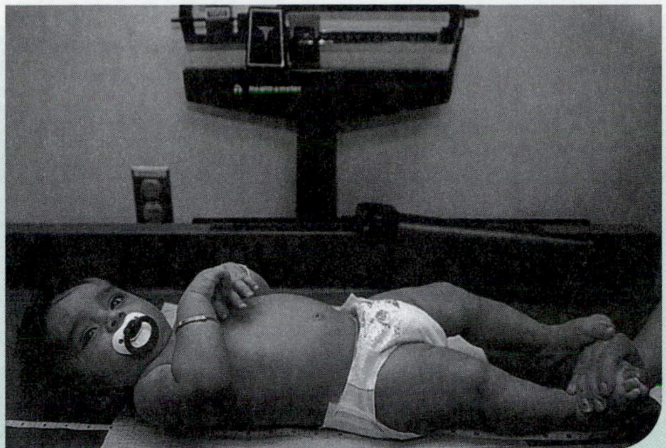

FIGURE 17-12 Measuring the length of an infant from the top of the head to the base of the heels.

11. Tell the measurements to the parent or caregiver.
12. Discard the paper towel.
13. Perform hand hygiene.

CHARTING EXAMPLE

2/14/XX weight 16 lb 3 oz, length 30 inches .... M. King, CMA (AAMA)

Patient Education

Patient education is an important part of the medical assistant's responsibilities. Patients have the right to receive instruction and information on how to care for themselves and manage their own health needs.

Most patient education occurs with adult patients, and it is important to understand how this patient population learns best. If adult patients actively participate in their education, they are likely to learn at a more rapid rate and retain more of the information being taught. Role playing and demonstrations are methods that work especially well with adult learners.

For additional examples of patient teaching methods, see Chapter 7.

MAINTENANCE AND DISEASE PREVENTION

Promoting healthy habits such as maintaining a healthy weight, exercising regularly, not smoking, and limiting consumption of alcohol all fall under patient education for health maintenance and disease prevention (Procedures 17-7 and 17-8). As a medical assistant, you can encourage patients to continue to maintain their healthy habits and help them identify those that are not healthy. Once the nonhealthy habits have been identified, you can provide educational information in the form of brochures, videos, and Internet Web sites that the patient can visit.

WELLNESS GUIDELINES

- Keep a positive attitude.
- Cherish your values.
- Exercise your mind, body, and spirit.
- Control your stress.
- Soothe your fears.
- Think happy thoughts.
- Stay active.
- Challenge your mind.
- Forgive and forget.
- Avoid dangerous drugs.
- Watch your sugar intake.
- Walk briskly.
- Enjoy the outdoors.
- Maintain a healthy weight.
- Eat a well-balanced diet.
- Rinse fresh fruits and vegetables before eating.
- Practice cleanliness.
- Take medications as directed.
- Stop smoking.
- Lower your blood pressure and cholesterol.
- Learn to breathe deeply.

procedure
17-7

DEMONSTRATE PATIENT INSTRUCTION FOR TESTICULAR SELF-EXAMINATION

Objective: With the necessary materials, you will be able to instruct the patient on performing a testicular self-examination correctly.

EQUIPMENT AND SUPPLIES

- pamphlet with instructions for performing an at-home testicular exam

METHOD

1. Wash your hands. Gather equipment and supplies.
2. Identify the patient and guide him to the treatment area.
3. Instruct the patient to:
   - Take a warm bath or shower to relax the scrotum. In the clinical setting, the patient should take several deep breaths.
   - Observe the contour of the scrotum. If one testicle is slightly larger or lies somewhat lower than the other, this is considered normal (Figure 17-13).
   - Elevate the right leg to the level of a toilet, chair, or bed to expose the right testicle.
   - With the left hand, lightly support the right testicle. With the right hand, palpate the right testicle for hardness, lumps, or anything unusual (Figure 17-14).
   - Reverse the process by elevating the left leg to examine the left testicle. Support the left testicle with the right hand and, with the left hand, palpate the left testicle.
4. If the patient finds any abnormalities or has any questions, he should contact the physician.

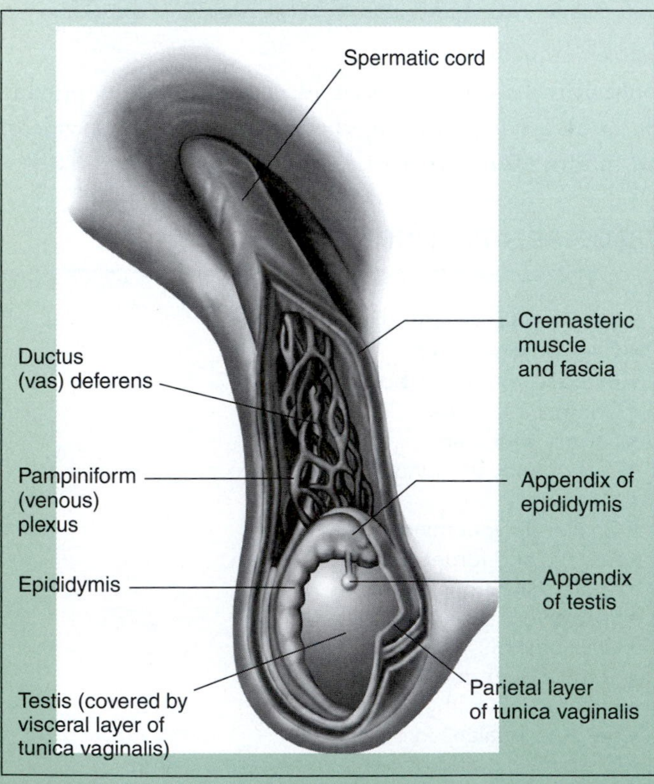

FIGURE 17-13 Illustration of normal scrotum.

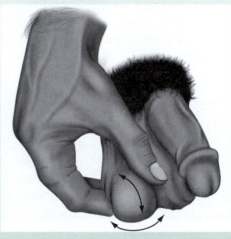

FIGURE 17-14 Palpate the testicle for hardness, lumps, or anything unusual.

CHARTING EXAMPLE

02-28-XX 9:25 A.M. Patient given written and verbal testicular self-exam instructions. Patient demonstrated correct technique and understanding of the importance of monthly self-examinations. .... Erin Janson, RMA (AMT)

Source: Medical Assisting: Foundations and Practices by M. S. Frazier, C. Malone, and C. Morgan, Upper Saddle River, NJ: Pearson Education, Inc., 2010, p. 703. Reprinted with permission.

procedure

17-8

INSTRUCT THE PATIENT IN BREAST SELF-EXAMINATION

Objective: With the necessary materials, you will be able to instruct the patient in the performance of breast self-examination correctly.

EQUIPMENT AND SUPPLIES

- patient chart
- educational materials such as patient brochures or breast models

METHOD

1. Wash your hands and gather the necessary supplies.
2. Escort the patient to the patient education area.
3. Emphasize the following habits for the monthly self-exam.
   a. Premenopausal women should perform the examination about one week after the menstrual period, when the breasts are not swollen. Postmenopausal women should select a specific date of the month.
   b. Perform a visual inspection while standing in front of a mirror. With the arms hanging at the sides, above the head, or forward, away from the body, or with the hands positioned on the hips, observe for bilateral similarities or differences, for color or texture changes in the skin and nipples, and for nipple discharge (Figure 17-15).
   c. Examine each breast in side-lying and flat positions, starting with the same breast each time (Figure 17-16). For the flat position, place a pillow under the shoulder on each side.
   d. Palpate each breast with the fingertip pads of the opposite hand, using a dime-sized, circular motion (Figure 17-17). Use the same search pattern of vertical strip, wedge, or circle search for both breasts.

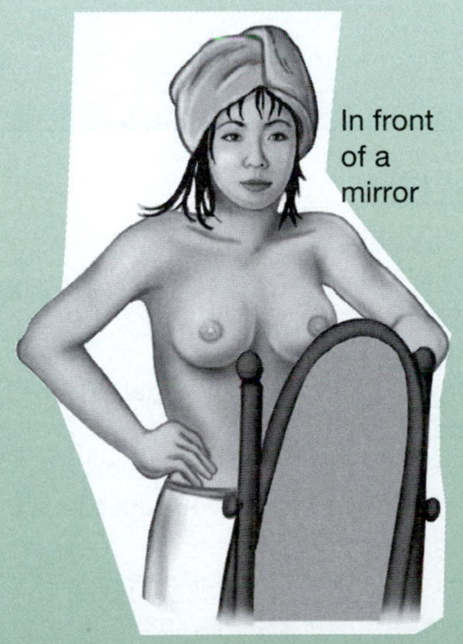

FIGURE 17-15 Perform a visual inspection while standing in front of the mirror.

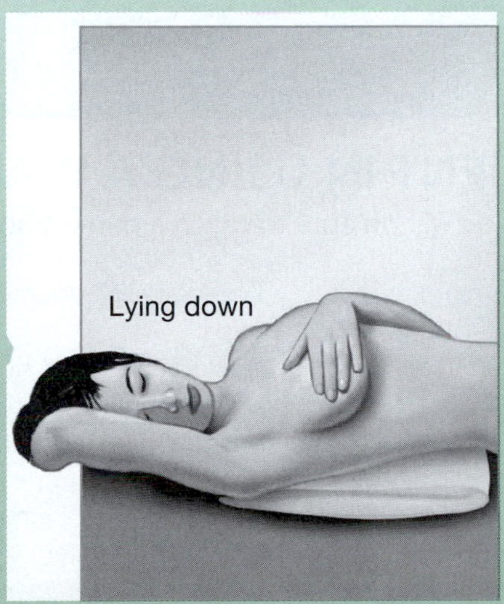

FIGURE 17-16 Patient in side-lying position for breast self-exam.

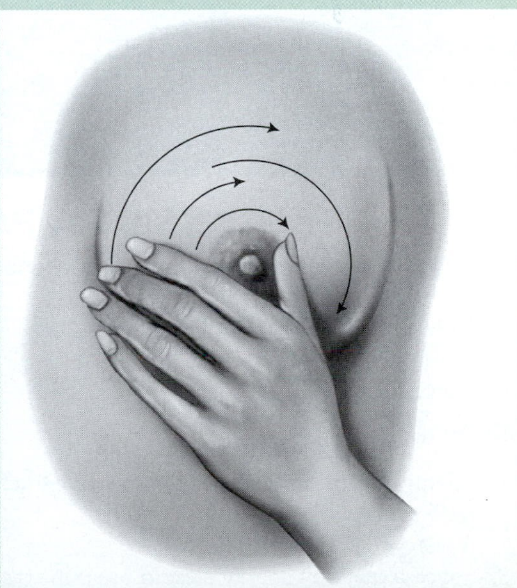

FIGURE 17-17 Palpate each breast in a circular motion.

e. Finish the breast examination by squeezing for nipple discharge and palpating the breast into the axillary area.
f. Report any abnormalities or changes to the physician.
4. Document your patient instruction in breast self-examination. Note the patient's level of understanding.
5. Perform any necessary cleaning of teaching models and store for the next patient use.

CHARTING EXAMPLE

6/7/XX 11:00 A.M. Patient given written materials, verbal instruction, and demonstration on breast self-examination. Patient gave return demonstration correctly without questions. .... Edward Lee, RMA (AMT)

Source: Medical Assisting: Foundations and Practices by M. S. Frazier, C. Malone, and C. Morgan, Upper Saddle River, NJ: Pearson Education, Inc., 2010, p. 1000. Reprinted with permission.

USE AND CARE OF PATIENT EQUIPMENT

Wheelchair

If it is determined that a patient needs to use a wheelchair, it is important to ensure that the wheels are locked and the footplates are folded back before the patient sits in the chair. When the patient is ready to be seated in the wheelchair, he or she should back into the seat, supporting the body on the armrests while lowering the body into the seat. Figure 17-18 shows how to move a wheelchair down a ramp, and Procedure 17-9 provides the necessary steps in order to assist a patient who is learning to use a walker.

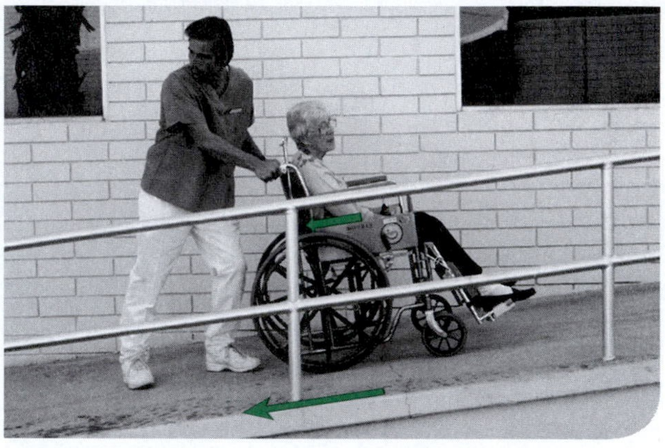

FIGURE 17-18 Wheelchairs are moved down a ramp backward.

Walker

procedure 17-9

ASSIST A PATIENT IN USING A WALKER

Objective: With the necessary materials, you will be able to teach a patient how to use a walker correctly.

EQUIPMENT AND SUPPLIES

- walker
- gait belt

METHOD

1. Identify the patient and explain why instruction in using a walker is necessary.
2. Wash your hands.
3. Place a gait belt snugly around the patient's waist. Tuck any excess belt length under the belt near the hip.
4. Position the patient inside the walker. Adjust the height of the walker as needed. The patient's arms should be flexed at a 30-degree angle when resting on the hand grips.
5. Stand behind and slightly to the side of the patient, with an underhand grip on the gait belt.
6. Instruct the patient to move the walker directly ahead until the back supports of the walker are even with the patient's toes (Figure 17-19).
7. Instruct the patient to grip the handles firmly and step toward the walker with the stronger leg first, then the other leg.
8. Repeat: The patient moves the walker first, then moves toward the walker.

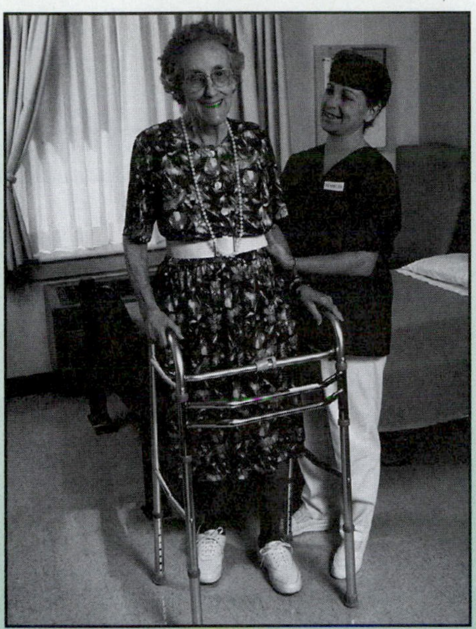

9. Watch the patient for signs of fatigue. Some walkers are equipped with platforms on which the patient can sit to rest.

CHARTING EXAMPLE

08/23/XX 10:45 A.M. Patient assisted with use of her new walker. Patient practiced ambulating around the clinic. Patient states she is "comfortable" using the walker on her own. .... Steve Sanders, RMA (AMT)

FIGURE 17-19 Using a walker for support.

Source: Medical Assisting: Foundations and Practices by M. S. Frazier, C. Malone, and C. Morgan, Upper Saddle River, NJ: Pearson Education, Inc., 2010, p. 978. Reprinted with permission.

Crutches

Several types of crutches are shown in Figure 17-20. Procedure 17-10 discusses the necessary steps when assisting a patient who is learning to use crutches.

PATIENT-ADMINISTERED MEDICATION

Medication errors are very common and are mostly preventable. Medical assistants can educate patients regarding the proper storage, preparation, and administration of their medications and help prevent medication errors.

Inhalers

Metered-dose inhalers (MDIs) are self-administered and allow delivery of a premeasured dose of prescribed medication via a pressurized container. The MDI consists of a pressurized canister that contains approximately 200 doses and a mouthpiece. When the MDI is used correctly, the medication goes directly into the respiratory tract to help dilate the airways.

For patients who have difficulty using the inhaler correctly, a spacer may be used. The spacer traps the medication released from the inhaler, and then the patient inhales the medication from the spacer.

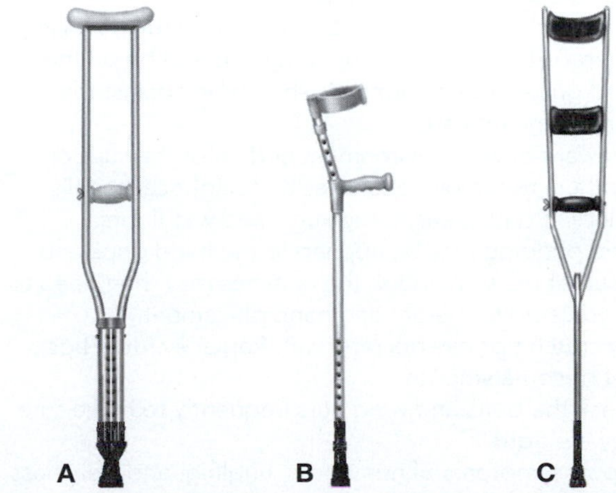

FIGURE 17-20 Types of crutches: (A) Axillary crutch. (B) Lofstrand or forearm crutch. (C) Canadian or elbow crutch.

procedure 17-10

ASSIST A PATIENT WITH CRUTCH WALKING

Objective: With the necessary materials, you will be able to assist a patient with crutch walking correctly.

EQUIPMENT AND SUPPLIES

- crutches correctly fitted to the patient

METHOD

1. Inspect the crutches for correctly fitted arm pads, tight wing nuts, and comfortable handgrips.
2. Instruct the patient to relax the injured knee and keep it slightly bent to avoid touching the foot to the ground.
3. Instruct the patient in the crutch-walking gait ordered by the physician.
4. Have the patient practice taking several steps to ensure correct technique.

CHARTING EXAMPLE

08/23/XX 10:45 A.M. Patient instructed on proper crutch walking and how to inspect the crutches for wear and tear. Patient correctly demonstrated knowledge of crutch use. . . . . Maurice Ellis, RMA (AMT)

Source: Medical Assisting: Foundations and Practices by M. S. Frazier, C. Malone, and C. Morgan, Upper Saddle River, NJ: Pearson Education, Inc., 2010, p. 976, Reprinted with permission.

PATIENT INSTRUCTION: GUIDELINES FOR WALKING WITH CRUTCHES

General Guidelines

- Practice arm strengthening exercises regularly before and during the early stages of crutch walking.
- Practice the crutch gait prescribed by the physician before leaving the medical office, physical therapy department, outpatient treatment center, or convalescent aid supplier.
- Keep the back straight to maintain correct body posture, prevent back strain, and maintain balance.
- Look ahead when walking. Do *not* look at your feet.
- Nonskid shoes will provide stability when crutch walking.
- When crutch walking, body weight should be on the hand grips, and the armrests should be against the sides of the rib cage.
- Be aware of your environment and enlist the support of others to remove obstacles that might cause falls, including dark areas, throw rugs, and wet floors.
- Extra padding may be applied to the hand grips and shoulder rests, although the crutches may then need to be adjusted for height and hand placement.
- Dry crutch tips can become wet. Replace crutch tips that become smooth.
- Check the bolts and wing nuts frequently to make sure they are tight.
- Report symptoms of numbness, tingling, and weakness in the arms, wrists, or hands.

Four-Point Gait (Figure 17-21)

Start in the tripod position (crutch 4 to 6 inches in front of the foot and 4 to 6 inches to the lateral aspect) with your feet approximately a foot apart for balance (you may widen the base distance if you have a large frame). The sequence of steps is:

- Right crutch forward.
- Left foot forward.
- Left crutch forward.
- Right foot forward.
- Repeat.

Three-Point Gait (Figure 17-22)

Start in the tripod position with the feet base distance apart. The sequence of steps is:

- Move the affected leg forward with the crutches.
- Balancing on the crutches, move the unaffected leg forward.
- Repeat.

Two-Point Gait (Figure 17-23)

Start in the tripod position with the feet base distance apart. The sequence of steps is:

- Move the left crutch and right foot forward at the same time.

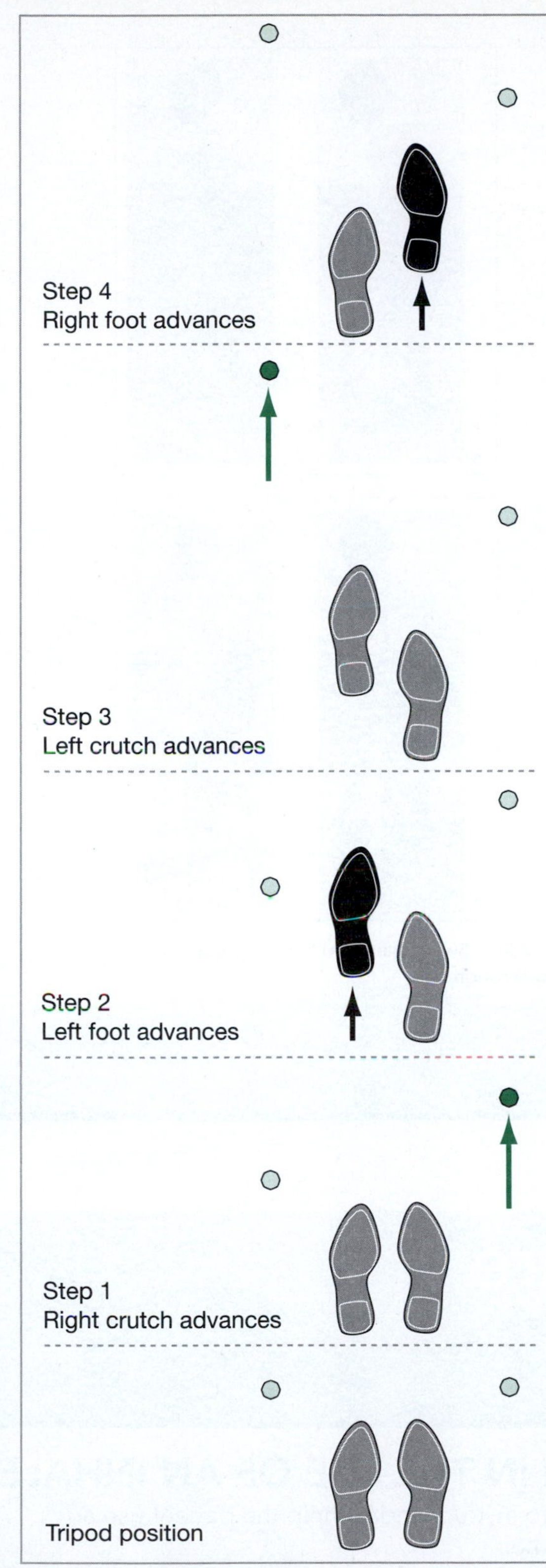

FIGURE 17-21 **Four-point gait.**

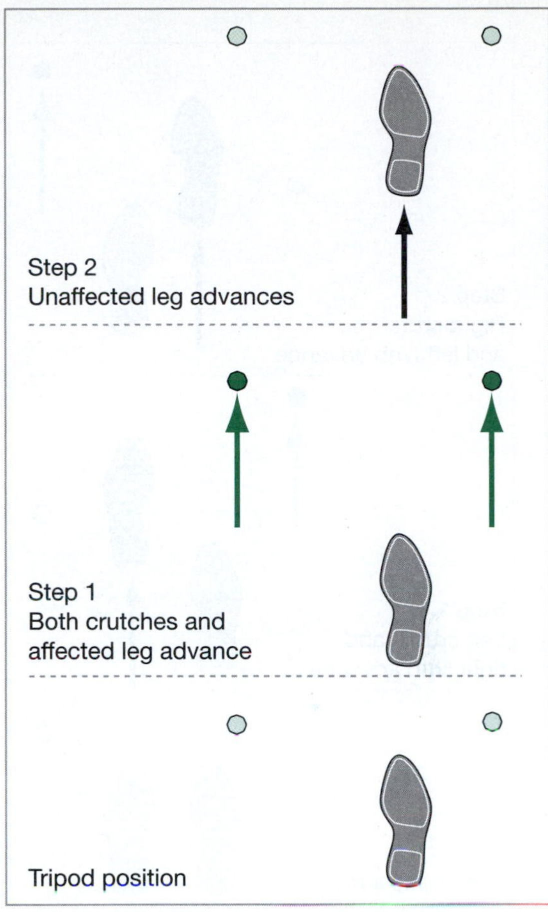

FIGURE 17-22 **Three-point gait.**

- Move the right crutch and left foot forward at the same time.
- Repeat.

Swing Gait (Figure 17-24)

Start in the tripod position with the feet base distance apart. The sequence of steps for the swing-to gait is:

- Move both crutches forward.
- Lift and swing the extremities to the crutches.
- Repeat.

For the swing-through gait:

- Move both crutches forward.
- Lift and swing the extremities to and past the crutches.
- Repeat.

(continued)

(Continued)

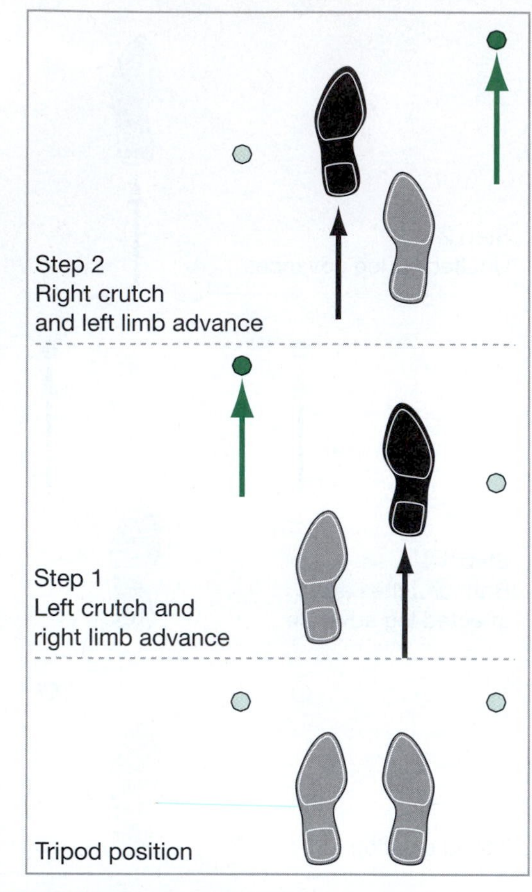

FIGURE 17-23 Two-point gait.

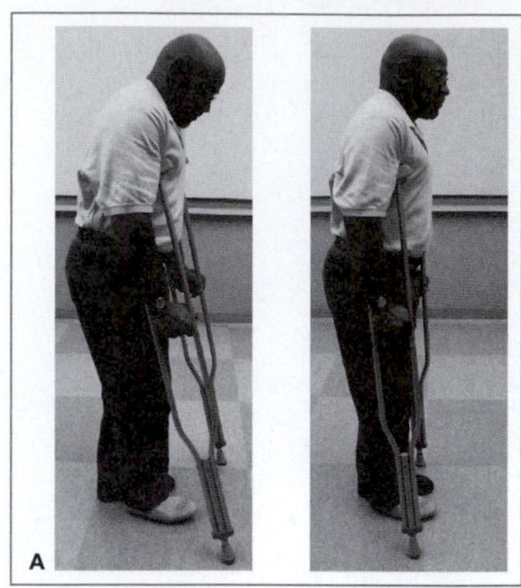

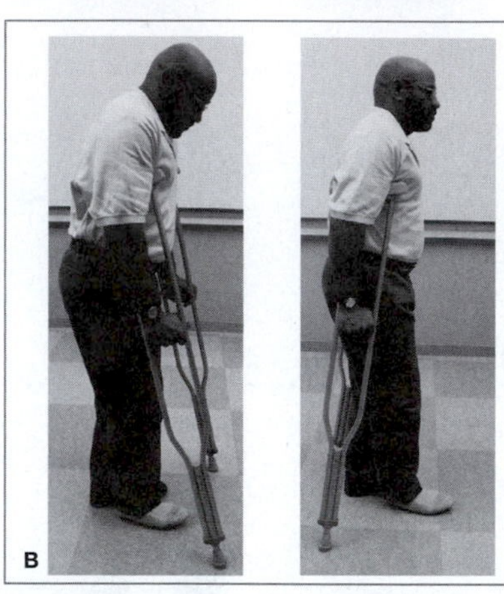

FIGURE 17-24 Swing gaits: (A) Swing-to gait. (B) Swing-through gait.

Source: Medical Assisting: Foundations and Practices by M. S. Frazier, C. Malone, and C. Morgan, Upper Saddle River, NJ: Pearson Education, Inc., 2010, p. 973. Reprinted with permission.

procedure 17-11

DEMONSTRATE PATIENT INSTRUCTION IN THE USE OF AN INHALER

Objective: With the necessary materials, you will be able to instruct and/or help the patient use an inhaler for the first time.

EQUIPMENT AND SUPPLIES

- patient's prescription inhaler
- patient's chart

METHOD

1. Wash your hands and gather the equipment.
2. Identify and guide the patient to the treatment area.

3. Give the patient the following instructions.
   - Shake the canister thoroughly.
   - Hold the canister upright within 2 inches of the mouth. Place the mouthpiece in your mouth, sealing the opening with your lips (Figure 17-25).
   - Activate the inhaler (usually by pressing the canister down) to spray (Figure 17-26).

Breathe slowly but deeply after the medication is delivered.
   - Hold your breath for as long as possible, up to 10 seconds.
   - Begin breathing normally again.
   - Follow the physician's instructions for immediate repeat use.
4. Document the patient's ability to follow instructions. Inform the physician if the patient has any problems with self-administration. Give the patient backup written instructions.

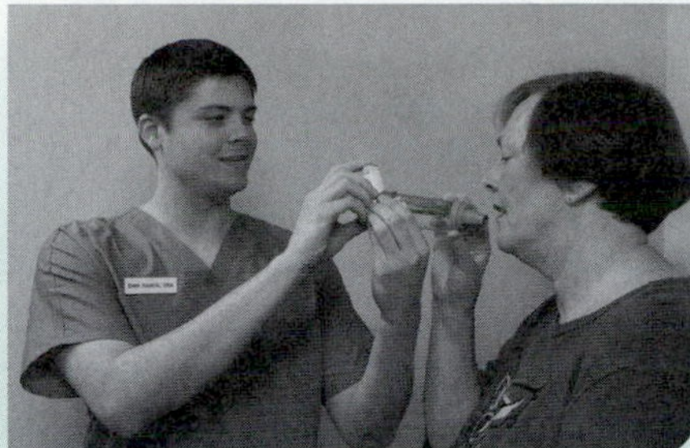

FIGURE 17-25 Patient with inhaler held upright.

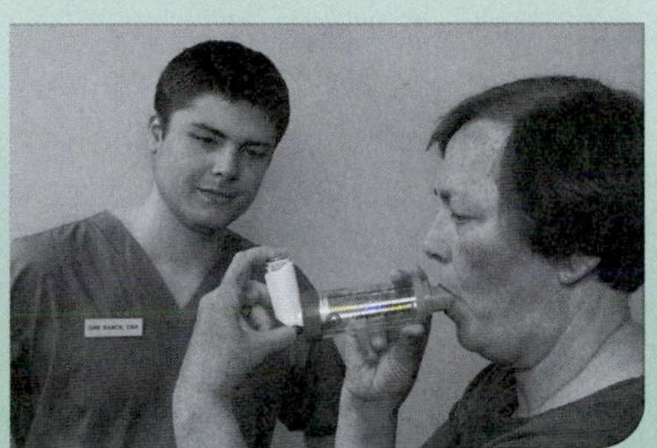

FIGURE 17-26 Activate the inhaler.

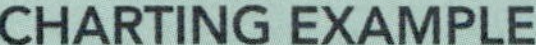

CHARTING EXAMPLE

11/23/XX 2:30 P.M. Pt demonstrated correct use of the inhaler with instruction. Written instructions were given with the office's phone number. Pt states that medication has helped make breathing easier. · · · · · · · · · · · Parker Clay, CMA (AAMA)

Source: Medical Assisting: Foundations and Practices by M. S. Frazier, C. Malone, and C. Morgan, Upper Saddle River, NJ: Pearson Education, Inc., 2010, p. 787. Reprinted with permission.

In order to ensure that the medication is administered as ordered, patient teaching is very important (see Procedure 17-11).

Nebulizers

Figure 17-27 shows photos of nebulizers. Refer to Procedure 17-12 for information on how to provide patient instruction on the proper use of a nebulizer.

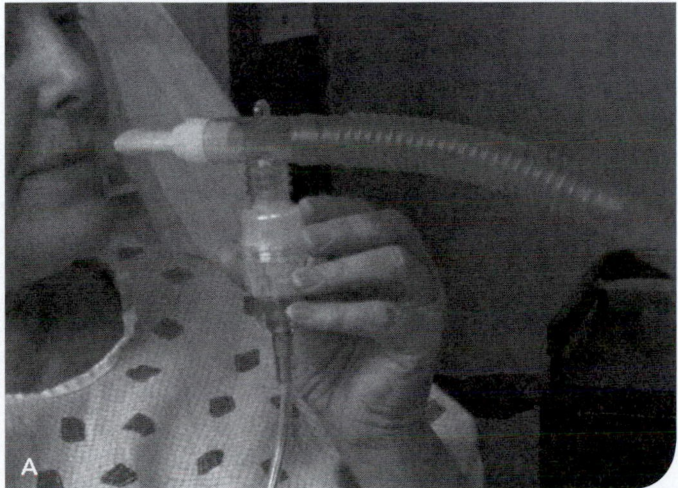

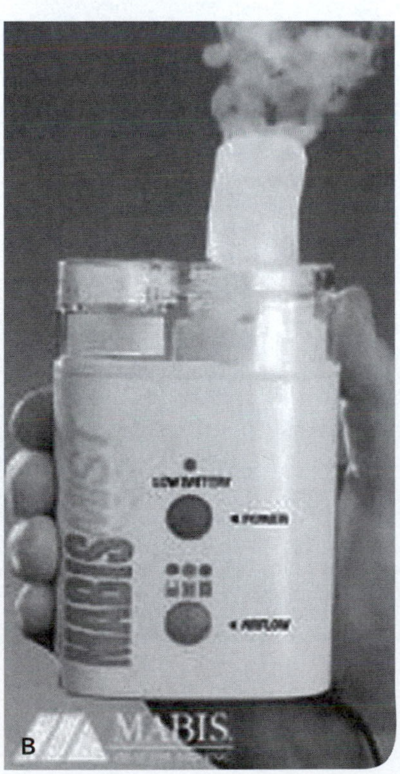

FIGURE 17-27 (A) Nebulizer. (B) Ultrasonic nebulizer.

procedure 17-12

DEMONSTRATE PATIENT INSTRUCTION IN THE USE OF A NEBULIZER

Objective: With the necessary materials, you will be able to assist the patient in the use of a nebulizer.

EQUIPMENT AND SUPPLIES

- compressor
- nebulizer with mask and tubing
- medications
- patient's chart

METHOD

1. Wash your hands. Gather equipment and supplies.
2. Identify the patient and guide him or her to the treatment area.
3. Obtain vital signs.
4. Wash your hands again.
5. Prepare the nebulizer cup with medication(s) as ordered and/or prescribed (Figure 17-28).
6. Turn on the compressor (Figure 17-29).
7. Instruct, or help, the patient to hold the mask while the medication is being delivered.
8. Continue treatment until no medication remains in the nebulizer. Monitor the patient's pulse every 5 minutes throughout the treatment (Figure 17-30). If the pulse rises to 120 beats per minute or the patient's condition worsens, *stop the treatment and tell the physician.*
9. Dispose of used materials in the appropriate containers.
10. Wash your hands.
11. Document the patient's vital signs at the beginning, middle, and end of the treatment. Also describe the patient's signs and symptoms at the beginning and end of the treatment.

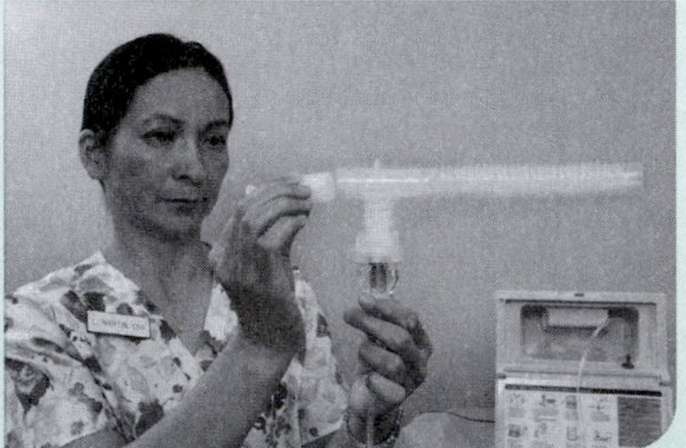

FIGURE 17-28 Prepare the nebulizer cup with medication(s) as ordered and/or prescribed.

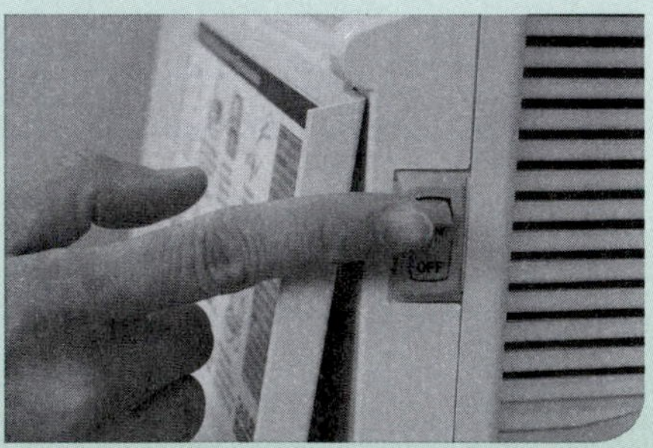

FIGURE 17-29 Turn on the compressor.

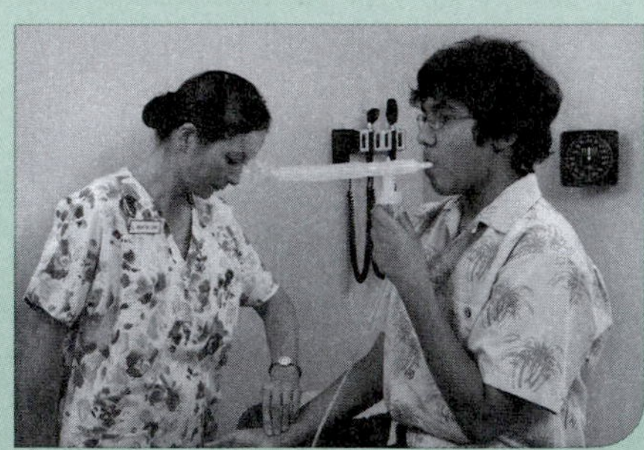

FIGURE 17-30 Monitor the patient's pulse.

CHARTING EXAMPLE

12/27/XX 2:45 P.M. Instructions given to pt's wife to perform the nebulizer treatment. She demonstrated the procedure correctly. She described the correct frequency and symptoms to observe and demonstrated the correct procedure for counting a radial pulse. .... Susan Tucker, RMA (AMT)

Source: Medical Assisting: Foundations and Practices by M. S. Frazier, C. Malone, and C. Morgan, Upper Saddle River, NJ: Pearson Education, Inc., 2010, p. 788. Reprinted with permission.

Insulin

Often it will be the medical assistant who provides instruction for the diabetic patient on how to administer daily insulin injections. When providing education on patient administration of insulin, you will need to follow the guidelines for subcutaneous injections found in Chapter 21 as well as the blood glucose testing guidelines found in Procedure 20-18. The patient must rotate the injection sites (Figure 17-31).

It is especially important that patients understand how to prepare and administer their medication accurately. In addition, they need to understand the connection between their glucometer reading and the amount of insulin to be administered.

Most pharmaceutical companies have printed patient education material available.

Oxygen

It may be necessary for patients to be placed on oxygen in order for them to continue the activities of daily living. In an outpatient or home setting, oxygen is usually delivered via nasal cannula and is prescribed for three primary reasons:

- Decrease the work of breathing.
- Decrease the work of the heart.
- Reverse or prevent low blood oxygen levels.

It is important that patients understand that they should not adjust the flow rate of oxygen without the physician's direction. Doing so may cause the patient's condition to worsen.

Patients should also be instructed to avoid flammable substances such as oil-based lubricants, smoking materials, and open gas or heat sources.

If the patient needs to moisten dry lips or nostrils, only water-soluble lubricants should be used. Refer to Procedure 17-13 for guidelines on administering oxygen.

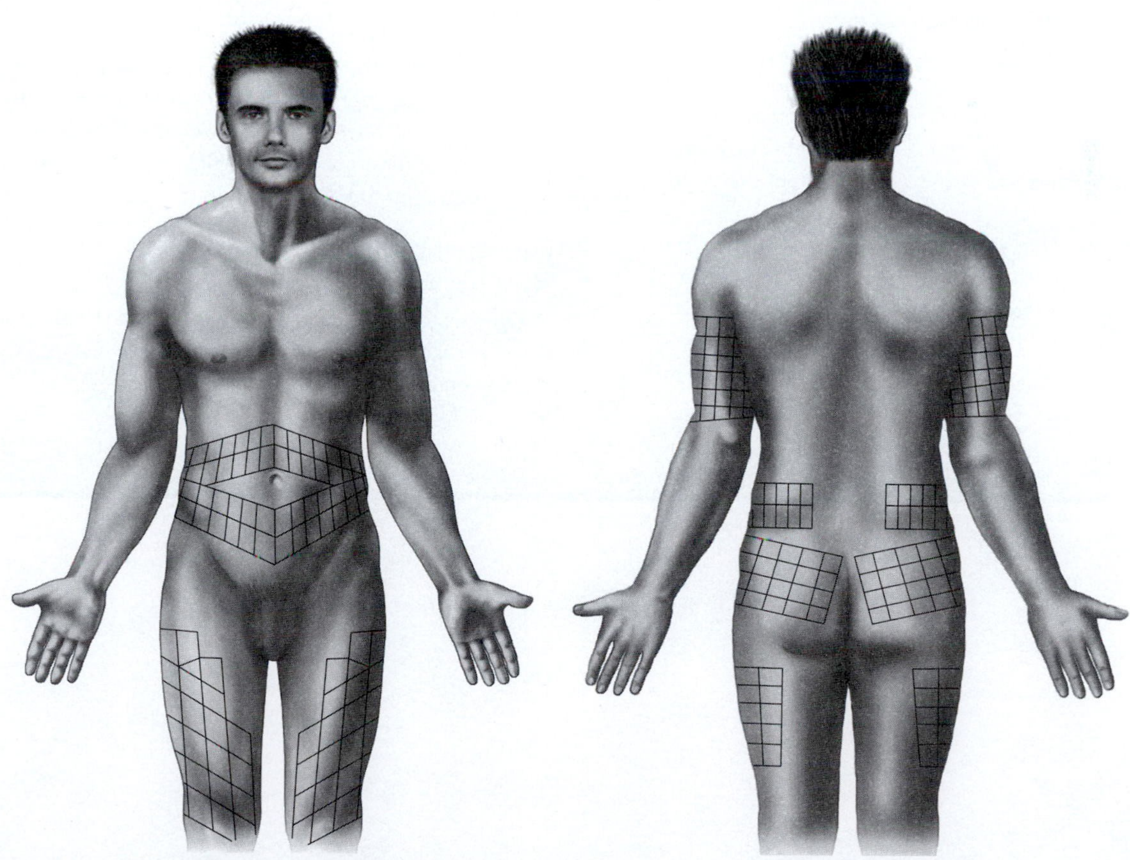

FIGURE 17-31 Rotation of sites for administering insulin.

procedure 17-13

ADMINISTERING OXYGEN

Objective: With the necessary materials, you will be able to administer oxygen therapy to an adult.

EQUIPMENT AND SUPPLIES

- portable oxygen tank
- pressure regulator
- oxygen flow meter
- sterile, prepackaged, disposable nasal cannula with tubing
- gloves
- oximeter
- patient chart

METHOD

1. Gather all needed equipment.
2. Wash your hands.
3. Identify the patient and confirm the physician's order for oxygen therapy.
4. Check the pressure reading on the oxygen tank to make sure that it contains enough oxygen.
5. Start the flow of oxygen by opening the cylinder.
6. Attach the cannula tubing to the flow meter. Adjust the oxygen flow to the physician's order.
7. Hold the cannula tips over the inside of your wrist, without touching the skin, to determine if the oxygen is flowing.
8. Don gloves if necessary. You may prefer to wear gloves with patients who demonstrate a chronic cough, a nasal drip, or another situation of potential exposure.
9. Place the tips of the nasal cannula into the patient's nostrils. Wrap the tubing behind the patient's ears (Figure 17-32).

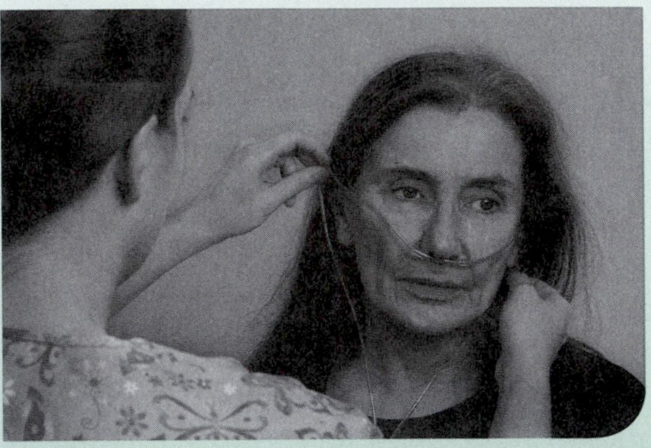

FIGURE 17-32 Adjust the tubing around the back of the patient's ears.

10. Instruct the patient to breathe normally through the mouth and nose. Some patients instinctively hold their breath or avoid breathing through the nose when an object is placed in the nostrils.
11. Check the patient's oxygen level with an oximeter. Place the probe over the index finger and record the reading. If necessary, have the patient take a short walk to verify that the oxygen flow rate is sufficient for activity.
12. Document the procedure in the patient's chart.

CHARTING EXAMPLE

10/25/XX 11:30 A.M. Patient evaluated for oxygen use. Patient tested on 2 lpm [liters per minute] continuous flow while at rest. 4 lpm needed for activity to maintain 90% blood oxygen saturation. Order for O_2 two lpm rest/four lpm with exertion faxed to Apria Home Health Care. . . . .
. . . . Connie Hughes, CMA (AAMA)

17 APPLICATION

Directions: Select the best answer for each of the following questions. Check your answers in the Answer Key at the end of the book.

1. "Bob, how would you describe your pain?" is an example of what type of interview question?
   a. Reflecting
   b. Open-ended
   c. Close-ended
   d. Intrusive
   e. Indirect

2. The patient's past history should include the following information:
   a. Allergies
   b. Occupation
   c. Marital status
   d. Medications
   e. A and D

3. Social history will include all of the following except:
   a. Childhood diseases
   b. Smoking history
   c. Occupation
   d. Marital status
   e. Diet and exercise habits

4. During the physician's review of systems (ROS), if the patient says that he or she does not tolerate temperature changes very well, this might suggest that something is happening within which body system?
   a. Respiratory
   b. Cardiovascular
   c. Neurologic
   d. Endocrine
   e. Musculoskeletal

5. Which of the following is not one of the six C's of charting?
   a. Clarity
   b. Comprehensive
   c. Conciseness
   d. Chronological
   e. Confidentiality

6. All of the following are considered vital signs except:
   a. Temperature
   b. Pulse
   c. Respirations
   d. Blood pressure
   e. Weight

7. The normal rectal temperature (Fahrenheit) for an adult is:
   a. 96.8
   b. 97.6
   c. 98.6
   d. 99.6
   e. None of the above

8. When you take a patient's blood pressure and you hear a swishing or whooshing sound, this is known as which Korotkoff phase?
   a. Phase I
   b. Phase II
   c. Phase III
   d. Phase IV
   e. Phase V

9. When measuring a child's temperature using the axillary method, the thermometer should remain in the child's armpit for:
   a. 2 minutes
   b. 4 minutes
   c. 6 minutes
   d. 8 minutes
   e. 10 minutes

10. The preferred method for measuring body temperature in a patient who is able to follow instructions is:
    a. Temporal artery
    b. Tympanic
    c. Axillary
    d. Rectal
    e. Oral

11. The average pulse rate for an older adult is:
    a. 120–160 bpm
    b. 80–120 bpm
    c. 80–100 bpm
    d. 60–80 bpm
    e. 50–65 bpm

12. When measuring a radial pulse, which of the following statements is not considered proper procedure?
    a. Ask the patient to place the arm in a comfortable position.
    b. The patient's arm should be at waist level with the palm down.
    c. Start counting the pulse when the second hand on the watch is at 3, 6, 9, or 12.
    d. Count the pulse for 1 full minute.
    e. The number will always be an even number.

13. The popliteal pulse may be located:
    a. In the inner aspect of the elbow
    b. At the side of the head
    c. In the groin
    d. Behind the knee
    e. On top of the foot slightly lateral to midline

14. The normal respiratory range for a newborn is _____ breaths per minute:
    a. 18–24
    b. 20–30
    c. 22–40
    d. 30–50
    e. 40–60

15. Which of the following blood pressure readings is considered to be prehypertensive?
   a. > 140/90
   b. 120/80 to 139/89
   c. 119/79 to 139/89
   d. 129/84 to 140/89
   e. 124/86 to 139/89

16. Essential hypertension is best described as:
   a. Elevated blood pressure associated with other conditions, such as renal disease or pregnancy
   b. Rapidly developing elevated blood pressure that may become fatal if not treated immediately
   c. Slow-onset elevated blood pressure without symptoms
   d. Primary hypertension of unknown cause
   e. Temporary fall in blood pressure that occurs when the patient moves rapidly from a lying to a standing position

17. When measuring a patient's blood pressure, which of the following statements is not correct?
   a. Blood pressure may be taken while the patient is lying down.
   b. If the patient's arm is below heart level, the blood pressure reading will be lower than normal.
   c. Never take a blood pressure reading through clothing.
   d. The sphygmomanometer should be placed 1 to 2 inches above the brachial artery.
   e. The level of mercury should be pumped 20 to 30 mmHg above the point at which the radial pulse is no longer palpable.

18. The pulse rate in a normal, healthy adult is approximately:
   a. 80 bpm
   b. 60 bpm
   c. 65 bpm
   d. 70 bpm
   e. 55 bpm

19. ______________ respirations per minute is considered to be normal.
   a. 16 to 20
   b. 35 to 45
   c. 8 to 12
   d. 10 to 14
   e. None of the above

20. The term describing a rattling breath sound is ______________:
   a. Stridor
   b. Stertorous
   c. Rales
   d. Rhonchi
   e. Cheyne-Stokes

21. When teaching a patient how to use a walker correctly, which of the following statements is not true?
   a. Position the patient inside the walker.
   b. Place a gait belt around the patient's waist.
   c. The patient's hands should be on the handgrip, with the elbows flexed at a 30 degree angle.
   d. The patient should move toward the walker and then move the walker.
   e. Instruct the patient to bring the stronger foot forward, even with the weaker foot.

22. When instructing a male patient on the proper technique for testicular self-exam, which of the following statements is not correct?
   a. Take a warm bath or shower to relax the scrotum.
   b. If one testicle is slightly larger, or lies somewhat behind or lower than the other, this is considered abnormal.
   c. The patient should palpate the testicle for lumps, hardness. or anything unusual.
   d. Any abnormalities should be reported to the physician.
   e. It is recommended that men perform testicular self-exams monthly.

23. Which of the following correctly lists the proper procedure for a four-point gait?
   a. Move both crutches forward; lift and swing the extremities to the crutches.
   b. Move the left crutch and right foot forward at the same time; move the right crutch and left foot forward at the same time.
   c. Move both crutches forward; lift and swing the extremities to and past the crutches.
   d. Move the affected leg forward with the crutches, balancing on the crutches, and move the unaffected leg forward.
   e. Move the right crutch forward, left foot forward, left crutch forward, right foot forward.

24. Which of the following statements about MDIs is not correct?
   a. They are self-administered.
   b. A pressurized canister is used.
   c. Medication goes directly into the respiratory tract.
   d. A spacer may be used.
   e. The canister contains approximately 300 doses of premeasured medication.

25. If a patient is using a nebulizer, you should monitor the patient's pulse every _____ minute(s).
   a. 5
   b. 4
   c. 3
   d. 2
   e. 1

18 Exam Room Equipment, Examinations, and Procedures

CONTENTS

Equipment Operation

It is important that a medical assistant knows how to use and care for equipment used within the medical office.

AUTOCLAVE

The autoclave is one of the most effective methods used to sterilize instruments and other supplies, such as gauze, used during in-office procedures and surgeries. The autoclave has two separate compartments. The outer compartment surrounds the inner compartment, where the sterilization occurs. By reducing the air in the inner chamber, it allows pressure to build, and the pressure (15 to 17 pounds per square inch [psi]) causes the distilled water to reach a temperature of 250°F. Once this temperature is reached, the water converts to steam, penetrates the wrapping on the instruments, and kills all microorganisms and bacterial spores. The temperature must be maintained for a minimum of 15 minutes.

Sterilization Indicators

Sterilization indicators should be used with each load autoclaved. This will help eliminate the question of whether or not the load was sterilized. Sterilization indicators show, either by melting or by changing color, that the proper temperature has been achieved. The most common indicators are autoclave tape and sterilization indicator strips.

The CDC recommends keeping accurate records of all loads autoclaved and the results of quality control measures. See Procedures 18-1 and 18-2.

procedure 18-1

WRAPPING AND LABELING INSTRUMENTS FOR AUTOCLAVING

Objective: Wrap and label instruments properly.

EQUIPMENT AND SUPPLIES

- wrapping material
- instrument(s) for autoclaving
- sterilization indicator strips
- autoclave tape
- indelible-ink pen
- label

METHOD

1. Wash your hands.
2. Place a square of wrapping material on the table so that it appears as a diamond shape when you look at it. Be sure that the wrapping material is large enough to cover the entire article being wrapped.
3. Place the item in the center of the wrapping material. If hinged items are included, be sure that the instrument is in the open position. If sharp instruments are being autoclaved, wrap the tip in a piece of gauze to prevent puncture through the material.
4. Place the indicator strip in the center of the packet.
5. Fold the bottom point of the wrapping material up and over the instruments. Fold a small portion of the point back over so that it can be used to pick up the paper when it is unwrapped (Figure 18-1A).
6. Fold the right side of the wrapping paper over until it covers the instrument(s). Fold a small portion of the point back over, as in the previous step.
7. Fold the left side of the wrapping paper over until it covers the instrument(s). Fold a small portion of the point back over, as in the previous step (Figure 18-1B).
8. Now fold up the bottom of the package. Continue folding until you have reached the top point (Figure 18-1C).
9. Be sure that the pack is folded snugly.
10. Secure the package with a piece of autoclave tape (Figure 18-1D).
11. Label the package with the name of the item(s) inside, your initials, and the date.
12. If bags are used for the autoclaving procedure, place the item and an indicator strip inside the bag. (If the item has a sharp point, wrap the point in a piece of gauze.)
13. Seal the bag. Label the bag with the name of the item(s) inside, your initials, and the date.

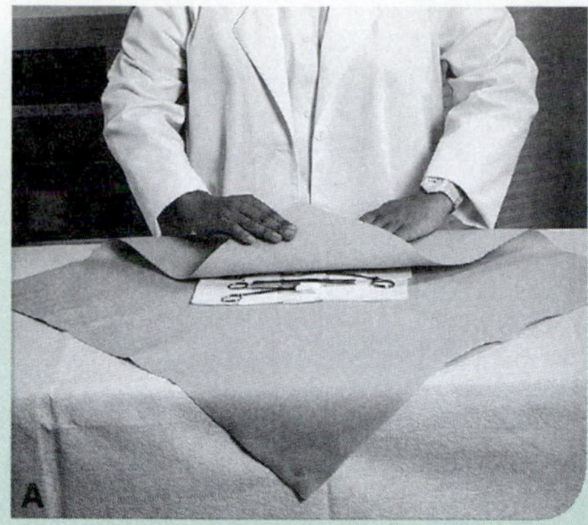

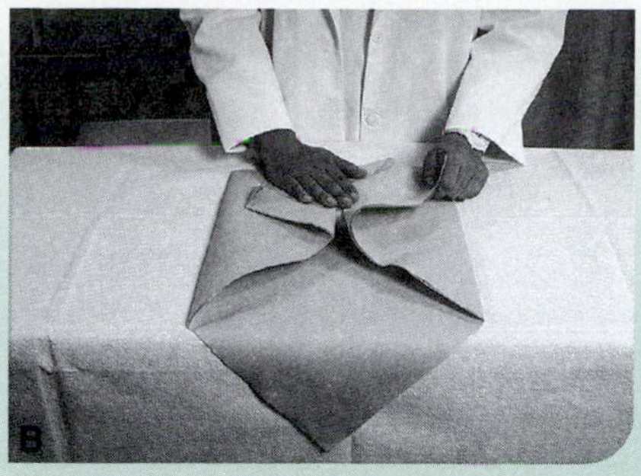

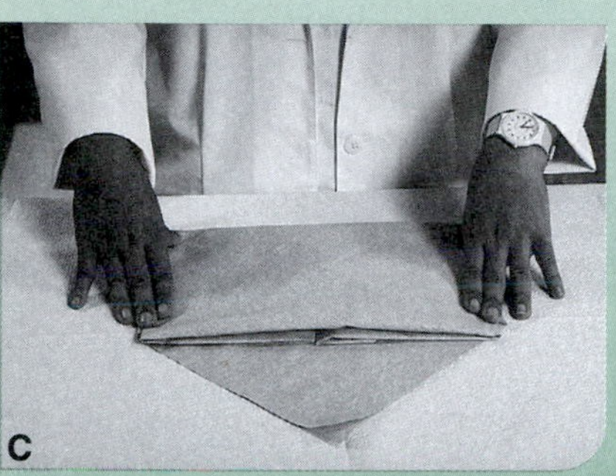

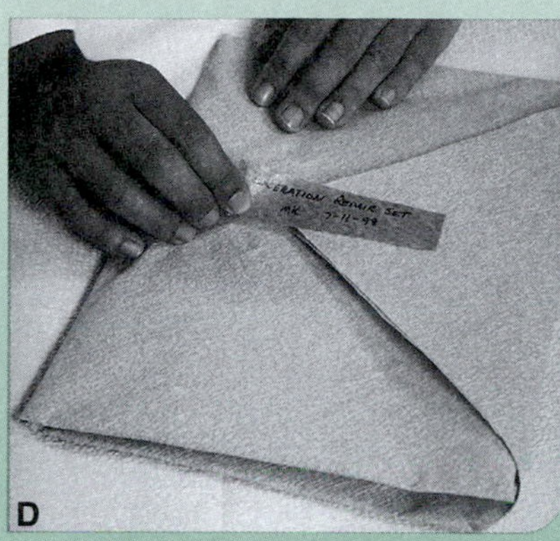

FIGURE 18-1 (A) Place the item in the center of the wrapping material with the hinges open and fold the bottom up over the instrument. (B) Fold the right side of the paper until it covers the item and make a small flap; next, proceed in the same way with the left side. (C) Fold up the bottom of the package. (D) Use a piece of autoclave tape to secure the package.

procedure 18-2

STERILIZING INSTRUMENTS IN AN AUTOCLAVE

Objective: Sterilize instruments in an autoclave to prevent the spread of pathogens.

EQUIPMENT AND SUPPLIES

- autoclave
- instruments sanitized and wrapped for autoclaving
- distilled water
- autoclave directions

METHOD

1. Check the level of water in the autoclave reservoir. Add distilled water as needed to the fill line (Figure 18-2A).
2. Load the autoclave. Trays and packs should be loaded on their sides. Containers should be loaded on their sides with the lids off or ajar. Mixed loads are loaded with hard objects on bottom racks and softer items on top racks. Keep large packs 2 to 4 inches apart and smaller packets 1 to 2 inches apart.
3. Read the manufacturer's instructions and follow them exactly. Most autoclaves follow similar protocols.

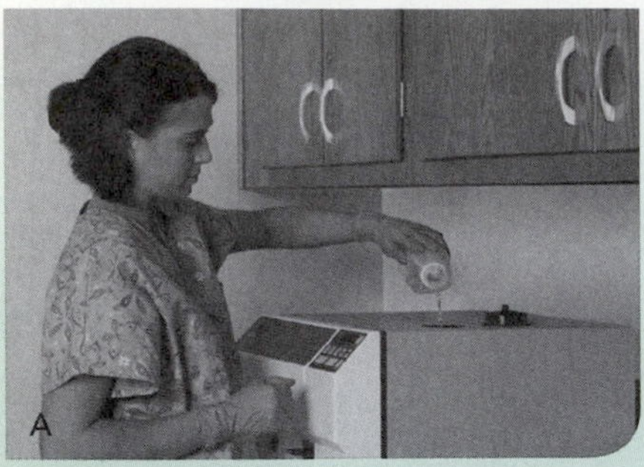

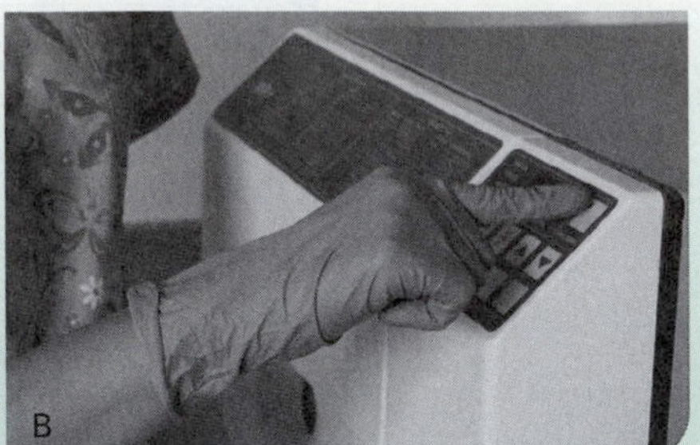

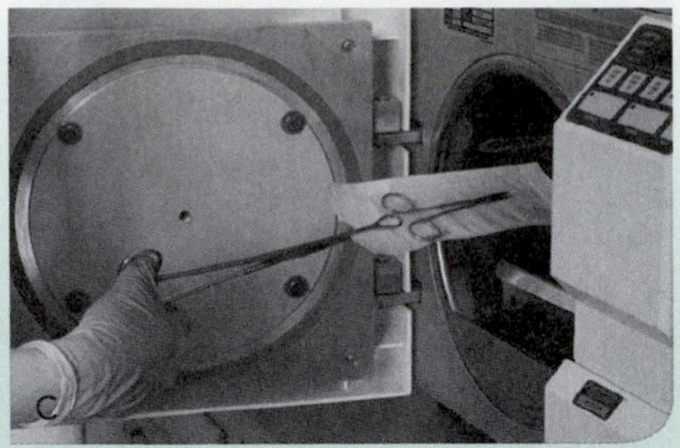

FIGURE 18-2 **(A) Check the level of water in the autoclave and add water as needed. (B) Properly set the autoclave according to the manufacturer's instructions. (C) Remove the instruments to a clean container using the sterile transfer forceps.**

   a. Turn the control knob to FILL and observe carefully with the door open until the water reaches the chamber fill line.
   b. Turn the knob to the autoclave position (Figure 18-2B). This shuts off the water.
   c. Close and lock the door.
   d. When pressure reaches 15 to 17 psi and the temperature reaches 250°F to 270°F, set the timer for the required time. Typical timing is 30 minutes for wrapped trays and packages and 15 minutes for unwrapped items. Always check the manufacturer's suggested times and the facility's protocol.
4. When the timing is complete, turn the control knob to VENT.
5. When the pressure reaches zero, open the chamber door about 1 inch and allow the items in the autoclave to dry completely before removing them (about 30 to 45 minutes).
6. Turn the autoclave knob to OFF.
7. Remove the wrapped items and check the autoclave tape on the outside for color change. Store the items in a dry closed cabinet for use. Unwrapped items must be removed using sterile transfer forceps and must be placed on a sterile field or in a sterile storage area (Figure 18-2C).
8. Record the date, time, and types of items autoclaved in the log and initial it.

EQUIPMENT USED FOR PHYSICAL EXAMINATIONS

Endoscope	• Instrument used to look into a hollow organ or body cavity • Used to examine the larynx, bladder, colon, sigmoid colon, stomach, abdomen, and some joints
Exam Table	• Typically, the physician will examine most patients on the examination table. • Several styles of exam tables are available; the type of exam table found in the office will most likely reflect the physician's medical specialty. • Some exam tables are equipped with hydraulics that allows the physician to elevate and lower the patient by operating the foot controls.
Ophthalmoscope	• Instrument used to examine the interior of the eye • Light is focused through a magnifying lens onto the interior surface of the eye to check for abnormalities.
Otoscope	• Instrument used to examine the ears • Light is focused through a speculum into the outer ear and onto the tympanic membrane. • Additional speculums may be used to view other structures, such as the nose.
Oximeter	• Instrument used to measure oxygen saturation in arterial blood • Clipped to the bridge of the nose, forehead, earlobe, or fingertip

(*Continued*)

Scales	• Used to measure the patient's weight • May be calibrated in either kilograms or pounds
Sphygmo-manometer	• Also known as the *blood pressure cuff* • Instrument used for measuring the pressure the blood exerts against the walls of the artery Types of Sphygmomanometers • *Aneroid:* has a round dial that contains a scale calibrated in millimeters and a needle to register the reading • *Mercury:* not used as often as the aneroid due to the presence of mercury; may be found on walls; contain a column of mercury that rises as the bulb is pressed • *Electronic:* does not require a stethoscope and provides a digital readout on a lighted display Components of the Sphygmomanometer • *Manometer:* scale that registers the pressure reading • *Inflatable rubber bladder:* when the bulb is pumped, it causes the rubber bladder to inflate and temporarily constrict blood circulation in the arm. • *Cuff:* soft material that covers the rubber bladder and is placed against the patient's skin • *Bulb:* has a thumbscrew attached to a control valve that allows inflation and deflation of the cuff
Stethoscope	• Diagnostic instrument used to amplify sounds in the body such as the heart, lungs, and abdomen Components of the Stethoscope: • *Chest piece:* portion that is placed over the site where the sound is to be heard • *Diaphragm:* disc-like sound sensor that picks up both low- and high-pitched sound frequencies • *Bell:* hollow curved bell- or cup-shaped sound sensor that may have one, two, or three "heads" that are useful in picking up cardiovascular sounds • *Flexible tubing:* rubber or plastic tubing that carries the sound from the patient to the binaurals • *Binaurals:* Rigid small metal tubes that connect the tubing to the earpieces • *Spring mechanism:* flexible external metal spring that holds the binaural steady • *Earpieces:* molded plastic tips that attach to the end of the binaurals and are placed in the ears prior to listening to the patient's body sounds
Thermometer	• Instrument used for measuring body temperature Types of Thermometers • *Nonmercury:* available in two shapes: long, slender tip (oral thermometer); stubby, pearl-shaped tip (oral, axillary, or rectal thermometer) • *Electronic:* battery operated, with a digital window for viewing and reading • *Tympanic membrane:* also known as an *aural thermometer*; detects heat waves within the ear canal near the eardrum • *Temporal artery:* scanner that, when stroked gently across the forehead, measures the heat emitted through the skin from the temporal artery • *Chemical disposable:* uses liquid dots or heat-sensitive bars. When applied to the forehead, the dots/bars change color.

SUPPLIES USED FOR PHYSICAL EXAMINATIONS

TYPICAL EXAMINING ROOM EQUIPMENT AND SUPPLIES

Equipment/Supply	Use
Alcohol Wipes	Used to disinfect and cleanse skin before injections and phlebotomy
Balance Scale	Used to take patient's weight and height
Bandages (Small)	Applied after taking a blood sample and some injections

(*continued*)

(*Continued*)

Equipment/Supply	Use
Batteries and Light Bulbs	Extra batteries and light bulbs required for lighted equipment
Betadine (or Other Topical Antiseptic)	Used to disinfect skin before minor surgery
Biohazardous Waste Container	Closed rigid container with biohazardous labeling and appropriate red waste bags
Cotton Balls (Sterile and Nonsterile)	Used to apply antiseptic or to clean the skin
Cotton-Tipped Swabs (Sterile and Nonsterile)	Used to clean recessed areas, to apply medications and lubricant, and to obtain specimens from the throat and other orifices
Drapes	Disposable paper or cloth sheet used to cover the patient during the examination
Emesis Basin	Kidney-shaped receptacle for body drainage, such as sputum, and for used instruments
Fixative Spray	Used to preserve slides
Gauze Dressings (4 × 4 or 3 × 4)	Applied to dress small wounds
Gloves (Nonsterile Disposable)	Worn by all staff to protect against microorganisms and blood-borne pathogens
Gloves (Sterile Disposable)	Worn when performing minor surgery and handling sterile materials
Gooseneck Lamp	Movable light used to focus on a body area for increased visibility
Hydrogen Peroxide (H_2O_2)	Used to clean open wounds
Irrigation Syringe	Used to wash cerumen (earwax) out of the ear canal or to irrigate wounds
Lubricant	Water-soluble gel applied to the physician's glove, speculum, or rectal thermometer to reduce friction during insertion; prevents damage to delicate mucous membranes
Soap Dispenser	Used to dispense germicidal soap for handwashing between examinations of patients
Sphygmomanometer	Machine used to measure blood pressure
Tape	Used to secure dressings
Tape Measure	Used to measure lesions, head circumference, and body areas
Thermometers (Various Types)	Used to measure temperature
Tissues	Used to wipe body secretions
Tongue Depressor	Wooden blade used to hold down patient's tongue while examining the mouth and throat
Vaginal Speculum	Instrument used to expand the vaginal opening to view the cervix

Preparation in the Exam and Treatment Rooms

One of the most important responsibilities the medical assistant may have is to ensure that exam rooms and treatment areas are clean and well stocked, as this affects patient care and perceptions as well as enabling productive work flow. Ordering supplies and stocking exam room supplies are ongoing procedures that must be performed throughout the day.

PREPARING THE EXAM AND TREATMENT ROOM

Preparing for the next patient may begin before the patient currently in the room leaves. While the physician is talking with the patient, the medical assistant may begin gathering necessary supplies for the next patient that might not be stored in the exam or treatment room where the medical assistant will be. Once the current patient leaves the exam room, the medical assistant must quickly but efficiently clean the room and set it up for the next patient (Procedure 18-3).

procedure

18-3

CLEANING THE EXAMINATION ROOM

Objective: Clean an examination room to the instructor's specifications.

EQUIPMENT AND SUPPLIES

- disinfectant
- paper towels
- disposable gloves
- examination table
- pillow
- disposable gown

METHOD

1. Perform hand hygiene.
2. Put on a clean pair of disposable gloves.
3. Roll the soiled disposable gown into a ball shape and dispose of it in the appropriate waste container.
4. Roll the soiled examination table paper into a ball shape and dispose of it in the appropriate waste container.
5. Remove the soiled pillow cover and dispose of it in the appropriate waste container.
6. Remove any other soiled items or equipment from the examination room.
7. Clean the examination table and cabinet surfaces with disinfectant and paper towels (Figure 18-3).
8. Dispose of soiled paper towels in the appropriate waste container.

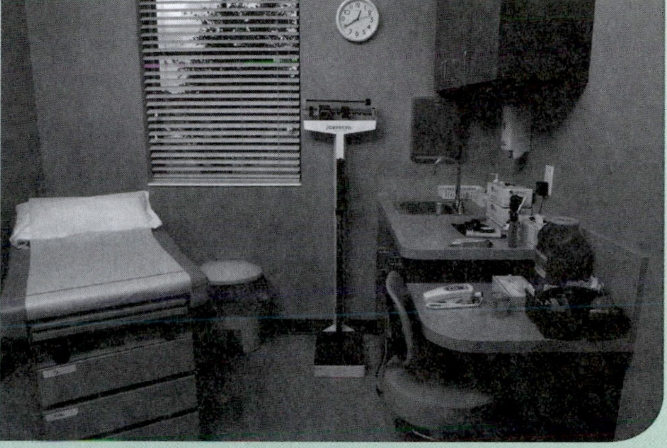

FIGURE 18-3 Examination room.

9. Remove the soiled gloves and dispose of them in the appropriate waste container.
10. Perform hand hygiene.
11. Put clean paper on the examination table.
12. Put a new pillow covering over the pillow.
13. Make sure that the examination room is clean and clutter and odor free.

STOCKING SUPPLIES

Most staff restock their exam and treatment rooms at the end of the day to make sure that everything is in place for the following day and that there are enough supplies for all procedures scheduled that day. Other offices may have staff arrive early and restock before the first patients are seen. Rescheduling appointments due to supply deficiencies reflects poorly on the office and affects patient care.

When restocking supplies, it is important to keep in mind the first in, first out (FIFO) rule. This means that the oldest items should be the first ones used. To follow this rule, new supplies should be stored behind older supplies.

Examinations

During a physical examination, the medical assistant will help the physician by performing the following tasks:

- Position and drape the patient and assist the patient onto the table if necessary.
- Hand instruments, equipment, and supplies to the physician as necessary.
- Document and label specimens.
- Reassure the patient.
- Witness the physician's and patient's behavior,
- Assist in carrying out treatment plans as assigned by the physician.
- Schedule diagnostic tests as ordered by the physician.

TYPES AND METHODS OF EXAMINATION

Inspection	Visual examination of the exterior surface of the body
Palpation	Using the hands to feel the skin and accessible underlying organs and tissues
Percussion	Using the fingertips to tap the body lightly but sharply to gain information about the position and size of the underlying body parts Two fingers of one hand are placed on the patient's skin and then struck with the index and middle finger of the other hand, which produces sound.
Auscultation	Listening to sounds within the body, such as those made by the heart, lungs, stomach, and bowels A stethoscope is usually used during this method of examination.
Mensuration	Use of special tools to measure the body or specific parts *Examples*: scale, tape measure, or calipers
Manipulation	Passively assessing the range of motion (ROM) in a joint

BODY PART, METHOD OF EXAMINATION, AND EQUIPMENT USED DURING THE GENERAL PHYSICAL EXAMINATION

Area	Body Part	Method/Equipment
Head	Skull, hair, scalp	Inspection and palpation
Ears	Ear canals, eardrum	Inspection with otoscope and tuning fork
Eyes	Visual acuity	Vision chart, Snellen eye chart Inspection with ophthalmoscope
Nose	Nasal passages	Inspection with otoscope and nasal speculum
Mouth and Throat (Pharynx)	Mucous membranes, lips, gums, teeth, tongue, pharynx	Inspection with laryngeal mirror, flashlight, tongue blade Palpation and inspection
Neck	Thyroid gland, trachea, and cervical lymph nodes; carotid artery	Palpation, auscultation, and inspection
Back and Spine	Muscles, spinal cord	Inspection, palpation, and percussion
Chest and Lungs	Heart, lungs	Stethoscope Inspection, percussion, palpation, and auscultation
Breasts	Breast tissue, nipples	Palpation
Heart	Heart sounds, apical pulse	Auscultation with stethoscope
Abdomen	Bowel sounds Symmetry Presence of air masses, enlargement Uterus	Auscultation Inspection Percussion, palpation Palpation Stethoscope
Inguinal Area	Inguinal nodes hernia	Palpation
Genitalia	*Female:* cervix and vagina *Male:* penis, scrotum, prostate gland	Inspection using vaginal speculum Palpation
Rectal Area	Anus Rectum	Inspection Inspection using proctoscope
Legs	Circulation Pulse sites	Inspection Palpation
Musculoskeletal System	Muscle strength Gait abnormalities	Inspection Palpation
Neurological Examination	Reflexes	Percussion hammer, pinwheel

PATIENT POSITIONING

Depending on the examination or procedure the physician will be performing, the medical assistant will need to instruct the patient on how to lie on the table in order for the physician to be able to access the exam or procedure site (Figures 18-4 through 18-13).

DRAPING

In order to help protect the patient's privacy and keep the patient warm during exams and procedures, it is important to ensure that the patient has been properly draped. Typically, drapes are smaller than bed sheets, but they may be made of the same material or of disposable paper. See Figures 18-4 to 18-13 for proper draping technique.

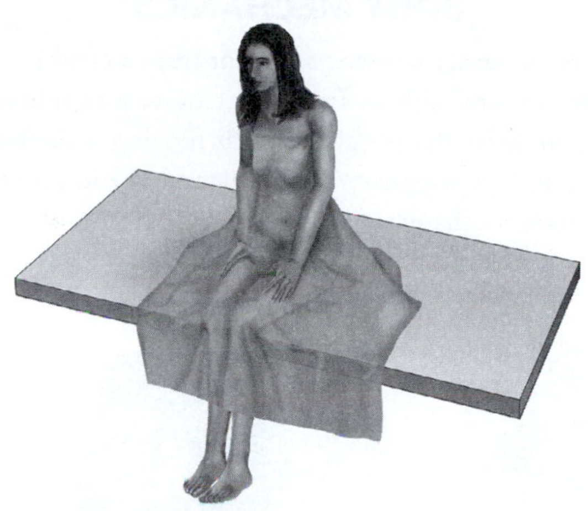

FIGURE 18-4 Sitting position.

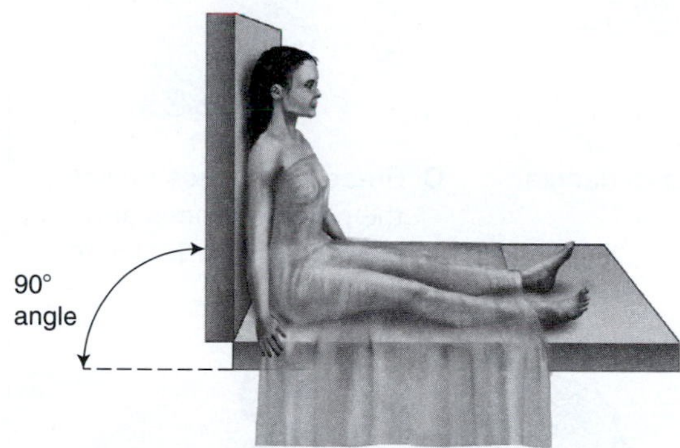

FIGURE 18-5 Fowler's position.

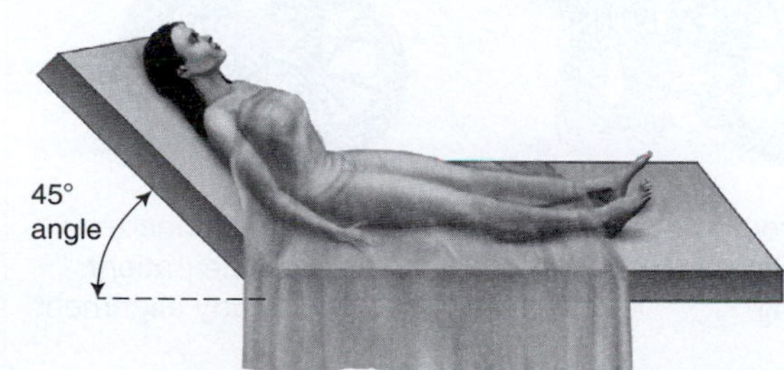

FIGURE 18-6 Semi-Fowler's position.

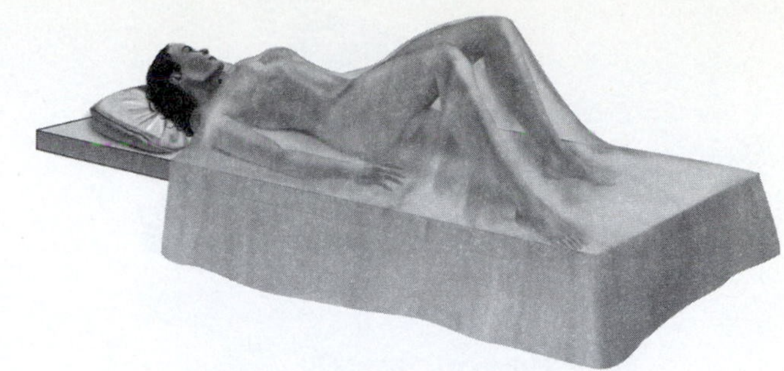

FIGURE 18-7 Dorsal recumbent position.

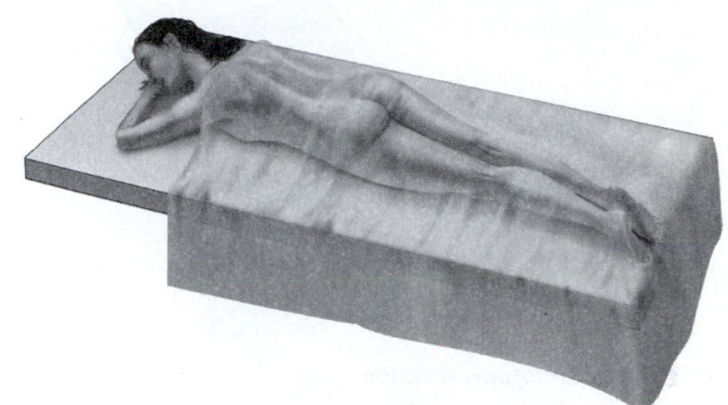

FIGURE 18-8 Prone position.

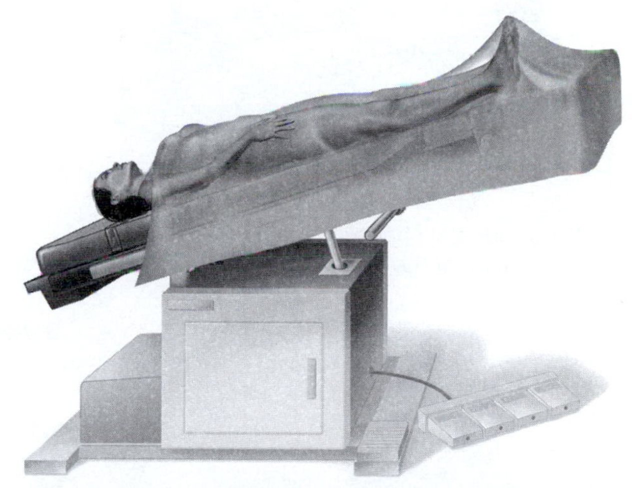

FIGURE 18-9 Trendelenburg position.

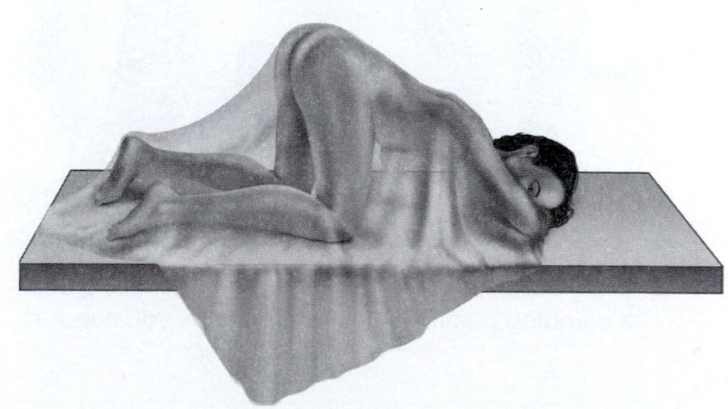

FIGURE 18-10 Knee-chest position.

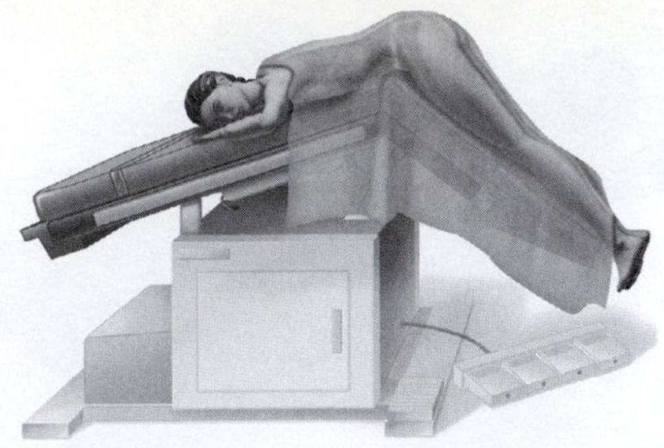

FIGURE 18-11 Jackknife position.

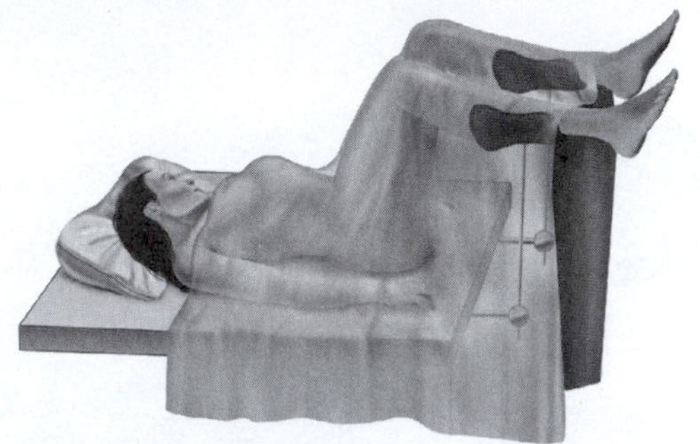

FIGURE 18-12 Lithotomy position.

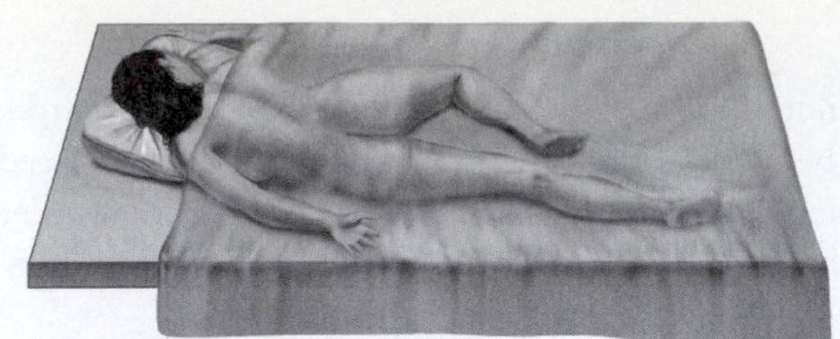

FIGURE 18-13 Sims' position.

During sterile procedures, sterile drapes must be used to protect the surgical site from contamination. Some sterile drapes are *fenestrated*, which means that they have a hole. The hole allows access to the surgical site while keeping the surrounding area sterile.

BODY MECHANICS

It may be necessary to assist a patient from a chair or wheelchair to an exam table or from a sitting to a standing position, or to assist the physician with moving a patient, For this reason, it is necessary to understand the importance of proper body mechanics. See Figure 18-14.

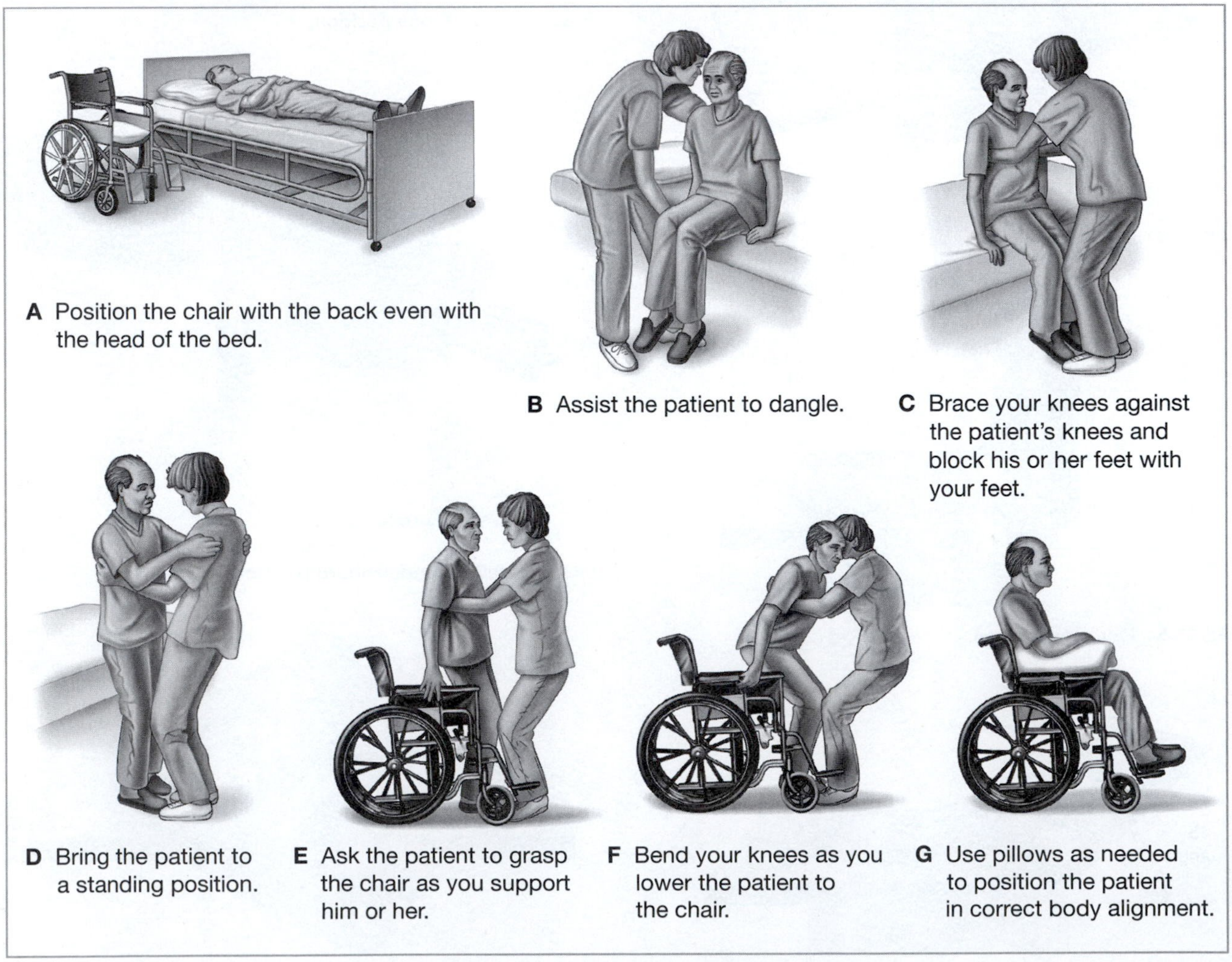

A Position the chair with the back even with the head of the bed.

B Assist the patient to dangle.

C Brace your knees against the patient's knees and block his or her feet with your feet.

D Bring the patient to a standing position.

E Ask the patient to grasp the chair as you support him or her.

F Bend your knees as you lower the patient to the chair.

G Use pillows as needed to position the patient in correct body alignment.

FIGURE 18-14 (A–G) Assisting the patient to transfer from the bed or examining table to a wheelchair.

The following guidelines should be followed:

- Prior to assisting the patient, know the patient's level of functioning both physically and mentally and assess the patient's ability to support his or her own weight. It may be necessary to ask another staff member for assistance.
- If the patient is getting up from the wheelchair, ensure that the brakes for the wheelchair are engaged prior to assisting the patient.
- Remove armrests and leg attachments from the wheelchair prior to transfer. This will help minimize the number of obstacles to work around.
- Face the patient, move your feet apart to shoulder width, and put one foot slightly forward. Assist the patient with standing by bending at the knees and help lift the patient with your legs.
- Never twist your body. If you need to turn, use your whole body.

SEQUENCE OF PHYSICAL EXAMINATION PROCEDURES

1. Registration	Receptionist/medical assistant
2. History	Receptionist/medical assistant
3. Urine specimen	Medical assistant or laboratory technician
4. Blood specimen	Medical assistant or laboratory technician
5. Vital signs	Medical assistant
6. Weight and height	Medical assistant
7. Visual acuity	Medical assistant
8. Electrocardiogram	Medical assistant
9. X-ray	X-ray technician (provided that the X-ray room is available; otherwise, the X-ray is completed before the patient's visit)
10. Preparation of the patient	Medical assistant

Procedures

The medical assistant may be expected to assist the physician during procedures performed in the office. The procedures will vary widely, depending on the specialty of the physician.

EYE AND EAR PROCEDURES (PROCEDURES 18-4 AND 18-5)

procedure 18-4

PERFORM EYE IRRIGATION

Objective: With the necessary materials, you will be able to irrigate the patient's eye safely and correctly.

EQUIPMENT AND SUPPLIES

- irrigating solution
- sterile basin
- irrigating syringe
- protective gear (gown, face shield, disposable gloves)
- towels
- kidney-shaped basin
- tissues
- patient chart

METHOD

1. Wash your hands. Gather equipment and supplies.
2. Identify the patient and guide him or her to the treatment area.
3. Record the patient's history and main complaint.

4. Review the physician's order for the patient's name, the volume and name of the irrigating solution, and which eye to irrigate.
5. Ask the patient about medication allergies. Explain the entire procedure.
6. Check the label of the irrigating solution against the physician's order before pouring it into the sterile basin for irrigation.
7. Wash your hands.
8. Put on the gown, face shield, and gloves before proceeding with irrigation.
9. Ask the patient to lie or sit down with the head tilted toward the eye to be irrigated. Place a towel and the kidney-shaped basin next to the patient's face to catch irrigating fluid.
10. With your dominant hand, fill the irrigating syringe with the prescribed irrigating solution.
11. With your nondominant hand, press with a tissue against the patient's cheekbone beneath the eye to expose more of the eye surface.
12. While holding the syringe approximately ½ inch from the eye, gently direct the fluid toward the inside surface of the lower conjunctiva and from the inner to outer corner of the eye (Figure 18-15).
13. Continue irrigating until the prescribed volume is used. Depending on the cause and symptoms, the physician may order further irrigation.
14. When irrigation is complete, dry the area around the affected eye with tissues.
15. Remove your protective clothing and place it in the proper laundry and waste containers.
16. Wash your hands.

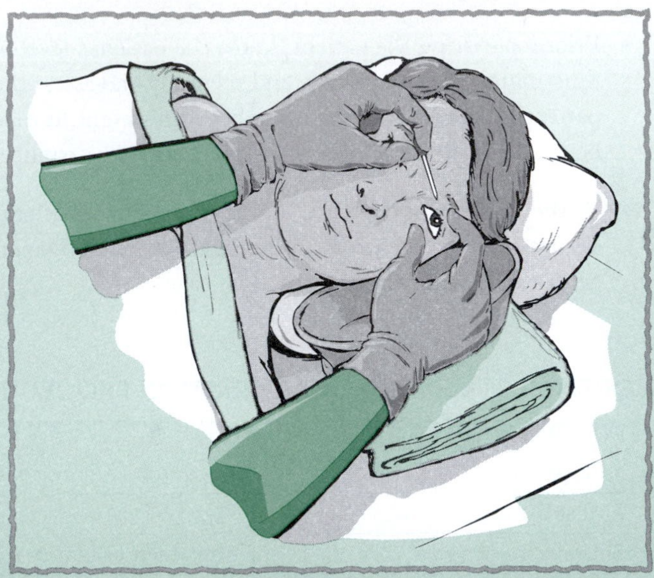

FIGURE 18-15 Irrigation of the eye.

17. Document the patient's tolerance of the procedure, the amount and kind of irrigating solution, and the eye irrigated.

CHARTING EXAMPLE

07/15/XX 2:45 P.M. Fussy 8-year-old pt presents with sand in both eyes from a sibling scuffle in the family's sandbox. Per physician's order, each eye was irrigated per procedure with 180 cc normal saline with holding assistance from mother. Both right and left conjunctival sacs and cornea are clear after irrigation. Child stated that both eyes now feel better. . . . . Ann Maynard, CMA (AAMA)

Source: Medical Assisting: Foundations and Practices by M. S. Frazier, C. Malone, and C. Morgan, Upper Saddle River, NJ: Pearson Education, Inc., 2010, p. 805. Reprinted with permission.

procedure 18-5

PERFORM EAR IRRIGATION

Objective: With the necessary materials, you will be able to irrigate the patient's ear safely and correctly.

EQUIPMENT AND SUPPLIES

- irrigating solution
- sterile basin
- irrigating syringe
- towels
- cotton ball(s)
- patient chart

METHOD

1. Wash your hands. Gather equipment and supplies.
2. Identify the patient and guide him or her to the treatment area. Explain the entire procedure.
3. Check the label of the irrigating solution when you take it from the shelf and against the physician's order.

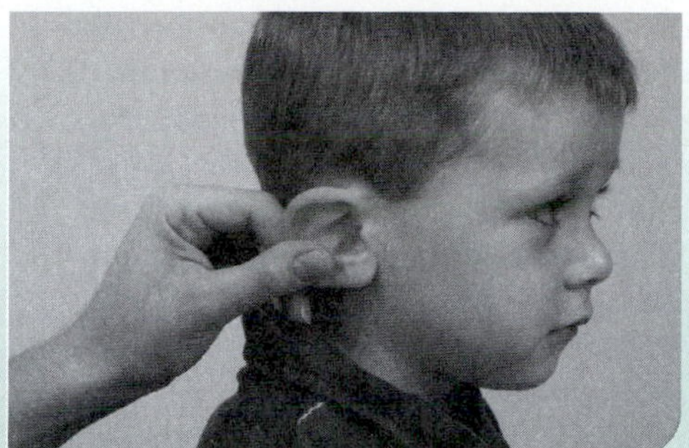

FIGURE 18-16 Proper holding position of the ear lobe for children.

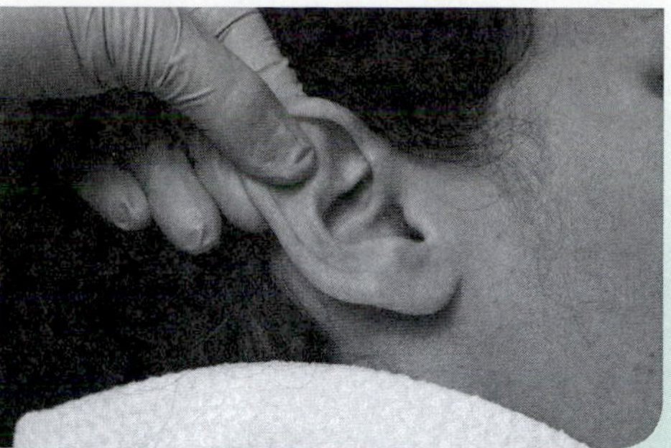

FIGURE 18-17 Proper holding position of the outer ear for adults.

4. Position the patient in a sitting position and instruct him or her to lean the head toward the side to be irrigated.
5. Check the condition of the external auditory canal with the otoscope.
6. Drape a towel across the patient's shoulder, under the ear.
7. Fill the irrigating syringe with prescribed solution.
8. Place the basin under the ear and against the skin. Instruct the patient or other office personnel to hold the basin in place.
9. For a child under 3 years, gently pull the auricle down and back (Figure 18-16). For a child over 3 years or an adult, gently pull the auricle ear up and back (Figure 18-17).
10. Gently place the tip of the irrigating syringe into the external auditory canal and point to the side or top. Do *not* point directly toward the tympanic membrane.
11. Instill the irrigating solution with gentle pressure on the plunger of the syringe.
12. Place the irrigation basin aside.
13. Use the otoscope to determine if more irrigation is needed.
14. Repeat the procedure until the desired results are obtained. If the patient experiences discomfort or other difficulties, report to the physician.
15. After irrigation, instruct and/or assist the patient to lie down with the head tilted toward the irrigated ear.
16. Place a towel under the head to catch the drainage.
17. Help the patient to a sitting, then standing position. Assess the patient for light-headedness or dizziness. Escort the patient to the waiting room.
18. Clean the treatment area and remove reusable equipment to the utility cleaning area.
19. Wash your hands.
20. Document the patient's tolerance and the results of the procedure.

CHARTING EXAMPLE

10/09/XX 9:30 A.M. Otoscope showed moderate amount of cerumen present in the rt external auditory canal. Ear irrigation was done. Pt stated no additional discomfort. Post-otoscopic examination shows clear auditory canal with pearly gray membrane visible. Pt states she can hear better with the rt ear. .... Liam Marks, RMA (AMT)

Source: Medical Assisting: Foundations and Practices by M. S. Frazier, C. Malone, and C. Morgan, Upper Saddle River, NJ: Pearson Education, Inc., 2010, p. 812. Reprinted with permission.

GASTROENTEROLOGY PROCEDURES (PROCEDURE 18-6)

procedure 18-6

ASSIST WITH A COLON ENDOSCOPIC/COLONOSCOPY EXAM

Objective: With the necessary materials, you will be able to set up an exam room and assist the physician with a colon endoscopic procedure.

EQUIPMENT AND SUPPLIES

- two pairs of nonsterile gloves
- instrument for viewing, depending on procedure being performed
- water-soluble lubricant
- patient drapes and gown
- sterile cotton-tipped applicators, for collection of fecal samples

- suction device
- sterile biopsy forceps
- disposable or sterile rectal speculum
- specimen containers with lab requisition form, as needed
- disposable tissue
- biohazard container
- patient chart

METHOD

1. Gather all needed supplies.
2. Identify the patient and explain the procedure. Verify that the patient has followed pre-exam instructions regarding foods, medications, and activities to avoid, such as enemas. The patient should be asked to empty the bladder prior to the exam.
3. Give the patient drapes and a gown and instructions on proper gown opening placement.
4. Take the patient's vital signs.
5. Assist the patient to the table and position him or her for the exam.
6. Wash your hands and put on gloves.
7. Assist the physician by handing him or her supplies as requested. To ease equipment entry into the anal canal, the physician will use an anal speculum. A suction device may be required to remove any fecal matter that obstructs the physician's view. If polyp tissue samples are needed, the physician will use sterile biopsy forceps.
8. To ease any discomfort, instruct the patient to breathe slowly and deeply. Observe the patient for any change in vitals, increased pain level, or other undue reactions.
9. After the physician has collected the necessary samples, you will place them in sterile specimen containers.
10. When the physician has completed the examination, cleanse the patient's anal area with tissues.
11. Remove the gloves, wash your hands, and assist the patient into a recovery position.
12. While the patient is resting, recheck vital signs. Invasive procedures often cause a drop in blood pressure.
13. Once the blood pressure is stable, allow the patient to get off the exam table and get dressed.
14. Complete laboratory forms. Seal the specimen containers in an appropriate biohazard-labeled transport bag.
15. When the patient has been released from the room, wash your hands, put on new gloves, and disinfect the area. A disposable speculum should be discarded into a biohazardous container; a stainless steel speculum should be prepared for autoclaving.
16. Document the procedure in the patient's chart.

CHARTING EXAMPLE

08/05/XX 7:30 P.M. Assisted in colon endoscopic procedure. Patient vital signs monitored and remained stable. Patient reported no feelings of faintness, dizziness, or discomfort following the procedure. Specimens collected and sent to laboratory. .... Anita Estrada, RMA (AMT)

Source: Medical Assisting: Foundations and Practices by M. S. Frazier, C. Malone, and C. Morgan, Upper Saddle River, NJ: Pearson Education, Inc., 2010, p. 939. Reprinted with permission.

GYNECOLOGIC PROCEDURES (PROCEDURES 18-7 AND 18-8)

procedure 18-7

ASSIST THE PHYSICIAN IN THE PERFORMANCE OF A PELVIC EXAMINATION AND PAP TEST

Objective: With the necessary materials, you will be able to assist the physician during the performance of a pelvic examination and Pap test.

EQUIPMENT AND SUPPLIES

- patient chart
- examination gloves
- water-soluble lubricant
- physician's gown and eye protection
- vaginal speculum

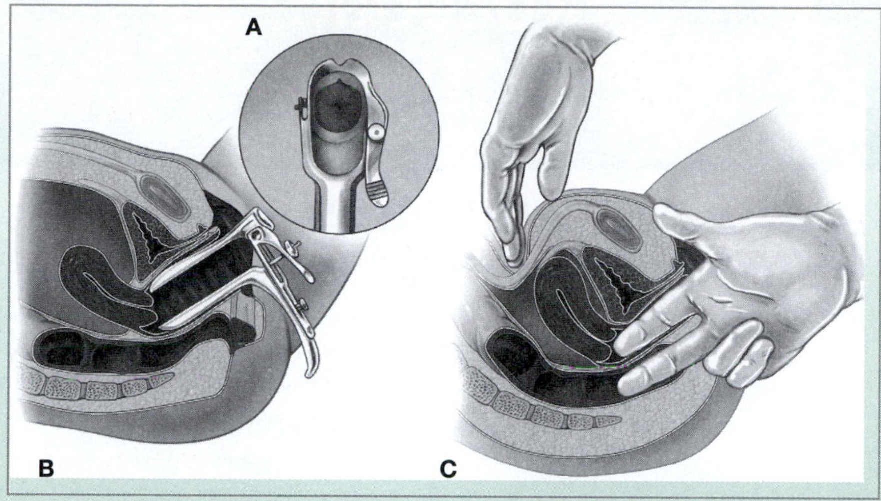

FIGURE 18-18 **(A, B) The physician performs a pelvic examination of a female patient using a vaginal speculum. (C) Bimanual technique.**

- gooseneck or other light source
- slide container, glass slides, marker to label slides, and slide fixative for Pap smear
- cervical/spatula scraper
- cotton-tipped applicators
- lab requisition form

METHOD

1. Wash your hands and assemble the equipment. Label the slide containers with patient information. Label the frosted edge of each slide with patient information and the location from which the specimen was taken.
2. Identify the patient and escort her to the examination room. Obtain the mensuration required by the physician (usually weight, temperature, blood pressure, pulse, and respirations).
3. Interview the patient for the following information:
   a. chief complaint (reason for visit)
   b. medications and known allergies
   c. start date of last menstrual period
   d. date of most recent Pap smear
4. Explain the procedure to the patient.
5. Before the procedure, assist the patient to the bathroom to void.
6. When the patient returns to the examination room, instruct her to remove clothing from the waist down. Assist as necessary. Provide a drape for the body from the waist down. If a breast examination is also to be performed, the patient will need to completely disrobe. Provide a gown cover for the chest area as well. The patient may sit on the examination table or lie comfortably until the physician arrives.
7. When the physician is present, assist the patient into a supine/dorsal recumbent position if a breast exam is to be performed. Slide the patient toward the stirrups and into the lithotomy position for the remainder of the pelvic examination and the Pap test.
8. Observe the patient's tolerance of the procedure and hand the slides, cervical/spatula scraper, and cotton-tipped applicators to the physician for the Pap smear. After the physician has placed the specimen on the slides, immediately spray or apply ethyl alcohol liquid fixative. Give the physician water-soluble lubricant for the pelvic examination (Figure 18-18).
9. When the procedure has been completed, assist the patient to a sitting position. Leave the room to allow her to dress in private, or assist if necessary.
10. Remove the used implements to the cleaning area. Dispose of disposable and biohazardous materials in the appropriate containers. Wash your hands.
11. Transport the labeled specimen to the laboratory, or arrange for transport, with the appropriate lab requisitions. Assist the patient with the scheduling of additional procedures, if necessary.
12. Document the patient's response to the procedure, any future appointments, and other patient information, including prescriptions or patient instruction.

CHARTING EXAMPLE

03/29/XX 2:30 P.M. Explained procedure to patient. Patient sent to bathroom to empty bladder. Patient required no assistance during examination. Instructions given to call office in two weeks for results and/or appointment in two weeks. Patient filled out reminder postcard for next year's appointment. . . . . Kimberly Rainer, RMA (AMT)

Source: Medical Assisting: Foundations and Practices by M. S. Frazier, C. Malone, and C. Morgan, Upper Saddle River, NJ: Pearson Education, Inc., 2010, p. 1001. Reprinted with permission.

procedure

18-8

ASSIST WITH CRYOSURGERY

Objective: With the necessary materials, you will be able to assist with a cryosurgery.

EQUIPMENT AND SUPPLIES

- gloves
- patient drapes
- light source
- liquid nitrogen
- vaginal speculum
- sterile specimen container (if needed)
- patient chart

METHOD

1. Verify the patient's identification.
2. Explain the procedure to the patient.
3. Wash your hands and put on gloves.
4. If necessary, assist the patient in undressing from the waist down. Provide proper patient drapes.
5. When the patient is undressed and draped, assist her into the lithotomy position.
6. Assist the physician as needed.
7. Reassure the patient that as the probe moves over the affected tissue and the liquid nitrogen freezes and kills the tissue, she will feel some discomfort, similar to menstrual cramping. The discomfort should not be unbearable, however.
8. After the procedure, assist the patient to a seated position and help her dress as needed.
9. Clean and disinfect the room.

PATIENT EDUCATION

Instruct the patient in post-cryosurgery care:

- Expect a heavy discharge for up to four weeks. It should have a clear, watery consistency.
- Cleanse the perineal area often.
- Use only sanitary napkins, not tampons or other devices that must be inserted, such as silicone cups.
- Remain on full cervical/pelvic rest for four weeks—no douching, tampon use, or sexual intercourse.
- Report any signs of infection such as vomiting, foul-smelling discharge, pain, or fever.
- The next menstrual cycle will be heavier than usual. This is normal.

CHARTING EXAMPLE

04/28/XX 9:41 A.M. Cryosurgery performed for chronic cervicitis. Patient reported slight cramping for 20–30 minutes and was monitored. Vital signs remained stable and patient was released home. Patient received postoperative care instructions, both verbal and written. .... Diane Edwards, CMA (AAMA)

Source: Medical Assisting: Foundations and Practices by M. S. Frazier, C. Malone, and C. Morgan, Upper Saddle River, NJ: Pearson Education, Inc., 2010, p. 1005. Reprinted with permission.

ORTHOPEDIC PROCEDURES

Cast Equipment and Materials

TYPES OF CASTS

Short Arm Cast (SAC)	• Extends from the fingers to just below the elbow • Used for fractures of the wrist or forearm
Long Arm Cast (LAC)	• Extends from the fingers to the axilla, with a bend at the elbow • Used for fracture of the upper arm
Long and Short Leg Casts (LLC and SLC)	• Extends from the thigh to the toes (LLC) or from below the knee to the toes (SLC) • Usually include an embedded walking heel

The following equipment is required for casting:

- Bandage roll or tape
- Container of warm water
- Stockinette
- Webril (sheer wadding)
- Padding rolls
- Bandage scissors
- Rubber gloves
- Sponge rubber

TYPES OF CASTING MATERIAL

Plaster Casts	• Applied wet around a stockinette liner with cotton padding over the limb • Use a wet bandage roll impregnated with calcium sulfate • Heavier than synthetic casts • May soften or crumble with moisture • Can crack or break • Easily molded to the body part, so immobilization is more effective • Less expensive than synthetic casts	**Synthetic Casts**	• Formed by using tape with either fiberglass, polyester, or cotton in the tape • Lighter than plaster casts • Not affected by moisture • Dry faster than plaster casts • Less likely to dent and create a pressure area • Not flexible • More expensive • Do not mold to the body part • Rough surface can tear clothing and scratch the skin

PATIENT INSTRUCTIONS: CAST CARE

Immediate Care Instructions

- Elevate the casted limb above heart level for the first 24–48 hours to prevent swelling and reduce pain.
- Move the toes or fingers frequently to maintain joint and muscle mobility.
- Cold dry therapy in the form of ice bags may be applied at the local area of injury for 20 minutes per hour to reduce swelling. The cast should be protected from water damage.
- With a plaster cast, avoid weight-bearing activity for 24 hours. With a synthetic cast, avoid activity for one hour.

General Care Instructions

- To avoid injuring the skin, do not force anything under the cast.
- Keep the cast dry. If the synthetic cast becomes wet, blot it dry, then sweep a blow-dryer on low or cool setting back and forth across the area.
- Check the skin around the cast for signs of redness, sores, or swelling. Report any such findings to the physician.
- Do not trim or break the cast. Notify the physician about any broken or loose areas.
- Follow the exercise instructions prescribed by the physician or physical therapist to maintain muscle tone while the extremity is immobilized.
- Follow the schedule for return appointments.
- Report the following symptoms:
  - Numbness or tingling in the fingers or toes.
  - Blue, pale, or cold fingers or toes.
  - Increased pain or swelling that is not helped with elevation or rest.
  - Pain or burning under the cast.
  - Drainage or foul odor coming from the cast.
  - Sores around the edge of the cast.
  - Fever, chills, nausea, or vomiting.

Source: Medical Assisting: Foundations and Practices by M. S. Frazier, C. Malone, and C. Morgan, Upper Saddle River, NJ: Pearson Education, Inc., 2010, p. 964. Reprinted with permission.

procedure 18-9

ASSIST WITH A LUMBAR PUNCTURE

Objective: With the necessary materials, you will be able to assist the physician with a lumbar puncture to obtain CSF.

EQUIPMENT AND SUPPLIES

- lumbar puncture kit: iodine antiseptic, iodine applicator, adhesive bandages, spinal puncture needle, 4 testing tubes
- patient drape
- BP cuff, sized appropriately for the patient
- manometer
- xylocaine 1–2%
- syringe and needle for anesthetic
- sterile gloves
- gauze sponges
- fenestrated drape

METHOD

1. Identify the patient and explain the procedure. Reinforce the need for postoperative care.
2. Verify that the patient has signed a consent form and that it has been filed in the chart.
3. Have the patient empty his or her bowel and bladder.
4. Obtain the patient's vital signs.
5. Wash your hands, put on gloves, and set up a tray using sterile technique.
6. With the iodine in the kit, disinfect the puncture site (L3 and L4).
7. Have the patient lie on his or her left side and curl into the fetal position. Provide drapes for patient comfort.
8. Assist the physician as necessary in swabbing the patient with antiseptic and placing a fenestrated drape.
9. Assist the physician in aspirating the xylocaine.
10. To avoid potential trauma to the spinal cord, assist the patient in maintaining the fetal position.
11. While the physician is taking a pressure reading, remind the patient to breathe evenly and avoid talking. If the physician requests, assist the patient in straightening his or her legs to get a true pressure reading.
12. Place a gauze pad with firm pressure over the puncture site to absorb any bleeding.
13. After the fluid has been collected, tighten the sample tubes and fill out a lab order form. Correctly label the samples for analysis.
14. Move the patient to the recovery area.
15. Clean and disinfect the treatment area.
16. Remove the gloves and wash your hands.
17. Document the procedure in the patient's chart.

CHARTING EXAMPLE

09/23/XX 9:00 A.M. Lumbar puncture performed by Dr. J. Lee. 3 vials of CSF obtained and sent to laboratory for testing. Patient tolerated procedure well, BP remained stable, checked every 15 minutes for 3 hours postprocedure. Patient was given verbal and written instructions to increase fluid intake, remain flat for 3–4 hours, and report any headaches, fever, bleeding, numbness, paralysis, or tingling. .... Kathleen Graham, RMA (AMT)

procedure 18-10

PERFORM URINE COLLECTION WITH A PEDIATRIC URINE COLLECTION BAG

Objective: With the necessary materials, you will be required to collect a urine specimen in a urine collection bag.

EQUIPMENT AND SUPPLIES

- urine collection bag for newborn or pediatric patient
- sterile gloves
- sterile container with label
- cotton balls
- prepackaged sterile cleansing swabs or towelettes
- laboratory requisition form
- patient chart

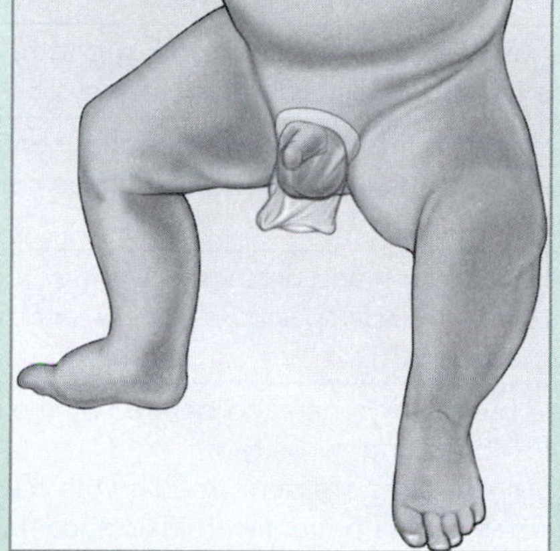

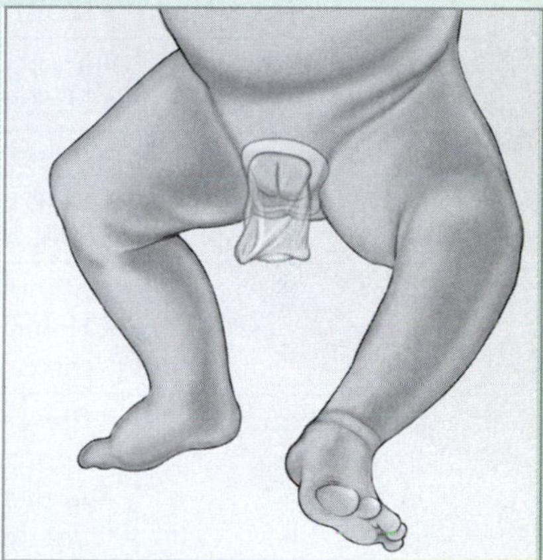

FIGURE 18-19 Applying urine collection bags on a male and female infant.

METHOD

1. Wash your hands. Gather the equipment and supplies.
2. Identify the parent or guardian with the child and guide them to the treatment area. Explain the procedure to the parent or guardian.
3. Put on sterile gloves.
4. Remove the diaper and dispose of it in the appropriate container.
5. Wipe the child's genital area with sterile towelettes or cleansing swabs. For boy infants, wipe around and away from the urinary meatus. For girl infants, wipe from the clitoris toward the rectal area. Repeat the wipe with a separate towelette or cleansing swab a second and third time to cleanse the area immediately surrounding the urinary meatus, then cleanse the wider surrounding area.
6. Dry the cleansed area with dry cotton balls.
7. Remove the adhesive tabs of the urine collection bag and apply the bag to the genital area securely, without gaps between the tabs and the skin (Figure 18-19).
8. Diaper the child.
9. Wash your hands.
10. Instruct the parent or guardian to encourage the infant or toddler to drink or nurse.
11. Recheck the diaper every 20 minutes until a specimen is obtained in the bag.
12. Wash your hands and put on sterile gloves.
13. Remove the urine collection bag. Place the bagged urine specimen in the sterile cup and cover the container tightly.
14. Diaper the child.
15. Remove the gloves and wash your hands.
16. Prepare the container label and laboratory requisition.
17. Transport or arrange for transport of the specimen to the laboratory.
18. Document the procedure in the child's chart.
19. Dispose of biohazardous materials in the proper containers.
20. Clean the area.
21. Wash your hands.

CHARTING EXAMPLE

09/27/XX 2:35 P.M. One-year-old female with history of 101° fever for two days. Mother states child is fussy, not drinking, and urine is darker than normal. Urine collection bag applied per physician order and office procedure. .... Shane Washington, RMA (AMT)

09/27/XX 3:15 P.M. Urine collection bag removed and placed in sterile urine cantainer. Urine is dark yellow and smells strong. Laboratory requisition sent with labeled urine specimen. .... Shane Washington, RMA (AMT)

Source: Medical Assisting: Foundations and Practices by M. S. Frazier, C. Malone, and C. Morgan, Upper Saddle River, NJ: Pearson Education, Inc., 2010, p. 1032. Reprinted with permission.

PHYSICAL THERAPY MODALITIES

Some physicians may refer patients to physical therapy for a variety of reasons, including instruction in the use of assistive devices and thermodynamic applications; however, some physicians may ask the medical assistant to provide this instruction.

PHYSICAL THERAPY MODALITIES

Therapy	Description and Purpose
Cryotherapy	• Also known as *cold therapy* • Constricts blood vessels; slows circulation to affected area; reduces swelling, inflammation, and pain; decreases body temperature • Dry cryotherapy: ice collars, ice-filled gloves, or other forms of commercial or improvised ice bags • Moist cryotherapy: cold compresses
Exercise therapy	• Improves joint flexibility, muscle tone, strength, and mobility • Should be monitored by a physician or physical therapist
Hydrotherapy	• Affected part is immersed in a whirlpool or container of water • Water exercise takes place in swimming pools or spas, directed by a physical therapist trained in hydrotherapy
Massage	• Stimulates circulation and promotes healing • Helps to relieve muscle spasms, soreness, and tightness, and to restore motion and function to the body part
Range of motion (ROM) exercises	• Prescribed by the physician and defined by the physical therapist • Improve flexibility and mobility • Active ROM exercises are performed by the patient without assistance; passive ROM exercises are performed by the patient with assistance from another person
Thermotherapy	• Increases circulation to the area for greater comfort and healing • Moist thermotherapy: hot soaks or compresses • Dry thermotherapy: heat lights, infrared lights, light bulbs, and heating pads
Ultrasound	• Vibrates tissues, generates heat, promotes circulation

Source: Medical Assisting: Foundations and Practices by M. S. Frazier, C. Malone, and C. Morgan, Upper Saddle River, NJ: Pearson Education, Inc., 2010, p. 968. Reprinted with permission.

UROLOGY PROCEDURES (PROCEDURES 18-11 AND 18-12)

procedure 18-11

PERFORM CATHETERIZATION OF A FEMALE PATIENT

Objective: With the necessary materials, you will be able to catheterize a female patient correctly.

EQUIPMENT AND SUPPLIES

- lighting source, preferably a gooseneck lamp
- sterile specimen container
- sterile drapes
- sterile catheterization kit or straight catheter
- sterile K-Y gel or other lubricant
- sterilized Mayo stand
- sterile gloves, two pairs

- nonsterile latex gloves
- biohazardous waste receptacle
- several 2 × 2 sterile gauze squares (minimum of 6)
- Betadine or other iodine solution
- maxipad or pantyliner
- patient chart
- lab order forms

METHOD

1. Gather all needed supplies to bring into the room. Generally, the patient will already be disrobed and covered with a drape. Bringing all supplies into the room in one trip avoids opening the door more than once while your patient is in a potentially embarrassing position.
2. Explain the procedure to the patient and obtain verbal permission to begin touching her.
3. If the patient is not unclothed, explain the correct dorsal recumbent position and draping.
4. Position the gooseneck lamp so that it is directed at the genital area but do not turn it on, as it may heat up quickly and make the patient uncomfortable.
5. Wash your hands and put on nonsterile gloves. Open the catheterization kit.
6. Ask the patient to keep her knees apart and take slow deep breaths while lifting her hips off the table surface.
7. When her hips have cleared the surface, slide a sterile drape beneath her by encircling the corners with your hands. Avoid touching the patient or the table with your hands.
8. Open a second sterile drape and place it over the patient's genital area, making sure that the vulvar area is exposed.
9. Place the insertion portion of the kit on the sterile drape you placed under the patient's hips between her knees.
10. Remove the gloves and wash your hands.
11. Following sterile technique, put on sterile gloves.
12. Soak the 2 × 2 gauze pads in Betadine or other iodine solution.
13. Open the sterile lubricant and place it on the sterile field on the Mayo stand. Open the remaining items, including the sterile container, and place them on the tray.
14. Cleanse the patient with the Betadine-soaked gauze squares. Separate the labia with the thumb and index finger of your nondominant hand (Figure 18-20). With your other hand, take a gauze square and wipe one side of the labia from top to bottom in *one pass*. Throw the square away (Figure 18-21). Take another square, repeat on the other side, and discard. Do not let the hand that is separating the labia touch and thereby contaminate your other hand.
15. With a third gauze square, cleanse the urinary meatus with a circular motion, working from the inside to the outside. Discard the square.
16. With your dominant hand, pick up the catheter, your thumb and index finger approximately 3 inches from the end to be inserted.

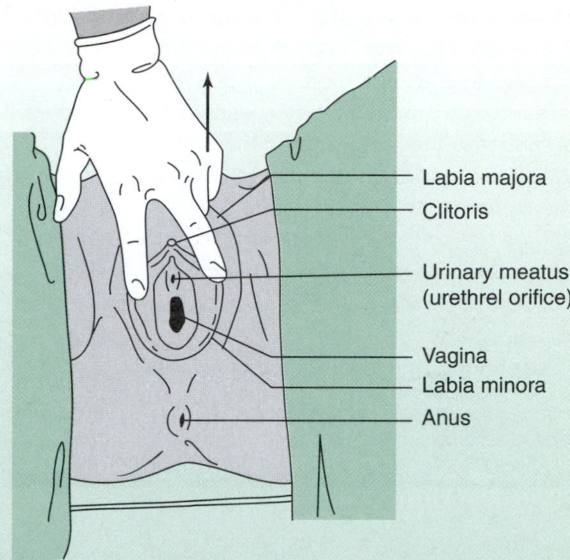

FIGURE 18-20 Separate the labia with the thumb and index finger of your nondominant hand.

17. Dip the insertion end of the catheter into the sterile lubricant. Make sure the opposite end of the catheter is in the collection portion of the kit's tray.
18. Thread the catheter into the urinary meatus approximately 2 to 3 inches, until urine begins to flow into the collection tray.
19. If you meet resistance when threading the catheter, do not force it in. Resistance can be an indication of a problem. Remove the catheter and notify the physician.
20. After a small amount of the urine has flowed into the collection tray, move the end of the catheter into the sterile collection container.

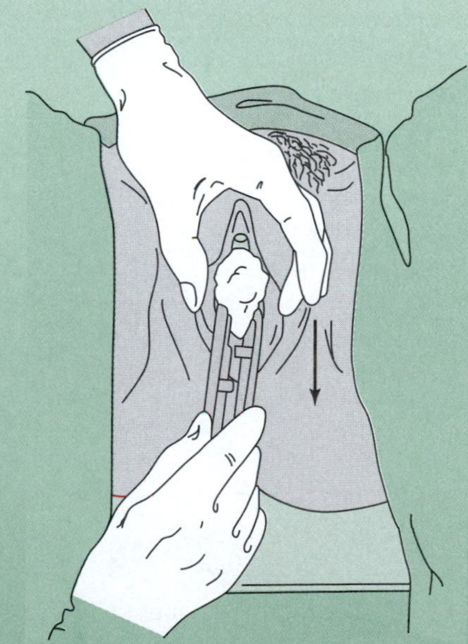

FIGURE 18-21 When cleansing the urinary meatus, move the swab downward.

21. Measure the urine that has flowed from the bladder. Emptying more than 500 ml at one time may cause the bladder to spasm. If more than 500 ml has been released, clamp the catheter, wait 10 to 15 minutes, and release the remainder of the urine.
22. When the bladder is completely empty, gently remove the catheter.
23. Secure the collection container's lid in place and prepare the paperwork for laboratory testing.
24. Remove all supplies and dispose of them in a biohazardous container.
25. Assist the patient in sitting up and dressing if necessary.
26. Inform the patient that the Betadine used to cleanse the labia may stain her undergarments, and offer her a maxi-pad or pantyliner to protect her clothing.
27. Document the procedure in the patient's chart.

CHARTING EXAMPLE

05/23/XX 9:25 A.M. Sterile urine sample obtained through catheterization. Patient tolerated procedure well and does not report any pain, tingling, or burning. Urine sample sent to laboratory for culture and sensitivity testing. .... Mary Brady, CMA (AAMA)

Source: Medical Assisting: Foundations and Practices by M. S. Frazier, C. Malone, and C. Morgan, Upper Saddle River, NJ: Pearson Education, Inc., 2010, p. 690. Reprinted with permission.

procedure 18-12

PERFORM CATHETERIZATION OF A MALE PATIENT

Objective: With the necessary materials, you will be able to catheterize a male patient correctly.

EQUIPMENT AND SUPPLIES

- lighting source, preferably a gooseneck lamp
- waterproof underpad
- sterile specimen container
- sterile catheterization kit or straight catheter
- sterile drapes
- sterile K-Y gel or other lubricant
- sterilized Mayo stand
- sterile gloves, 2 pairs
- nonsterile latex gloves
- biohazardous waste receptacle
- several 2 × 2 sterile gauze squares (minimum of 6)
- Betadine or other iodine solution
- fenestrated drape
- patient chart
- lab order forms

METHOD

1. Wash your hands. Collect all the needed supplies and bring [them] into [the] patient's room.
2. Explain the procedure to the patient and explain that it will be necessary to remove all articles of clothing from the waist down.
3. Assist the patient, if needed, into the supine position.
4. Wash your hands and put on nonsterile gloves.
5. Following sterile technique, open the catheterization kit and place the items on the sterile field on the Mayo stand.
6. Wrap the corners of the sterile underpad over your hands and place it over the patient's thighs, sliding it under the penis (Figure 18-22).

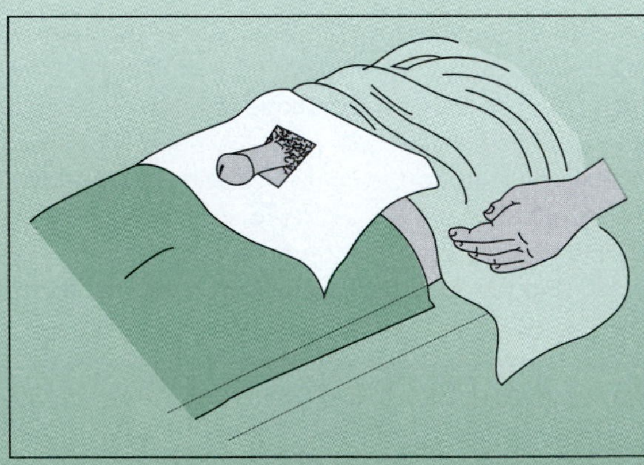

FIGURE 18-22 Place the sterile underpad over the patient's thighs, sliding it under the penis.

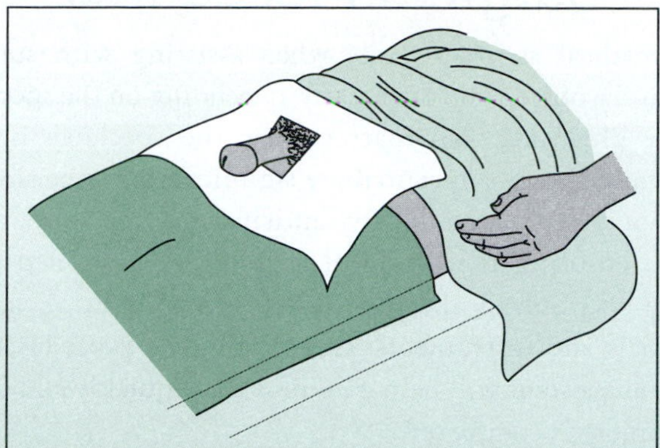

FIGURE 18-23 Place a fenestrated drape over the genital area so that the penis is exposed.

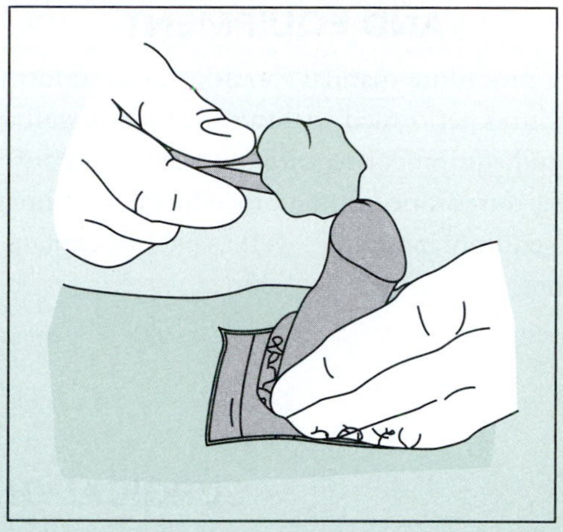

FIGURE 18-24 Clean around the meatus in a circular motion.

7. Remove the gloves, wash your hands, and put on sterile gloves.
8. Being careful not to touch the patient or the table, place a fenestrated drape over the genital area so that the penis is exposed (Figure 18-23).
9. Soak the 2 × 2 gauze pads in Betadine and place them on the patient's thighs for easy access.
10. With your nondominant hand, grasp the penis below the glans and hold it upright. If the patient is uncircumcised, retract the foreskin to expose the meatus.
11. With your dominant hand, cleanse the meatus with a gauze square in a circular motion, working from the inside to the outside (Figure 18-24). Discard the gauze.
12. Repeat step 11 a total of three times, using a fresh gauze square each time you cleanse.
13. Dip the insertion tip of the catheter into lubricant to cover the 7 or 8 inches that will be inserted into the penis. Place the opposite end of the catheter in the collection tray.
14. Hold the penis firmly at a straight, upward angle to straighten the urethra for easier insertion.
15. Ask the patient to constrict the penis muscles in the same manner as when trying to urinate. While he is doing this, gently thread the catheter into the penis until urine begins to flow, generally 6 to 8 inches (Figure 18-25).
16. *Never* force the catheter. If you meet resistance, discontinue the procedure and notify the physician.
17. After a small amount of the urine has flowed into the collection tray, move the end of the catheter into the sterile collection container.
18. Measure the urine that has flowed from the bladder. Emptying more than 500 ml at one time may cause the bladder to spasm. If more than 500 ml has been released, clamp the catheter, wait 10 to 15 minutes, and release the remainder of the urine.
19. When the bladder is completely empty, gently remove the catheter.

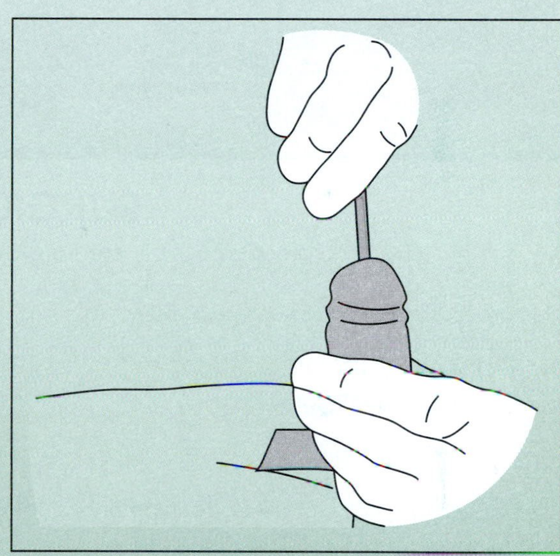

FIGURE 18-25 Gently thread the catheter into the penis until urine begins to flow, generally 6 to 8 inches.

20. Secure the collection container's lid in place and prepare the paperwork for laboratory testing.
21. Remove all supplies and dispose of them in a biohazardous container.
22. Assist the patient in sitting up and dressing if necessary.
23. Inform the patient that the Betadine used to cleanse the glans may transfer to his undergarments and stain them.
24. Document the procedure in the patient's chart.

CHARTING EXAMPLE

04/04/XX 9:25 A.M. Sterile urine sample obtained through catheterization. Patient tolerated procedure well and does not report any pain, tingling, or burning. Urinary sample sent to laboratory for culture and sensitivity testing. . . . . Joseph Baker, RMA (AMT)

Source: Medical Assisting: Foundations and Practices by M. S. Frazier, C. Malone, and C. Morgan, Upper Saddle River, NJ: Pearson Education, Inc., 2010, p. 691. Reprinted with permission.

INSTRUMENTS, SUPPLIES, AND EQUIPMENT

The office procedure manual should contain information on the procedures performed within the office as well as list the supplies and equipment required for each procedure. See the above procedures for common procedures, instruments, supplies, and equipment used as well as patient explanation and instructions.

Surgical Procedures

The medical assistant's role when assisting with surgery within the office will vary greatly, depending on the specialty of the physician. No matter what the specialty is, the medical assistant can contribute significantly to the smooth functioning of surgery. By anticipating the physician's needs, ensuring that surgical asepsis is maintained both before and during the procedure, and accounting for all materials and instruments used during the procedure, the medical assistant will help determine how quickly and safely the surgery is completed.

SURGICAL GLOVING (PROCEDURE 18-13)

procedure 18-13

SURGICAL GLOVING

Objective: Apply sterile gloves without a break in sterile technique.

Note: This procedure follows a surgical hand scrub.

EQUIPMENT AND SUPPLIES

- double-wrapped sterile glove pack

METHOD

1. Assemble equipment and check the tape or seal for the expiration date and condition of the pack.
2. Place the pack on a flat surface at waist height with the cuffed end of the gloves toward you.
3. Open the outside wrapper by touching only the outside of the pack. Leave the opened wrapper in place to provide a sterile work field.
4. Open the inner wrapper without reaching over the pack or touching the inside of the wrapper. Pull the inner wrapper edges to each side without touching the inside of the pack (Figure 18-26A).
5. Using the thumb and fingers of your left hand (if you are right-handed), pick up the glove on the right side of the pack by grasping the folded inside edge of the cuff (Figure 18-26B). The glove can be dangled slightly off the sterile packing material for easier insertion.
6. Pull the glove onto your right hand using only the thumb and fingers of the left hand (Figure 18-26C). Do not allow your fingers to touch the rest of the glove.

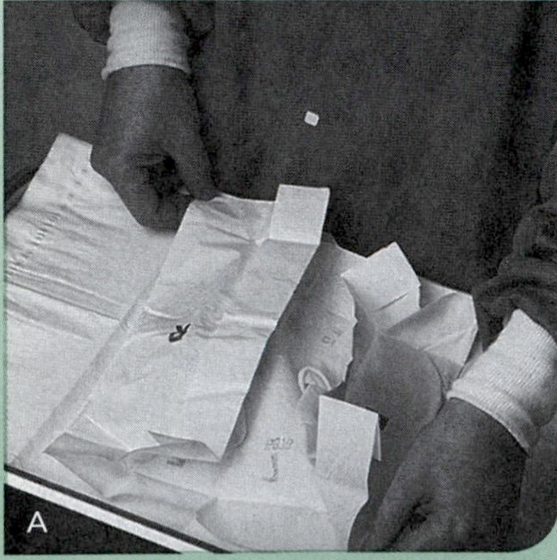

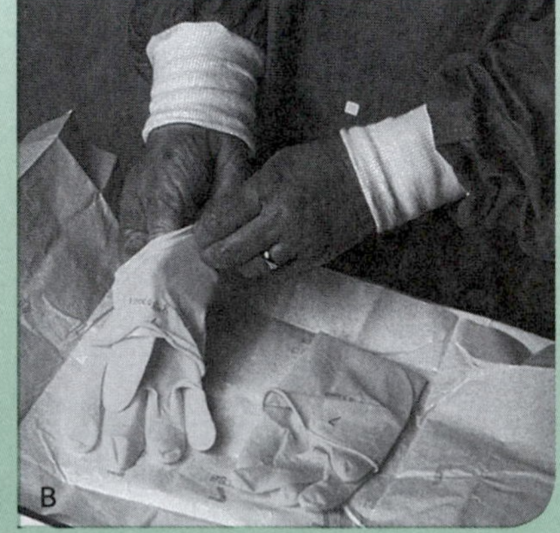

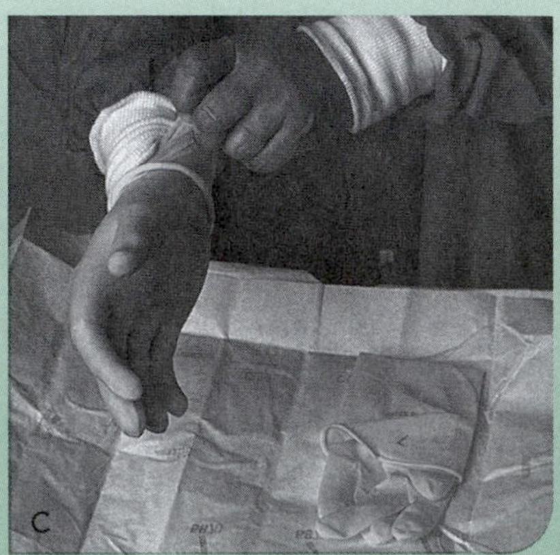

FIGURE 18-26 (A–C) Sterile gloving and glove removal technique.

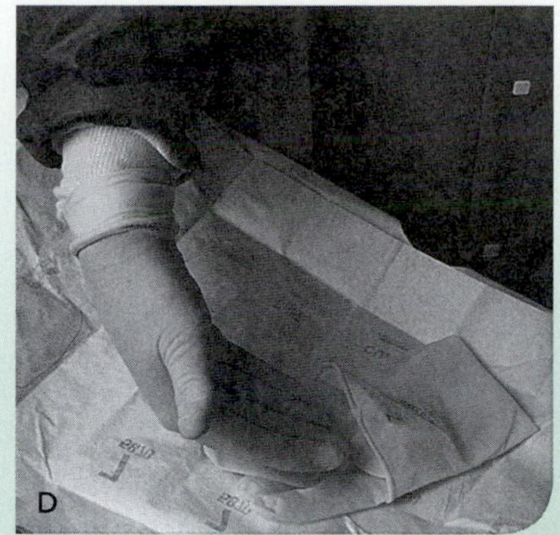

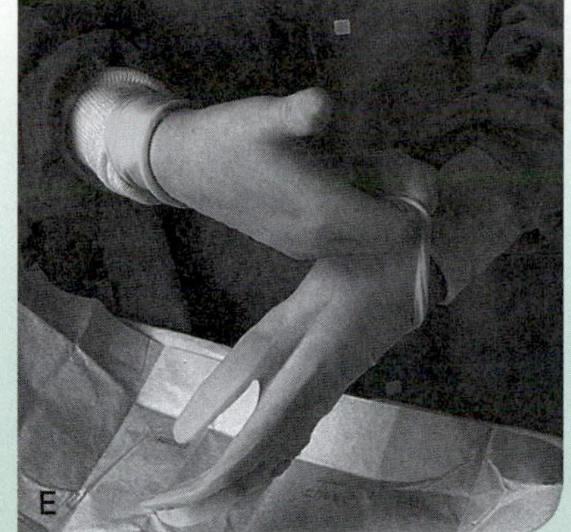

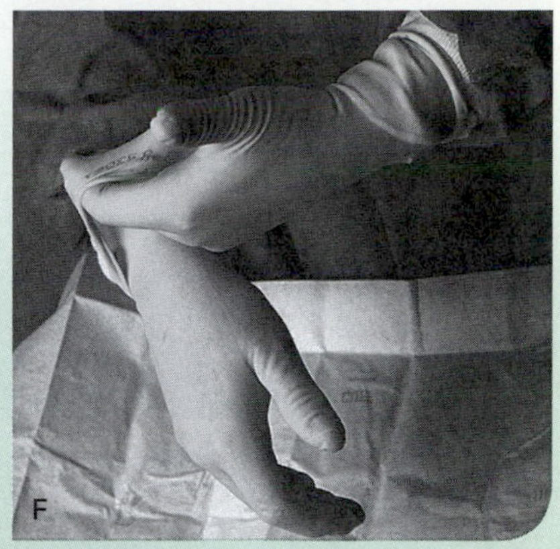

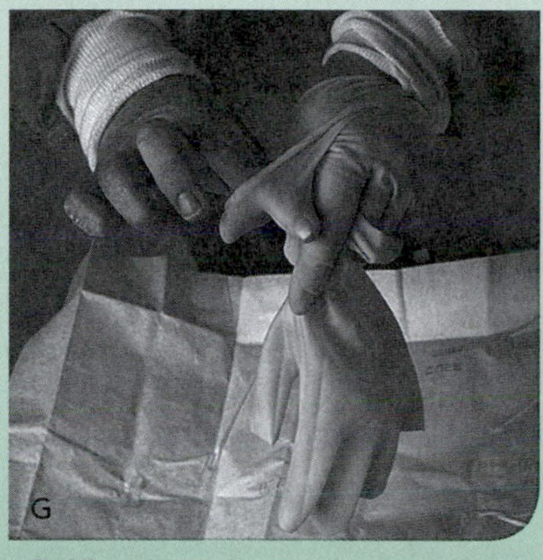

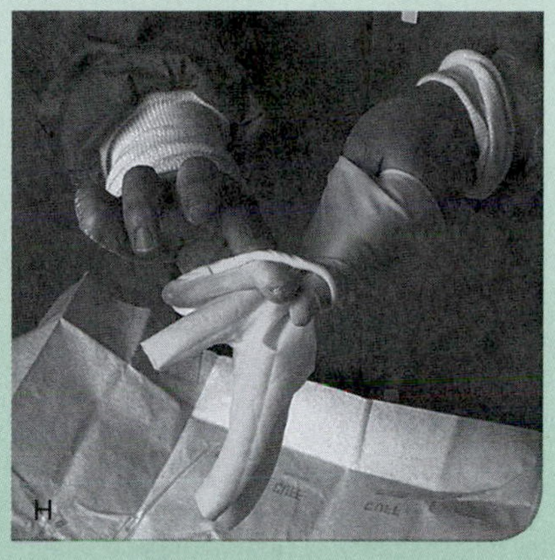

FIGURE 18-26 (*continued*) **(D–H).**

7. Place the fingers of the right-gloved hand under the cuff of the left glove and pull it onto the left hand and up over the left wrist (Figure 18-26D).
8. With the gloved right hand, place your fingers under the cuff of the left glove and pull it up over the left wrist (Figure 18-26E). The thumb should not touch the cuff.
9. After the gloves are in place, the fingers can be adjusted, if necessary, by using the gloved hands.
10. Removing gloves (Figures 18-26F–H): Remove the first glove by grasping the edge of that glove (with the fingers of the other gloved hand) and pull the first glove over the hand, inside out. Discard the first glove into the proper biohazard waste container. Remove the other glove by grasping the edge of the cuff with your fingers (from the ungloved hand) and pull it down over the hand, inside out. Discard the gloves appropriately.

SURGICAL INSTRUMENTS

Instruments used within the medical office are typically categorized based on their use and fall into one of the following categories (Figures 18-27 through 18-36):

INSTRUMENT CATEGORIES

Category	Example(s)
Cutting	Scalpel or knife
Dissecting	Scissors
Grasping and Clamping	Forceps
Dilating and Probing	Probe, trocar, punch
Visualizing	Scope, speculum

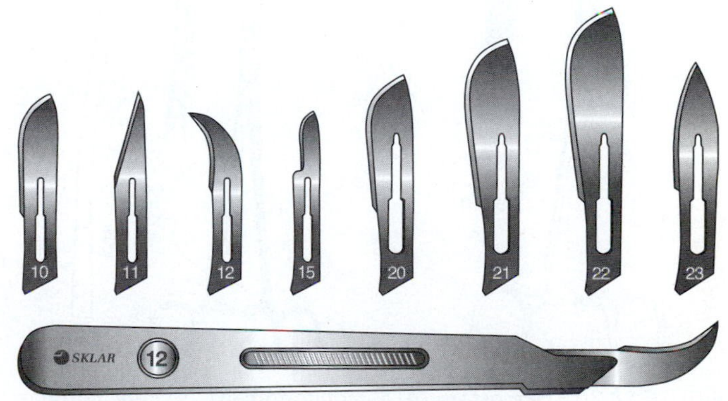

FIGURE 18-27 A variety of scalpels and blades.

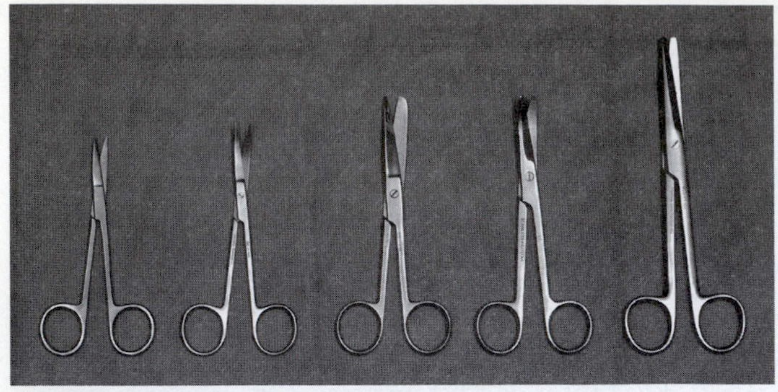

FIGURE 18-28 A variety of types of scissors.

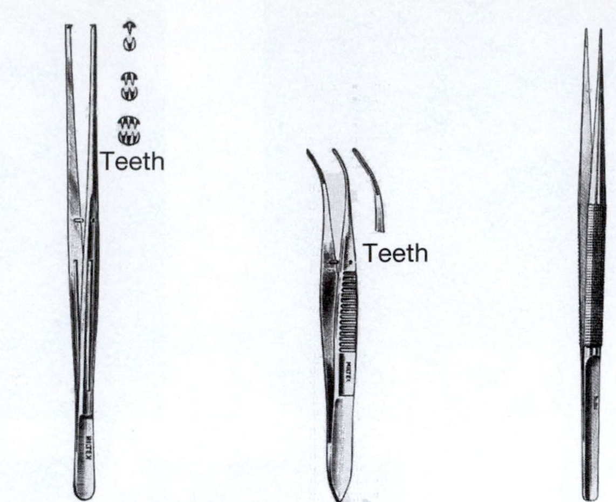

FIGURE 18-29 Types of forceps.

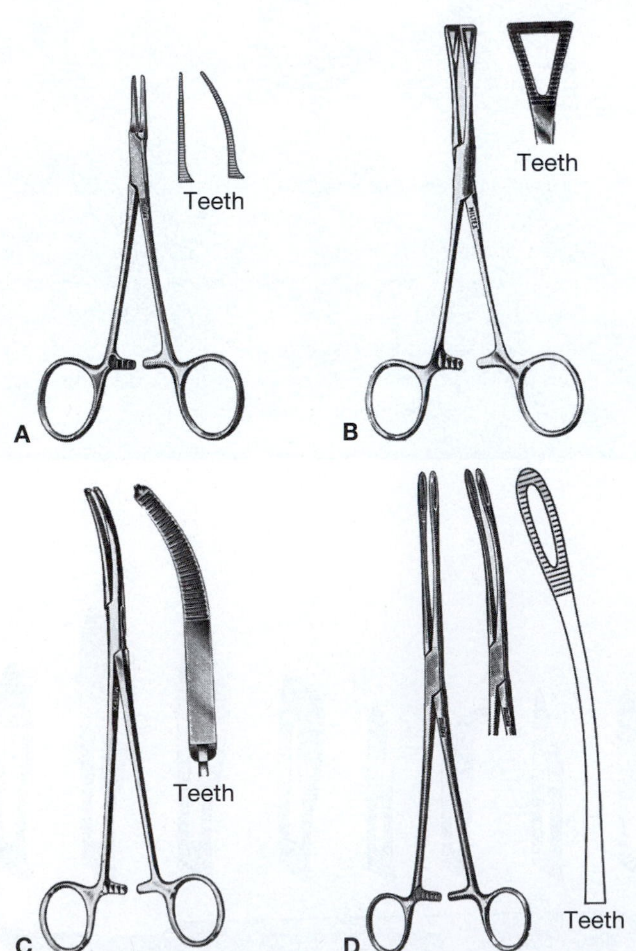

FIGURE 18-30 Hemostats: (A) Mosquito forceps. (B) Pennington hemostatic forceps. (C) Curved forceps. (D) Sponge forceps.

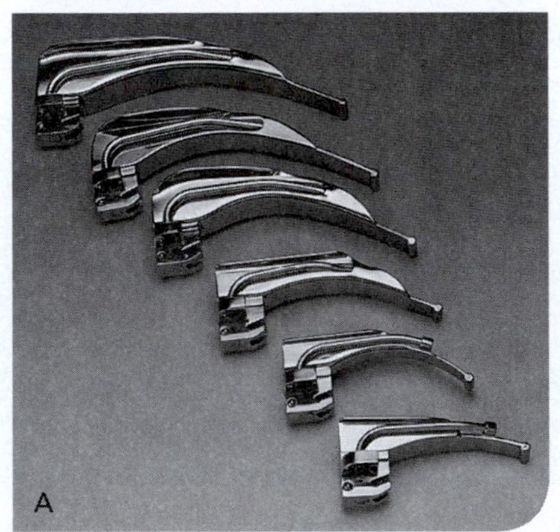

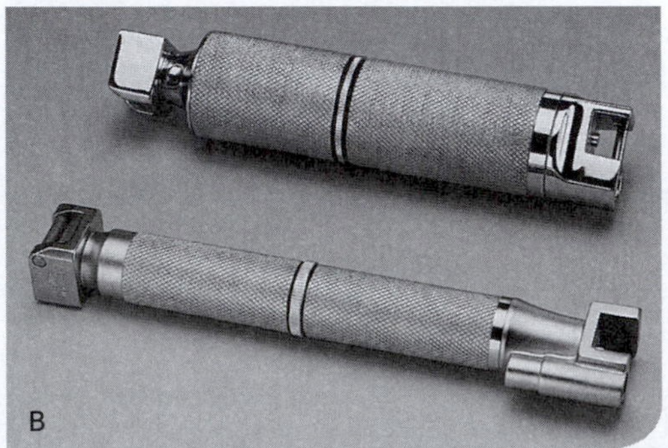

FIGURE 18-31 Laryngoscopes: (A) Scopes. (B) Handles.

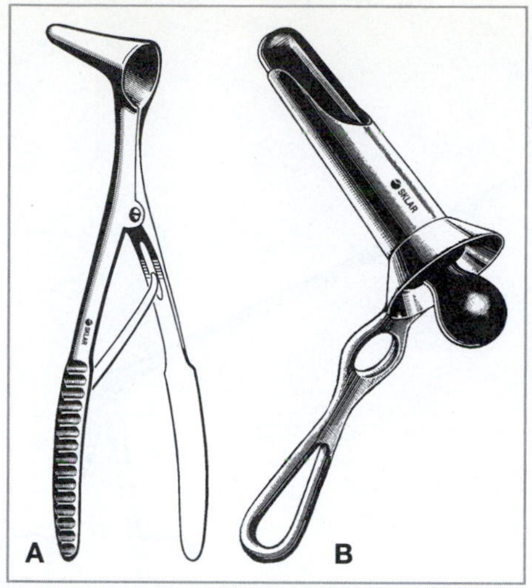

FIGURE 18-32 Specula: (A) Vienna nasal speculum. (B) Ives-Fanster rectal speculum.

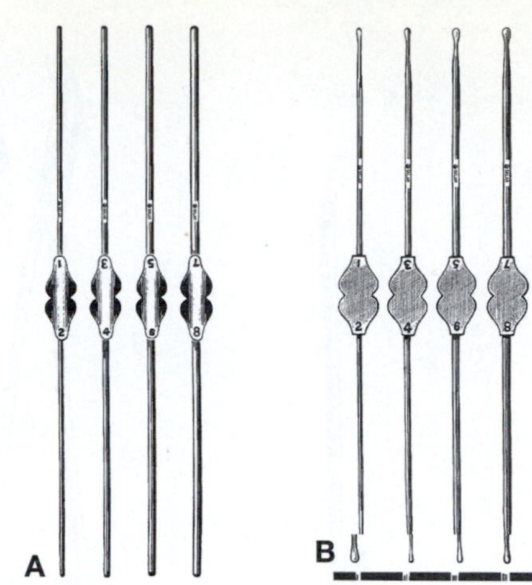

FIGURE 18-33 Lachrymal probes: (A) Bowman probe. (B) Williams probe.

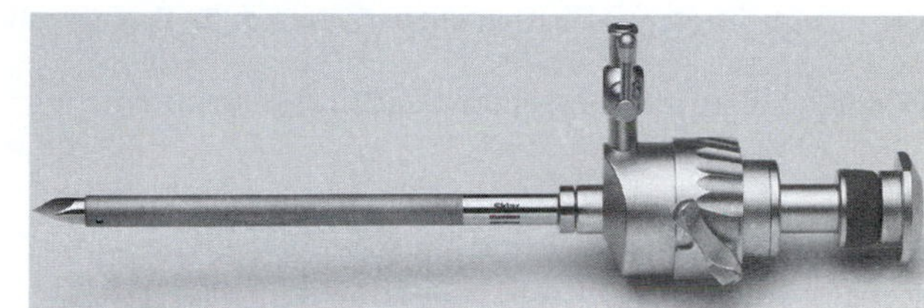

FIGURE 18-34 Trocar.

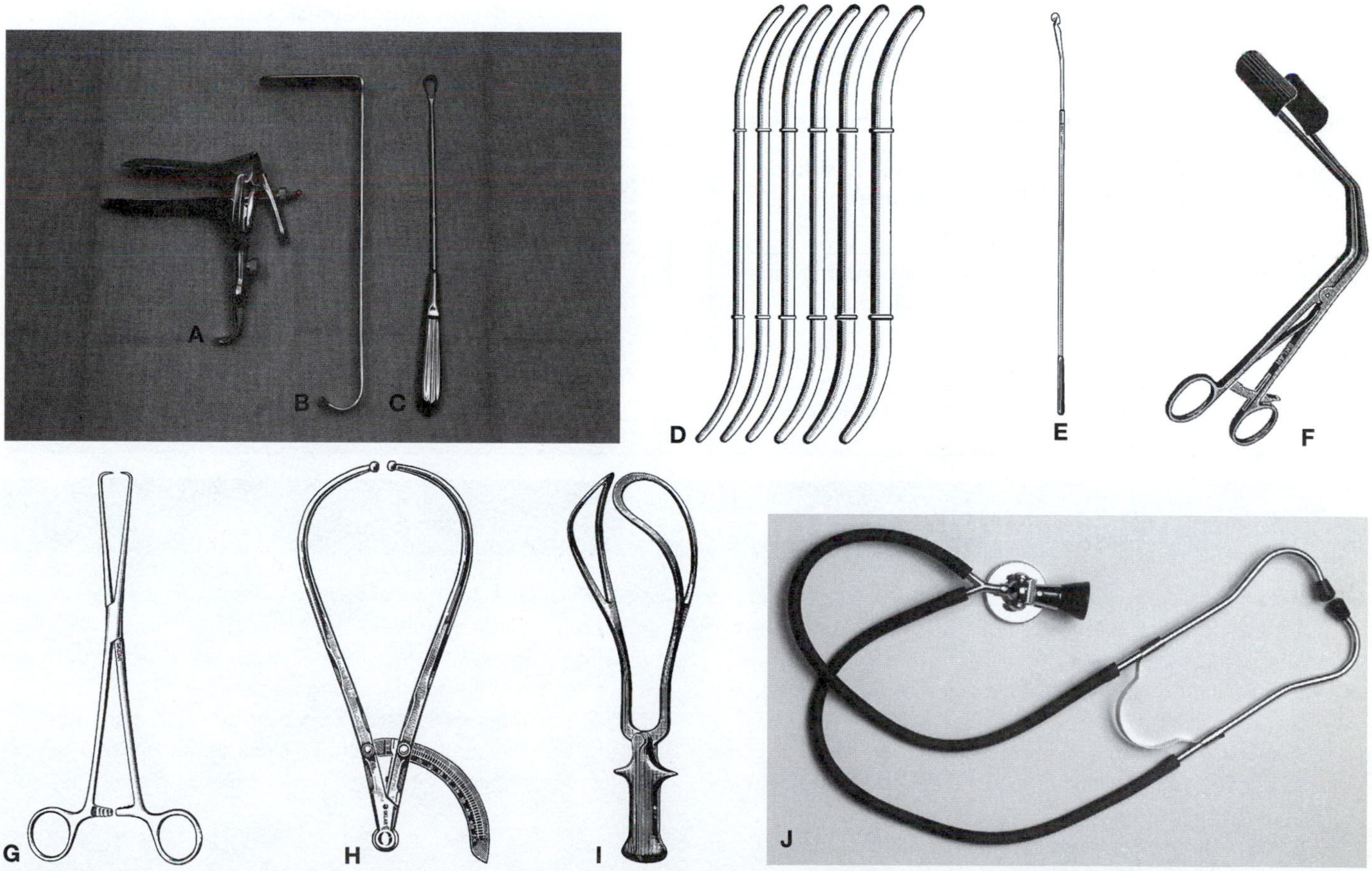

FIGURE 18-35 Gynecological instruments: (A) Vaginal speculum. (B) Retractor. (C) Uterine curette. (D) Uterine dilators. (E) IUD extractor forceps. (F) Lateral vaginal retractor. (G) Schroeder uterine tenaculum forceps. (H) Martin pelvimeter. (I) De Lee OB forceps. (J) Bowles obstetrical stethoscope.

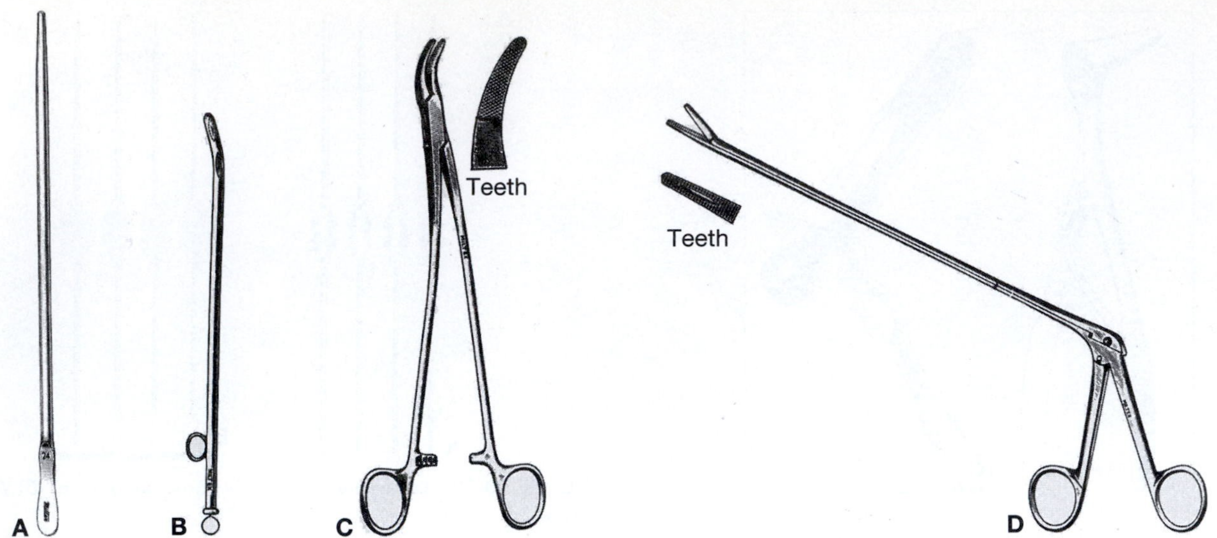

FIGURE 18-36 **Urological instruments: (A) Sound. (B) Female catheter. (C) Needle holder. (D) Urethral forceps.**

Box 18-1 lists guidelines for handling instruments.

SURGICAL NEEDLES/SUTURE

Suture needles are available in different shapes, and the area being sutured will help determine which needle to use.

NEEDLES

Straight	Used when there is enough room to suture and a curved needle is not required Needle holder not required
Curved	Allows the surgeon to go in and out of tissue when there is not enough room to suture using a straight needle Requires a needle holder
Swaged	Needle and suture combined in one length

Suture is the thread that is used to approximate a surgical incision or wound and is either absorbable or nonabsorbable.

SUTURES

Absorbable Suture	Also known as *catgut* or *Vicryl* Does not have to be removed because enzymes within the body tissues break down the material Typically used: • With internal organs • With subcutaneous tissue • For tying off blood vessels
Nonabsorbable Suture	Used on skin surfaces Requires removal Examples: • Silk: expensive but dependable • Nylon: elastic and strong • Steel: strongest; used for major surgery • Polyester: second strongest • Cotton: weakest

Box 18-1 Handling Instruments

- Instruments should be rinsed, cleaned, and scrubbed with a brush as soon after use as possible to prevent hardening of blood and tissue materials.
- Handle instruments carefully. Do not throw them into the basin for cleaning.
- Avoid allowing large numbers of instruments to become tangled. They are difficult to separate and could damage your protective gloves.
- Sharp instruments should remain separated from other instruments.
- Delicate instruments, such as those with lenses, should be handled separately.
- Instruments with ratchets should be stored open to maintain their good working condition.
- Check all instruments for defects before sterilizing them. All tips on the instruments should close tightly, scissors should cut evenly, and the cutting edges should be smooth.

Suture is measured by gauge or diameter and stated in terms of 0s, decreasing in size. For example, 0 is the thickest and 6-0 is the smallest. Surgeons may use 2-0 suture because it is thicker, but plastic surgeons may use 6-0 suture on the face to minimize scarring. See Procedures 18-14 and 18-15.

SUTURE USE, SIZE, AND TYPE OF MATERIAL

Use	Gauge	Type of Material
Blood Vessels	3-0 to 0	Chromic gut
	3-0	Cotton
	3-0 to 0	Silk
Eyelid	6-0 to 4-0	Silk
	6-0 to 5-0	Polyester
Fascial	2-0 to 0	Chromic gut
	2-0 to 0	Silk
	2-0 to 0	Cotton

Use	Gauge	Type of Material
Muscle	3-0 to 0	Plain gut
	3-0 to 0	Chromic gut
	3-0 to 0	Silk
Skin	6-0 to 2-0	Nylon
	5-0 to 3-0	Polyethylene
	5-0 to 2-0	Stainless steel

procedure 18-14

ASSISTING WITH SUTURING

Objective: Assist with suture repair of an incision or laceration using sterile technique.

EQUIPMENT AND SUPPLIES

- Mayo stand
- side stand
- anesthetic
- sterile transfer forceps
- sterile saline
- waste container/plastic bag
- biohazard waste container
- sharps container
- sterile gloves (two pairs)
- sterile pack(s) (patient drape, towel pack with four towels, 4 × 4 gauze sponge pack)
- scalpel blades pack (Nos. 10 and 15)
- needle and syringe pack
- suture and needle pack (according to the physician's preference)
- two sterile basins
- suture pack (scalpel handle, needle holder, thumb forceps, two scissors three hemostats)

METHOD

1. Use a sterile scrub and gloving procedure.
2. Stand across from the physician.
3. Place two sponges ready for the physician near the wound site.
4. Assist by using additional sponges to keep the wound dry.
5. Pass instruments, such as scissors, to the physician using a firm snap of the handle into his or her hand without letting go until the physician has grasped it firmly.
6. The blade is placed into the scalpel using a hemostat.
7. Hand the scalpel to the physician with the blade edge down to avoid cutting the physician.
8. Continue to use sponges to keep the wound free of drainage.
9. Pass all instruments to the physician as requested. Try to anticipate the next instrument that the physician may need, such as another hemostat or scissors for cutting a suture.

10. Pass the toothed forceps to the physician if laceration edges need to be grasped.
11. Mount the needle in the needle holder and pass them as one unit to the physician, taking care to keep the suture within the sterile field. Pass the needle holder with the needle pointing outward. Hold the suture with the other hand, and do not let go of it until the physician sees it.
12. Using the suture scissors, prepare to cut the suture as directed by the physician (usually ⅛ to ¼ inch from the knot).
13. Sponge the closed wound once with a sponge and discard it.
14. Repeat this step with each suture.
15. Apply a layer of sterile dressing over the wound, such as a sterile gauze pad. The medical assistant may use forceps if preferred. The sterile dressing should extend a minimum of 2 inches past all edges of the wound.
16. Apply a second layer of gauze over the wound site.
17. Add a final third layer of wound dressing, such as a SurgiPad.
18. Secure the edges of the dressing with paper tape or a similar product. Some physicians prefer that the wound be covered with a clear, waterproof membrane such as Telfa. Paper tape is often used because it contains a less intense adhesive, lowering the risk of adverse skin reactions.
19. After they are used, place all soiled instruments on the sterile field if they will be used again; discard others in the instrument basin.
20. When the procedure is complete, remove your gloves and perform hand hygiene before assisting the patient.
21. Allow the patient to rest and recover from the anesthetic. Periodically check the patient's vital signs according to your office policy.
22. Provide clear oral and written postoperative instructions for the patient. Make sure that the patient is stable before he or she leaves the office.
23. Clean, sanitize, and sterilize the instruments. Clean and sanitize the room in preparation for the next patient.
24. Perform hand hygiene.

CHARTING EXAMPLE

2/14/XX 1:00 P.M. Cleansed wound with antiseptic. Assisted physician with suturing. Pt. instructed on wound care, signs and symptoms of infection, and given follow-up appointment.
.... M. King, CMA (AAMA)

The physician will chart the details of the surgical procedure.

procedure 18-15

REMOVING SUTURES

Objective: Remove sutures using proper sterile technique, following the physician's order.

EQUIPMENT AND SUPPLIES

- suture removal pack (suture scissors, sterile gauze squares, thumb forceps, skin antiseptic, sterile gloves, bandages, biohazard waste container)

METHOD

Removal of Sutures

1. Perform hand hygiene.
2. Assemble the equipment and check the expiration date on the pack.
3. Identify the patient.
4. Explain the procedure to the patient, and assist him or her into a comfortable position.
5. Perform hand hygiene.
6. Remove the old dressing using proper technique.
7. Perform hand hygiene.
8. Open the suture or staple removal pack using proper technique.
9. Apply sterile gloves using proper technique.
10. Cleanse the wound as needed.
11. Place a gauze square next to the wound for placement of sutures or staples as they are removed.
12. Grasp the knot of the suture with thumb forceps and lift gently (Figure 18-37).
13. Insert the suture scissors and cut the suture at skin level. Pull out the suture.
14. Place the cut suture on the gauze.
15. Repeat these steps until all sutures are removed.
16. Count the sutures to make sure that all have been removed.

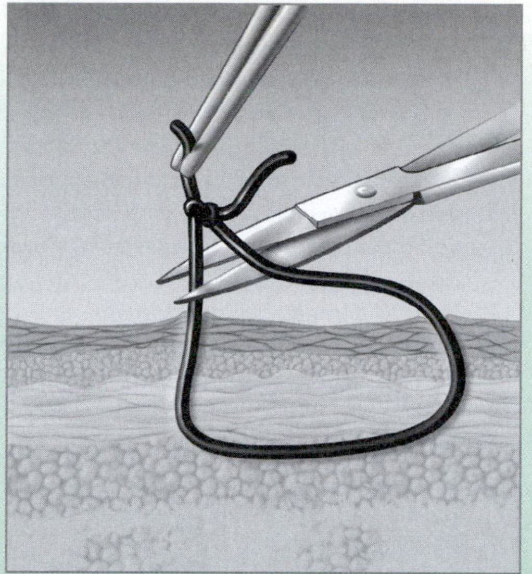

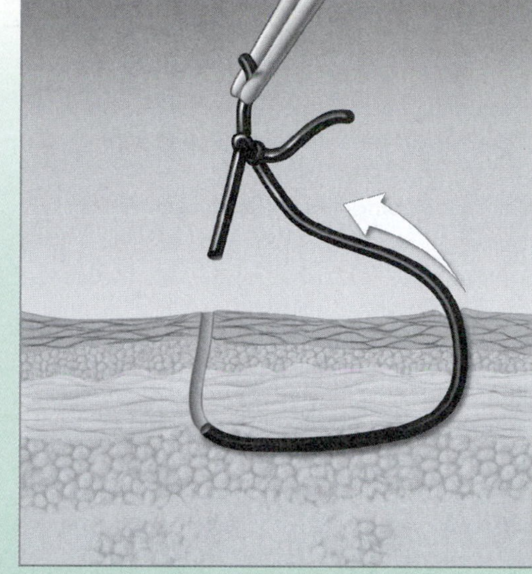

FIGURE 18-37 Removal of sutures.

Removal of Staples

1–10. Perform steps 1 through 10 above.

11. Place the lower tips of a sterile staple remover under the staple.
12. Squeeze the handles together until they are completely closed. (Pressing the handles together causes the staple to bend in the middle and pulls the edges of the staple out of the skin.) Do not lift the staple remover when squeezing the handles.
13. When both ends of the staple are visible, gently move the staple away from the incision site.
14. Hold the staple remover over a disposable container, release the staple remover handles, and release the staple.
15. Place the staple on the gauze, repeat these steps until all staples are removed, and count the number of staples to ensure that all have been removed.

Closing Steps for Removal of Sutures or Staples

16. Clean the wound with antiseptic and allow it to dry.
17. Dress the wound as ordered.
18. Properly dispose of equipment and supplies.
19. Remove gloves and perform hand hygiene.
20. Instruct the patient on wound care.
21. Document the procedure, including the condition of the wound, the number of sutures or staples removed, and patient instructions on wound care.

CHARTING EXAMPLE

2/14/XX 11:00 A.M. Removed sutures and cleansed wound with antiseptic. Wound healing well. Pt. instructed on wound care. . . . . M. King, CMA (AAMA)

ASSISTING WITH MINOR SURGERY (PROCEDURE 18-16 AND BOX 18-2)

procedure 18-16

ASSISTING WITH MINOR SURGERY

Objective: Prepare all materials and equipment for immediate use in a surgical procedure using sterile technique.

EQUIPMENT AND SUPPLIES

- Mayo stand
- side stand
- transfer forceps and container
- sharps container
- waste container/plastic bag
- biohazard waste container
- anesthetic

- alcohol swab
- sterile specimen container, depending on the type of surgery
- sterile pack (two pairs of sterile gloves, towel pack, 4 × 4 sponge pack, patient drape, needle pack, and suture materials)
- instrument pack(s), including towel clamp pack
- syringe pack
- two sterile basin packs

METHOD

1. Perform hand hygiene.
2. Open sterile tray packs on the Mayo stand and side stand. Use sterile wrapper to create a sterile field. The wrapper will hang over the edge of the tray.
3. Use sterile transfer forceps to move instruments on the tray or to place equipment from packets. Materials in peel-away packets should be flipped onto the tray.
4. Open the sterile needle and syringe unit and drop it gently onto the sterile field. Take care not to reach over the sterile field.
5. Open the sterile drape packs and towel clamp packs.
6. Open a set of sterile gloves for the physician.
7. After the tray is ready, with all equipment open and arranged, pull the edge of the sterile towel across the tray, using sterile transfer forceps. The sterile towel will provide a protective covering for the sterile tray until the procedure begins. Do not leave the room once the tray is set up (Figure 18-38).
8. When the physician has donned the sterile gloves, remove the sterile towel covering the tray of instruments.
9. Remove the towel by standing to one side and grasping the two distal corners, then lifting the towel toward you so that you do not reach over the unprotected sterile field.

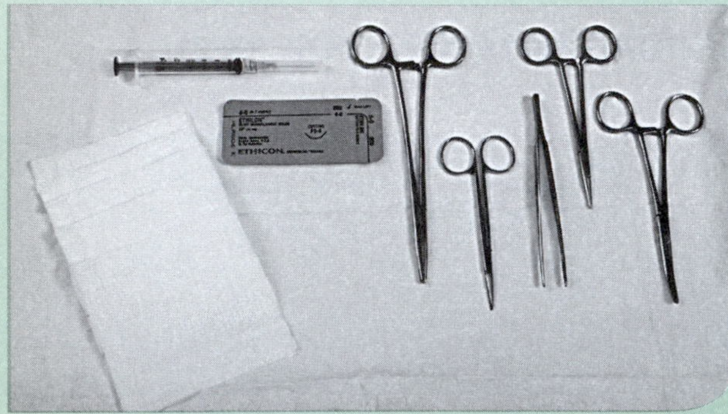

FIGURE 18-38 Sterile instrument setup.

10. Cleanse the vial of anesthetic with a sterile alcohol swab and hold it upside down in the palm of your hand, with the label facing toward the physician. Hold it steady while the physician draws up the anesthetic.
11. Stand to one side of the patient and assist the physician as requested. Provide additional supplies as needed. If you assist by handing instruments directly to the physician, you must perform a surgical scrub and wear a sterile gown and gloves.
12. Hold all containers for specimens, drainage, or contaminated 4 × 4s. Wear nonsterile gloves to protect yourself from contact with drainage.
13. Collect and place all soiled instruments in a basin out of the patient's view.
14. Place all soiled gauze sponges (4 × 4s) and dressings in a plastic bag. Do not allow wet items to remain on a sterile field.
15. Immediately label all specimens as they are obtained. Close all specimen containers tightly.
16. Periodically reassure the patient by quietly asking how he or she is doing. Do not touch the patient with soiled gloves.
17. When the procedure is complete, wash your hands before assisting the patient. The patient will often be moved to a recovery area so that the surgical area can be cleaned.

To dispose of soiled dressings, use the following steps:

   a. Remove gloves.
   b. Place one hand into the empty plastic bag.
   c. Using the hand covered with the plastic bag, pick up all the soiled materials. With the other hand, pull the outside of the bag over the soiled dressings.
   d. Dispose of the bag in a biohazard waste container.
   e. Perform hand hygiene and document the procedure.

18. Allow the patient to rest and recover from the anesthetic. Periodically, check the patient's vital signs according to your office policy.
19. Provide clear oral and written postoperative instructions for the patient. Make sure that the patient is stable before he or she leaves the office.
20. Send the specimen(s) to the laboratory with a requisition slip.
21. Clean, sanitize, and sterilize the instruments. Clean and sanitize the room in preparation for the next patient.
22. Perform hand hygiene.

CHARTING EXAMPLE

11/8/20XX 9:00 A.M. The physician will chart the details of the surgical procedure.· J. Wall, RMA (AMT)

Box 18-2 Guidelines for Surgical Asepsis

A sterile item can touch only another sterile item.

- If a sterile item touches a nonsterile item, it is contaminated.
- If a clean item touches a sterile item, it is contaminated.
- A sterile packet that is torn, wet, or punctured is contaminated.
- A sterile packet is contaminated after the date on the packet.
- If you are unsure of sterility, consider the item contaminated.
- Skin is always considered contaminated. It cannot be sterilized, only disinfected.

A sterile item on a sterile field must be within your field of vision and above your waist.

- If you cannot see an item, it is contaminated.
- If items or your hands are below your waist, they are contaminated.
- If you turn your back on a sterile field, it is contaminated.
- If you leave a sterile field unattended, it is contaminated.

Airborne microorganisms contaminate sterile fields.

- Do not place sterile fields in a draft.
- Avoid extra movements near the sterile field.
- Do not talk, cough, sneeze, or laugh over a sterile field.
- Wear a mask if you need to talk during a procedure.
- Do not reach over a sterile field.
- Avoid spills on a sterile field. A wet field is contaminated.

The edges of a sterile field are contaminated.

- If an item touches any part of the 1-inch border around the sterile field, it is contaminated.

Sterile gloves must touch only sterile items.

- Do not touch the outside of sterile gloves with bare hands.
- Sterile gloves are contaminated if punctured. Remove and dispose of the item and gloves, rescrub, and reglove.

Sterile packets may be touched on the outside with bare hands.

- Outer wrappings are considered contaminated.
- Open sterile packets away from you to avoid contaminating the packet by touching your clothing.
- Never rewrap an unused sterile packet. The unused items must be resanitized, rewrapped, and reautoclaved.

Be honest if you make an error or suspect that you have made an error.

- Remove the contaminated item and correct the error.
- Report contamination to your superior.

18 APPLICATION

Directions: Select the best answer for each of the following questions. Check your answers in the Answer Key at the end of the book.

1. Regarding sterilizing instruments in an autoclave, which of the following statements is not true?
   a. Only distilled water should be used.
   b. Trays and packs should be loaded on their side.
   c. Unwrapped sterile items must be removed with clean transfer forceps.
   d. Typical timing for wrapped trays and packages is 30 minutes.
   e. Typical timing for unwrapped items is 15 minutes.

2. A/An ________ is an instrument used to examine the ears.
   a. Ophthalmoscope
   b. Otoscope
   c. Endoscope
   d. Sphygmomanometer
   e. Oximeter

3. Which portion of the stethoscope is the small metal tube that connects the tubing to the earpieces?
   a. Diaphragm
   b. Bell
   c. Binarual
   d. Chest piece
   e. Sound sensor
4. The _____ of the stethoscope is a disc-like sound sensor that picks up high- and low-pitched sound frequencies.
   a. Diaphragm
   b. Bell
   c. Earpiece
   d. Cuff
   e. Bulb
5. Which of the following is not a true statement regarding the physical therapy modality cryotherapy?
   a. Increases circulation to the area for greater comfort and healing
   b. Reduces swelling
   c. Reduces inflammation
   d. Decreases body temperature
   e. An ice collar is an example of cryotherapy.
6. ________________ is used to examine the larynx, bladder, and stomach.
   a. Ophthalmoscope
   b. Otoscope
   c. Endoscope
   d. Sphygmomanometer
   e. Oximeter
7. Which of the following is not a characteristic of plaster casts?
   a. Use a wet bandage roll impregnated with calcium sulfate
   b. Can crack or break
   c. Easily molded to the body part
   d. Lighter than synthetic casts
   e. May soften or crumble with moisture
8. Which of the following exam room supplies is typically used to preserve slides?
   a. Hydrogen peroxide
   b. Lubricant
   c. Irrigation syringe
   d. Cotton-tipped swab
   e. Fixative spray
9. Which type of sphygmomanometer has a round dial that contains a scale calibrated in millimeters?
   a. Manometer
   b. Electronic
   c. Aneroid
   d. Mercury
   e. None of the above
10. A tympanic thermometer is also known as a/an __________ thermometer.
    a. Nonmercury
    b. Electronic
    c. Aural
    d. Oral
    e. Temporal artery
11. When providing immediate cast care instructions, the patient should be told to elevate the casted limb above heart level for:
    a. 10 hours
    b. 12 hours
    c. 24 hours
    d. 36 hours
    e. 24–36 hours
12. Which of the following correctly lists the sequence of physical exam procedures?
    a. Blood specimen, urine specimen, vital signs, weight and height EKG, X-ray
    b. Urine specimen, blood specimen, vital signs, weight and height EKG, X-ray
    c. Vital signs, urine specimen, blood specimen, weight and height EKG, X-ray
    d. Weight and height, vital signs, urine specimen, blood specimen, EKG, X-ray
    e. Vital signs, weight and height, urine specimen, blood specimen, EKG, X-ray
13. The method of examination that assesses the range of motion (ROM) in a joint is:
    a. Auscultation
    b. Mensuration
    c. Manipulation
    d. Percussion
    e. Inspection
14. ________________ is a type of examination whereby the hands are used to feel the skin and accessible underlying organs and tissue.
    a. Manipulation
    b. Inspection
    c. Palpation
    d. Mensuration
    e. Percussion
15. When a patient is in a supine position with the knees bent, this is known as:
    a. Fowler's position
    b. Semi-Fowler's position
    c. Trendelenburg position
    d. Doral recumbent position
    e. Lithotomy position

16. Which of the following statements regarding handling instruments is incorrect?
   a. Sharp instruments should remain separated from other instruments.
   b. Instruments with ratchets should be stored closed in order to maintain their good working condition.
   c. Tips on instruments should close tightly.
   d. Cutting edges should be smooth.
   e. Instruments should be scrubbed with a brush as soon as possible to prevent hardening of blood.

17. Which of the following sutures is used most often on muscle?
   a. 2-0
   b. 3-0
   c. 4-0
   d. 5-0
   e. 6-0

18. Regarding surgical asepsis, which of the following statements is incorrect?
   a. Airborne microorganisms contaminate sterile fields.
   b. Open sterile packets toward you to avoid contaminating them.
   c. Do not place sterile fields in a draft.
   d. Do not talk over a sterile field.
   e. A wet field is contaminated.

19. Absorbable suture is typically used for:
   a. Skin surface in incisions
   b. Internal organ incisions
   c. Tying off blood vessels
   d. A and C
   e. B and C

20. Which of the following sutures is considered to be absorbable?
   a. Vicryl
   b. Silk
   c. Nylon
   d. Polyester
   e. Cotton

21. An example of a surgical instrument used to grasp and/or clamp is:
   a. Scalpel or knife
   b. Scissors
   c. Forceps
   d. Trocar
   e. Speculum

19 Diagnostic Testing

CONTENTS

Electrocardiogram

An electrocardiogram (more commonly known as an EKG or ECG) is a recording of electrical activity of the heart. The physician may order this test as part of an annual routine physical exam or if there are unusual sounds in the heart, or arrhythmias, or if the patient is complaining of any symptoms associated with heart conditions and diseases. See Procedure 19-1 and Figures 19-1 and 19-2.

procedure 19-1

RECORDING A 12-LEAD EKG

Objective: Perform an EKG without assistance.

EQUIPMENT AND SUPPLIES

- EKG machine with sensors, patient cable, and power cord
- EKG paper
- electrolyte, if needed
- alcohol
- screwdriver for adjustments, if needed
- patient gown, if needed

METHOD

1. Perform hand hygiene.
2. Assemble necessary supplies.
3. Attach and plug in the power cord.
4. Verify that the machine is operational and positioned properly.

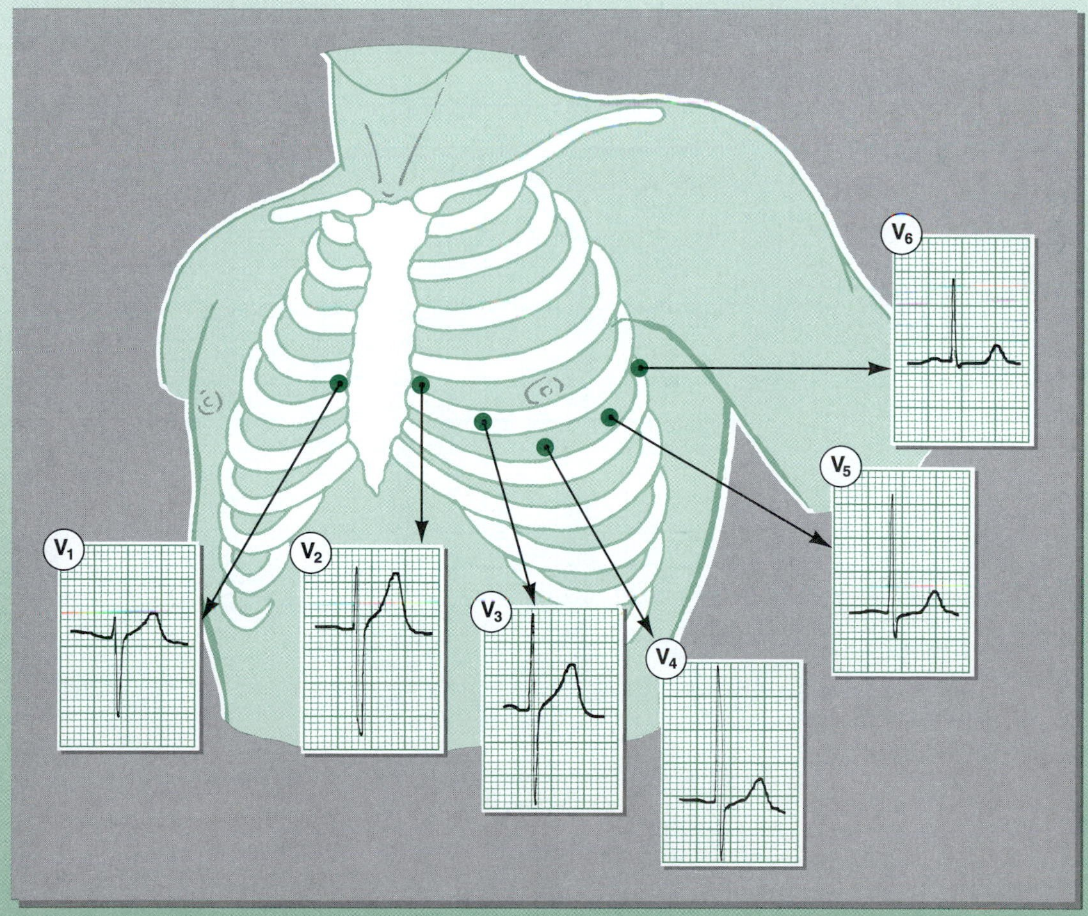

FIGURE 19-1 Electrode placement for chest leads V1–V6.

5. Identify, interview, and instruct the patient on the procedure.
6. Offer female patients gowns to be worn, with the opening down the front.
7. Position the patient flat on the table, with a pillow under the head and one under the knees if needed.
8. Prepare the electrode sites and attach the electrodes. Limb electrodes should be applied over the fleshy part of the inner aspects of the lower legs and on the upper part of the forearms. Chest leads should be applied as illustrated in Figure 19-1.
9. Connect the patient cable.
10. Instruct the patient to relax, breathe normally, and refrain from speaking.
11. Standardize the machine.
12. Adjust the stylus to the center of the paper or the center of each channel.
13. Record. For automatic machines, depress AUTO-RUN; for manual machines, select the leads in sequence and use RUN 25. Use your problem-solving skills if you encounter artifacts.
14. Mark the leads, if necessary.
15. Remove the sensors; wipe electrolyte from the patient's skin, if used.
16. Politely dismiss the patient, aiding the patient in getting up and dressed, if necessary.
17. Perform hand hygiene.
18. Clean the machine, straps, and sensors according to the manufacturer's instructions.
19. Mount the EKG if necessary and transfer patient information.
20. Chart the procedure in the patient's record. Sign or initial your work.

CHARTING EXAMPLE

3/11/XX 2:10 P.M. 12-lead ECG performed and given to Dr. Salpega to read. .... W. Short, CMA (AAMA)

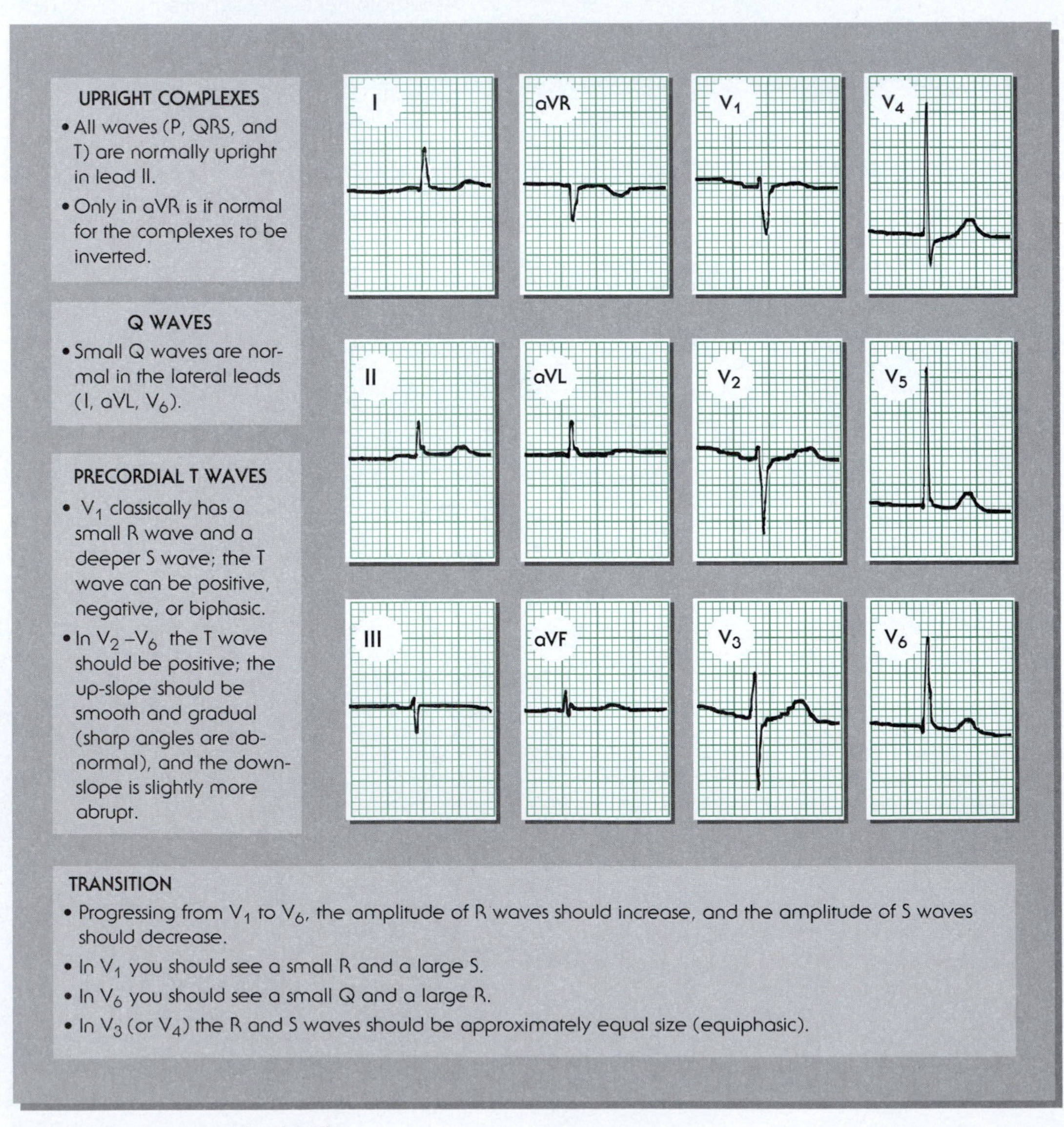

UPRIGHT COMPLEXES
• All waves (P, QRS, and T) are normally upright in lead II.
• Only in aVR is it normal for the complexes to be inverted.
Q WAVES
• Small Q waves are normal in the lateral leads (I, aVL, V_6).
PRECORDIAL T WAVES
• V_1 classically has a small R wave and a deeper S wave; the T wave can be positive, negative, or biphasic.
• In V_2–V_6 the T wave should be positive; the up-slope should be smooth and gradual (sharp angles are abnormal), and the down-slope is slightly more abrupt.
I
aVR
V_1
V_4
II
aVL
V_2
V_5
III
aVF
V_3
V_6
TRANSITION
• Progressing from V_1 to V_6, the amplitude of R waves should increase, and the amplitude of S waves should decrease.
• In V_1 you should see a small R and a large S.
• In V_6 you should see a small Q and a large R.
• In V_3 (or V_4) the R and S waves should be approximately equal size (equiphasic).

FIGURE 19-2 Features of a normal 12-lead EKG.

EQUIPMENT

Several types of EKG machines are available, both manual and computerized. Manual machines require someone to move the chest sensor and record from each lead, then move the sensor again. Computerized EKG machines automatically switch the sensors from lead to lead, so the leads do not have to be moved. No matter what machine is used, it is important to make sure that the machine has been properly calibrated. A properly calibrated EKG machine will move the paper at a speed of 25 mm per second, and the stylus will move 10 mm for every 1 mV of electrical input.

In addition to the EKG machine, special standardized graph paper is required (Figures 19-3). The horizontal line records the time and the vertical line records the amplitude. The paper is divided into 5 × 5 mm squares. Each square is the equivalent of 0.20 second and is made up of smaller 1 × 1 mm squares. Each square is the equivalent of 0.04 second.

PLACEMENT OF LEADS

The EKG machine records the cardiac cycle through electrodes or sensors placed on the patient's bare skin. In order for the electrical activity to be transmitted to the EKG machine, three leads are required:

- Positive
- Negative
- Ground

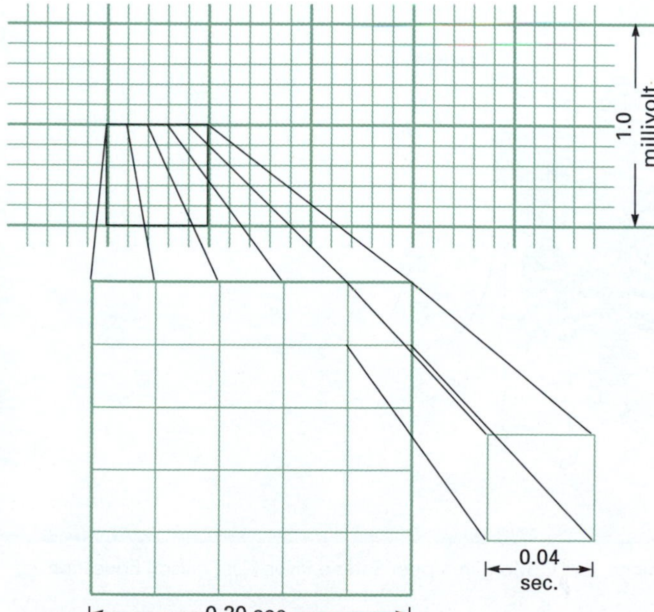

FIGURE 19-3 EKG paper and markings.

LIMB LEADS The limb leads are placed over the fleshy area of each limb and are usually identified by color and lead number

Right Arm (RA)	White
Left Arm (LA)	Black
Right Leg (RL)	Green
Left Leg (LL)	Red

CHEST LEADS In order to properly place the chest leads, also known as *precordial leads*, you must first find the third intercostal space at the sternum

Lead	Placement
V1	Fourth intercostal space to the right of the sternum
V2	Fourth intercostal space to the left of the sternum
V3	Midway between the fourth and fifth intercostal spaces and halfway between the base of the sternum and the left nipple
V4	Over the fifth intercostal space and in line with the left nipple
V5	Same line midway between the left nipple and the midpoint of the axilla
V6	Over the intercostal space at the axilla midpoint

EKG WAVEFORMS

When performing an EKG, each cardiac cycle is represented as a pattern of waves that correspond to certain electrical activities within the heart, such as atrial and ventricular contraction followed by relaxation of each atrium and ventricle (Figure 19-7).

EKG LEADS

Limb Leads (Figure 19-4)

Lead I: Records electrical activity from right arm to left arm

Lead II: Records electrical activity from right arm to left leg

Lead III: Records electrical activity from left arm to left leg

Augmented Leads (Figure 19-5)

aVR: Records electrical activity away from midpoint between left arm and left leg to left arm (across heart to right shoulder)

aVL: Records electrical activity from midpoint between right arm and left leg to left arm (across heart to left shoulder)

aVF: Records electrical activity from midpoint between right arm and left arm to left leg (across heart toward feet)

Chest or Precordial Leads (Figure 19-6)

V1: Records electrical activity between center of heart and the chest wall where V1 electrode is placed

V2: Records electrical activity between center of heart and chest wall where V2 electrode is placed

V3: Records electrical activity between center of heart and chest wall where V3 electrode is placed

V4: Records electrical activity between center of heart and chest wall where V4 electrode is placed

V5: Records electrical activity between center of heart and chest wall where V5 electrode is placed

V6: Records electrical activity between center of the heart and chest wall where V6 electrode is placed

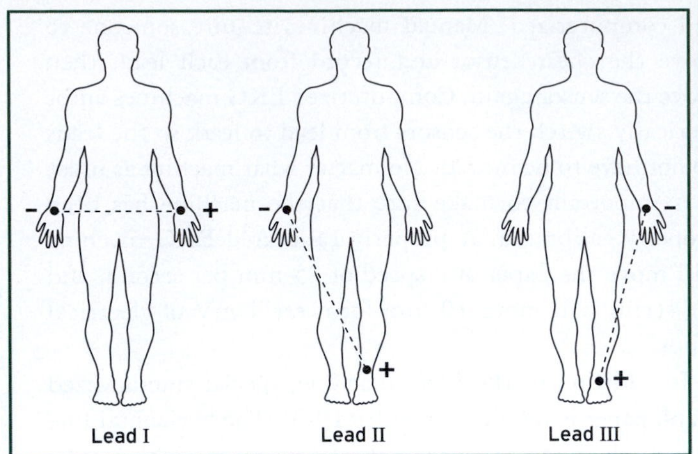

FIGURE 19-4 The limb leads.

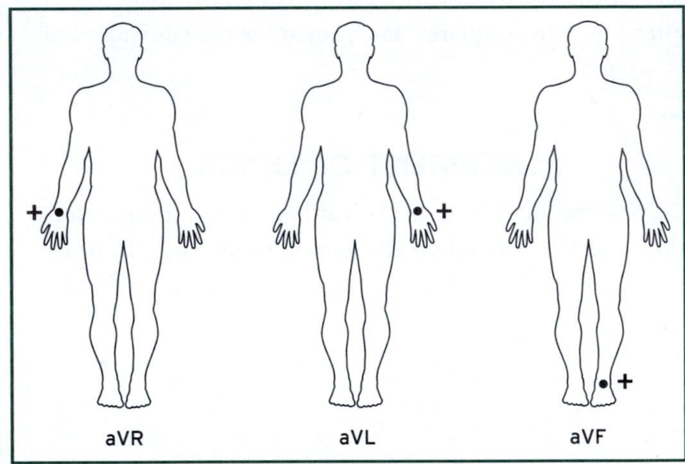

FIGURE 19-5 The augmented leads.

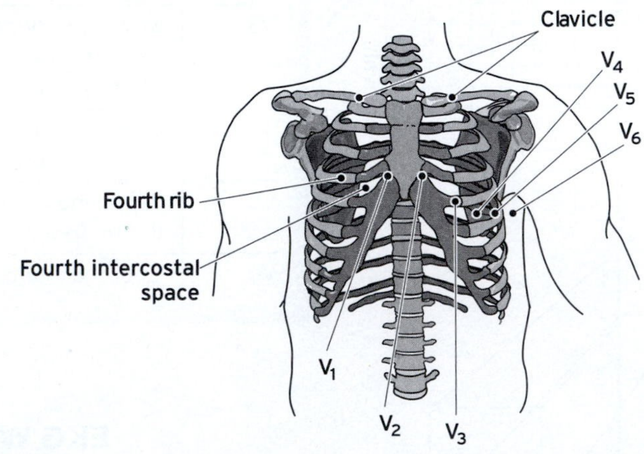

FIGURE 19-6 The precordial leads.

Source: Medical Assisting: Foundations and Practices by M. S. Frazier, C. Malone, and C. Morgan, Upper Saddle River, NJ: Pearson Education, Inc., 2010, p. 745. Reprinted with permission.

EKG TERMS: WAVES

Wave	Represents
P	Contraction of the atria via firing of the sinoatrial (SA) node
PR Interval	Time between impulse to SA node (P wave) and when it travels through the atria to the ventricles
QRS Complex	Impulse from the bundle of His through the ventricles
ST Segment	Ventricles depolarized and repolarization (recovery) begins
T	Repolarization of the ventricles

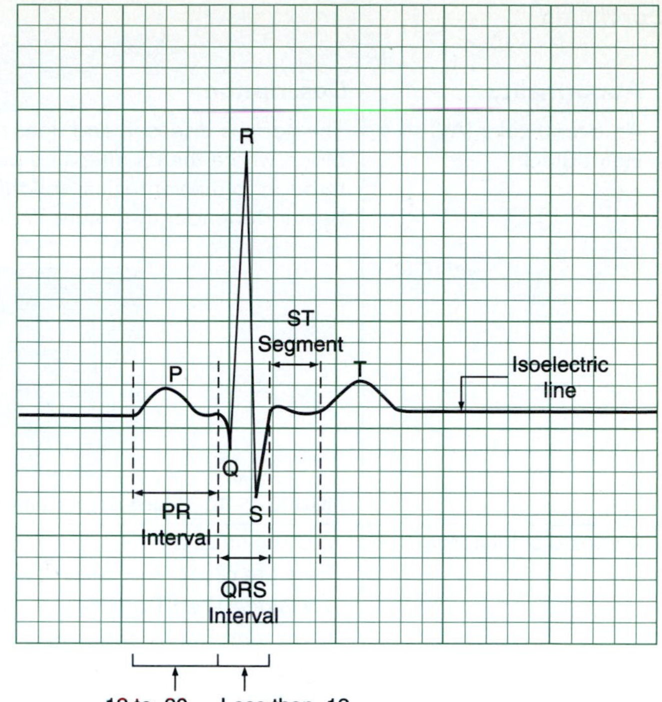

FIGURE 19-7 EKG waveforms.

The following table shows abnormalities caused by cardiac pathology.

ABNORMALITIES CAUSED BY CARDIAC PATHOLOGY

Abnormality	Description
Atrial Fibrillation	There are as many as 350 irregular P waves and 130–150 irregular QRS complexes per minute (Figure 19-8). **FIGURE 19-8 Atrial fibrillation.**
Atrial Flutter	This rapid fluttering of the upper chambers looks like the pattern of teeth on a saw on the EKG. The atrial rate is 250–350 per minute. Not all of the impulses are conducted through the AV node because they are coming too fast. There is some blockage at the AV node. This is one type of heart block (Figure 19-9). **FIGURE 19-9 Atrial flutter.**

(continued)

(Continued)

Abnormality	Description
Atrioventricular (AV) Heart Block	The node is diseased and does not conduct the impulse well. There are three types: first-degree block, where the PR interval is prolonged; second-degree block, where some waves do not pass through to the ventricles; and third-degree or complete AV block, where the atria and ventricles beat independently (Figure 19-10). 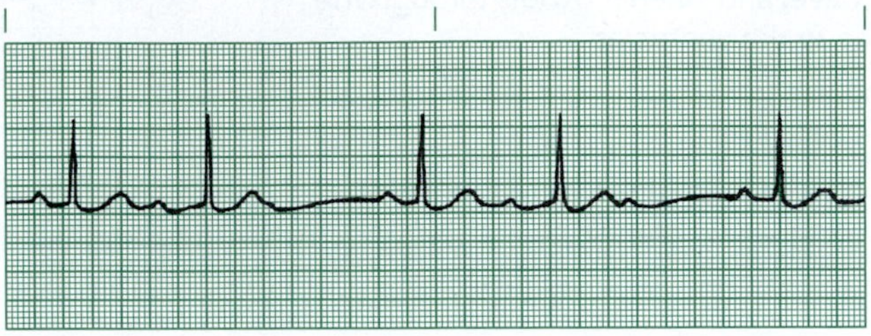 **FIGURE 19-10 Third-degree heart block.**
Myocardial Infarction	Also known as *MI* There are broad and deep Q waves. *Old injury:* The ST segment is usually depressed below the baseline. *New injury:* The ST segment is usually elevated above the baseline. *Angina pectoris* is the name for the syndrome of pain and oppression in the anterior chest due to heart tissue being deprived of oxygen. If this pain lasts for 20–30 minutes, suspect a myocardial infarction in which the heart tissue is actually dying.
Paroxysmal Atrial Tachycardia	Also known as *PAT* This is a common arrhythmia, usually seen in young adults with normal hearts. There are no visible P waves because they are hidden by the T wave of the previous cycle. The atrial rate is 140–250 per minute. In many ways, it looks like repeated PACs on the EKG.
Premature Atrial Contractions	Also known as *PACs* A P wave occurs earlier than expected, usually from a source outside the sinus node. Therefore, P waves are distorted.
Premature Ventricular Contractions	Also known as *PVCs* The wide QRS complexes occur without preceding P waves. They may be caused by electrolyte imbalance, stress, smoking, alcohol, or toxic reactions to drugs. They also occur in a majority of patients who have had a heart attack (Figure 19-11). 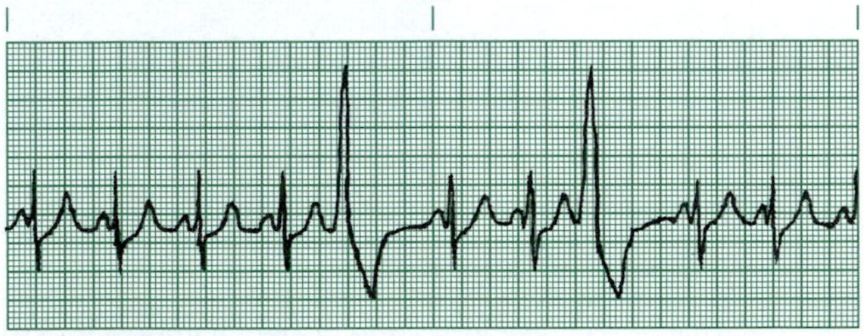 **FIGURE 19-11 Multifocal PVCs.**
Sinus Arrhythmia	Normally seen in children and young adults; all aspects of the EKG are normal except the irregularity. The space between QRS complexes is not equal. The heart rate increases on inspiration and decreases on expiration.
Sinus Bradycardia	There are fewer than 60 bpm; cycles are normal (Figure 19-12). 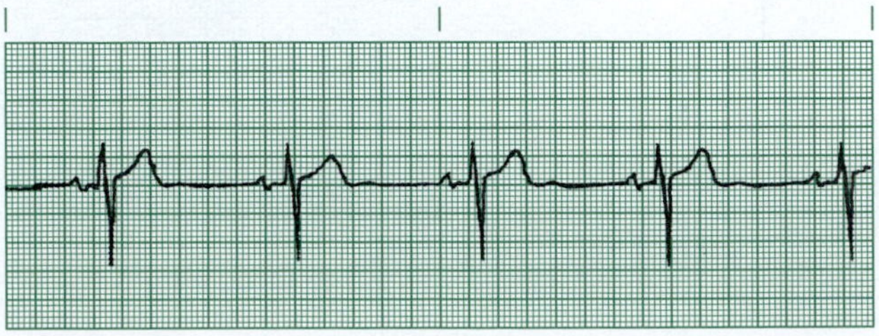 **FIGURE 19-12 Sinus bradycardia.**

(Continued)

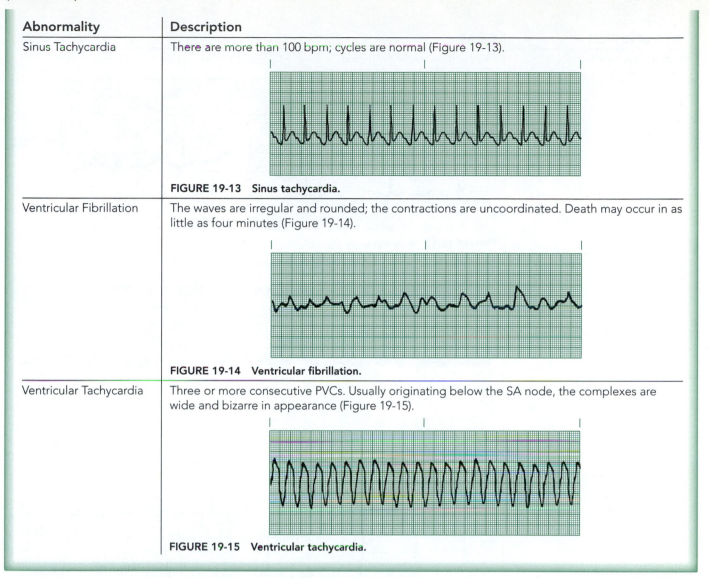

Abnormality	Description
Sinus Tachycardia	There are more than 100 bpm; cycles are normal (Figure 19-13). 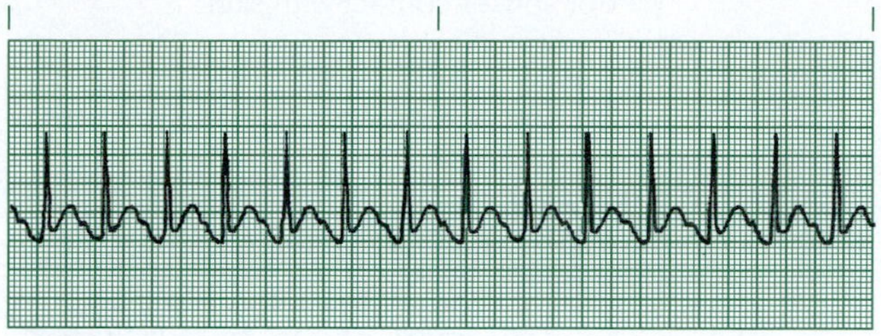 **FIGURE 19-13 Sinus tachycardia.**
Ventricular Fibrillation	The waves are irregular and rounded; the contractions are uncoordinated. Death may occur in as little as four minutes (Figure 19-14). 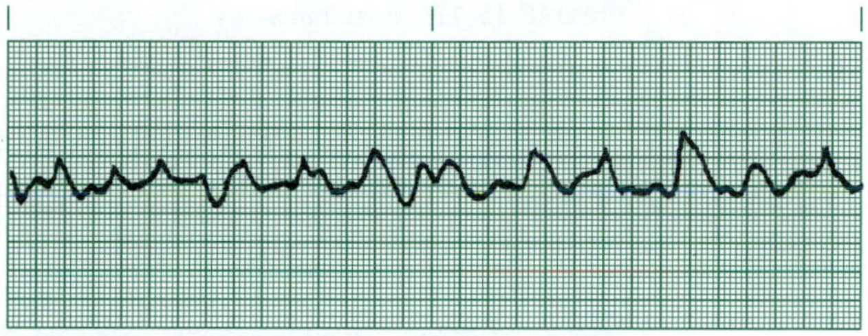 **FIGURE 19-14 Ventricular fibrillation.**
Ventricular Tachycardia	Three or more consecutive PVCs. Usually originating below the SA node, the complexes are wide and bizarre in appearance (Figure 19-15). 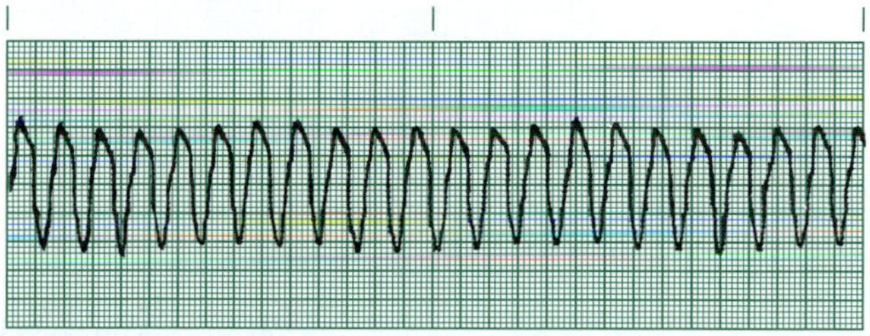 **FIGURE 19-15 Ventricular tachycardia.**

ARTIFACTS Artifacts are caused by electrical activity from sources other than the heart.

Type of Artifact	Cause
Somatic Tremor (Figure 19-16)	Tense muscles or a muscle contraction 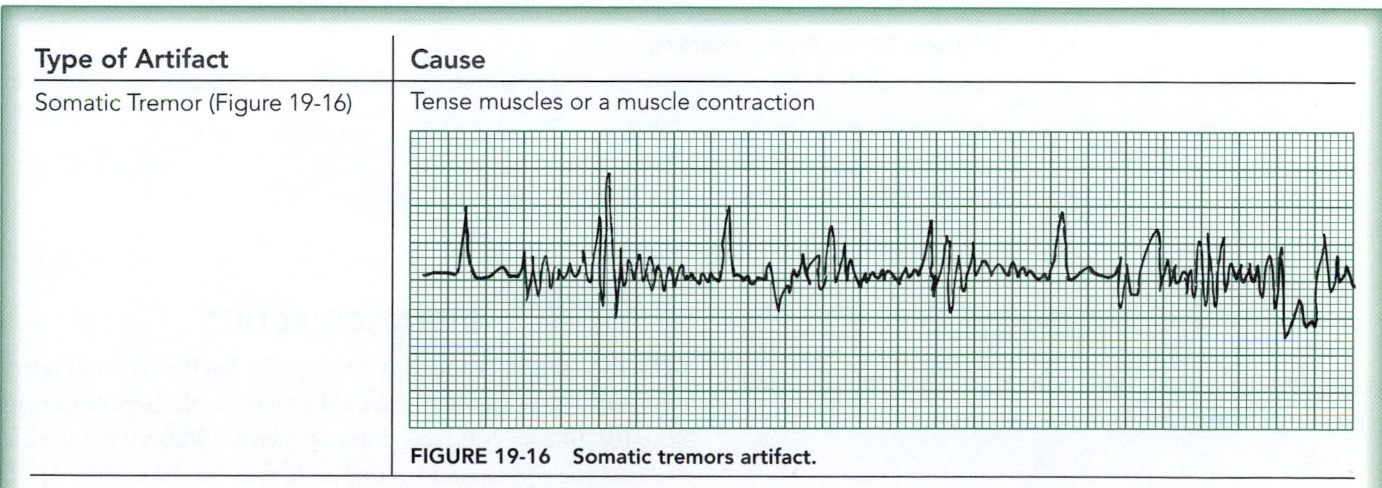 **FIGURE 19-16 Somatic tremors artifact.**

(continued)

(*Continued*)

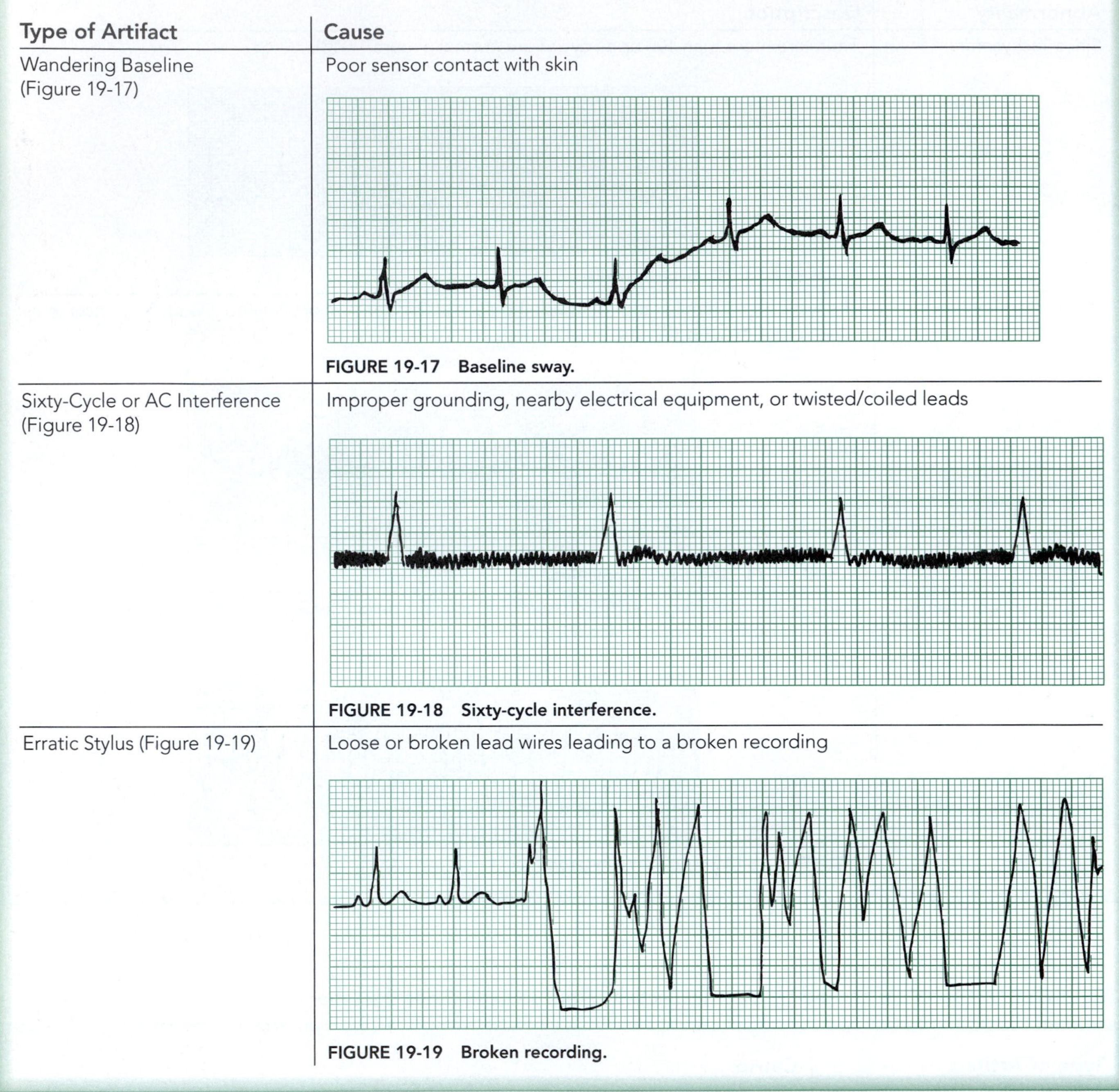

Type of Artifact	Cause
Wandering Baseline (Figure 19-17)	Poor sensor contact with skin **FIGURE 19-17 Baseline sway.**
Sixty-Cycle or AC Interference (Figure 19-18)	Improper grounding, nearby electrical equipment, or twisted/coiled leads **FIGURE 19-18 Sixty-cycle interference.**
Erratic Stylus (Figure 19-19)	Loose or broken lead wires leading to a broken recording **FIGURE 19-19 Broken recording.**

Vision

Vision testing may be done within the medical office and is typically performed by a medical assistant.

DISTANCE ACUITY

Distance acuity is measured using the Snellen chart (Figure 19-20). The person with normal vision should be able to read the top line at 200 feet. Someone with 20/20 vision is able to read the corresponding line at 20 feet. See Procedure 19-2.

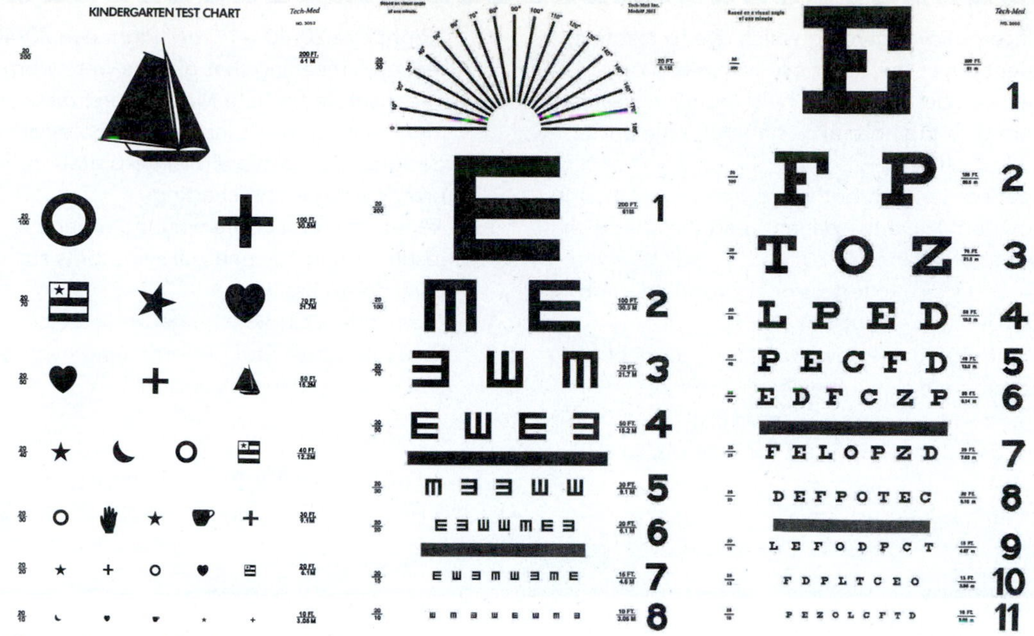

FIGURE 19-20 Different types of Snellen eye charts.

procedure 19-2

TESTING VISUAL ACUITY USING A SNELLEN EYE CHART

Objective: Screen a patient for distance acuity using a Snellen eye chart.

EQUIPMENT AND SUPPLIES

- Snellen eye chart placed at a distance of 20 feet
- eye shield or occluder
- pointer
- pen and paper
- alcohol and gauze

METHOD

1. Assemble equipment.
2. Review the physician's order.
3. Perform hand hygiene and identify the patient.
4. Explain the procedure.
5. Determine the patient's ability to recognize letters. If the patient is unable to read letters, use the necessary chart to accommodate the patient's abilities.
6. Place the patient 20 feet from the Snellen eye chart, either seated or standing, as long as the chart is at eye level (Figure 19-21).
7. Follow office policy regarding testing with or without corrective lenses.

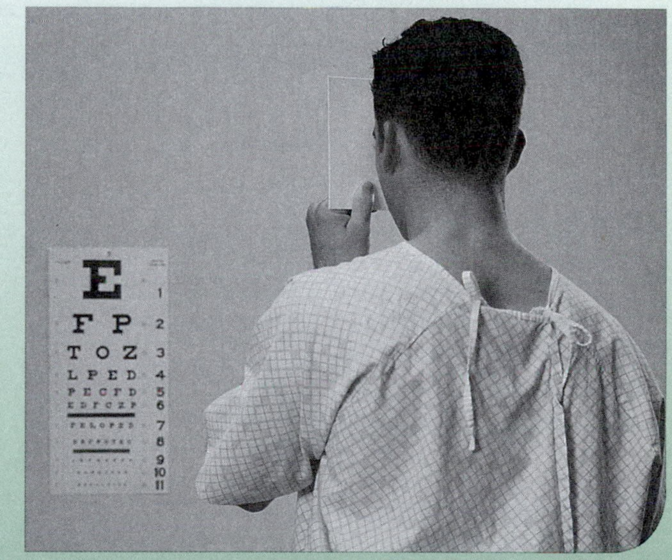
FIGURE 19-21 Test of distance vision using the Snellen eye chart.

8. Following office policy regarding which eye to test first, have the patient cover the other eye with a cup or occluder. The occluder should be held in such a way as not to interfere with the normal position of a patient's glasses.
9. Instruct the patient to keep both eyes open even though one eye is covered. Have the patient read the lines with both eyes first at a distance of 20 feet.
10. Use a pointer and point to letters or appropriate symbols in random order.
11. Starting with the 20/70 line, ask the patient to identify each line and proceed down the chart to the last line the patient can read without error. Observe for signs of squinting or tilting the head, which indicate difficulty identifying letters.
12. Record the ratio numbers adjacent to the line the patient can read without error. If there is an error, note it (e.g., "Right eye 20/40—1"; or "Right eye 20/40—1 with correction," meaning that glasses were worn during testing). The Institute for Safe Medication Practices (ISMP) recommends using words instead of abbreviations for eye designations to avoid misinterpretation. Follow office protocol regarding charting.
13. Repeat the procedure with the other eye and record the result, noting any unusual symptoms such as squinting or blinking excessively.
14. Clean the occluder with gauze and alcohol.
15. Remove gloves and perform hand hygiene.
16. Document the results accurately.

CHARTING EXAMPLE

2/14/XX 4:00 P.M. Snellen eye test. Rt eye 20/30. Lt eye 20/30. Both eyes 20/30. . . . . M. King, CMA (AAMA)

NEAR VISION ACUITY

Near vision acuity testing is measured using the Jaeger card. This test is performed if the patient complains of having difficulty reading or performing other close tasks such as threading a needle. The card is held at a normal reading distance, and if the patient is able to read paragraph J2, he or she is said to have 20/20 vision. See Procedure 19-3.

procedure 19-3

SCREENING FOR NEAR VISION ACUITY

Objective: Screen near vision acuity using the Jaeger system.

EQUIPMENT AND SUPPLIES

- Jaeger near vision acuity card
- paper and pen

METHOD

1. Perform hand hygiene.
2. Review the physician's order.
3. Assemble equipment.
4. Identify the patient and introduce yourself.
5. Explain the procedure.
6. In a well-lit room, have the patient hold the Jaeger card at a distance of 14 to 16 inches.
7. Ask the patient to read aloud, with both eyes open, the smallest paragraph or line possible without error (Figure 19-22).
8. Document the results accurately, noting any unusual symptoms, such as squinting.

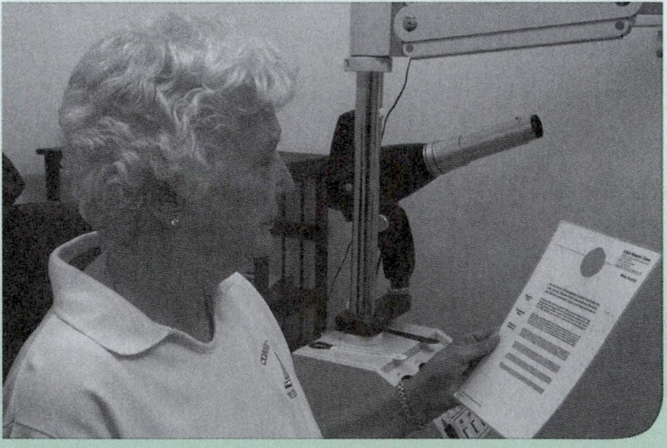

FIGURE 19-22 A patient using a near vision acuity card.

CHARTING EXAMPLE

09/11/XX Pt performed near vision acuity screening reading without error—J2. . . . . L. Mckay, RMA (AMT)

procedure 19-4

PERFORM A SNELLEN EYE EXAM ON A CHILD

Objective: Perform a Snellen eye exam for distance acuity on a child.

EQUIPMENT AND SUPPLIES

- Snellen E eye chart and oculator
- pencil and paper
- mark on floor at a distance of 20 feet from the chart

METHOD

1. Assemble equipment.
2. Introduce yourself and identify the patient.
3. Explain the procedure to the patient and parent or caregiver.
4. Perform hand hygiene.
5. Ask the child to indicate which way the legs on the E are pointing to make sure that the child understands the directions.
6. If the child understands, position him or her in front of the Snellen E chart at a distance of 20 feet.
7. Make sure that the child is comfortable.
8. Ask the child to hold the oculator over his or her first eye and remind the child to keep both eyes open (Figure 19-23).
9. Point to the *E*s on the chart. Make sure that the child is pointing in the same direction as the *E* on the chart. Proceed until you have the results from the first eye.
10. Repeat the procedure with the other eye.
11. Document the procedure and record the results using written words (*not* OS, OD, OU).
12. Compliment the child and caregiver on how well the child performed.

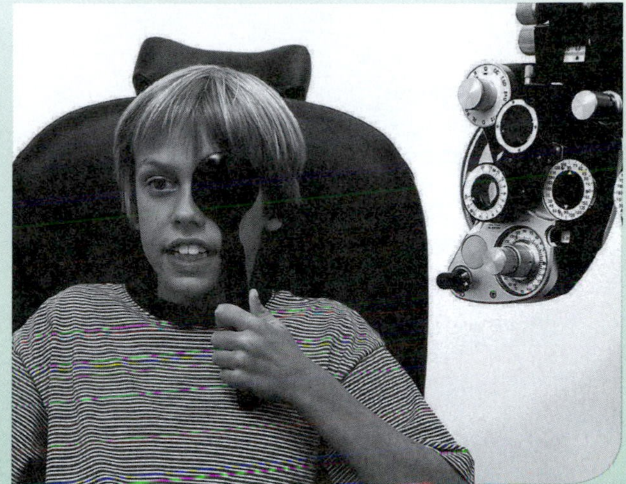

FIGURE 19-23 Testing distance visual acuity using the Snellen eye chart.

13. Perform hand hygiene.
14. Sanitize and replace equipment.

CHARTING EXAMPLE

4/1/10/XX Visual acuity using Snellen E chart Right eye 20/20; Left eye 20/30; Both eyes 20/20 .... M. King, CMA (AAMA)

ISHIHARA COLOR VISION EXAM

Color vision testing is performed to determine whether a patient has difficulty distinguishing one color from another (Procedure 19-5). The most common color vision defect is the inability to distinguish between red and green.

procedure 19-5

SCREENING FOR COLOR VISION ACUITY

Objective: Screen a patient for color vision defects.

EQUIPMENT AND SUPPLIES

- Ishihara screening book/cards
- paper and pen

METHOD

1. Perform hand hygiene.
2. Review the physician's order.
3. Assemble equipment.
4. Identify the patient and introduce yourself.
5. Explain the procedure.
6. Have the patient assume a comfortable position, and tell the patient to keep both eyes open.
7. In a well-lit room, have the patient identify, at a distance of 30 inches, the number that is formed by the colored dots on each card or page within three seconds per page or card.
8. If the patient is unable to identify the numbers, have the patient trace the number with his or her finger.
9. Score each plate as it is read. (Figure 19-24 is an example of one color plate.) If the patient is able to identify the number, then record the number seen after the plate number (e.g., Plate 1:7). If the patient is unable to identify the number on a plate, record the plate number and mark an X next to it.

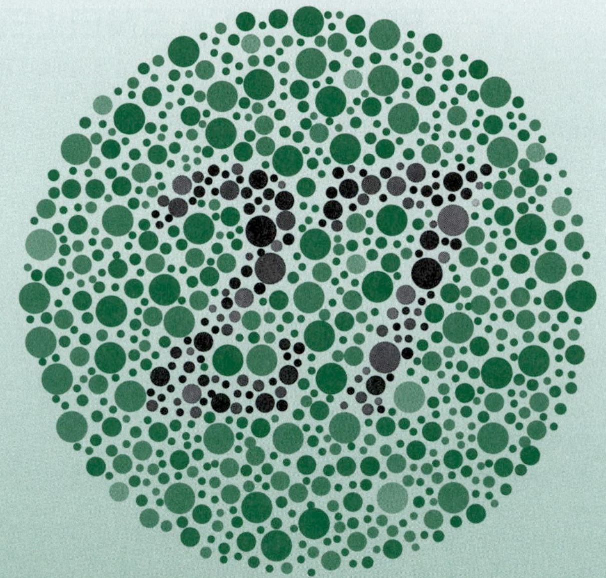

FIGURE 19-24 One page of a color vision chart.

10. Note any unusual symptoms.
11. Document the results accurately.

CHARTING EXAMPLE

2/14/XX 3:00 P.M. Ishihara eye chart normal. . . . . M. King, CMA (AAMA)

Hearing

Several tests are used to evaluate hearing acuity, including using a tuning fork as well as an audiometer (Procedure 19-6). Tuning forks provide a rough hearing assessment; however, if it is determined that a more definitive test is required, an audiometer would be used.

procedure 19-6

ASSISTING WITH AUDIOMETRY

Objective: Perform an audiometric test without error.

EQUIPMENT AND SUPPLIES

- audiometer with headphones
- quiet room or small, enclosed cubicle
- patient's record
- pen

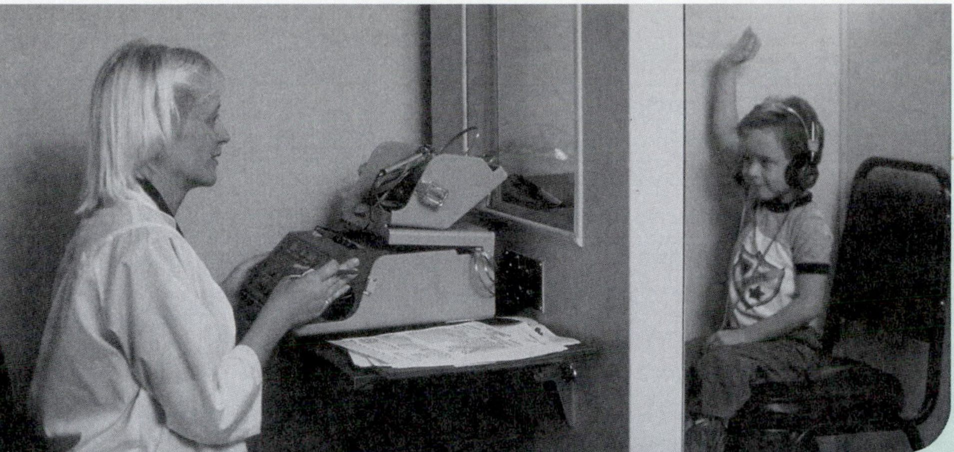

FIGURE 19-25 Performing a hearing test on a child.

METHOD

1. Check the physician's orders.
2. Perform hand hygiene.
3. Prepare equipment.
4. Test the equipment and make sure that the power is on.
5. Identify the patient and explain the procedure.
6. Establish the signal response that the patient will give if no automatic button is available; nodding the head or holding up a finger are acceptable signals (Figure 19-25).
7. Have the patient assume a comfortable position.
8. Place the headphones over the patient's ears.
9. Begin with low-frequency sound and watch the patient for an indication that the sound has been heard; push the button to record if the machine does not do it automatically.
10. Gradually increase the frequency until the test is completed in the first ear.
11. Proceed to the other ear and repeat the entire procedure.
12. Remove the headphones.
13. Clean the equipment following the manufacturer's instructions.
14. Perform hand hygiene.
15. Document the procedure appropriately.

CHARTING EXAMPLE

2/14/XX 9:00 A.M. Audiometry test administered in both ears. Results given to Dr. Williams. ········ M. King, CMA (AAMA)

Respiratory Exams

Respiratory testing may be conducted for a variety of reasons, including assessment of drug therapies and to assist in diagnosing patients with respiratory diseases and conditions.

PULMONARY FUNCTION TEST

Pulmonary function tests (PFTs) are performed to evaluate lung volume and capacity. Spirometry measures how much air can be held in the lungs and how quickly that air can be expelled (Procedure 19-7).

PULMONARY FUNCTION TESTS

Lung Function	Definition
Expiratory Reserve Volume	Also known as *ERV* Maximum volume of air left that can be exhaled after a normal expiration
Forced Vital Capacity	Also known as *FVC* Amount of air that can be forcefully exhaled from a maximum inhalation
Functional Residual Volume	Also known as *FVR* Amount of air left in the lungs after a normal expiration
Inspiratory Capacity	Also known as *IC* Maximum amount of air that can be inspired after a normal expiration

(*continued*)

(*Continued*)

Lung Function	Definition
Maximal Volume Ventilation	Also known as *MVV* Maximum volume that the patient can breathe in and out in one minute
Residual Volume	Also known as *RV* Volume of air left in lungs after forced expiration
Total Volume	Also known as V_T Amount of air inspired and expired in a normal respiration
Vital Capacity	Also known as *VC* Maximum amount of air that can be expired after a maximum inspiration

procedure 19-7

PERFORMING A SPIROMETRY TEST TO MEASURE FORCED VITAL CAPACITY

Objective: Perform a forced vital capacity test.

EQUIPMENT AND SUPPLIES

- functioning spirometry machine
- nose clip
- patient mouthpiece
- disinfectant
- biohazard waste container
- paper and pencil
- scale for height and weight
- sphygmomanometer and blood pressure cuff

METHOD

1. Perform hand hygiene.
2. Assemble all equipment.
3. Calibrate the spirometer as necessary according to the manufacturer's instructions.
4. Identify the patient.
5. Ask whether the patient has prepared for the test by not smoking and not using a bronchodilator for the preceding six hours.
6. Inquire about the patient's general health at present.
7. Explain and demonstrate the procedure to the patient.
8. Weigh the patient, measure the patient's height, and record the results.
9. Measure the patient's vital signs and record them.
10. Explain the proper positioning and, if necessary, assist with loosening any tight clothing.
11. Start the machine and enter the needed data.
12. Review the procedure with the patient. Be sure that the patient knows that it is necessary to breathe forcibly several times into the spirometer.
13. Have the patient place the mouthpiece in his or her mouth and seal the lips around it (Figure 19-26A).

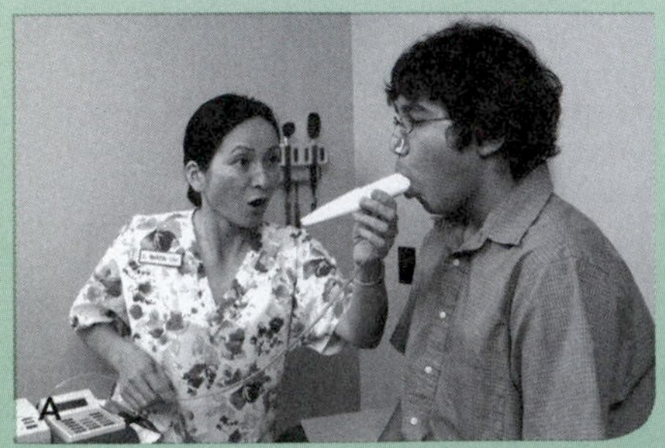

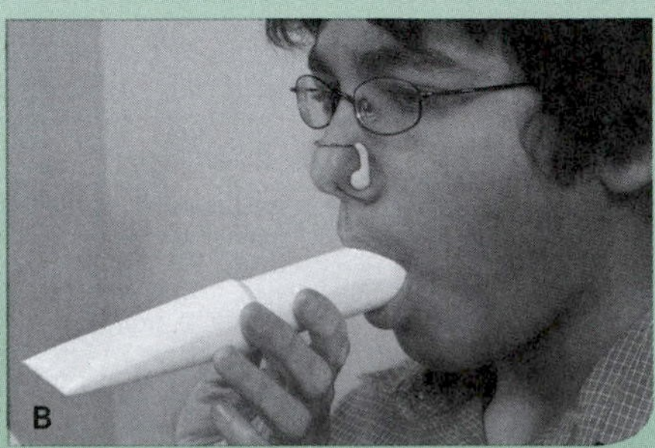

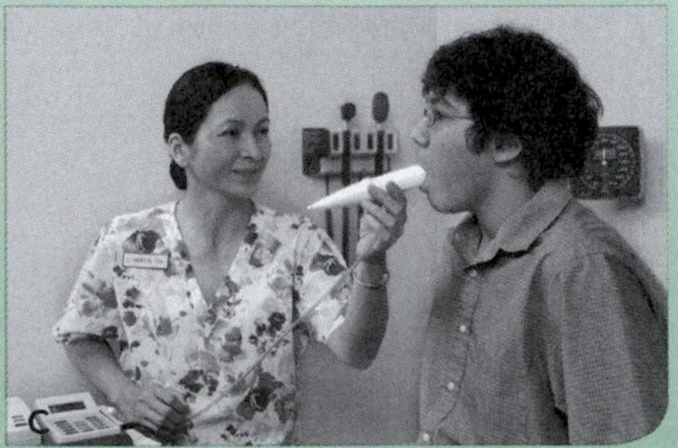

FIGURE 19-26 (A) The patient must close the lips tightly around the mouthpiece. (B) Place the nose clip on the patient's nose. (C) Direct the patient to blow the air out into the mouthpiece as hard and fast as possible.

14. Apply nose clips (Figure 19-26B).
15. Have the patient inhale deeply.
16. Push the start button at the same time as you give the following instruction to the patient.
17. Encourage the patient to blast breath out as hard, fast, and long as possible (Figure 19-26C).
18. Make recommendations to improve the outcome, if necessary.
19. Obtain the second set of maneuvers.
20. Obtain the third set of maneuvers.
21. Continue until you have three acceptable outcomes. You may facilitate up to eight attempts, if needed, to obtain three good trials. Some computerized machines will select the best attempt and print it.
22. Remove the nose clip and ask the patient to remain until the physician reviews the results.
23. Give the physician the trial information.
24. Record the results in the patient's chart.
25. Clean the tubing and dispose of the mouthpieces using standard precautions and following the manufacturer's directions.

CHARTING EXAMPLE

3/12/XX 8:30 A.M. Spirometry performed, with three good results submitted to Dr. Penningworth. .... K. Christianson, CMA (AAMA)

SPIROMETER

A spirometer is a diagnostic tool used to measure and record the volume of air exhaled in a specific amount of time (Figure 19-27).

PEAK FLOW METER

Peak flow meters are used to measure the patient's ability to move air into and out of the lungs. Most physicians will ask the patient to use the peak flow meter daily, in addition to the times when attacks occur, and record the results (Procedure 19-8). The information gathered will help the physician determine a baseline and proper treatment plan for that particular patient.

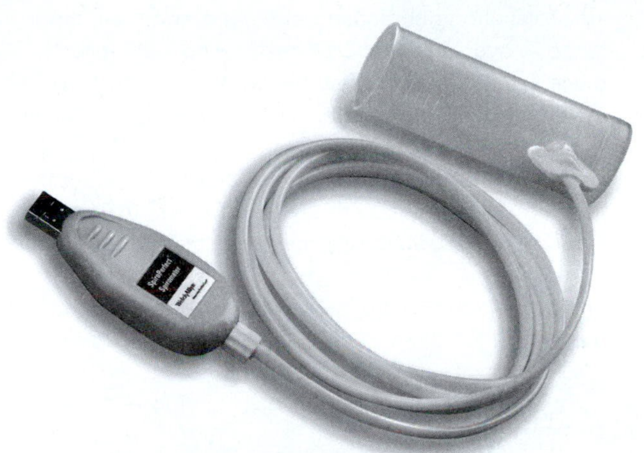

FIGURE 19-27 One type of spirometer.
Courtesy of Welch Allyn.

procedure 19-8

TEACHING PEAK FLOW MEASUREMENT

Objective: To instruct the patient to correctly monitor peak flow and record the results.

EQUIPMENT AND SUPPLIES

- peak flow meter
- documentation diary/chart
- diagram of lungs and breathing processes
- pen
- patient's record

METHOD

1. Perform hand hygiene.
2. Assemble a peak flow meter with a disposable mouthpiece or an individual peak flow meter for the patient's use at home.

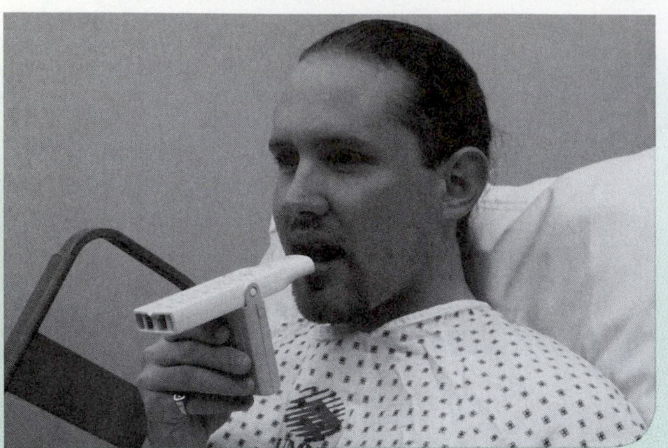

FIGURE 19-28 Peak expiratory flow rate (PEFR) measurement.

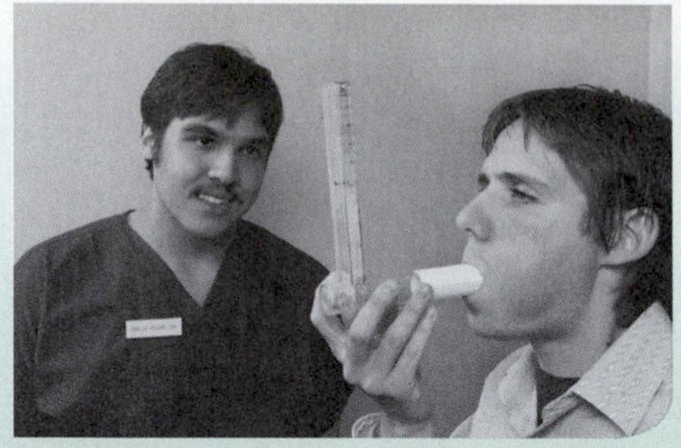

FIGURE 19-29 Ask the patient to exhale as hard and fast as possible.

3. Identify the patient and explain the procedure. Include an explanation of breathing processes and their importance to overall health. Demonstrate how the mouthpiece fits and explain what the numbers on the side mean. The peak flow meter should always be set at zero to start.
4. Have the patient place the mouthpiece in the mouth and form a tight seal with the lips. Explain that better results may be obtained if the patient stands during the test.
5. The patient should be instructed to stand, take as deep a breath as possible, place the mouthpiece in the mouth without biting down on it, and exhale as completely and forcibly as possible (Figures 19-28 and 19-29).
6. Instruct the patient to note the number on the machine where the sliding gauge stopped and to record the results. Reset the meter to zero. Repeat the test three times. This reading indicates the PEFR.
7. The patient should follow the physician's orders concerning when and how often each day to perform this procedure. The best result is documented on a chart or in the diary.
8. Demonstrate how to wash the mouthpiece with soap and water without submerging the peak flow meter.
9. Document the instruction.
10. Perform hand hygiene.

CHARTING EXAMPLE

05/16/XX 9:30 A.M. Pt. instructed on use of peak flow meter and recording of results. Returned demonstration easily, verbally confirmed understanding. Peak flow charting form given. Pt. to perform procedure 3× twice/day in A.M. and P.M. Results today: 380 LPM. .... R. Negri, CMA (AAMA)

NEBULIZER

A nebulizer may be used to treat breathing difficulties (Figure 19-30). If a handheld nebulizer is used, a small amount of aerosolized liquid medication is placed in a chamber. The patient puts the nebulizer in the mouth and breathes deeply for 8 to 10 minutes.

Radiology

The medical assistant may be responsible for scheduling radiologic procedures and providing the patient with written instructions regarding preparation and what will occur during the procedure (Procedure 19-9).

SAFETY

People are constantly exposed to low levels of natural radiation. The level of radiation a patient is exposed to during a radiologic procedure is typically less than the natural radiation.

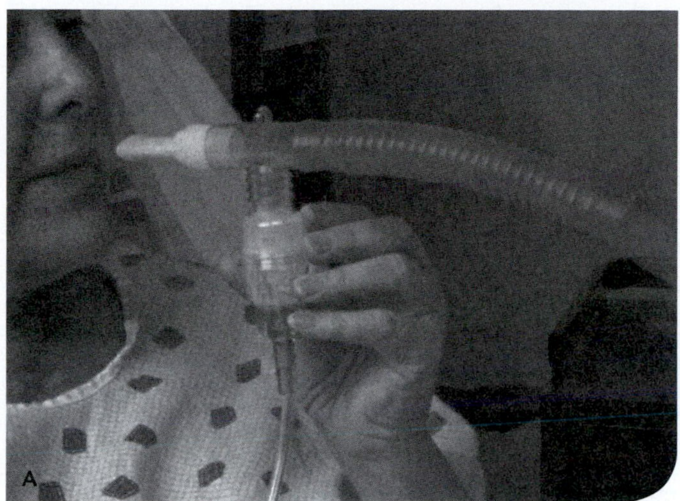

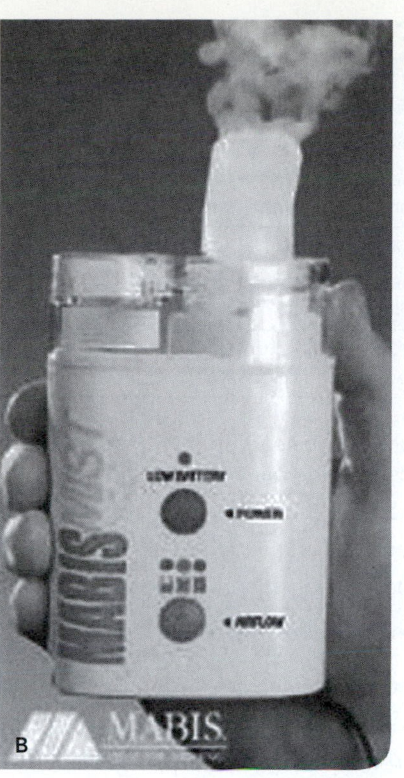

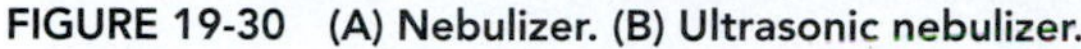
FIGURE 19-30 (A) Nebulizer. (B) Ultrasonic nebulizer.

procedure 19-9

PROCEDURE FOR A GENERAL X-RAY EXAMINATION

Objective: Assist with a radiologic procedure under the supervision of a physician or radiologic technologist.

EQUIPMENT AND SUPPLIES

- order for X-ray examination
- dosimeter badge
- appropriate X-ray equipment—X-ray film, holder, and machine
- processing equipment
- drape
- lead patient shield

METHOD

1. Check the X-ray examination order.
2. Check necessary X-ray equipment as needed.
3. Identify the patient.
4. Determine patient compliance with procedure preparation instructions.
5. Explain the procedure to the patient.
6. Instruct the patient to remove all clothing appropriate for the procedure.
7. Ask the patient to remove all jewelry and metal objects as needed for the procedure.
8. The following steps will most likely be performed by a radiologic technologist.
9. Position and drape the patient correctly.
10. Align the X-ray tube and cassette at the correct distance and set the controls.
11. Ask the patient to hold his or her breath as necessary.
12. Leave the room and stand behind the lead shield to take the X-ray(s).
13. Ask the patient to take a comfortable position while all X-rays are processed and reviewed.
14. Instruct the patient to dress if the X-rays are satisfactory.
15. Label the X-rays and place them in an envelope according to office procedures.
16. Document appropriately.

CHARTING EXAMPLE

05/05/XX 7:00 A.M. Chest X-ray done. · · · M. King CMA (AAMA)

RADIOLOGY POSITIONS

Position	Description
Anterioposterior	Also known as *AP* The X-ray beam is directed from front to back. The patient may be standing or supine. The patient's front will face the X-ray equipment, and the patient's back will be near the film plate.
Posterioanterior	Also known as *PA* The X-ray beam is directed from back to front. The patient will be standing upright. The patient's back will face the X-ray equipment, and the patient's front will be near the film plate.
Oblique	The patient is turned at an angle to the film plate so that the X-ray beam can be directed at areas that would be hidden on an AP, PA, or lateral X-ray.
Lateral	The X-ray beam is directed toward one side of the body. In the right lateral (RL) position, the patient's right side is near the film plate, and the left side is near the X-ray equipment. In a left lateral (LL) position, the patient's left side is near the film plate.
Axial	The X-ray tube is angled to direct a ray along the axis of the body or body part. *Cephalad angulation:* The X-ray beam is directed at an angle from the feet toward the head. *Caudal angulation:* The X-ray beam is directed from the head toward the feet.

In order to help protect personnel, anyone in the medical field working around radiation should be using lead aprons, shields, and gloves. Personnel also wear a film badge or dosimeter on the outside of their clothing. The dosimeter cumulatively records the level and intensity of radiologic exposure. See Boxes 19-1 and 19-2 for guidelines on maintaining personnel and patient safety.

Box 19-1 Guidelines for Maintaining Personnel Safety

- Wear a film badge on outer clothing at all times when exposed to any form of X-rays. Do not wear a patient gown or lead shield over the badge. These badges are submitted for routine—usually weekly—evaluation of the level of radiation exposure.
- Health care personnel should stay behind a lead shield in a lead-lined room when the X-ray equipment is in use.
- A sign or lighted display should be visible, and the X-ray room door should be closed when X-ray equipment is in use.
- Nonessential personnel should leave the X-ray room.
- All equipment should be inspected on a frequent, routine basis to check for radiation leakage.
- The patient should not be held or supported during radiologic procedures. There are devices that can be used to hold and position the patient.
- If it is necessary to remain in the room with the patient, the attendant should wear a protective lead apron and lead-lined rubber gloves. The attendant should face the patient, with the lead apron between the patient and the attendant.
- Periodic blood tests may be required by facilities to determine the presence of blood abnormalities from radiation exposure.

Box 19-2 Guidelines for Maintaining Patient Safety

- Ask if the patient has recently been exposed to X-rays from other examinations or through work-related activities.
- If the patient is female, inquire about the possibility of a pregnancy. If the patient is pregnant, report this to the physician before scheduling or assisting with any X-ray procedure. Due to liability concerns, it is important to obtain a release, or even a pregnancy test, prior to some X-ray procedures.
- Advise female patients of the potential radiation risk before X-rays are taken.
- Place a lead shield over the abdominal and reproductive organs of patients who are of childbearing age, or pregnant, or children.
- Patients must be carefully positioned to obtain an accurate image.

Note: Perform this procedure only if you have been fully instructed and trained and are authorized to do so in your state.

PATIENT PREPARATION

X-ray procedures requiring patient preparation are listed in table below.

X-RAY PROCEDURES REQUIRING SPECIAL PREPARATIONS

Procedure	Preparation
Angiogram	No breakfast before a morning examination; no lunch before an afternoon examination
Barium Enema (Lower GI)	Perform enemas until the bowel return is clear on the evening before the examination; a rectal suppository may be ordered in the morning or a cathartic such as 2 oz of castor oil or citrate of magnesia at 4 P.M. the day before the X-ray; clear liquids and gelatin for dinner, nothing by mouth (NPO) after midnight
Barium Meal (Upper GI)	NPO after midnight
Bronchogram	NPO
Cholecystogram (GB Series)	Light supper of nonfatty food such as fruits and vegetables without butter or oil the evening before the X-ray; gallbladder tablets (prescribed by the physician) are taken with water after supper; NPO except for water until X-ray is performed the following day
Computerized Tomography	Also known as *CT* NPO for 4 hours before the X-ray if a contrast medium is used
Intravenous Cholangiogram	NPO
Intravenous Pyelogram	Also known as *IVP* Three Dulcolax tablets or 2 oz castor oil at 4 P.M. the day before the X-ray; light supper; NPO after midnight
Myelogram	NPO
Retrograde Pyelogram	Enemas or laxatives on the evening before the X-ray; NPO for eight hours before the procedure
Ultrasound	May require a full bladder or laxatives, depending on the type of ultrasound

PATIENT INSTRUCTION

Boxes 19-3 and 19-4 give guidelines for GI series.

Box 19-3 Guidelines for Upper GI Series

- The patient should not eat or drink after midnight since the stomach must be empty for this procedure. Not even water should be swallowed while brushing the teeth. The physician may order that no morning medications be taken.
- The patient should be instructed not to smoke since this can stimulate gastric secretions.
- The patient will have to undress and put on a patient gown.
- A barium sulfate drink is prepared for the patient. This may be flavored, but it will still retain a slightly chalky taste.
- The patient will stand in front of the fluoroscopic screen while drinking the mixture. The radiologist will observe the progress of the barium as the patient drinks.
- The patient is then placed on an X-ray table that will tip into various positions for additional views. Permanent X-rays are taken while the patient is instructed to hold his or her breath.
- The procedure may last for several hours, during which time the barium will move out of the stomach and into the small intestine.
- The patient may resume normal eating after the examination but should be reminded to drink water to assist in flushing out the remaining barium, as it may cause constipation. The stool may remain chalky for a couple of days.

Box 19-4 Guidelines for Lower GI Series

The colon and rectum need to be free of stool for a clear view of the area on the X-ray.

Day Before the Examination

- The patient may be instructed to follow a low-residue diet for several days before the test. On the morning before the test, he or she will change to an all-liquid diet (such as water and clear soup) because NO solid foods may be taken until after the procedure.
- A cathartic, such as castor oil or citrate of magnesia, may be ordered to be taken at 4 P.M. the day before the procedure. Enemas must be performed until the return fluid is clear.

Day of the Examination

- The patient must undress and wear a gown for the procedure. Another cleansing enema may be given before the procedure.
- The patient lies on his or her side on the X-ray table while the technician administers an enema of barium sulfate. The patient is asked to retain or hold the enema within the rectal and colon area.
- The patient is then moved or tipped into different positions on the table while the radiologist observes the flow of barium on the fluoroscope. Radiographs (X-rays) are taken periodically during the procedure.
- The patient is asked to expel the barium into the toilet. Then a final X-ray is taken of the empty bowel.
- The patient may return to a regular diet after this procedure. Whitish stools may be present for one or two days after the procedure. The patient should be encouraged to drink water to flush out the remaining barium with stool.

19 APPLICATION

Directions: Select the best answer for each of the following questions. Check your answers in the Answer Key at the end of the book.

1. Each 5 × 5 mm square on the EKG paper is the equivalent of _________ second.
   a. 0.04
   b. 0.40
   c. 0.02
   d. 0.20
   e. 0.25

2. The color of the left leg limb lead is:
   a. White
   b. Black
   c. Green
   d. Red
   e. Blue

3. The contraction of the atria via firing of the SA node is reflected as the _______ in an EKG.
   a. P wave
   b. PR interval
   c. QRS complex
   d. ST segment
   e. T wave

4. A wandering baseline artifact is most likely due to:
   a. Tense muscles
   b. Poor sensor contact with skin
   c. Improper grounding
   d. Twisted coils
   e. Broken lead

5. The proper placement for a V2 EKG precordial lead is:
   a. Midway between the fourth and fifth intercostal spaces to the left of the sternum
   b. The fourth intercostal space to the right of the sternum
   c. Over the intercostal space at the axilla midpoint
   d. The fourth intercostal space to the right of the sternum
   e. Over the fifth intercostal space, in line with the left nipple

6. When screening an adult for near vision acuity, the patient should hold the Jaeger card at what distance?
   a. 20 feet
   b. 30 inches
   c. 14–16 inches
   d. 20 inches
   e. 30 feet

7. Which of the following PFTs measures the volume of air left in the lungs after forced expiration?
   a. Vital capacity
   b. Expiratory reserve volume
   c. Forced vital capacity
   d. Total volume
   e. Residual volume

8. The radiology position that allows the X-ray beam to be directed from back to front is:
   a. Anterioposterior
   b. Posterioanterior
   c. Oblique
   d. Lateral
   e. Axial

9. Which of the following procedures may require a full bladder or laxatives?
   a. Lower GI series
   b. Upper GI series
   c. Myelogram
   d. Ultrasound
   e. Cholecystogram

10. The most common color vision defect is the inability to distinguish between:
    a. Red and blue
    b. Orange and red
    c. Red and green
    d. Green and blue
    e. Yellow and orange

11. In order for the electrical activity to be transmitted to the EKG machine, how many leads are required?
    a. One
    b. Two
    c. Three
    d. Four
    e. Five

12. When performing a vision test using the Snellen chart, you should start with the __________ line and ask the patient to identify each line and proceed down the chart to the last line the patient can read without error.
    a. 20/70
    b. 20/60
    c. 20/50
    d. 20/40
    e. 20/30

13. When screening for color vision acuity, how far away should the card/page be?
    a. 20 feet
    b. 20 inches
    c. 14 feet
    d. 14–16 inches
    e. 30 inches

14. Which of the following PFTs measures the maximum volume of air left that can be exhaled after normal expiration?
    a. Vital capacity
    b. Expiratory reserve volume
    c. Forced vital capacity
    d. Total volume
    e. Residual volume

15. When the X-ray tube is angled to direct a ray along the axis of the body or body part, this is known as the ______________________ position.
    a. Anterioposterior
    b. Posterioanterior
    c. Oblique
    d. Lateral
    e. Axial

16. Which of the following X-ray procedures does not require the patient to be NPO?
    a. Upper GI series
    b. CT
    c. IVP
    d. Ultrasound
    e. Intravenous cholangiogram

17. Which of the following statements is not correct regarding an upper GI series?
    a. The patient should not eat or drink after midnight.
    b. The patient will have to undress and put on a gown.
    c. A barium sulfate drink is prepared for the patient.
    d. The patient may smoke up to one hour prior to the study.
    e. The procedure may last for several hours.

18. Which of the following statements is not correct regarding a lower GI series?
    a. Enemas must be used until the return fluid is clear.
    b. The patient may be instructed to follow a low-residue diet for several days before the test.
    c. The patient lies on his or her side on the X-ray table while the technician gives an enema of barium sulfate.
    d. The patient may return to a regular diet after this procedure.
    e. Whitish stools may be present for 7 to 10 days after the procedure.

19. A properly calibrated EKG machine will move the paper at a speed of _____ mm/second.
    a. 5
    b. 10
    c. 15
    d. 20
    e. 25

20 Laboratory Procedures

CONTENTS

LABORATORY TERMINOLOGY

Laboratory testing usually falls into one of two categories: qualitative and quantitative testing.

Qualitative Test	Performed to determine whether or not a substance is present Results reported out as either positive or negative *Example:* Qualitative human chorionic gonadotropin (hCG) test reported out as positive or negative and indicates whether or not the patient is pregnant
Quantitative Test	Performed to determine whether or not a substance is present and the amount of the substance Results reported out using numerical values *Example:* Quantitative hCG test reported out as a numerical value and indicates the level of pregnancy hormone present

HEMATOLOGY TERMINOLOGY

Blood Gas	Levels of oxygen and carbon dioxide in the blood Also determines the acidity (pH) of the blood, as well as oxygen saturation and bicarbonate levels
Formed Elements	Also known as *blood cells* Consists of red blood cells, white blood cells, and platelets
Hematology	Study of blood and blood-forming tissues
Hematopoiesis	Normal formation and development of blood cells
Phagocytes	Cells that destroy worn-out cells and bacteria
Phagocytosis	Process that allows neutrophils to surround, swallow, and digest bacteria
Plasma	Liquid portion of blood Contains fibrinogen, which converts to fibrin during the clotting process
Whole Blood	Plasma, red blood cells, white blood cells, and platelets

FORMED ELEMENTS

Red Blood Cells	Erythrocytes	Also known as *RBCs* Contain hemoglobin
	Hemoglobin	Carries oxygen away from the lungs to the tissues Carries carbon dioxide from the body back to the lungs to be exhaled
White Blood Cells	Leukocytes	Also known as *WBCs* Defend against infection Larger than red blood cells Three types of granular white blood cells: • Neutrophils • Eosinophils • Basophils Two types of nongranular white blood cells: • Lymphocytes • Monocytes
	Neutrophils	Also known as *polymorphonuclear leukocytes (PMNs)* and *segs* Granules in cytoplasm Most common WBC Combat infection by phagocytosis

(continued)

(Continued)

	Eosinophils	Granules in cytoplasm Respond to allergies and inflammation
	Basophils	Granules in cytoplasm Contain histamine and heparin
	Lymphocytes	*No granules* in cytoplasm Produce antibodies against bacteria, viruses, and pollens
	Monocytes	*No granules* in cytoplasm Largest cells in the blood Assist in phagocytosis
Platelets	Thrombocytes	Smallest cells in the blood Assist in clotting of blood

SEROLOGY/IMMUNOLOGY TERMINOLOGY

Agglutination	Antigen/antibody reaction that occurs when an antigen clumps together with an antibody
Antibody	Defends the body against infection and is developed as a result of a specific antigen
Antigen	Stimulates the body's immune response
Immune	Resistant to an infectious disease
Immune Response	Response of the immune system to an antigen; triggers antibody production
Immunology	Study of the body's reaction to antigens
Serology	Study of blood serum and antigen/antibody reactions
Serum	Plasma minus fibrinogen

Patient Preparation for Laboratory Testing

The physician's order(s) for laboratory testing is the first step in the testing process. As the medical assistant, you will need to know whether the physician wants the results immediately (stat) or whether the normal reporting time frame is acceptable.

You will also need to know whether any type of preparation is required by the patient before the specimen is collected. For example, if the physician is ordering a fasting lipid profile, the patient will need to be NPO for 8 to 12 hours before the specimen is collected. It may be necessary to schedule the test for another day if the patient has had something to eat or drink recently.

Methods of Specimen Collection (Box 20-1)

BLOOD

In addition to gloves, equipment required for blood collection may include the items in the following table.

Butterfly Needle	Consists of a very small needle attached to tubing. A vacuum tube or syringe may be attached to the tubing. May be used for venipuncture on small or fragile veins
Evacuation Tube System	Consists of a plastic holder, an attachable needle, and vacuum tubes The needle has two pointed ends. One end has a retractable sheath. This is the end that is screwed into the plastic holder. When the vacuum tube is pushed into the plastic holder, the sheath covering is pushed back and the needle punctures the tube, allowing blood to flow into the tube. This is the fastest and most efficient system for performing venipuncture.
Micropipette	Very small calibrated glass tubes used to collect small volumes of blood samples
Sharps Container	Puncture-proof, rigid, locked container labeled with an international biohazard sticker. Any disposable sharps, such as needles and scalpels, must be placed in a sharps container. When the container is two-thirds to three-quarters full, it should be closed, replaced, and disposed of properly.
Sterile Lancet	Used for capillary punctures and when only a small amount of blood is required for testing, such as fingerstick glucose, and hematocrits. The lancet consists of a very small double-sided/edged scalpel and is typically loaded into an automatic spring-loading mechanism.
Needle and Syringe	This method for performing venipuncture may be used if veins are fragile or there is concern that the vein may collapse if the vacuum tube method is used. The same preparation steps used for the evaculation tube method are followed; however, a needle of appropriate gauge is attached to a syringe, and the blood is extracted by slowly pulling back on the plunger as the syringe fills. The collected blood is then transferred to the appropriate vacuum tube.
Tourniquet	Soft, flat vinyl/rubber tubing, usually 1 to 1½ inches wide and 12 to 16 inches long A blood pressure cuff may also be used as a tourniquet. Used to make the veins more prominent and easier to locate for venipuncture
Vacuum Tube	Also known as an *evacuated tube* Glass vacuum tubes with different additives and correlated colored rubber tops are used to collect blood specimens. When the needle punctures the rubber top, the vacuum helps draw the blood into the tube.

Box 20-1 Guidelines for Specimen Collection

The basic rules for specimen collection are:

1. Confirm the identity of the patient by asking the patient to state his or her name and spell it, if necessary.
2. Screen the patient to determine if pretest preparation was followed.
3. Collect a specimen prior to beginning antibiotic treatment.
4. Collect a sufficient quantity of material for testing.
5. Use only the appropriate collection technique by observing proper cleaning and aseptic procedures to control contamination.
6. Use only sterile containers.
7. Select the proper containers for collection that comply with the reference laboratory's or outside laboratory's requirements.
8. Ensure that the collection container is tightly closed and appropriately sealed to avoid leakage and contamination of the specimen and any surface with which the container may come in contact.
9. Label the specimen accurately at the time of collection with the following information:
   a. Patient's full name
   b. Date
   c. Time of collection
   d. Type of specimen
   e. Antibiotic treatment in use, if any
   f. Your initials
10. Fill out the requisition form for the reference laboratory and double-check that the information matches the label.
11. Deliver the specimen promptly to the laboratory and document it. Otherwise, maintain proper storage until the specimen can be picked up or transported appropriately.

Note: Cerebrospinal fluid always requires immediate delivery.

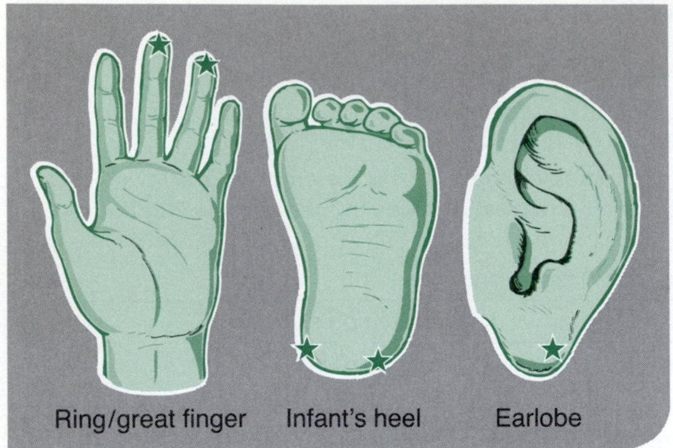

FIGURE 20-1 Capillary puncture sites.

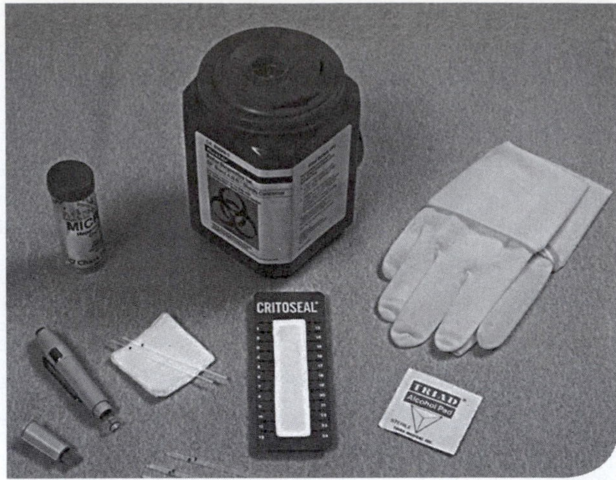

FIGURE 20-2 Capillary puncture equipment.

As a result of the Needlestick Safety and Prevention Act, OSHA standards have become more strict and require employers to solicit employees' input for identifying, evaluating, and implementing safer medical devices, including needles. Offices must make safe needle devices available for employees to use. These devices reduce the possibility of needlestick injuries.

Capillary Puncture

Capillaries are microscopic blood vessels and can easily be punctured when small amounts of blood are required for testing (Figures 20-1 and 20-2). The most common site used is the finger and is known as a *fingerstick* (Figure 20-3). See Procedure 20-1.

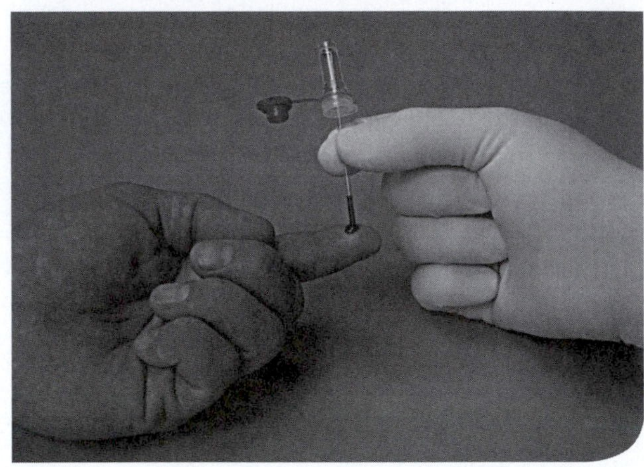

FIGURE 20-3 A fingerstick is useful for obtaining small amounts of blood.

procedure 20-1

PERFORMING A CAPILLARY PUNCTURE (MANUAL)

Objective: Perform a capillary stick using a lancet or spring-loaded lancet following correct aseptic technique and obtain an adequate sample.

EQUIPMENT AND SUPPLIES

- biohazard sharps container
- gloves
- alcohol sponge
- 2 × 2 gauze square or cotton balls
- lancet or spring-loaded lancet
- capillary tubes
- sealing clay
- ammonia ampules
- bandage
- lab coat

Note: Lancets come in a variety of sizes and needle gauges for specific purposes. The majority of capillary punctures performed on adults, requiring only a few drops of blood, can be performed with needle gauges 21G, 25G, or 28G. Pediatric collections and microcollections will require specific lancets and blades.

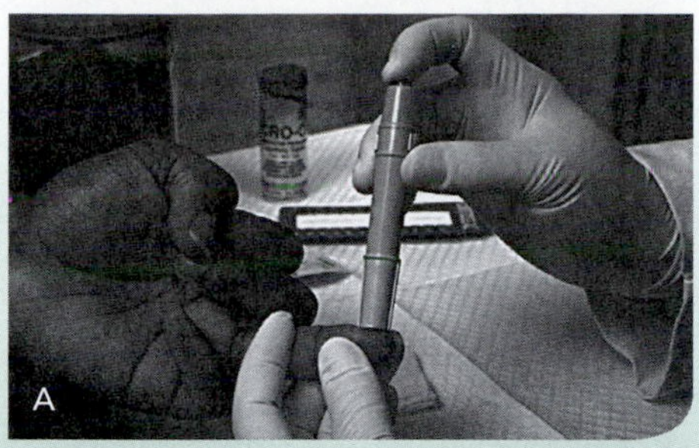

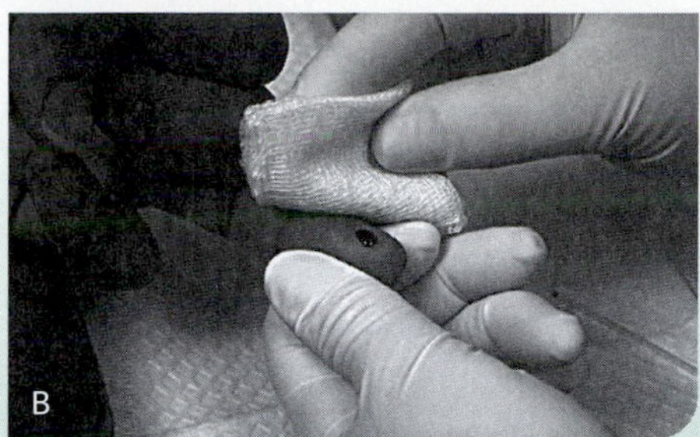

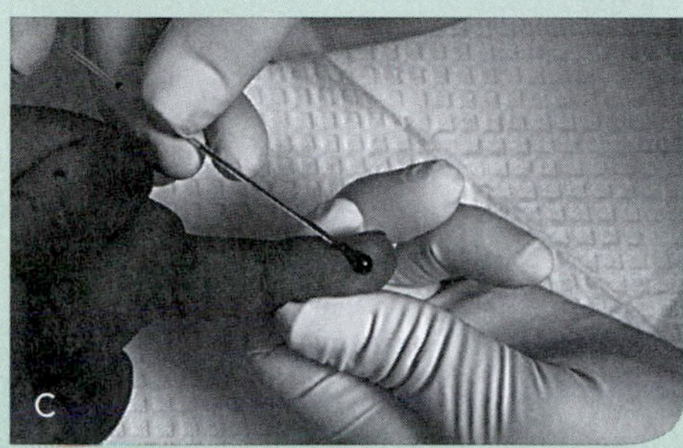

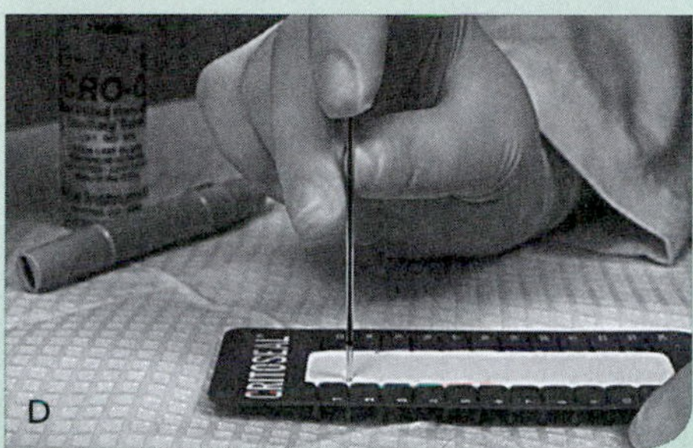

FIGURE 20-4 (A–D) Capillary puncture procedure.

Note: Follow standard precautions and safety guidelines. Take care to avoid splashing or spilling blood. Wipe up all spills using the guidelines established by OSHA.

METHOD

1. Perform hand hygiene.
2. Assemble equipment.
3. Identify the patient and explain the procedure. Have the patient sit or lie down.
4. Apply gloves.
5. Select either the ring or great finger on the nondominant hand. Wipe the site with an alcohol sponge. Let the alcohol evaporate.
6. Remove the plastic protective tip to expose the lancet.
7. Grasp the patient's hand and gently squeeze the finger 1 inch below the chosen puncture site.
8. Puncture the site using a quick, jabbing motion across the fingerprints to obtain a full round drop of blood (Figure 20-4A). Do not puncture the direct center of the finger pad since the skin is generally tougher there. Immediately discard the lancet in a sharps container. (A spring-loaded lancet may also be used.)
9. Wipe away the first drop of blood with a gauze square or cotton ball (Figure 20-4B).
10. Obtain the sample using a microhematocrit capillary tube (Figure 20-4C). The finger may be gently massaged to increase blood flow. Seal one end of the capillary tube in a clay sealer (Figure 20-4D).
11. Apply clean gauze over the site and ask the patient to apply firm, continuous pressure until the bleeding stops.
12. Assess the patient and the site. Apply a bandage, if needed. Ask the patient if he or she is dizzy or lightheaded.
13. Remove gloves and perform hand hygiene.
14. Record the procedure in the patient's medical record.

CHARTING EXAMPLE

2/28/XX 1:30 P.M. Performed capillary puncture on left ring finger; no complications. . . . . M. Garcia, RMA (AMT)

Venipuncture

The most common venipuncture site is the antecubital space, which is the triangular area just below the bend of the elbow. The median cephalic is the vein of choice; however, depending on the patient's condition, other veins may be used (Figure 20-5). See Figure 20-6 for a venipuncture equipment demonstration and Procedure 20-2 for the procedure for performing venipuncture using the vacutainer method.

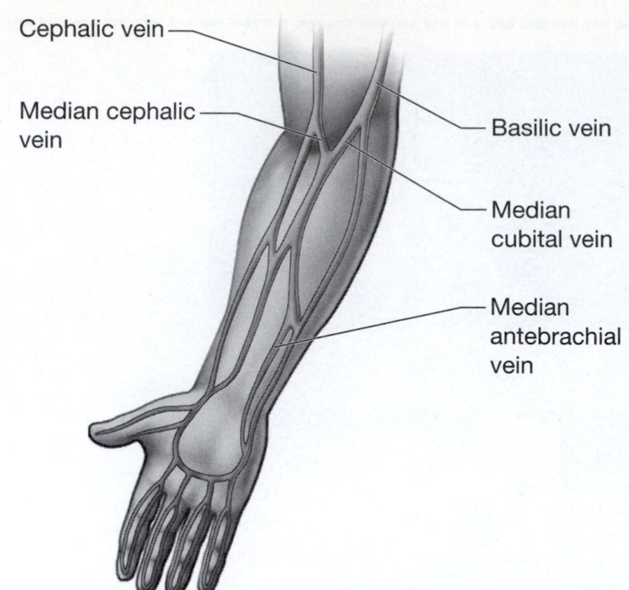

FIGURE 20-5 Anatomy of an arm for venipuncture.

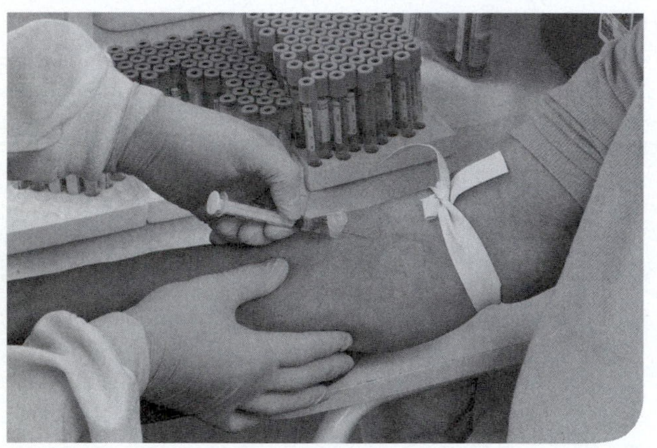

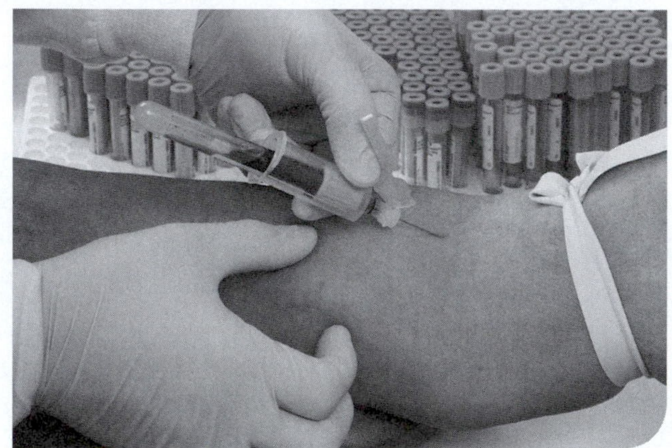

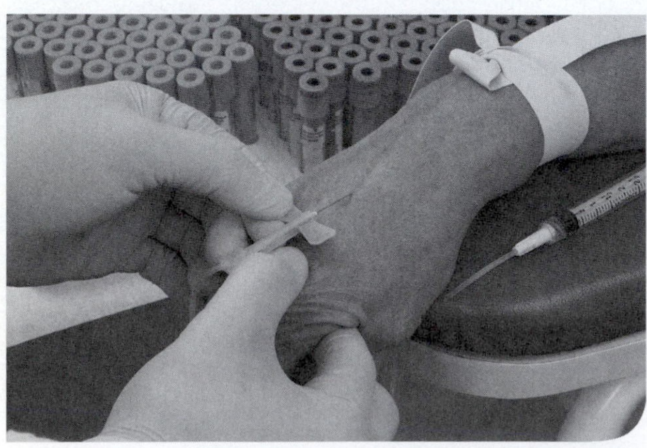

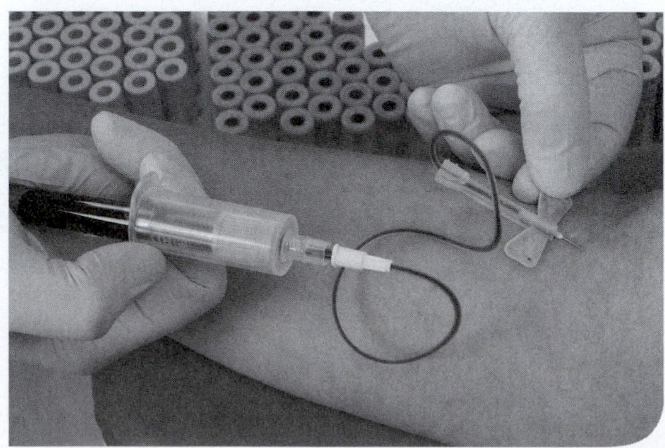

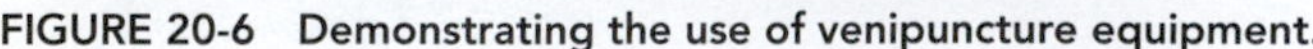

FIGURE 20-6 Demonstrating the use of venipuncture equipment.

procedure

20-2

PERFORMING VENIPUNCTURE USING THE VACUTAINER METHOD

Objective: Perform venipuncture by correctly assembling, locating, and entering a vein and withdrawing a blood sample.

EQUIPMENT AND SUPPLIES

- biohazard sharps container
- Vacutainer tubes
- multisample needle
- two or three 2-inch gauze squares
- alcohol pads
- examination gloves
- Vacutainer sleeve
- tourniquet
- bandage
- cotton balls
- adhesive
- ink pen
- lab coat
- patient record
- ammonia ampules

Note: Follow standard precautions and safety guidelines when working with blood samples. Take care to avoid splashing or spilling blood. Wipe up all spills using the guidelines established by OSHA.

METHOD

1. Perform hand hygiene.
2. Assemble equipment (Figure 20-7A).
3. Identify the patient and explain the procedure. Have the patient either sit or lie down.
4. Apply gloves.
5. Screw the Vacutainer needle into the plastic sleeve (Figure 20-7B). Insert the tube into the other end of the sleeve. The top of the colored stopper should reach the thin guide line on the sleeve. Do not press the tube. If the tube exceeds the line, discard the tube; it may not have a vacuum.
6. Apply the tourniquet about 2 inches above the antecubital space (Figure 20-7C). Place the middle of the tourniquet on the posterior (elbow) side of the arm. Crisscross the ends. While holding one end stable, tuck in the other end. This creates a tie that can be quickly released with one hand. In addition, the tourniquet should apply enough tension to engorge the vein with blood.
7. The arm should be in an extended position, with the palm facing up. Palpate the vein with your fingertips (Figure 20-7D). If a vein cannot be felt in one arm, try the other.
8. Wipe the site with an alcohol pad in a circular pattern, beginning at the insertion site (Figure 20-7E). Let the alcohol evaporate. Cleanse your gloved finger with alcohol in case you need to repalpate after the site is cleansed.
9. Anchor the vein by placing the thumb of the nondominant hand 2 inches below the insertion site and pulling the skin toward the hand.
10. While holding on to the tube's sleeve with your dominant hand, insert the needle smoothly and rapidly at a 15- to 20-degree angle with the bevel up (Figure 20-7F). The

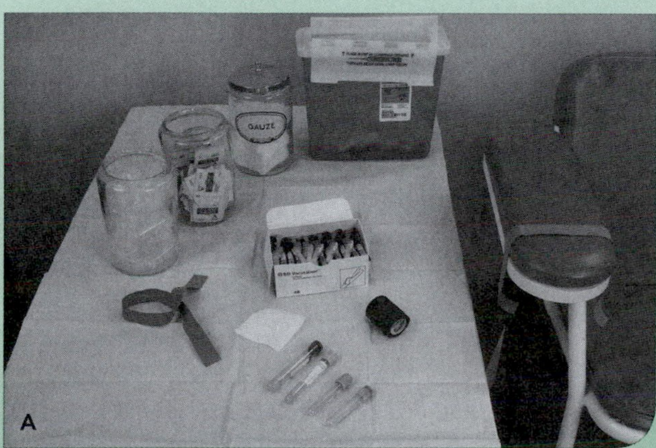

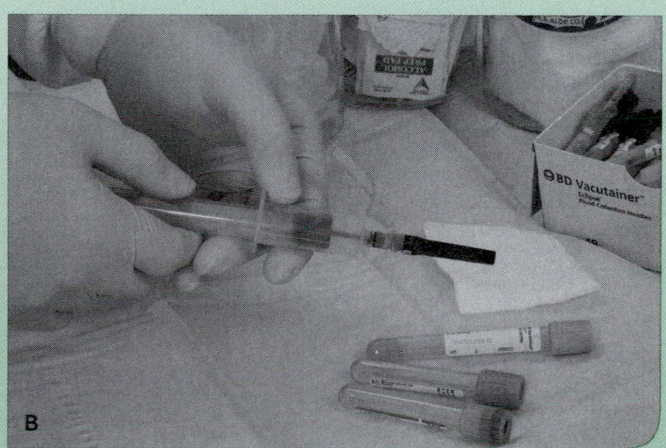

FIGURE 20-7 (A–B) Venipuncture procedure.

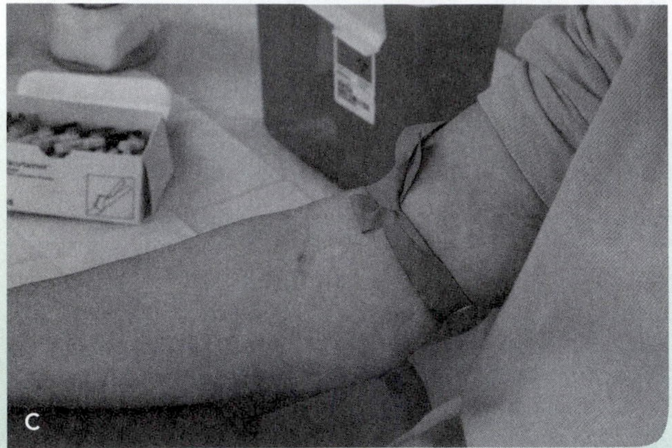

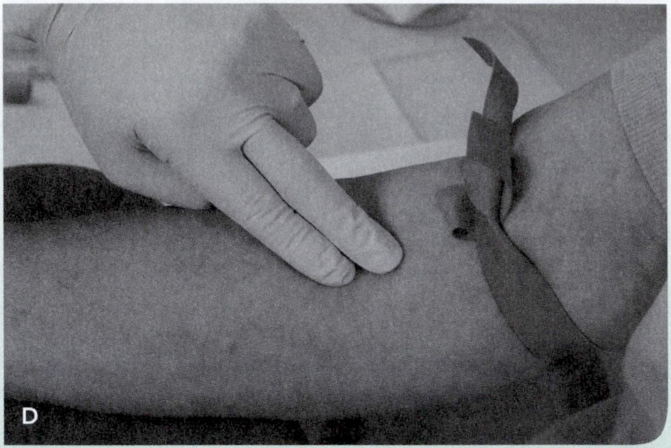

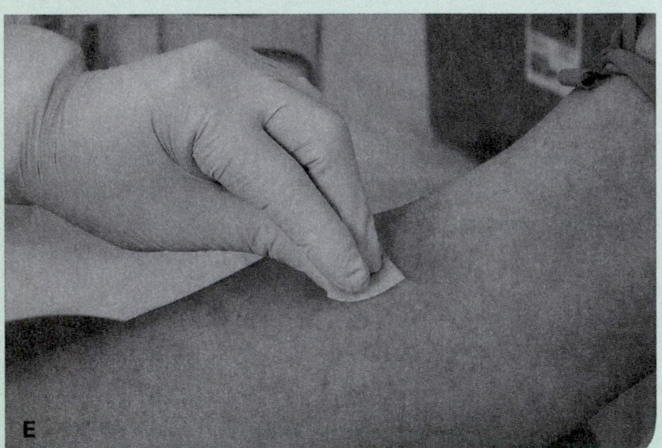

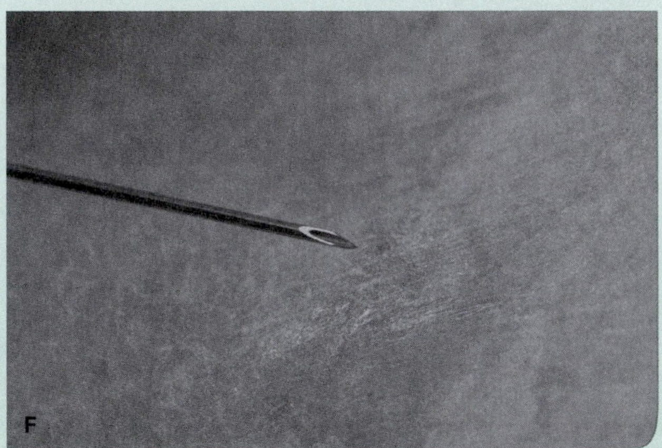

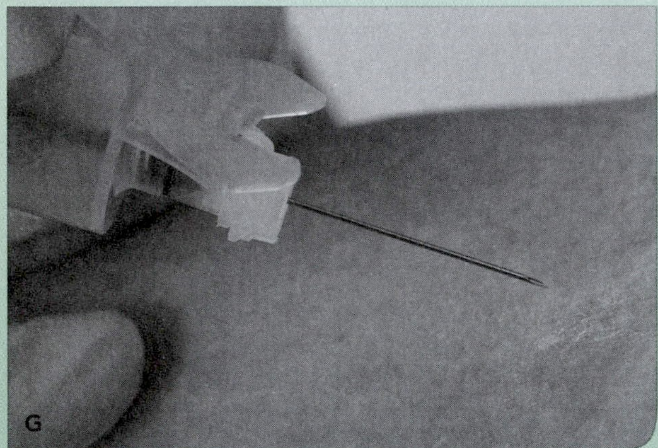

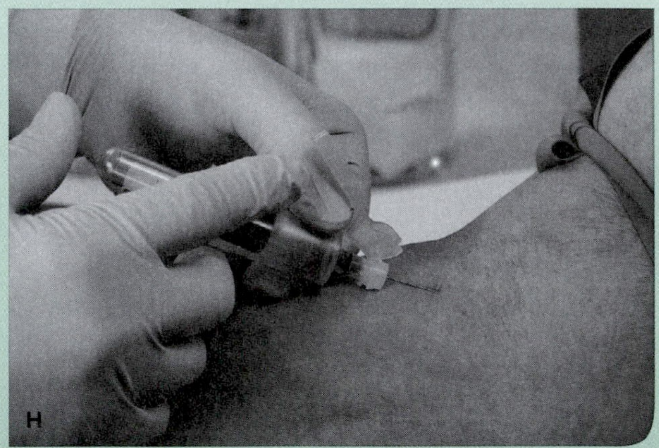

FIGURE 20-7 (C–H) (Continued)

needle needs to be inserted only just past the bevel. If it is inserted too far, it will puncture both vein walls. Also, keep the needle in line with the vein. The dominant hand is now considered *fixed*, meaning that you may not remove it from the tube sleeve until the procedure is over. All other movements must be done with the nondominant hand.

11. While the dominant hand is stabilizing the sleeve, use the nondominant hand to push the tube into the sleeve (Figure 20-7G). Use your thumb to push the tube, and hold the sleeve with the index and middle fingers on the flange (Figure 20-7H).
12. Allow the tube to fill. The vacuum will automatically fill the tube to the manufacturer's recommended level for the specific tube used. You should familiarize yourself with the adequate fill level of the individual tubes. Blood collection tubes may contain a weak vacuum due to processing errors, and you will need to redraw those specimens.

13. Remove the tube very carefully without moving the needle and apply a second tube if needed (Figure 20-7I). Gently roll the tube five or six times after removing it from the sleeve to allow the blood to mix with the additive. If both a red and a purple tube are needed, collect blood in the red tube that contains no additive first.
14. Release the tourniquet once the last tube has been inserted into the adaptor. Fill the last tube, remove it, swiftly remove the needle, and cover the site with a clean gauze pad (Figure 20-7J). Be careful not to push on the needle when covering the puncture site, since that may cause the needle to scratch the patient's arm. Gently invert the collection tube.
15. Immediately have the patient apply firm, continuous pressure using a cotton ball or gauze square.
16. Properly dispose of the needle in the biohazard container (Figures 20-7K–M).
17. Gently invert all tubes collected 8 to 10 times in a figure-eight pattern.
18. Assess the patient. Check the venipuncture site for bleeding; then apply some cotton and a strip of adhesive

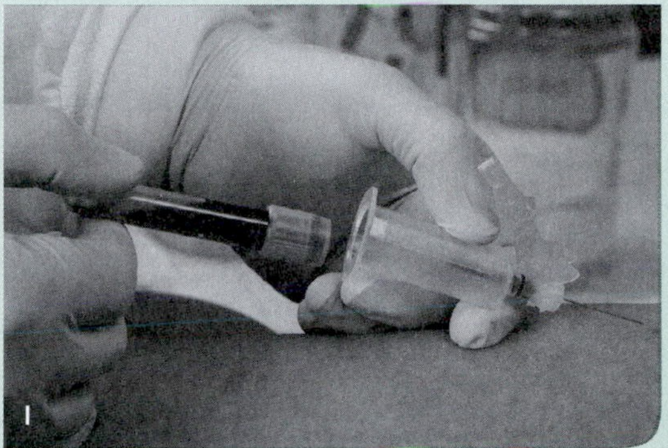

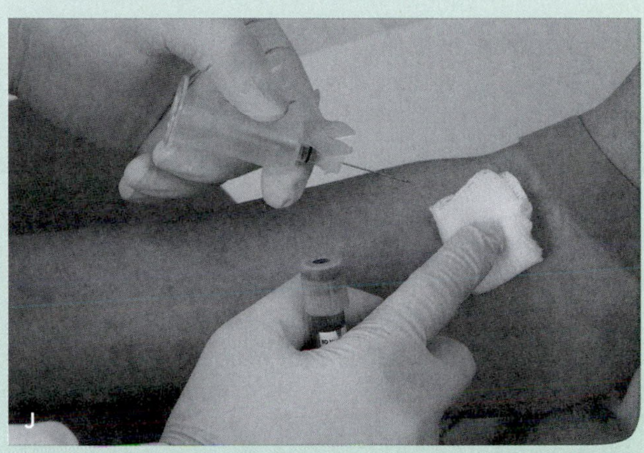

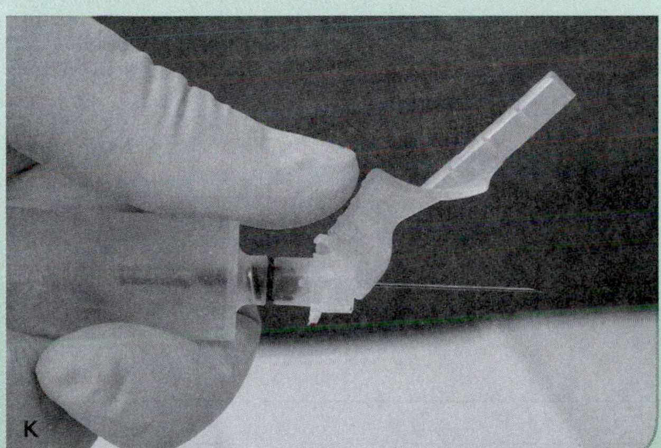

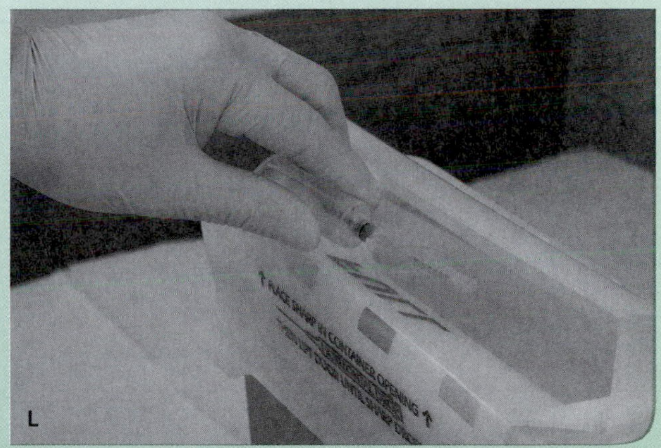

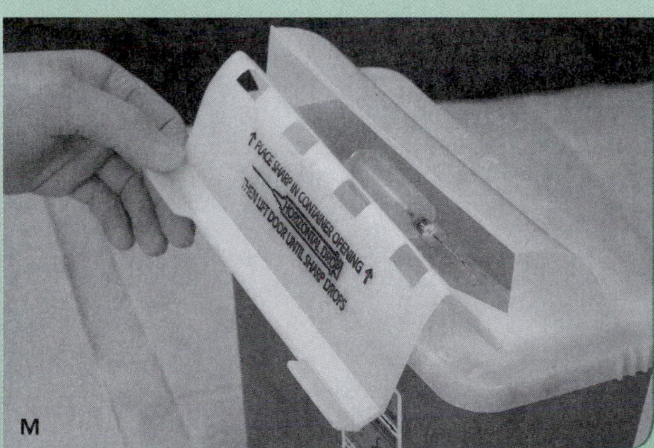

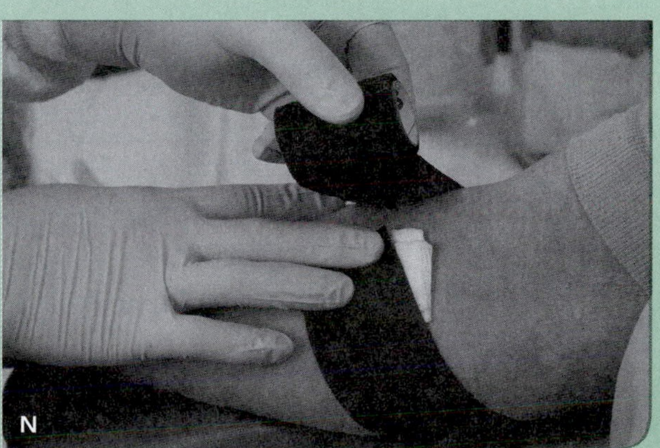

FIGURE 20-7 (I–N) (Continued)

or a bandage (Figure 20-7N). Ask if the patient is dizzy or lightheaded.

19. Label the tubes with the patient's name, date, time, ID number, specimen type, tests to be done, and the phlebotomist's initials. Fill out the laboratory requisition sheet (Figure 20-7O).
20. Remove gloves. Perform hand hygiene.
21. Record the procedure on the patient's medical record.

CHARTING EXAMPLE

2/28/XX 1.00 P.M. Withdrew 10 mL of blood from left arm; no complications. Sent blood to in-office lab for CBC. .... M. Garcia, RMA (AMT)

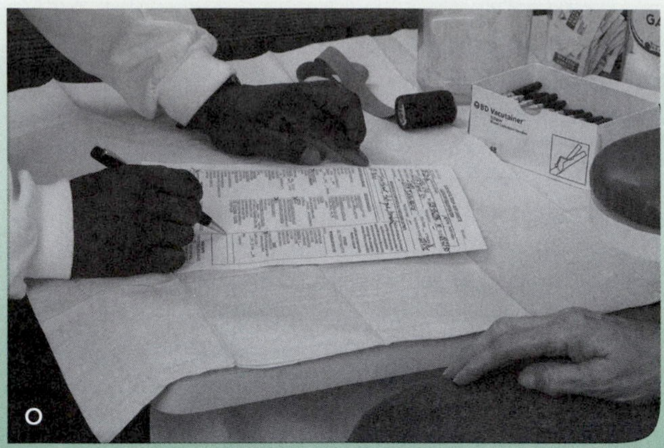

FIGURE 20-7 (O) (Continued)

Order of Draw

CLIA has established a recommended order of draw when using the vacuum tube method for venipuncture.

Vacuum tubes are available in the following sizes:

- 5 mL
- 7 mL
- 10 mL
- 15 mL

The minimum amount of blood required will depend on the test ordered. Check the laboratory testing manual to verify what is required.

ORDER OF BLOOD DRAW

Order of Draw	Vacutainer Color	Additive and Function	Laboratory Use
1	Yellow	Sodium polyanetholsulfonate (SPS) prevents clotting and stabilizes bacterial growth.	Cultures on blood or body fluid
2	Light blue	Sodium citrate removes calcium to prevent clotting.	Coagulation tests such as PT/INR and PTT
3	Red	None	Serum testing, serology, blood bank, blood chemistry
4	Red marbled	Silica is present to enhance clotting.	Serum testing
5	Green	Standard heparin (sodium/lithium/ammonium) prevents thrombin formation.	Blood chemistry such as whole blood tests and plasma testing
6	Light green	Lithium heparin and gel aid in plasma separation.	Plasma determination in chemistry tests
7	Lavender	Ethylenediaminetetraacetic acid (EDTA) removes calcium to prevent clotting.	Hematology such as CBC or glycosylated hemoglobin
8	Pink, white, or royal blue	Sodium heparin (may also be referred to as sodium EDTA) prevents thrombin formation and prevents clotting.	Chemistry for trace elements
9	Gray	Potassium oxalate and sodium fluoride to inhibit glycolysis (the chemical reaction of converting glucose into pyruvate) and remove calcium to prevent clotting.	Glucose tolerance tests and alcohol levels, chemistry tests
10	Dark blue (FDP)	Tube contains fibrin degradation product.	Detects if the patient has had a recent breakdown of clots, which may indicate several conditions such as blood clots in the legs (DVT [deep vein thrombosis], hepatic vein obstruction, PE [pulmonary embolus] or stroke

Source: Clinical Laboratory and Standards Institute, January 2004. Retrieved from http://www.clsi.org. Adapted with permission.

Blood Cultures

If the physician has ordered a blood culture, you need to use either a blood culture media set or a yellow-top vacuum tube. It is best if the blood can be drawn during febrile episodes, and two samples should be drawn. One specimen should be drawn from the right arm and the other from the left. Once drawn, the specimens should be delivered to the lab within two hours.

URINE (PROCEDURE 20-3)

procedure 20-3

COLLECTING A CLEAN-CATCH MIDSTREAM URINE SPECIMEN

Objective: Instruct both male and female patients to correctly obtain a contaminant-free, clean-catch midstream urine specimen.

EQUIPMENT AND SUPPLIES

- sterile midstream urine container
- antiseptic towelettes
- written patient instructions

METHOD

1. Perform hand hygiene.
2. Assemble equipment.
3. Identify and greet the patient.

Explain the procedure to a *male* patient as follows:

- Perform hand hygiene.
- Expose the penis. Pull the foreskin back if uncircumcised (and hold it back until the specimen has been collected).
- Cleanse each side of the urethral opening from top to bottom, using a separate antiseptic wipe, wiping in one direction only (Figure 20-8A). Cleanse across the top of the urethral opening with a third antiseptic, wiping in one direction only. Be certain to avoid having any body part touch the specimen container.
- Void a small amount of urine into the toilet (Figure 20-8B). Then void into the container, taking care not to touch the insides of the container (Figure 20-8C). Remove the container.
- Continue voiding the remainder of the urine into the toilet.
- Recap the container immediately, taking care not to contaminate the inside of the lid.
- Deliver the specimen as instructed.

Explain the procedure to a *female* patient as follows:

- Perform hand hygiene and remove underwear.
- Expose the urinary meatus by pulling apart the labia and holding the area open with the nondominant hand.
- Use the dominant hand to cleanse around one side of the urinary meatus from front to back with one antiseptic wipe (Figure 20-9A). Use the second wipe to cleanse the other side in the same manner. Using a third wipe, cleanse across the opening of the meatus itself. Continue holding the labia apart until the procedure is complete.
- Begin voiding into the toilet (Figure 20-9B). Place the container in position and void into it without touching the inside with your fingers (Figure 20-9C).
- Remove the container and continue voiding into the toilet.
- Wipe in the usual manner and cover the container with the lid, avoiding contaminating the inside of the lid.
- Deliver the specimen as instructed.

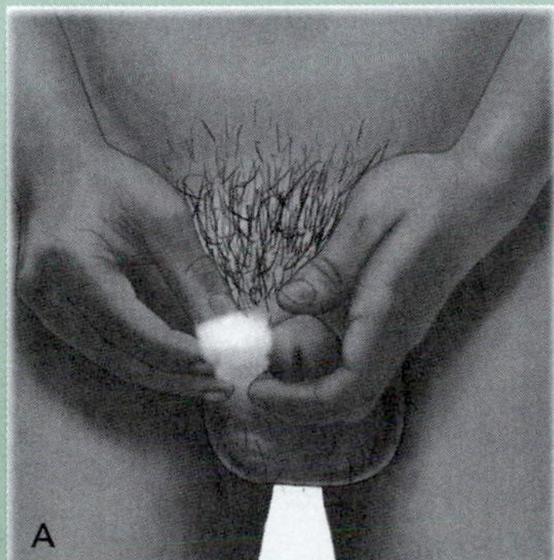

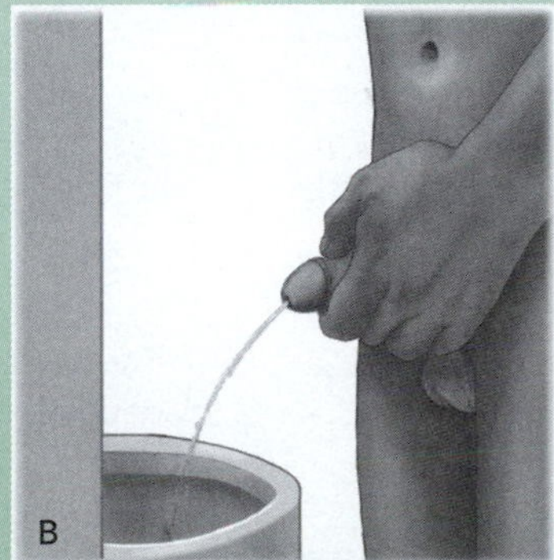

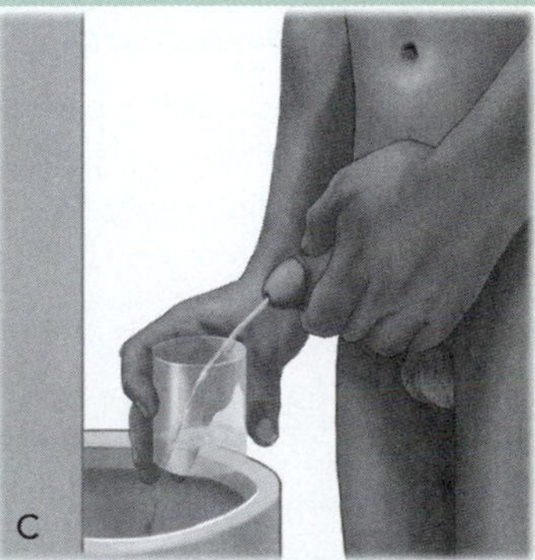

FIGURE 20-8 (A) The patient is instructed to cleanse the head of the penis in preparation for a clean-catch midstream urine collection. (B) Begin urinating into the toilet. (C) Continue urinating into the sterile cup provided for the clean-catch urine specimen.

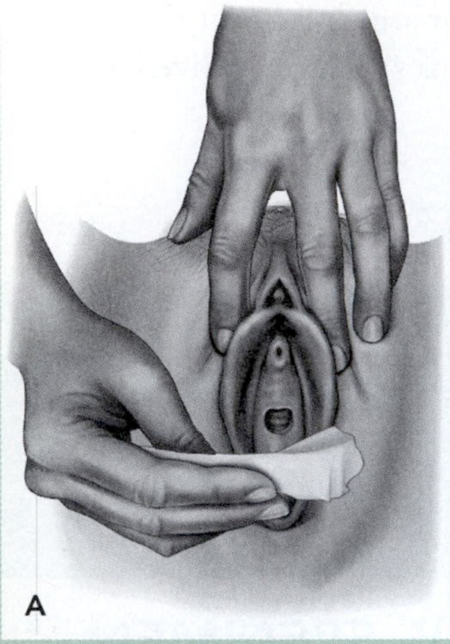

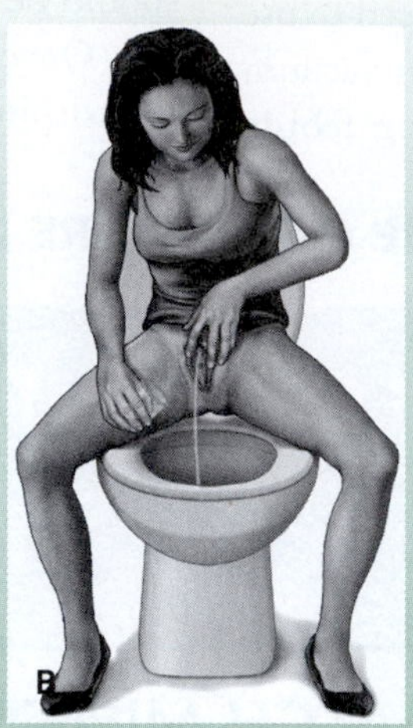

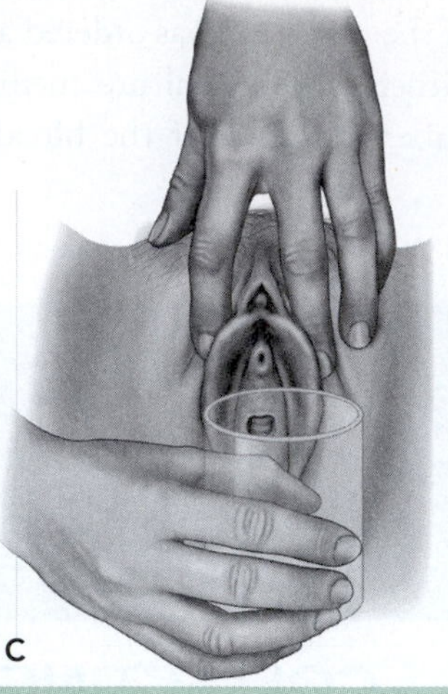

FIGURE 20-9 (A) Instruct the patient to spread the labia and expose the urinary meatus; then use towelettes to clean first one side from front to back and then do the same on the other side. (B) Begin urinating into the toilet. (C) Urinate into the sterile clean-catch container.

4. Label the specimen container.
5. Perform hand hygiene.
6. Document the chart appropriately.

CHARTING EXAMPLE

4/23/XX Clean-catch midstream urine specimen collected from patient at 11:00 A.M. Sent to lab for C&S. .... M. King, CMA (AAMA)

THROAT (PROCEDURE 20-4)

procedure 20-4

OBTAINING A THROAT CULTURE

Objective: Collect a throat or nasopharyngeal culture without contaminating the specimen.

EQUIPMENT AND SUPPLIES

- Culturette system
- laboratory requisition
- tongue depressor
- gloves
- biohazard waste container

Note: Follow standard precautions and safety guidelines when working with body fluid samples. Take care to avoid splashing or spilling body fluids. Wipe up all spills using the guidelines established by OSHA.

METHOD

1. Assemble equipment and the Culturette system.
2. Identify the patient and explain the procedure.
3. Perform hand hygiene and apply gloves.

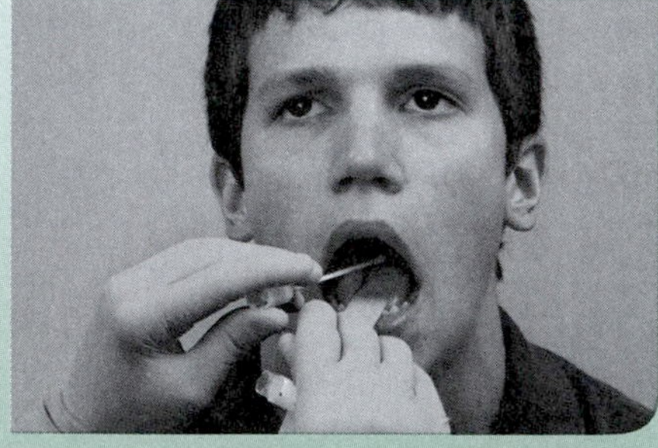

FIGURE 20-10 Swab the posterior pharynx between the tonsils.

4. Position the patient facing a light source, and have the patient open his or her mouth as wide as possible (Figure 20-10). The gag reflex may be diminished if the patient says "Aaaah."

5. Remove the sterile swab from the Culturette.
6. Depress the tongue, insert the swab, and roll it firmly across the back of the patient's throat or nasopharyngeal area where it is infected. Be careful not to contaminate the swab on the teeth, lips, tongue, or inside of the cheeks. Avoid touching the uvula to prevent gagging.
7. Insert the swab into a plastic vial. Crush the internal vial of transport medium, making sure that the swab is saturated.
8. Place the transport medium in a labeled mailing or transporting envelope and staple it shut if necessary. If the sample is being evaluated in the physician's office laboratory (POL), immediately inoculate the culture plate, and apply a bacitracin disk according to office procedure.
9. Remove and dispose of gloves.
10. Perform hand hygiene.
11. Document the procedure in the patient's record.

CHARTING EXAMPLE

2/14/XX 9:00 A.M. Throat culture obtained. Specimen labeled and sent to outside lab. (Specify the name of the lab.) .... M. King, CMA (AAMA)

STOOL (PROCEDURE 20-5)

procedure
20-5

OBTAINING A STOOL SPECIMEN FOR CULTURE AND SENSITIVITY

Objective: Instruct a patient how to collect a stool sample for culture and sensitivity in a sterile container using correct infection control procedures.

EQUIPMENT AND SUPPLIES

- sterile stool collection container
- bedpan or container for collection of stool
- tongue depressors
- sterile applicator sticks
- transportation/mailing container
- labels
- laboratory request form
- gloves
- biohazard waste container

Note: Follow standard precautions and safety guidelines when working with body fluid samples. Take care to avoid splashing or spilling body fluids. Wipe up all spills using the guidelines established by OSHA.

METHOD

1. Perform hand hygiene.
2. Assemble equipment.
3. Identify the patient and explain the procedure, giving written instructions as well. Do not overuse medical terminology, which might cause the patient to misunderstand your instructions.
4. Instruct the patient to defecate in a container or bedpan. If the patient is collecting a specimen at home, give the patient a sterile container and written instructions.
5. Using a sterile tongue depressor or applicator stick, take a small amount of stool from different parts of the specimen and place them in a container, making sure that no other contaminants are included (toilet paper, toilet water, urine, etc.).

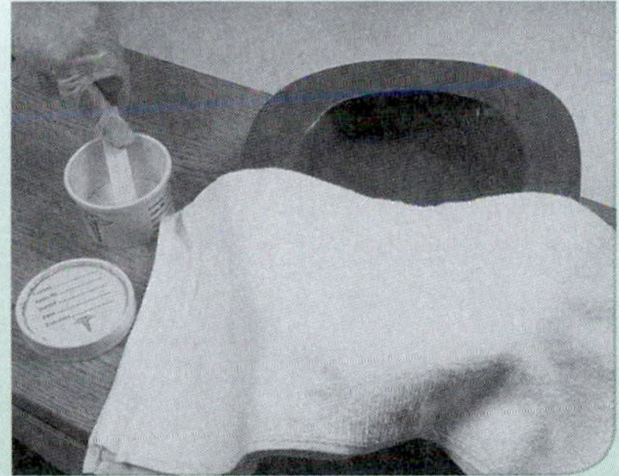

FIGURE 20-11 Equipment for collecting a stool specimen.

6. If the patient provides the stool specimen in a bedpan or other container, proceed using gloves as described above (Figure 20-11).
7. Fill out the lab request form and wrap it around the container, securing it with a rubber band.
8. Place the container in a proper mailing container.
9. Deliver or mail the specimen to the outside laboratory facility.

CHARTING EXAMPLE

2/14/XX 9:00 A.M. Stool specimen obtained C&S. Specimen labeled and sent to outside lab. (Specify the name of the lab.) .... M. King, CMA (AAMA)

procedure 20-6

OBTAINING A SPUTUM SPECIMEN FOR CULTURE

Objective: Collect a sputum specimen without contaminating it.

EQUIPMENT AND SUPPLIES

- sterile labeled sputum container with lid
- lab requisition form
- gloves
- biohazard waste container

Note: Follow standard precautions and safety guidelines when working with body fluid samples. Take care to avoid splashing or spilling body fluids. Wipe up all spills using the guidelines established by OSHA.

METHOD

1. Identify the patient.
2. Explain the procedure and give written instructions that the patient can take home, if necessary. Explain that he or she should breathe in and out deeply two to four times and perform a few low, deep coughs to raise sputum. This avoids getting only saliva. The first morning specimen, collected before eating or drinking, usually provides the best sample. The patient should do the following:
   a. Cough deeply, expel fluid into the center of the container, and close the lid immediately (Figures 20-12A, B).
   b. Make sure that no other fluids, such as tears, nasal mucus, or saliva, find their way into the cup.
   c. Fit the lid securely, then write the time and date the specimen was obtained.
   d. Bring the specimen to the physician's office as soon as possible, or place it in a refrigerator for no longer than two hours.
3. Perform hand hygiene and apply gloves.
4. Label the transport envelope with information, staple it shut, and transport the sample immediately.
5. Remove and dispose of gloves and perform hand hygiene.
6. Document the procedure in the patient's record.

CHARTING EXAMPLE

2/14/XX 10:30 A.M. Sputum specimen collected. Labeled and sent to outside lab. [Specify the name of the lab.] .... M. King, CMA (AAMA)

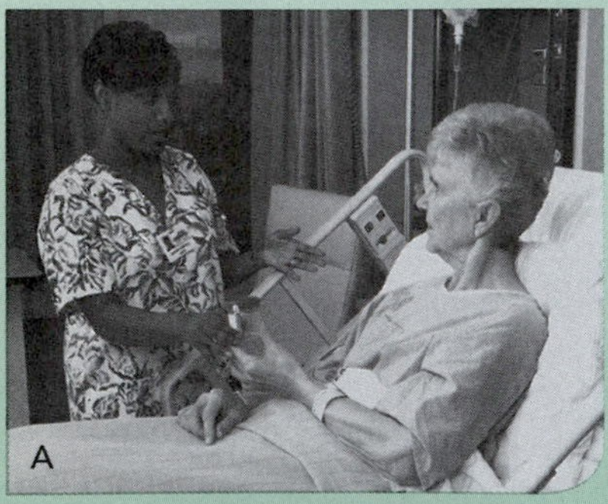

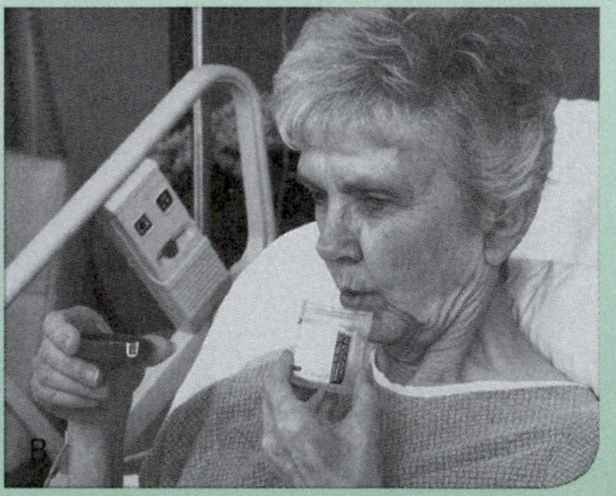

FIGURE 20-12 (A) Instruct the patient to cough deeply to bring up sputum. (B) Instruct the patient to obtain 1 to 2 teaspoons of sputum, then close and seal the container with the lid.

procedure 20-7

TAKING A WOUND CULTURE

Objective: Obtain a sample from a wound by using a swab technique without error.

EQUIPMENT AND SUPPLIES

- gloves
- culture tube with sterile swab and transport medium
- tape for dressing
- sterile water for cleansing the wound
- sterile 4 × 4 gauze dressing
- hazardous waste container
- bag for soiled dressing
- prepared label for culture tube or pen for labeling the tube

METHOD

1. Perform hand hygiene.
2. Assemble equipment.
3. Identify the patient and explain the procedure.
4. Apply gloves.
5. Remove the dressing, noting the amount and type of exudate, and place it in a bag.
6. Observe the wound for redness, crusting, swelling, and odor.
7. Place a sterile swab in the wound and rotate it back and forth. Place the swab in the sterile culture tube (Figure 20-13). Crush the ampoule of preservative that is in the culture tube and seal the tube. Label the culture tube with patient's name, identification number, source of the specimen, and date.
8. Remove gloves, perform hand hygiene, and apply sterile gloves.
9. Clean the wound using sterile water and 4 × 4 gauze squares.

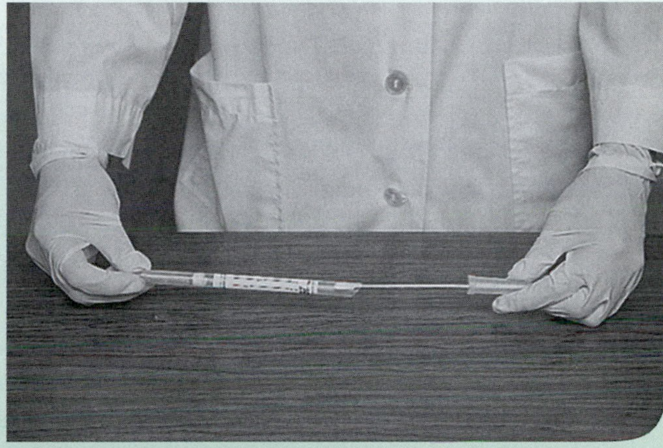

FIGURE 20-13 After obtaining the wound culture, push the tip of the swab into the liquid culture medium.

10. Apply sterile dressing over the wound.
11. Instruct the patient in wound care.
12. Remove gloves and dispose of them properly in a hazardous waste container.
13. Chart the procedure.

CHARTING EXAMPLE

2/14/XX 3:30 P.M. Small amount of exudate obtained from open wound on L. ankle using sterile swab. Tube labeled and sent to lab. Wound cleaned and dressed. Erythema surrounding wound site. No odor noted. Home care instructions given. .... M. King, RMA (AMT)

VAGINAL SPECIMENS

Obtaining vaginal specimens is outside the medical assistant's scope of practice. The licensed clinician will collect the specimen and then most likely give it to the medical assistant for completion of the lab requisition.

If *Chlamydia* or gonorrhea cultures have been ordered, it is important to ensure that the proper transport medium has been used.

CULTURES

The term *culture* refers to a process whereby a specimen of tissue or fluid is cultivated in a specific type of medium. Once the specimen has been allowed to grow for a set period of time, it is examined for bacteria.

The medical assistant's role is merely to obtain the specimen if it is within his or her scope of practice and then give it to the lab or lab technician to complete the culture process. Typically, a Culturette is used to obtain the specimen.

Culturette	Consists of a disposable clear plastic tube; inside the tube is a sterile cotton-tipped applicator swab and a sealed plastic vial of medium. Used to obtain specimens from the throat, genitourinary tract, nose, eyes, or wounds

CULTURE MEDIUM TERMINOLOGY

Culture Medium	Substance used to encourage growth of bacteria. The substance may be liquid, semisolid, or solid. If cultures are performed in the physician's office, the most often used medium is a semisolid medium.
Agar	Gelatin-like substance made from seaweed that is added to the culture medium to provide nutrition and a semisolid surface for the microbes to grow
Petri Dish/Plate	Covered glass or plastic dish that holds culture medium Once the petri dish has been inoculated with the microorganism, the lid should be replaced and the dish should be inverted and placed in the incubator, lid down.
Incubation	Occurs 24 to 48 hours after the petri dish has been inoculated and placed in the incubator
Sensitivity Testing	Once a microorganism has been identified within the culture, sensitivity testing can determine which antibiotic will be effective against that particular pathogen.

Processing of Specimens

When a specimen is collected, it is essential to label it with the patient's name, date and time of collection, specimen processing number, and source of the specimen either prior to or immediately following collection. The specimen should never be set down without a label, as there is a chance that it could be confused with another patient's specimen. If there is any possibility that a specimen has been mislabeled, it should not be tested.

Box 20-2 Culture Process for Identification of Microorganisms

Step 1: Inoculation
The specimen is aseptically transferred to plate and/or tube media.

Step 2: Incubation
The plate and/or tube media are placed in an appropriate environment to optimize the recovery of organisms—usually 35° to 37° Celsius, with increased CO_2 and humidity. Some exceptions, such as stool cultures, are not kept in elevated CO_2. Total incubation times range from 48 hours to four days. Each culture should be examined every 24 hours.

Step 3: Inspection
After the initial incubation of 24 hours, each plate is visually examined and any suspected pathogen is subcultured for purity and prepared for Step 4.

Step 4: Identification
Any suspected pathogen must be identified. A variety of manual and automated methods can be used to identify organisms to genus and species levels. Gram staining is an important part of this procedure. Enzymatic testing, carbohydrate assimilation testing, and antigen detection tests are other ways to identify organisms.

Source: Medical Assisting: Foundations and Practices by M. S. Frazier, C. Malone, and C. Morgan, Upper Saddle River, NJ: Pearson Education, Inc., 2010, p. 626. Reprinted with permission.

Box 20-3 Laboratory Requisition Information

- Physician's name, address, phone number, and account number
- Patient's full name, address, and phone number
- Patient's age, sex, and date of birth (DOB)
- Patient's complete insurance information
- All relevant diagnostic codes
- Diagnosis, if possible
- Source of the specimen
- If it is a fasting or nonfasting specimen
- Date and collection time
- Specific tests requested per physician's orders, including the five-digit procedure code
- Patient's present medications
- If the request is stat or regular

Once the specimen has been collected and properly labeled, it must be stored according to the recommendations of the laboratory testing the specimen. Some specimens must be centrifuged for a set amount of time and within a certain period of time following collection. Others may need to be refrigerated or frozen. The storage guidelines can be found in the laboratory's testing manual.

When it is necessary to send a specimen out for testing, a lab requisition must be completed (Box 20-3 and Figure 20-14).

Lab Services

IMPORTANT
Patient instructions
and map on back

PHYSICIAN ORDERS

Patient ______ (Last Name) ______ (First) ______ (M.I.) D.O.B. ______ M ☐ F ☐ Patient SS# ___ – ___ – ___
Address ______ City ______ Zip ______ Phone # ______
Physician ______
ATTACH COPY OF INSURANCE CARD
Diagnosis/ICD-9 Code ______
(Additional codes on reverse)

Date & Time of Collection: ______ ______
Drawing Facility ______

☐ 789.00 Abdominal Pain
☐ 285.9 Anemia (NOS)
☐ 414.9 Coronary Artery Disease (CAD)
☐ 250.0 DM (diabetes mellitus)
☐ 780.7 Fatigue/Malaise
☐ 272.0 Hypercholesterolemia
☐ 244.9 Hypothyroidism
☐ 272.4 Hyperlipidemia
☐ 401.9 Hypertension
☐ 483.9 URI (upper respiratory infection)

☐ ROUTINE
☐ ASAP
☐ STAT

☐ PHONE RESULTS TO: # ______
☐ FAX RESULTS TO: # ______
☐ COPY TO: ______

HEMATOLOGY
☐ 1021 CBC, Automated Diff (incl, Platelet Ct.)
☐ 1023 Hemoglobin/Hematocrit
☐ 1020 Hemogram
☐ 1025 Platelet Count
☐ 1150 Pro Time Diagnostic
☐ 1151 Pro Time, Therapeutic
☐ 1155 PTT
☐ 1315 Reticulocyte Count
☐ 1310 Sed Rate/ Westergren

URINE
☐ 1059 Urinalysis
☐ 1082 Urinalysis w/Culture if indicated
Urine-24 Hr ______ Spot ______
Ht. ______ Wt. ______
☐ 3033 Creatinine
☐ 3036 Creatinine Clearance (also requires blood)
☐ 3095 Protein
☐ 3096 Sodium/Potassium
☐ Microalbumin 24 Hr______ Spot______

SEROLOGY
☐ 8020 ANA (Antinuclear Antibody)
☐ 8040 Mono Spot
☐ 3494 Rheumatoid Factor
☐ 8010 RPR
☐ 5365 Rubella

CHEMISTRY
☐ 5550 Alpha Fetoprotein, Prenatal
☐ 3000 Amylase
☐ 3153 B12/Folate
☐ 3156 Beta HCG, Quantitative
☐ 3321 Bilirubin, Total
☐ 3324 Bilirubin, Total/Direct
☐ 3009 BUN
☐ 3159 CEA
☐ 3348 Cholesterol
☐ 3030 Creatinine, Serum
☐ 3509 Digoxin (recommend 12 hrs, after dose)
☐ 3515 Dilantin
☐ 3168 Ferritin
☐ 3193 FSH
☐ 3066 ▼ Glucose, Fasting
☐ 3061 Glucose, 1st Post 50 g Glucola
☐ 3075 ▼ Glucose, 2nd Post Glucola
☐ 3060 Glucose, 2nd Post Prandial (meal)
☐ 3049 ▼ Glucose Tolerance Oral GTT
☐ 3047 ▼ Glucose Tolerance Gestational GTT
☐ 3650 Hemoglobin, A1C

CHEMISTRY
☐ 5232 HBsAg
☐ 3175 HIV (Consent required)
☐ 3581 Iron & Iron Binding Capacity
☐ 3195 LH
☐ 3590 Magnesium
☐ 3527 Phenobarbital
☐ 3095 Potassium
☐ 3689 Prognancy Test Serum (HCG, qual)
☐ 3653 Pregnancy Test, Urine
☐ 3197 Prolactin
☐ 3199 PSA
☐ 3339 SGOT/AST
☐ 3342 SGPT/ALT
☐ 3093 Sodium/Potassium, Serum
☐ 3510 Tegretol
☐ 3551 Theophylline
☐ 3333 Uric Acid

MICROBIOLOGY
Source ______
☐ 7240 Culture, AFB
☐ 7200 Culture, Blood x ______
☐ Draw interval ______
☐ 7280 Culture, Fungus
☐ Culture, Routine
☐ 7005 Culture, Stool
☐ 7010 Culture, Throat
☐ 7000 Culture, Urine
☐ 7300 Gram Stain
☐ 7353 Occult Blood x ______
☐ 7365 Ova & Parasites x ______
☐ 7400 Smear & Suspension (includes Gram Stain/Wet Mount)
☐ 7060 Rapid Strep A Screen (______)
☐ 7065 Rapid Strep A Screen only
☐ 7030 Beta Strep Culture
☐ 5207 GC by DNA Probe
☐ 5130 Chlamydia by DNA Probe
☐ 5555 Chlamydia/GC by DNA Probe
☐ 7375 Wright Stain, Stool

Additional Tests ______

PANELS & PROFILES

☐ ✗ **3309 CHEM 12** Albumin, Alkaline Phosphatase, BUN, Calcium, Cholesterol, Glucose, LDH, Phosphorus, AST, Total Bilirubin, Total Protein, Uric Acid
☐ ▼ **3315 CHEM 20** Chem 12, Electrolyte Panel, Creatinine, Iron, Gamma GT, ALT, Triglycerides
☐ ▼ **3357 CARDIAC RISK PANEL** Cholesterol, HDL, LDL, Risk Factors, VLDL Triglycerides
☐ ✗ **3042 CRITICAL CARE PANEL** BUN, Chloride, CO2, Glucose, Potassium, Sodium
☐ **3046 ELECTROLYTE PANEL** Chloride, CO2, Potassium, Sodium
☐ ▼ **3399 EXECUTIVE PANEL** Chem 20, Iron, Cardiac Risk Panel CBC, RPR, Thyroid Cascade
☐ **5242 HEPATITIS PANEL, ACUTE** HAVIgMAb, HBsAg, HBsAb, HBcAb, HCVAb
☐ ▼ **3355 LIPID MONITORING PANEL** Cholesterol, Triglycerides, HDL, LDL, VLDL, ALT, AST
☐ **3312 LIVER PANEL** Alkaline,Phosphatase, AST, Total Bilirubin, Gamma GT, Total Protein, Albumin ALT
☐ ✗ **3083 METABOLIC STATUS PANEL** BUN, Osmolality (calculated), Chloride, CO_2 Creatinine, Glucose, Potassium, Sodium, BUN/Creatinine, Ratio, Anion Gap
☐ ✗ **3376 PANEL B** Chem 12, CBC, Electrolyte Panel
☐ ▼ **3382 PANEL D** Chem 20, CBC, Thyroid Cascade
☐ ✗ **3385 PANEL F** Chem 12, CBC, Electrolyte Panel, Thyroid Cascade
☐ ▼ **3391 PANEL G** Chem 20, Cardiac Risk Panel, CBC, Thyroid Cascade
☐ ▼ **3393 PANEL H** Chem 20, CBC, Cardiac Risk Panel, Rheumatoid Factor, Thyroid Cascade
☐ ▼ **3397 PANEL J** Chem 20, Cardiac Risk Panel
☐ **5351 PRENATAL PANEL** Antibody Screen, ABO/Rh, CBC Rubella, HBsAg, RPR
☐ 1059 with Urinalysis Routine
☐ 1062 with Urinalysis w/Culture if indicated
☐ ✗ **3102 RENAL PANEL** Matabolic Status Panel, Calcium, Phosphorus
☐ **3188 THYROID CASCADE** TSH, Reflex Testing

▼ – patient **required** to fast for 12-14 hours
✗ – patient recommended to fast 12-14 hours

LAB USE ONLY ______
☐ SST ☐ PLASMA
☐ PURPLE ☐ SERUM
☐ YELLOW ☐ SWAB
☐ BLUE ☐ SLIDES
☐ GREEN ☐ DNA PROBE
☐ GREY ☐ B. CULT BTLS
☐ URINE
☐ BLACK
☐ OTHER: ______
RECV. SPECIMEN: ☐ FROZEN
☐ AMBIENT ☐ ON ICE

Special Instructions/Pertinent Clinical Information ______
Physician's Signature ______ **Date** ______
These orders may be FAXed to: 449-5288 LAB 7060-500 (7/96)

FIGURE 20-14 Laboratory requisition slip.

LABORATORY EQUIPMENT The following laboratory equipment is typically found in a POL.

Autoclave	Sterilizes equipment and/or instruments
Centrifuge (Figure 20-15)	Separates specimens into layers by spinning
Hemoglobinometer	Measures hemoglobin levels
Incubator	Maintains a specific temperature and is used to encourage growth of throat and urine cultures
Microscope	Magnifies structures unseen by the naked eye
Photometer	Measures light intensity

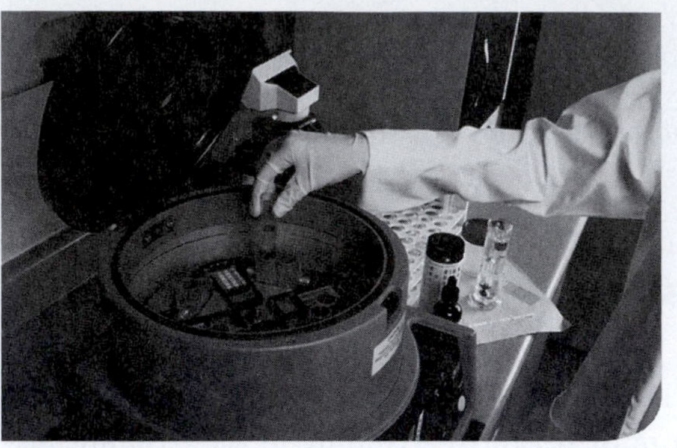

FIGURE 20-15 Example of a centrifuge used for blood and urine.

Types of microscopes are listed in following table.

TYPES OF MICROSCOPES

Type	Use	Magnification	Light	Stain
Compound or Bright Field	Most common type. Specimen is dark against an illuminated background.	Two magnification systems 100X to 1000X	Located below the specimen	Stained and unstained
Phase contrast	Thickness provides the contrast needed to see the live specimen. Thin areas are light; thick areas are dark. Background is dark.	100X to 1000X	Passes through or is deflected by the specimen	Unstained
Dark field	Light is deflected from the specimen, so the image is seen on a dark background.	100X to 1000X	Light source is projected from below. Condenser does not allow light to pass through the specimen. Light is directed at an angle.	Unstained
Fluorescence compound	Light rays are directed through a tube, a series of filters, a mirror, then through the ocular lens system, which illuminates the specimen on a black background.	100X to 1000X	Mercury lamp emits light rays.	Stained with special fluorescent stains. Colors range from bright yellow to orange to lime green.
Electron	Used to view ultramicroscopic organisms or individual cellular components. Image is formed on a screen, as in a television.	Up to 100,000 times normal size	Power source excites electrons through an electromagnetic field.	Stained and unstained

Source: Medical Assisting: Foundations and Practices by M. S. Frazier, C. Malone, and C. Morgan, Upper Saddle River, NJ: Pearson Education, Inc., 2010, p. 615 Reprinted with permission.

Figure 20-16 shows the parts of a microscope, and Procedure 20-8 explains how to use and clean a microscope.

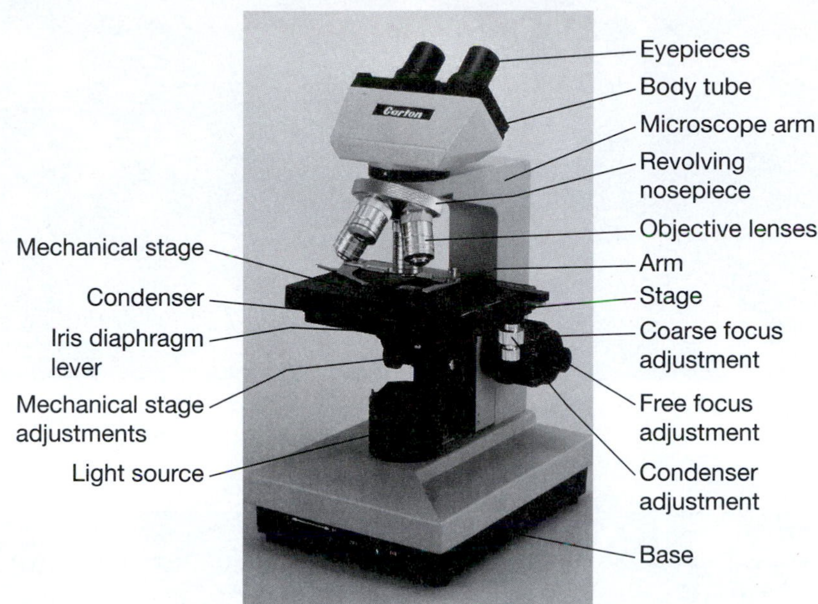

FIGURE 20-16 Binocular microscope with parts labeled.

procedure 20-8

USING AND CLEANING THE MICROSCOPE

Objective: Observe a slide under 10×, 40×, and oil immersion properly, and clean and store the microscope correctly.

EQUIPMENT AND SUPPLIES

- binocular compound microscope
- specimen slide
- lens paper
- lens cleaner
- dust cover for microscope

METHOD

1. Always carry the microscope with one hand on the arm and one hand under the base.
2. Make sure that the stage is in the down position before starting.
3. Clean the objectives with lens paper, starting with 10× and ending with oil immersion (Figure 20-17A).
4. Turn on the light and rotate the nosepiece until the 10× objective is directly over the slide (Figure 20-17B). Place the prepared slide on the stage (Figure 20-17C).
5. Use the coarse adjustment knob to raise the stage until the objective is close to the slide on the stage.
6. Look through the eyepiece and adjust the coarse focus knob until the microscope field is seen (a round circle of bright light).
7. Use the fine adjustment knob for a clearer image (Figure 20-17D).
8. Open the diaphragm and, if necessary, adjust the rheostat to focus.
9. Raise or lower the condenser to alter light refraction. The condenser is usually lowered when using 10× power (Figure 20-17E).
10. Observe the slide.
11. Change the objective to 40× and readjust as needed (Figure 20-17F). Move the objective and place a drop of oil on the slide before completing the turn to the oil immersion lens.

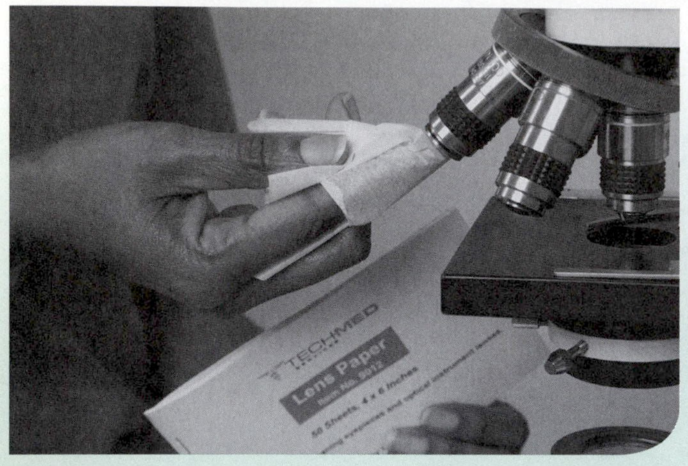

A

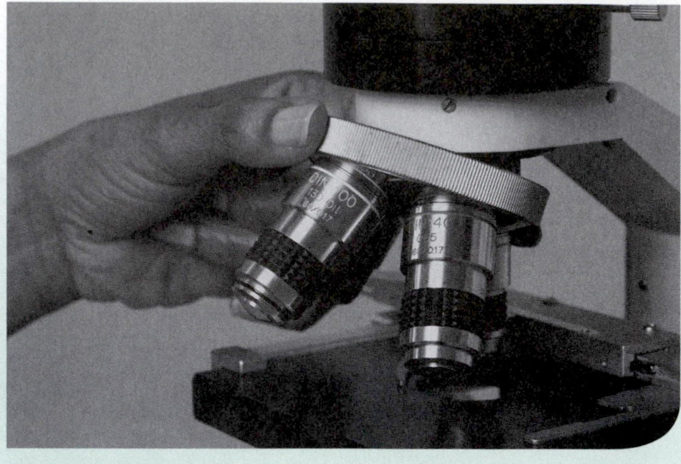

B

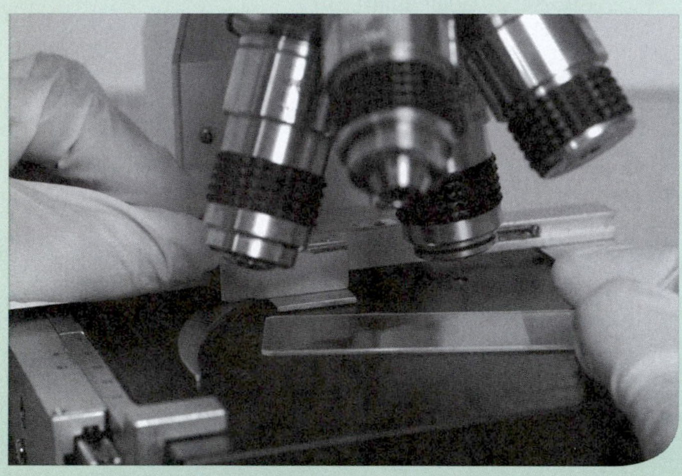

C

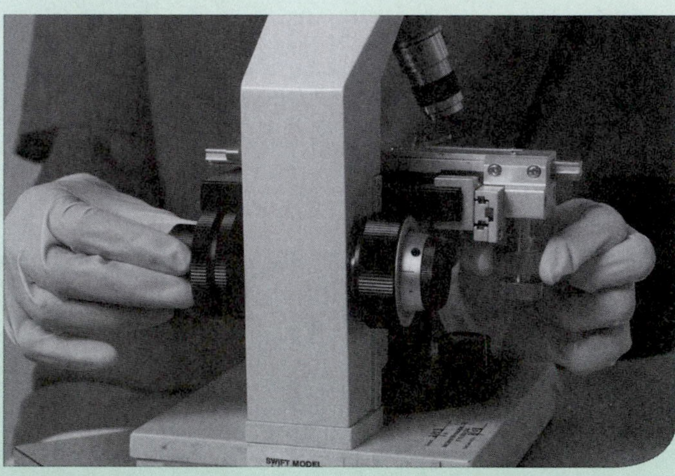

D

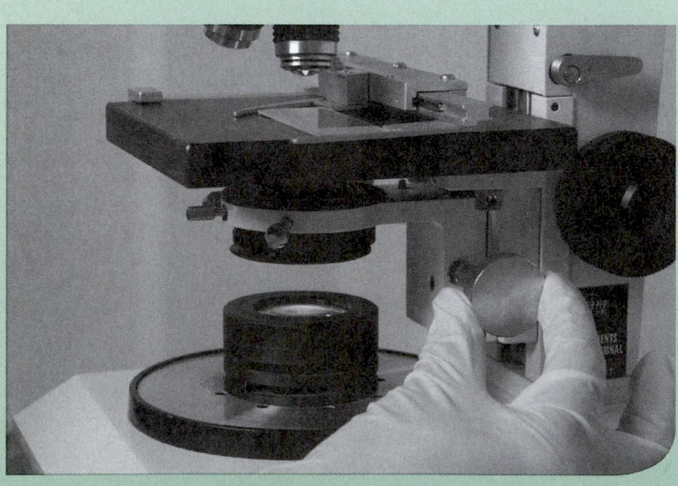

E

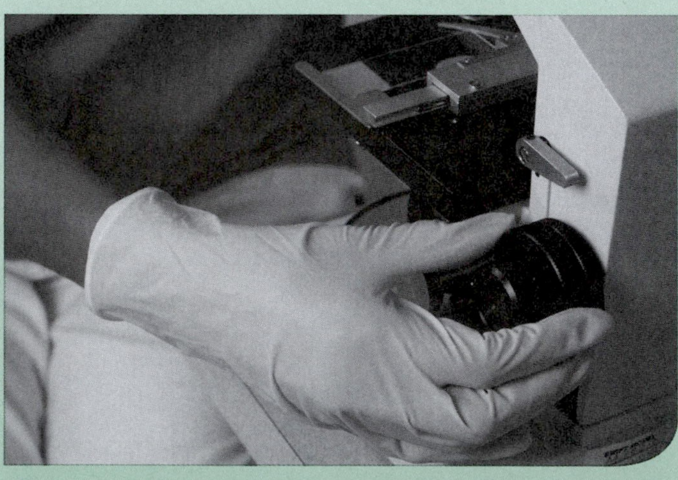

F

FIGURE 20-17 (A) Clean the objective with lens paper. (B) Rotate the nosepiece. (C) Place the slide on the stage. (D) Fine focus with the adjustment knob while moving the slide slightly with the mechanical slide controls. (E) The condenser height control is on the left, and the diaphragm control is on the right. (F) The mechanical stage control moves the slide up and down and back and forth.

12. When the focusing and examination are complete, lower the stage before removing the slide.
13. Turn off the light.
14. Clean the eyepieces and objectives with lens paper. Clean the oil immersion lens with lens cleaner.
15. Unplug the electrical cord and wrap it around the base.
16. Cover the microscope with a dust cover (Figure 20-17G).
17. Clean the slide and store it.

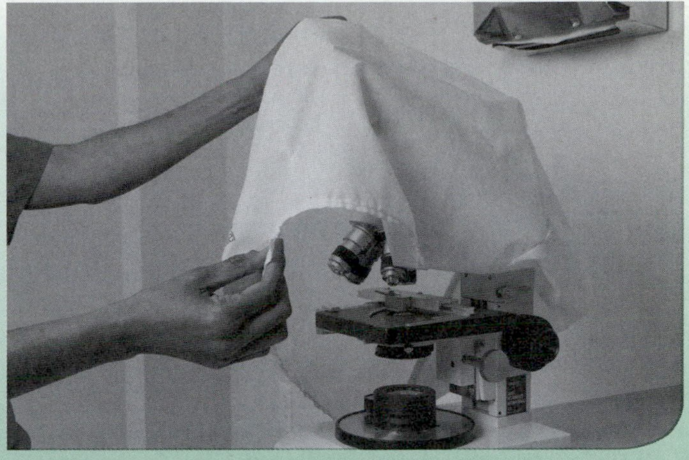

G

FIGURE 20-17 (G) After cleaning, always store the microscope with its protective cover. (Continued)

Performing Tests

CLIA

The Clinical Laboratory Improvement Amendment (CLIA) was established in 1988 by Congress in response to concerns over the accuracy of laboratory testing on human specimens. All laboratories testing human specimens are regulated by CLIA.

CLIA divides laboratories into three categories:

Outside Laboratory	Testing ranges from simple to very complex
Reference Laboratory	Testing is usually more complex than can be handled by an outside laboratory, and this laboratory handles those tests that are infrequently ordered.
Physician's Office Laboratory (POL)	Some tests ordered by the physician can be performed in the office.

CLIA classifies tests into the following categories:

Certificate of Waiver Tests (WTs)	Least complex and carries the least amount of risk if performed incorrectly Most of these tests have been approved by the Food and Drug Administration and are available over the counter to consumers. *Example:* Urine pregnancy test
Level I Tests	Moderately complex. Any lab performing Level I testing must be headed by a pathologist/MD or PhD. *Example:* CBC
Level II Tests	Highly complex Any lab performing Level II testing must be headed by an MD or PhD scientist. *Example:* cytology/histology testing

QUALITY CONTROL

Quality control (QC) monitors testing of specimens and helps to ensure reliable and consistent results. See Procedure 20-9.

QC TERMS

Control Samples	Samples that are similar to the testing specimen and have been previously tested with a known value
Reagents	Substances required for chemical reaction and/or used to detect the presence of another substance
Calibration	Use of a known standard to measure the accuracy of equipment
Maintenance	Keeping a written record of maintenance performed
Documentation	Written record of a test result, control result, or maintenance performed

procedure 20-9

QC FOR COLLECTING A BLOOD SPECIMEN

Objective: Perform a QC procedure while collecting a blood specimen.

EQUIPMENT AND SUPPLIES

- antiseptic cleaner
- biohazard waste container
- necessary sterile equipment
- specimen collection container
- disposable alcohol wipe
- disposable gloves
- appropriate requisition or paperwork required for collection
- pen or pencil
- patient's chart

METHOD

1. Review the request and verify the test ordered.
2. Prepare the equipment and work area.
3. Perform hand hygiene and apply gloves.
4. Identify the patient, explain the procedure, and make sure that he or she understands it.
5. Confirm that the patient has adhered to any pretest preparation requirements.
6. Collect the specimen properly, using the appropriate equipment and technique.
7. Use the appropriate collection container and the right preservatives.
8. Immediately label the specimen with the patient's name, date and time of collection, test's name, and the name of the person collecting the specimen.
9. Follow correct procedures for disposing of hazardous specimen waste and decontaminating the work area and equipment according to OSHA guidelines.
10. Remove gloves and dispose of them in the appropriate container. Perform hand hygiene. Dispose of all used needles and other equipment in a biohazard waste container.
11. Thank the patient and observe him or her for any signs or symptoms of an inappropriate response to the procedure.
12. Document the procedure in the patient's chart.
13. If the specimen is to be transported to an outside laboratory, prepare it for transport in the proper container, with all the appropriate information according to OSHA guidelines.

URINALYSIS

See Procedures 20-10, 20-11, and 20-12.

procedure 20-10

EVALUATING THE PHYSICAL CHARACTERISTICS OF URINE

Objective: Evaluate the physical characteristics of urine and properly record the results.

EQUIPMENT AND SUPPLIES

- urine specimen
- centrifuge tube
- laboratory slip
- personal protective equipment as needed

METHOD

1. Perform hand hygiene and apply gloves.
2. Label the centrifuge tube with the patient's name.
3. Mix the urine by carefully swirling it, avoiding spills.
4. Assess the color of the specimen and record observations, using appropriate terms: *straw, yellow, dark yellow, amber* (other colors if noted). See Figure 20-18 for examples of urines of different colors.
5. Assess and record the clarity of the urine using appropriate terms: *clear, slightly cloudy, cloudy*, or *turbid*. See Figure 20-19 for examples of urines of different clarity.
6. Clean the area.
7. Remove gloves and perform hand hygiene unless you are proceeding with complete urinalysis.
8. Document the results.

CHARTING EXAMPLE

4/23/XX Rand urine spec. collected. Clear, pale yellow. .... M. King, CMA (AAMA)

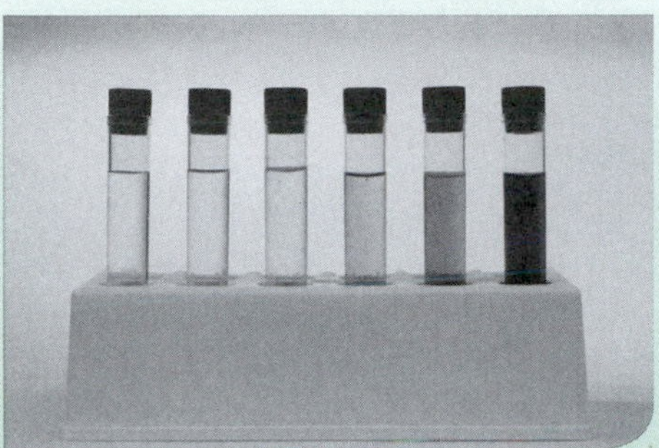

FIGURE 20-18 Colors of urine.

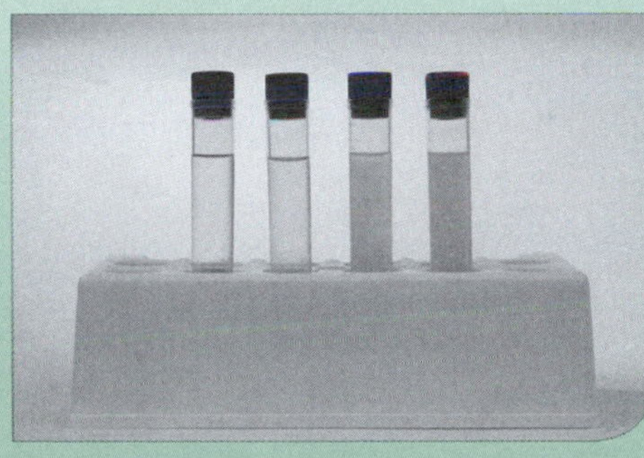

FIGURE 20-19 Appearance of urine (clear to very cloudy).

procedure 20-11

TESTING THE CHEMICAL CHARACTERISTICS OF URINE WITH REAGENT STRIPS

Objective: Perform chemical testing on urine using chemical reagent strips.

EQUIPMENT AND SUPPLIES

- urine specimen
- reagent test strips
- timer
- paper towel

- laboratory slip
- pen/pencil
- personal protective equipment as needed

METHOD

1. Perform hand hygiene and don personal protective gear.
2. Check the specimen for patient identity, date, and time of collection.
3. Check the expiration date on the chemical reagent strips.
4. Bring the specimen to room temperature and swirl it gently to mix it.
5. Dip the chemical reagent strip in the urine, making sure that all pads on the strip are moistened (Figure 20-20A).
6. Read each pad by comparing it to the chart on the side of the bottle, appropriately timing each test (Figure 20-20B). (Do not hold the test strip against the side of the bottle, as contamination will result.) Ignore color changes after the prescribed time has elapsed.
7. Record the results on the patient's laboratory slip.
8. Clean the work area, remove gloves, and perform hand hygiene.

CHARTING EXAMPLE

Note: Normally, a urine test slip would be used to record all results of chemical tests. Then, when the examination is complete and the physician has reviewed it, the test slip would be placed in the patient's chart.

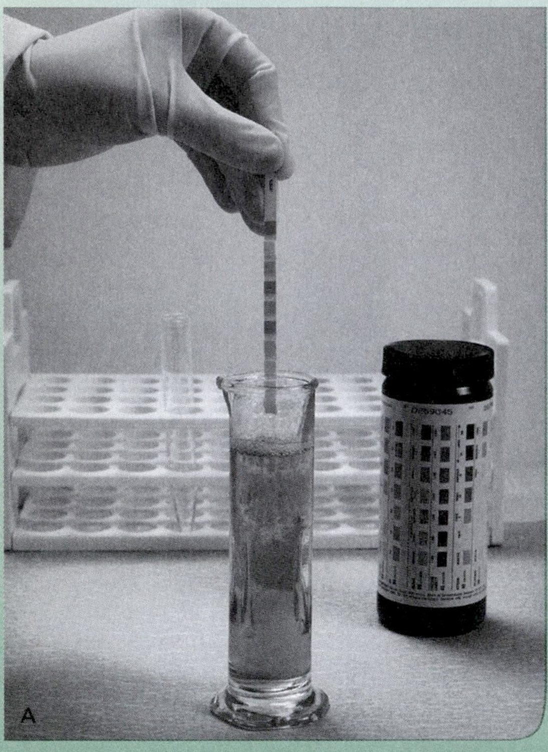

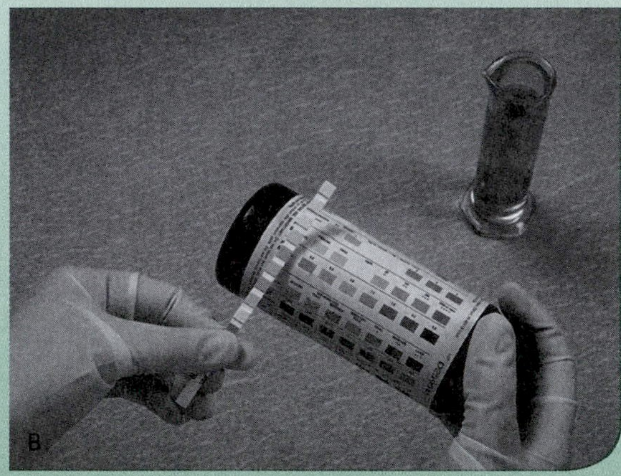

FIGURE 20-20 (A) Dip a reagent strip into urine and withdraw it. (B) Compare the color changes on the reagent strip to those on the chart on the side of the container without contaminating the container.

procedure 20-12

PREPARING A URINE SPECIMEN FOR MICROSCOPIC EXAMINATION

Objective: Perform microscopic examination of urine sediment for casts and cells.

EQUIPMENT AND SUPPLIES

- biohazard waste container
- body and body fluid protection—lab coat, goggles, non-sterile gloves
- capillary pipette
- centrifuge
- centrifuge tube
- microscope
- microscope slide
- paper, pen/pencil

- Sedi-stain (optional)
- urine specimen

Note: Medical assistants are not expected to perform a microscopic examination. They may be requested by the physician to prepare the specimen to step 11.

METHOD

1. Perform hand hygiene.
2. Apply gloves and protective clothing.
3. Assemble equipment and materials.
4. Mix the specimen gently to stir up the sediment that has settled to the bottom.
5. Place 10 mL of urine in the centrifuge tube. Place the cap on the tube. Place the tube in the centrifuge and balance this with another tube of 10 mL of water on the opposite side of the machine (Figure 20-21).
6. Set the centrifuge timer for five minutes.
7. After the centrifuge has stopped, remove the tube and pour off the supernatant fluid (the clear liquid left on the top of the specimen after centrifuging), leaving only the sediment (Figure 20-22).

Alternate Method: Some medical assistants prefer using stain (such as Sedi-stain) to help identify sediment more easily. Place 1 drop of the commercially prepared stain in the test tube.

8. Mix the sediment by holding the top of the tube and tapping the bottom with a finger, mixing well to ensure a correct reading.
9. Use a capillary pipette to transfer 1 drop of sediment to a clean slide (Figure 20-23).
10. Cover the drop of sediment with a cover slip.
11. Place the slide on the microscope stage.
12. Focus under low power and reduced light for casts and epithelial cells.
13. Carefully examine the slide for anything abnormal, paying close attention to the edges, which are where casts are seen if present.
14. Examine 10 to 15 fields using low power. Count the number of casts or other abnormalities seen in each field (Figure 20-24). If there is nothing in one field, then record 0 (zero). Average the count from the 10 to 15 fields for the final result.
15. Use the high-power magnification and adjust for more light, reviewing the 10 to 15 fields. Identify casts if present. Count RBCs, WBCs, round cells, transitional cells, and squamous epithelial cells. Average the count from the 10 to 15 fields for each formed element seen, and record appropriately.
16. Observe for crystals and identify them. Observe for bacteria, sperm, yeast, and parasites. Report them as few, moderate, or many.
17. Discard the urine according to OSHA guidelines.
18. Remove gloves and protective clothing, and dispose of them properly.
19. Perform hand hygiene.
20. Document the findings in the patient's record.
21. Clean the work area and equipment according to OSHA guidelines.

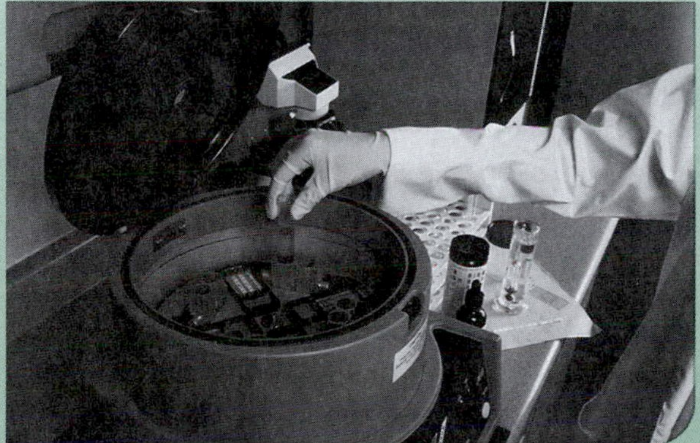

FIGURE 20-21 The centrifuge is used to spin urine specimens in preparation for a microscopic examination.

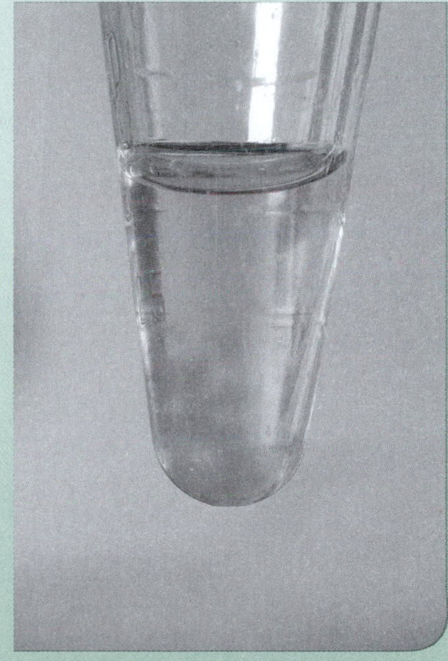

FIGURE 20-22 Pour out most of the liquid supernatant from the tube, but keep the sediment.

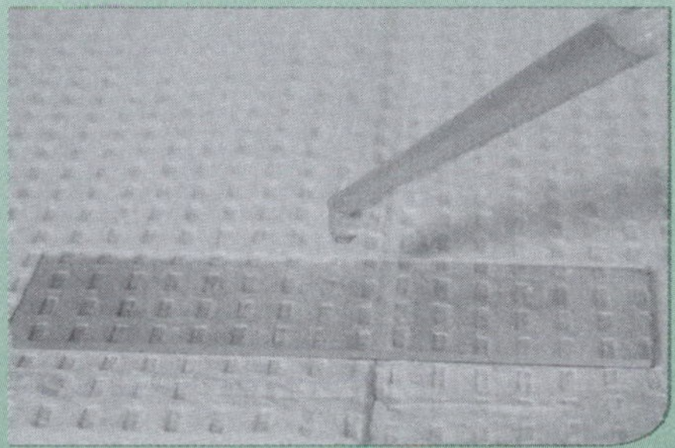

FIGURE 20-23 After mixing the sediment well, use a dropper to place 1 drop of urine on the slide.

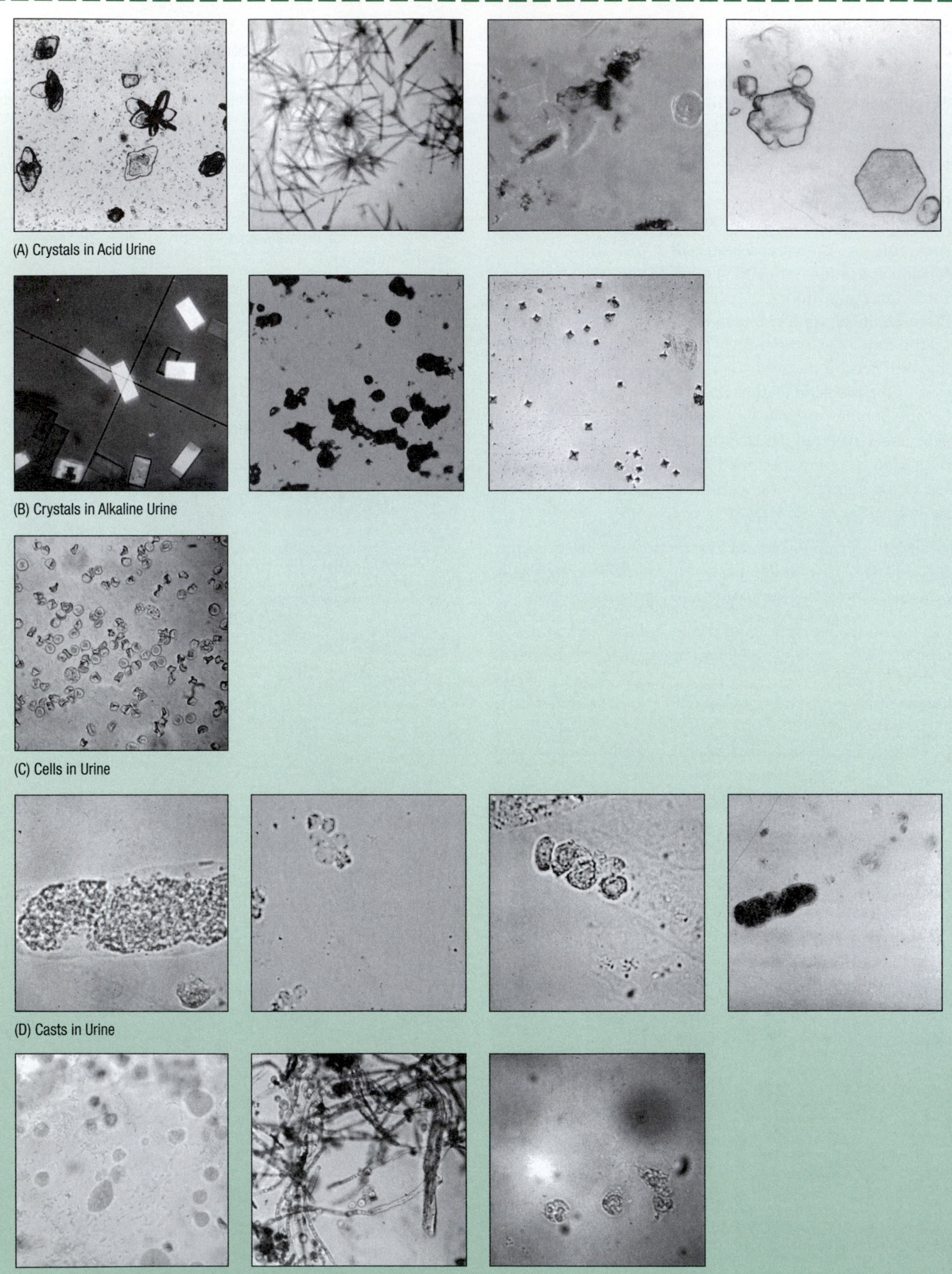

(A) Crystals in Acid Urine
(B) Crystals in Alkaline Urine
(C) Cells in Urine
(D) Casts in Urine
(E) Bacteria, Fungi, Parasites Found in Urine

FIGURE 20-24 Urine sediment chart.

NORMAL VALUES FOR URINALYSIS TESTING

Element	Normal Values
Color	Straw, pale yellow, yellow, darker yellow, amber
Appearance	Clear, slightly cloudy
Specific Gravity	1.010–1.030
Odor	Aromatic
Reaction/pH	4.6–7.9
Protein	Negative to trace

Element	Normal Values
Glucose	Negative
Ketones	Negative
Blood	Negative
Nitrites	Negative
Bilirubin	Negative
Urobilinogen	Less than 2 Ehrlich units/dL
Leukocytes	Negative

URINE MICROSCOPIC EXAMINATION TERMINOLOGY

Casts	Result from protein formation in the kidney tubules
Crystals	Formed by urinary salts when pH, temperature, or concentration changes occur Found in both alkaline and acidic urine

procedure 20-13

PERFORMING A URINE CULTURE

Objective: Inoculate a urine plate to aid in the identification of a urinary tract infection (UTI).

EQUIPMENT AND SUPPLIES

- lab requisition form
- clean-catch midstream (CCMS) urine specimen collected in a sterile container
- incinerator (electric or Bunsen burner)
- 1 μL loop
- agar plates (usually blood, MacConkey, and nutrient)
- gloves
- biohazard waste container

Note: Follow standard precautions and safety guidelines when working with body fluid samples. Take care to avoid splashing or spilling body fluids. Wipe up all spills using the guidelines established by OSHA.

METHOD

1. Assemble equipment and supplies.
2. Perform hand hygiene
3. Don gloves and face protection.
4. Verify that the name on the laboratory requisition and the specimen are the same.
5. With the lid on, swirl the urine sample to mix it.
6. Sterilize the loop and remove the lid, replacing it between inoculation of plates.
7. Inoculate each media plate in a pattern to allow for lawn technique, or use the colony count method to isolate colonies.
8. Label the bottom of the plates near the edges with the patient's name, date, and type of specimen.
9. Place media in the incubator with the agar side up for 24 hours.
10. Clean the area, remove and dispose of gloves, and perform hand hygiene.
11. Results will be interpreted (after incubation) by a physician or laboratory specialist.
12. Document the results appropriately.

CHARTING EXAMPLE

2/14/XX 11:00 A.M. Urine culture performed. . . . .
. . . . M. King, CMA (AAMA)

procedure 20-14

TESTING FOR OCCULT BLOOD

Objective: To test feces for occult blood.

EQUIPMENT AND SUPPLIES

- three occult blood slides
- applicators
- envelope
- timer
- patient's record
- pen
- gloves
- color developer

Note: Many test kits are available. Each one has its own set of directions, color developer, slides, and control monitors. The test kit directions should be followed exactly.

METHOD

1. Perform hand hygiene.
2. Apply gloves. Place a paper towel on the area to hold the slides.
3. Check the name and date on the occult blood slides.
4. Check the expiration date on the color developer. See Figure 20-25A for the supplies needed for occult blood testing.
5. Open the window flap on the back of the slide and apply 2 drops of the developer to Box A and Box B (Figure 20-25B).
6. Interpret the results in 30 to 60 seconds or according to the manufacturer's directions. A positive result will have blue color around the edge of the specimen; a negative result will have no color change visible. Any amount of blue color is positive.
7. Perform a test on positive and negative controls as required by the manufacturer for QC purposes.
8. Test the remaining slides in the same manner.
9. Dispose of all materials in a biohazard waste container. Clean the work area.
10. Remove gloves.
11. Perform hand hygiene.
12. Document the results in the patient's record.

CHARTING EXAMPLE

03/21/XX 10:30 A.M. Three occult blood rec'd. All tested neg. for occult blood. Dr. Chang notified of results. Pt. notified per Dr. Chang .... B. Negri, CMA (AAMA)

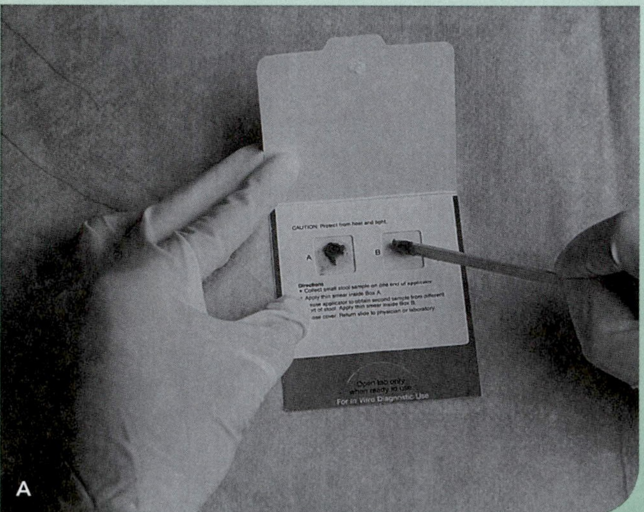

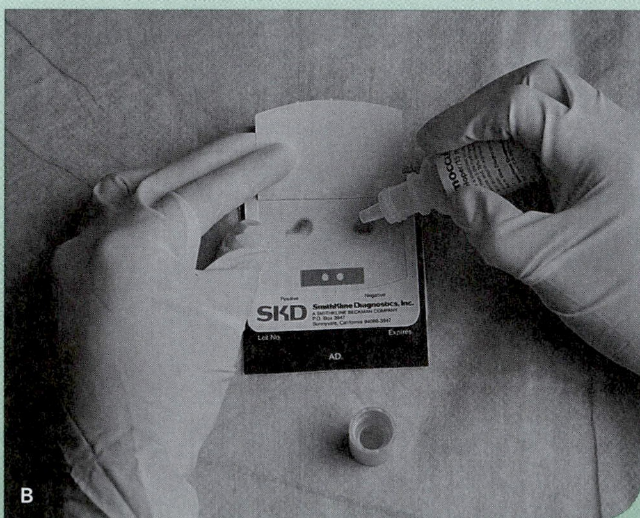

FIGURE 20-25 (A) Supplies needed for testing stool for occult blood. (B) Open the back flap of the slide and apply 2 drops of color developing fluid over each smear.

HEMATOLOGY

HEMATOLOGY TESTS

Hematocrit	Also known as *Hct* or *crit* • Can be measured manually or by an analyzer • Provides information about RBC volume • Low Hct may indicate anemia or hemorrhage • Elevated Hct may indicate dehydration or polycythemia • Normal for males: 40–50% • Normal for females: 35–45%
Hemoglobin	Also known as *Hgb* • Low Hgb may indicate iron-deficiency anemia • Elevated Hgb may indicate polycethemia • Normal for males: 14–18 g/dL • Normal for females: 12–16 g/dL • Can be measured either manually or by an automated blood analyzer
Erythrocyte Sedimentation Rate	Also known as *ESR* or *sed rate* • Rate at which RBCs settle to the bottom of a tube • Can be performed by either the Wintrobe or Westegren method • Elevated ESR may indicate inflammation, menstruation, pregnancy, or a malignant tumor • ESR is a screening test and is not intended to be used by itself, but rather in conjunction with other tests.
Red Blood Cell Count	Also known as *RBC count* • Low RBC may indicate anemia • Elevated RBC may indicate polycythemia • Normal for males: 5.0–6.0 million per mm^3 • Normal for females: 4.5–6.0 million per mm^3
White Blood Cell Count	Also known as *WBC count* • Low WBC may indicate a viral infection or an autoimmune deficiency • Elevated WBC may indicate infection or, if significantly elevated, leukemia • Adult normal range: 4500–11,000 • Can be measured either manually or by an automated blood analyzer
Platelets	Also known as *thrombocytes* • Low platelet level may indicate anemia, leukemia, or the use of chemotherapy • Elevated platelet level may indicate certain types of cancer, anemia, or polycythemia • Normal range: 150,000–400,000 per mm^3
Coagulation Tests	Consist of a prothrombin time (PT) and/or a partial thromboplastin time (PTT) • Identify bleeding problems Prothrombin Time (PT) • Evaluates blood's ability to clot • Used to determine if warfarin (Coumadin) is effective • Normal range: 10–12 seconds Partial Thromboplastin Time (PTT) • Used to determine if heparin is effective • Normal range: 30–45 seconds

COMMON LABORATORY TESTS AND THEIR NORMAL VALUES

Test	Result	Test	Result
Total Cholesterol	130–200 mg/dL	Chloride	98–106 mEq/L
Glucose	70–120 mg/dL	Carbon Dioxide (CO_2)	25–32 mEq/L
Triglycerides	40–150 mg/dL	White Blood Cell Count	5000–10,000/mm^3
Creatinine	0.7–1.4 mg/dL	Red Blood Cell Count	3.5–5.5 × 10/mm^3
Uric acid	3.5–7.5 mg/dL	Hemoglobin	12–16 g/dL
Blood Urea Nitrigen (BUN)	8–20 mg/dL	Hematocrit	35.5–49%
Sodium	132–142 mEq/L	Sedimentation Rate	0–10 mm/hr
Potassium	3.5–5.5 mEq/L	Platelet Count	150,000–400,000 per μL^3

procedure 20-15

PERFORMING A MICROHEMATOCRIT

Objective: Perform a microhematocrit on a capillary blood sample using proper aseptic technique.

EQUIPMENT AND SUPPLIES

- biohazard sharps container
- gloves
- capillary tubes
- sealing clay
- microhematocrit centrifuge
- whole blood
- hematocrit card or other reader

Note: Follow standard precautions and safety guidelines when working with blood samples. Take care to avoid splashing or spilling blood. Wipe up all spills using the guidelines established by OSHA.

METHOD

1. Perform hand hygiene and apply gloves.
2. Assemble equipment as shown in Figure 20-26A.
3. Fill two capillary tubes three-quarters full. The blood specimen can be obtained from a vacuum tube of anticoagulated blood using a plain capillary tube or directly from a fingerstick site using a heparinized capillary tube. Seal one end with the sealing clay.
4. Place the capillary tubes in the centrifuge with the sealed ends against the rubber gasket (Figure 20-26B). If more than one patient's blood is being tested, mark down the number of the slot the patient's tube is in. Spin for three to five minutes at 10,000 rpm. (Always check the manufacturer's recommendations for the proper time and speed.) After centrifuging, the sample will be separated into three layers:
   - The top layer is the plasma.
   - The middle layer, or the buffy coat, is made up of WBCs and platelets.
   - The bottom layer is packed RBCs.
5. Remove the tubes immediately after the centrifuge stops. If the tubes are not removed immediately, the layers of blood may begin to mix together.
6. Determine the results. Use the Hct card by placing the sealing clay just below the zero line on both tubes. Then, on both tubes, match the top of the plasma with the 100 line. Read the results on both tubes directly below the buffy coat. Then add the results together and divide by 2.
7. Discard the tubes into the sharps container.
8. Remove gloves and perform hand hygiene.
9. Record the value as a percentage on the patient's medical record.

CHARTING EXAMPLE

2/28/XX 1:45 P.M. Hct 47 percent. · · · · · M. King, CMA (AAMA)

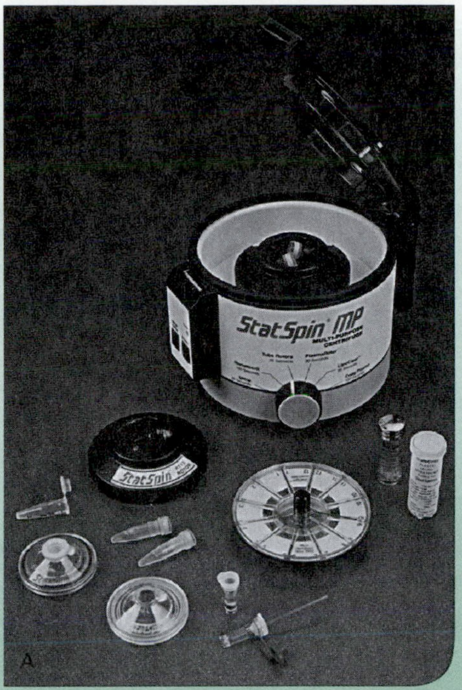

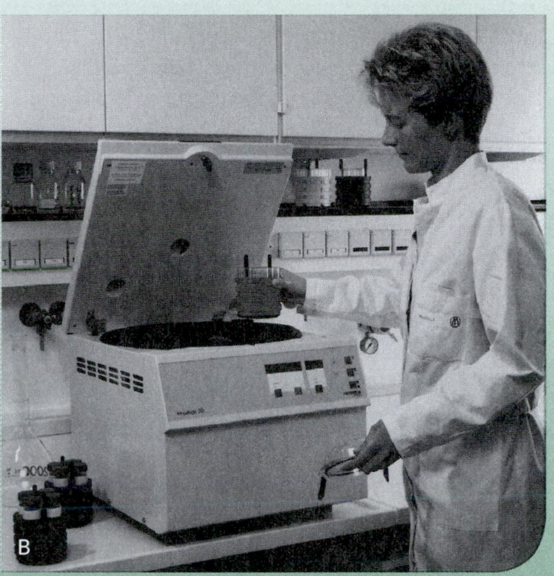

FIGURE 20-26 (A) Centrifuge and supplies. (B) loading a centrifuge.

procedure 20-16

DETERMINING HEMOGLOBIN LEVEL USING THE HEMOGLOBINOMETER

Objective: Perform a blood test to determine hemoglobin level using the hemoglobinometer.

EQUIPMENT AND SUPPLIES

- hemoglobinometer
- glass slide chamber
- hemolysis applicator (plastic or wooden)
- sterile manual or spring-loaded lancet
- cotton balls
- dry gauze square
- alcohol sponges
- gloves
- patient's record
- lab coat
- biohazard sharps container

Note: Follow standard precautions and safety guidelines when working with blood samples. Take care to avoid splashing or spilling blood. Wipe up all spills using the guidelines established by OSHA.

METHOD

1. Perform hand hygiene and apply gloves.
2. Gather the necessary equipment and supplies.
3. Clean the puncture site with an alcohol sponge.
4. Using a manual or spring-loaded lancet, obtain capillary blood.

5. Pull the glass chamber out of the hemoglobinometer and position the lower part of the slide so that it is slightly offset.
6. Place a large drop of capillary blood on the slide.
7. Wipe the puncture site with a cotton ball and provide the patient with a dry gauze square to apply mild pressure to the puncture. This should stop further bleeding.
8. Mix blood with the hemolysis applicator until the blood becomes clear.
9. Push the glass chamber into the clip and place it in the slot on the left side of the hemoglobinometer.
10. Hold the hemoglobinometer in your left hand at eye level while using your left thumb to turn on the light by depressing the bottom button. Look into the instrument to see a split green field.
11. Slide the button on the right side of the meter with your right thumb and index finger while looking into the meter until a matching green field occurs. Leave the sliding scale on the calibrated line where the solid green field appeared.
12. Read the hemoglobin value at the top of the scale. The results are read as grams of hemoglobin per 100 mL of blood (g/dL).
13. Wash the chamber and the reusable hemolysis applicator with a detergent solution, rinse, dry, and return to the instrument for the next test.
14. Remove gloves and perform hand hygiene. Discard gloves and nonreusable supplies in appropriate containers.
15. Record the results in the patient's record.

CHARTING EXAMPLE

1/18/XX 10:35 A.M. Patient's Hgb 9.2. · · · · M. Walling, RMA (AMT)

procedure 20-17

PERFORMING AN ERYTHROCYTE SEDIMENTATION RATE (ESR) TEST USING THE WINTROBE TUBE METHOD

Objective: Perform an ESR test using the Wintrobe tube method and aseptic technique.

EQUIPMENT AND SUPPLIES

- gloves
- whole blood (EDTA)
- Wintrobe tube
- Wintrobe rack
- ink pen
- patient's record
- lab coat
- biohazard sharps container

Note: Follow standard precautions and safety guidelines when working with blood samples. Take care to avoid splashing or spilling blood. Wipe up all spills using the guidelines established by OSHA.

METHOD

1. Perform hand hygiene and apply gloves.
2. Assemble equipment.
3. Obtain a whole-blood sample using a purple-top tube. Mix well. EDTA is the anticoagulant of choice.
4. Slowly fill the Wintrobe tube with blood. Avoid air bubbles.
5. Adjust the meniscus of the specimen to the zero line at the top of the tube.
6. Maintain the tube in an upright vertical position for one hour.
7. After one hour, record the number of RBCs that settle. Read the ESR on the same side of the tube as the zero line at the top.
8. Remove gloves and perform hand hygiene.
9. Record the procedure on the patient's medical record.

CHARTING EXAMPLE

2/28/XX 2:00 P.M. ESR (Wintrobe method) 10 fall of mm/hr. · M. Garcia, RMA (AMT)

BLOOD CHEMISTRY

Blood chemistry panels may be ordered as part of a screening or as a diagnostic tool. Serum is generally needed for most blood chemistry tests.

BLOOD CHEMISTRY TESTS

C-Reactive Protein	Also known as *CRP* • Serology blood test used in conjunction with other blood tests • Normally, the level of C-reactive protein detected in the blood is 0. • Used to measures levels of a particular protein produced in the liver during episodes of acute inflammation or infection • During bouts of inflammation or infection, the C-reactive protein level is typically >10 mg/dL.
Hemoglobin A1C	Blood test used to determine how well diabetes is being controlled The test averages blood sugar control over a 6- to 12-week period. The patient is required to fast before the blood is drawn. Currently, the American Diabetes Association recommends the following levels: • Diabetic's HgbA1C: <7%. • Nondiabetic's HgbA1C: 4–6% Diabetics are encouraged to have this test every three months to help determine if their diabetes is under control.
Lipid Profile	Helps determine the risk of heart disease or whether or not lipid-lowering medications are working Requires 12 hours of fasting prior to the blood draw The lipid profile consists of the following tests: • Total cholesterol • High density lipoprotein cholesterol (HDL-C), or "good cholesterol" • Low density lipoprotein cholesterol (LDL-C), or "bad cholesterol"
Liver Panel	Also known as the *liver function test* or *LFT* Helps detect, evaluate, and monitor liver disease or damage Consists of the following tests: • ALT/SGPT (alanine aminotransferase) • Albumin • Alkaline phosphatase • AST/SGOT(aspartate aminotransferase) • Bilirubin, direct • Bilirubin, total • Protein, total
Renal Panel	Also known as the *kidney function test* Used in the diagnosis and management of illnesses and injuries that cause changes in renal function Consists of the following tests: • Creatinine • BUN (blood, urea, nitrogen) • BUN:creatinine ratio • Albumin • Calcium • Carbon dioxide • Chloride • Glucose • Phosphorus • Potassium • Sodium

procedure

20-18

MONITORING BLOOD GLUCOSE LEVEL

Objective: Determine blood glucose level using a glucometer.

EQUIPMENT AND SUPPLIES

- sterile lancet
- testing strips
- glucometer
- examination gloves
- cotton balls
- alcohol sponges
- gauze squares
- pen
- lab coat
- patient's record

METHOD

1. Identify the patient and make sure that the patient has fasted if required.
2. Assemble equipment and supplies.
3. Perform hand hygiene and apply gloves.
4. Make sure that the glucometer has been turned on for the required amount of time and has been calibrated for accuracy according to the manufacturer's instructions.
5. Remove a plastic test strip from the container and place it in the glucometer in the designated slot. Ensure that the "Apply Blood" message appears on the screen (Figure 20-27A).
6. Perform a capillary puncture, preferably on the patient's finger, utilizing a sterile lancet.
7. After wiping away the first drop of blood with a cotton ball, gently touch the test strip to the second drop of blood that has formed on the patient's finger. The glucometer should automatically begin to count down the time that must elapse during the test. This is usually 30 seconds (Figure 20-27B).
8. At this time, provide the patient with a dry cotton ball to hold over the puncture site after wiping the site with an alcohol sponge.
9. The results of the blood glucose test will appear on the screen after the proper amount of time has elapsed. The blood glucose reading will remain on the glucometer until the unit has been turned off. Immediately remove the test strip and discard all used equipment.
10. Remove gloves and perform hand hygiene.

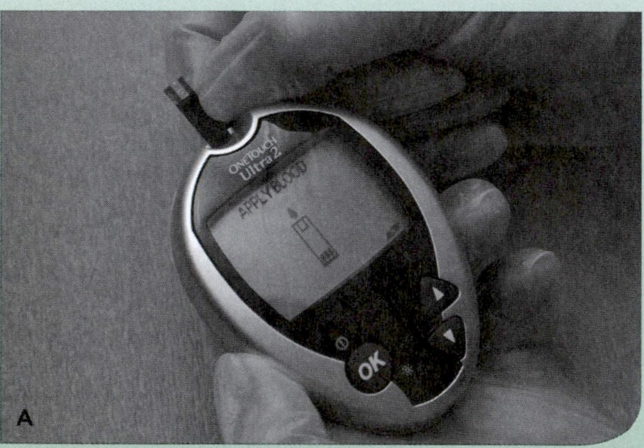

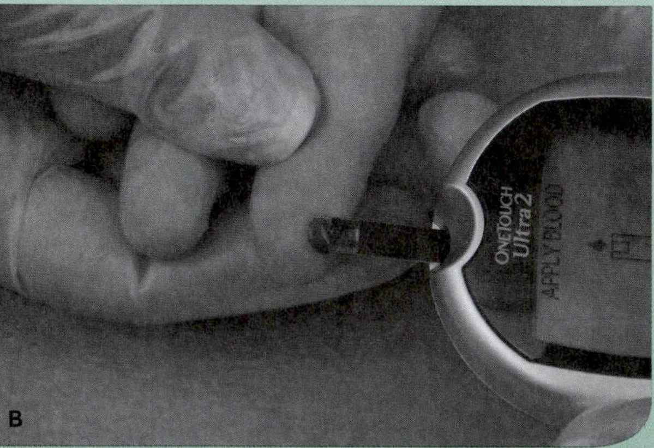

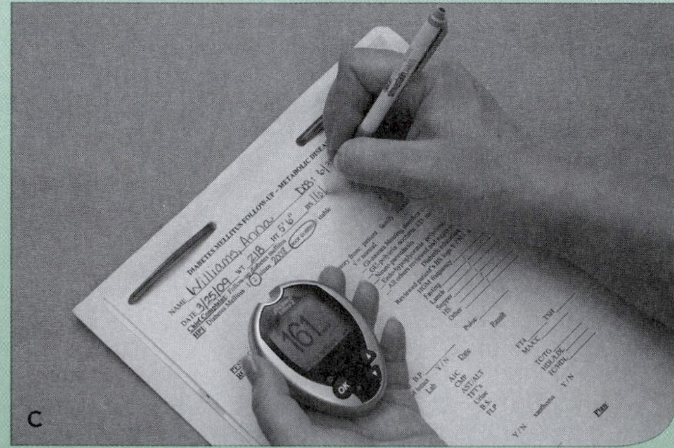

FIGURE 20-27 (A) Make sure that the monitor is turned on, and insert a test strip into the glucometer in the designated slot. (B) Touch the test strip to the second drop of blood that has formed on the patient's finger. (C) Record the blood glucose result in the patient's chart.

11. Record in the patient's chart the number of milligrams (mg) of glucose per deciliter (mg/dL) displayed on the glucometer screen (Figure 20-27C).

Note: Several different types of testing instruments may be used to perform this test. It is critical to follow the manufacturer's instructions for the testing equipment provided.

CHARTING EXAMPLE

2/28/XX 1:30 P.M. Random blood glucose performed; result 161 mg/dL. .... M. Garcia, RMA (AMT)

COMMON BLOOD CHEMISTRY TESTS

Test	Common Medical Abbreviation	Normal Adult Value	Description	Purpose of Test
Alanine Aminotransferase	ALT (SGPT)	<45 units/L	Liver enzyme; may also be found in kidneys	To detect liver disease or inflammation.
Albumin	No standard abbreviation	3.5–5.0 g/dL	A protein that normally constitutes 60% of plasma serum	To determine the effectiveness of specific medications, such as warfarin, because it binds to albumin. High levels may indicate dehydration; low levels may indicate drug toxicity in the liver.
Alkaline Phosphate	ALP	20–70 units/L	Enzyme found in all tissues; especially concentrated in the kidneys, bile, liver, bone, and placenta	Used to detect several conditions in the bone and liver and blocked bile ducts
Aspartate Aminotransferase	AST (SGOT)	<40 units/L	Enzyme found in all tissues; similar to ALT; found in cardiac muscle cells and red blood cells	Used to detect conditions of liver health
Blood Urea Nitrogen	BUN	7–18 mg/dL	Metabolic products of protein catabolism	Used to measure the amount of nitrogen in the blood, indicating renal function
Cholesterol	CH, Chol	Total count: <200 mg/dL; LDL <130 mg/dL; HDL >35 mg/dL	Lipids	Annual screening done to determine the presence of atherosclerosis and other cardiac-related diseases
Creatinine	Creat	0.2–0.8 mg/dL	The product of creatinine phosphate breaks down in muscle at a fairly constant rate, then filters out through the kidneys	Screening for renal function often used in combination with BUN Checked prior to contrast studies, such as CT, to assess the kidneys' ability to filter out contrast material
Glucose Tolerance Test	GTT	70–100 mg/dL	Carbohydrate	To determine how quickly the body is able to filter glucose to help diagnose diabetes, insulin resistance, and reactive hypoglycemia
Troponin I and T	No standard abbreviation	<0.4	A specific protein found only in cardiac muscle when it is damaged	Aids in the determination of myocardial infarction
Thyroid-Stimulating Hormone	TSH	5–6 units/mL	Peptide hormone produced by thyrotropic cells in the pituitary gland	Assessment of thyroid and pituitary function

(continued)

(Continued)

Thyroxine	T4	5–12 mcg/dL	Hormone secreted by the follicular cells of the thyroid gland	Assessment of the body's ability to control the metabolic processes in the body that influence physical development
Triglycerides	Trig	30–190 mg/dL	Dietary fat	Annual screening done to determine the presence of atherosclerosis and other cardiac-related diseases.
Uric Acid	UA	*Male:* 3.4–7.0 mg/dL *Female:* 2.4–6 mg/dL	Organic compound consisting of carbon, nitrogen, oxygen, and hydrogen	Diagnosis of several conditions, including gout, Lesch-Nyhan syndrome, cardiovascular disease, diabetes, metabolic syndrome, and multiple sclerosis (low levels)

IMMUNOLOGY

See Procedures 20-19, 20-20, and 20-21.

procedure 20-19

PERFORM RAPID GROUP A STREP TESTING

Objective: With the necessary materials, you will be able to perform rapid Group A strep testing correctly.

EQUIPMENT AND SUPPLIES

- labeled throat specimen
- Group A strep kit (controls may be included, depending on the kit)
- personal protective equipment
- timer
- biohazard waste container

METHOD

1. Wash your hands and gather supplies.
2. Verify that the name on the specimen container and the laboratory requisition form are the same.
3. Put on your personal protective equipment.
4. Label one extraction tube with the patient's name, one for the positive control, and one for the negative control.
5. Follow the directions for the kit according to the manufacturer's instructions.
6. Add the appropriate reagents and drops to each of the extraction tubes.
7. Insert the patient's swab into the labeled extraction tube and add the appropriate controls to each of the labeled extraction tubes.
8. To ensure accuracy, set the timer for the appropriate time.
9. Add the appropriate reagent and drops to each of the extraction tubes.
10. Mix the reagents with the swab and add three drops from the well-mixed extraction tube to the sample window of the Strep A test unit. Repeat this procedure for each control.
11. Set the timer for the time indicated by the manufacturer.
12. A positive or negative result appears within 5 minutes. Refer to the directions in the kit to differentiate between a negative or positive result.
13. Properly dispose of the equipment and supplies in a biohazard waste container.
14. Remove your personal protective equipment and wash your hands.
15. Document the procedure and results in the patient chart.
16. Sanitize the area.

CHARTING EXAMPLE

12/23/XX 4:50 P.M. QuickVue One Step Strep A test performed according to manufacturer's guidelines. Test results positive. Patient medication instructions reviewed. .... Pamela King, CMA (AAMA)

Source: Medical Assisting: Foundations and Practices by M. S. Frazier, C. Malone, and C. Morgan, Upper Saddle River, NJ: Pearson Education, Inc., 2010, p. 630. Reprinted with permission.

procedure 20-20

PERFORMING A MONO TEST

Objective: Perform a mono test.

EQUIPMENT AND SUPPLIES

- antiseptic cleaner
- biohazard waste container
- disposable lancet
- gloves
- capillary tube
- test tube
- mono test diluent
- mono test stick(s)
- blood specimen

METHOD

1. Perform hand hygiene.
2. Apply gloves.
3. Assemble equipment and supplies.
4. Perform a capillary puncture on the patient's finger.
5. Fill a capillary tube end to end, dispensing all of the blood into the test tube.
6. Slowly add 1 drop of diluent to the bottom of the test tube.
7. Mix.
8. Remove the test stick(s) from the container. Recap the container immediately.
9. Place the absorbent end of the test stick into the treated sample. Leave the test stick in the test tube.
10. Read the result at five minutes. Positive results may be read as soon as the red control line appears.
11. Discard used test tubes, lancet, and test sticks in the biohazard waste container.
12. Remove gloves and dispose of them correctly. Perform hand hygiene.
13. Document the findings in the patient record:
    Positive: A blue test line and a red control line indicate a positive result.
    Negative: A red control line but no blue test line indicates a negative result.

Note: Although the medical assistant is responsible for reporting abnormal results (or positive results in the case of a mono test) to the physician, interpreting such tests as being positive or negative is *not* within the scope of practice for the medical assistant as such and should never be done. The medical assistant is allowed only to report the findings of "positive" or "negative."

14. Clean the work area and equipment according to OSHA guidelines.

procedure 20-21

PERFORMING A URINE PREGNANCY TEST USING THE ENZYME IMMUNOASSAY (EIA) METHOD

Objective: Perform a urine pregnancy test for human chorionic gonadotropin (hCG) using an EIA test and interpret results correctly.

EQUIPMENT AND SUPPLIES

- patient's first A.M. urine specimen
- EIA test kit for hCG
- timer
- gloves
- laboratory report

METHOD

1. Perform hand hygiene and apply gloves.
2. Gather supplies and equipment.
3. Allow the testing materials and specimen to come to room temperature.
4. Label the test with the patient's name or ID number.
5. Label one area positive and one negative for controls.
6. Place the patient's urine on the test chamber following the manufacturer's directions.
7. Place the positive and negative controls in the correct areas (Figure 20-28).
8. Time the test according to the manufacturer's directions.
9. Interpret the results correctly.
10. Record the results on the patient's laboratory slip.
11. Record the positive and negative controls in the QC logbook according to office policy.
12. Dispose of equipment and perform hand hygiene.

CHARTING EXAMPLE

10/19/XX 4:00 P.M. Preg test pos. · · · · · M. King, CMA (AAMA)

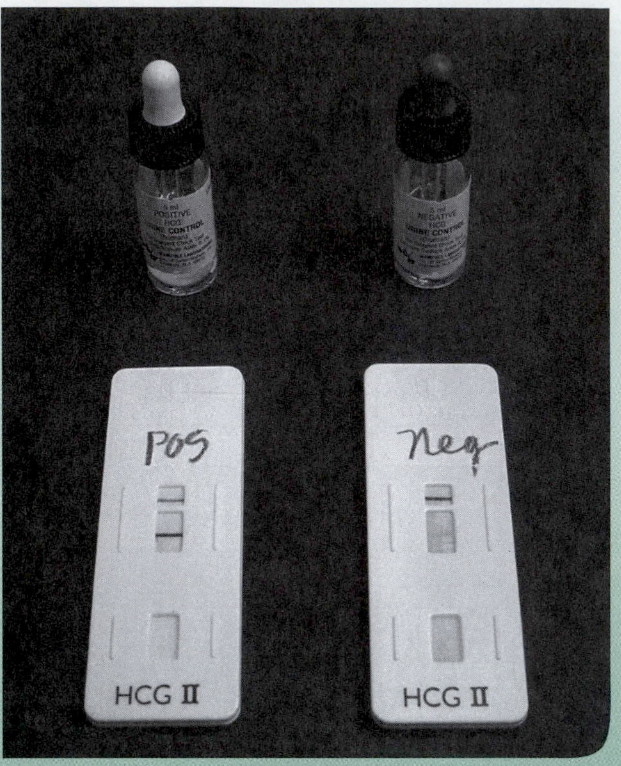

FIGURE 20-28 Urine pregnancy control test—positive and negative.

MICROBIOLOGY

MICROBIOLOGY TERMINOLOGY

Bacteria	Microorganisms, some capable of causing disease Classified by morphology and gram reaction
Fungi	Opportunistic pathogens that cause disease when the normal balance of flora is upset
Parasites	Organisms that infect living hosts and receive nourishment at the expense of their host without contributing to the host's survival
Protozoa	Parasites that are larger in size than bacteria Most live in the soil and receive nourishment from dead or decaying organic material
Viruses	Smallest known infection organisms that depend on living cells or other organisms for growth Cause many common diseases, such as colds, chickenpox, mumps, and warts

CLASSIFICATION OF BACTERIA ACCORDING TO MORPHOLOGY

Bacteria	Shape	Appearance	Examples
Coccus (plural: cocci)	Spherical	Often exist in pairs, groups, tetrads, or chains	*Staphylococcus* species *Streptococcus* species *Neisseria* species
Bacillus (plural: bacilli)	Rod-shaped	Parallel sides; different lengths and thickness depending on genus-specific characteristics	*Escherichia* species *Proteus* species *Campylobacter* species
Spirochetes	Spiral or cork-screw-shaped	Vary in length and thickness	*Treponema* species *Borrelia* species

Source: Medical Assisting: Foundations and Practices by M. S. Frazier, C. Malone, and C. Morgan, Upper Saddle River, NJ: Pearson Education, Inc., 2010, p. 619. Reprinted with permission.

PATHOGENIC MICROORGANISMS AND RESULTING DISEASES

Body Location	Pathogen	Disease
Respiratory System	*Streptococcus pyogenes* *Corynebacterium diphtheriae* *Mycobacterium tuberculosis* *Haemophilus influenzae* type B *Streptococcus pneumoniae*	Strep throat, scarlet fever Diphtheria Tuberculosis Influenza Pneumonia
Central Nervous System	*Neisseria meningitidis* Polioviruses Rabies virus	Meningitis Poliomyelitis Rabies
Genitourinary System	Herpes simplex viruses 1 and 2 *Candida albicans* (fungus) *Chlamydia trachomatis* *Escherichia coli*	Genital herpes Vaginitis Vaginitis Urinary tract infection
Integumentary System	*Staphylococcus aureus* *Varicella zoster* virus	Boils, carbuncles Chickenpox Scabies Lice
Gastrointestinal System	Hepatitis A, B, and C viruses *Salmonella enteritidis* *Escherichia coli*	Hepatitis A, B, and C Food poisoning *E. coli* diarrhea
Circulatory System and Blood, Immune System	*Streptococcus pyogenes* *Staphylococcus aureus* *Plasmodium falciparum, P. vivax, P. malariae, P. ovale* Human immunodeficiency virus Epstein-Barr virus *Borrelia burgdorferi*	Septicemia, endocarditis Malaria HIV/AIDS Infectious mononucleosis Lyme disease
Tissue	*Streptococcus pyogenes*	Necrotizing fasciitis

CLASSIFICATION OF MICROORGANISMS ACCORDING TO GRAM REACTION

Gram-positive	Gram-negative
Enterococcus faecalis	*Escherichia coli*
Streptococcus pyogenes or *Group A Streptococcus*	*Pseudomonas aeruginosa*
Staphylococcus epidermidis	*Klebsiella* species
Streptococcus agalactiae or *Group B Streptococcus*	*Salmonella* species
Streptococcus pneumoniae	*Shigella* species
Listeria monocytogenes	*Campylobacter* species
Clostridium perfringens	*Bacteroides* species
	Fusobacterium species

Source: Medical Assisting: Foundations and Practices by M. S. Frazier, C. Malone, and C. Morgan, Upper Saddle River, NJ: Pearson Education, Inc., 2010, p. 619. Reprinted with permission.

Gram Stain	Simple diagnostic test that identifies types of bacteria as either positive or negative based on whether or not the compounds in the cell walls stain or do not stain Gram-positive organisms retain color when stained and appear as blue/purple under the microscope Gram-negative organisms decolorize with ethyl alcohol and then take the counterstain Safranin (red) However, both gram-positive and gram-negative organisms stain with crystal violet

procedure 20-22

PERFORMING A GRAM STAIN

Objective: Prepare a slide for a Gram stain to differentiate a gram-positive organism from a gram-negative organism.

EQUIPMENT AND SUPPLIES

- Gram stain kit with decolorizer
- culture specimen
- slides
- Bunsen burner or methanol
- staining rack
- water wash bottle
- water
- immersion oil
- stopwatch
- gloves
- slide stand
- paper towels
- biohazard waste container

Note: Follow standard precautions and safety guidelines when working with body fluid samples. Take care to avoid splashing or spilling body fluids. Wipe up all spills using the guidelines established by OSHA.

METHOD

1. Perform hand hygiene and apply gloves.
2. Assemble equipment.
3. Make a smear, label it, air-dry the smear, and use heat or methanol to fix it.
4. Place the slide on the staining rack, smear side up.
5. Pour crystal violet solution all over the slide; let it stand for one minute (Figure 20-29A).

6. Tilt the slide to drain the excess crystal violet stain and rinse with water (Figure 20-29B).
7. Pour Gram iodine stain all over the slide; let it stand for one minute (Figure 20-29C).
8. Tilt the slide to drain the excess iodine and rinse with water.
9. Gently pour decolorizer with alcohol-acetone all over the slide for 15 seconds or until the color blue stops running (Figure 20-29D).
10. Rinse with water.
11. Pour safranine stain all over the slide and let it stand for 30 seconds (Figure 20-29E).
12. Tilt the slide to drain the excess safranine and rinse with water. Wipe the back of the slide (Figure 20-29F).
13. Stand the slide on end on a paper towel or in a slide drying rack, and air-dry it.

Note: Examination of a Gram-stained slide is beyond the scope of practice of the medical assistant. It should be performed by a physician or laboratory specialist.

14. Examine the slide under the microscope, using an oil immersion lens and oil.

CHARTING EXAMPLE

11/16/XX Gram stain of spec. from abscess of RT thigh prepared for physician to examine. · · · · M. King, CMA (AAMA)

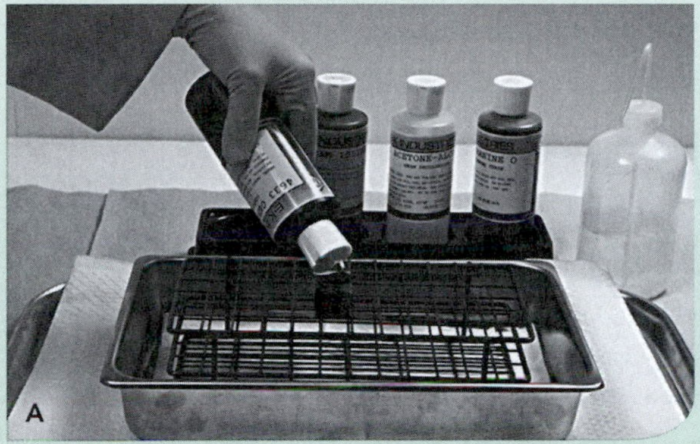

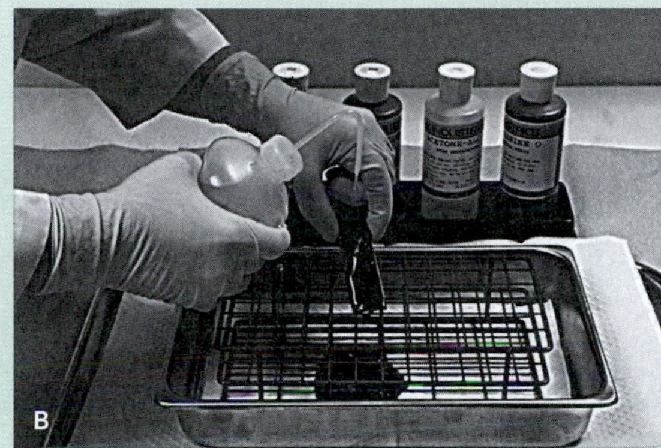

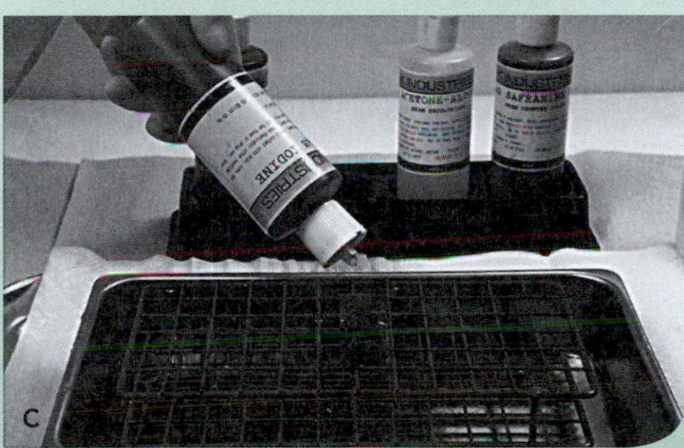

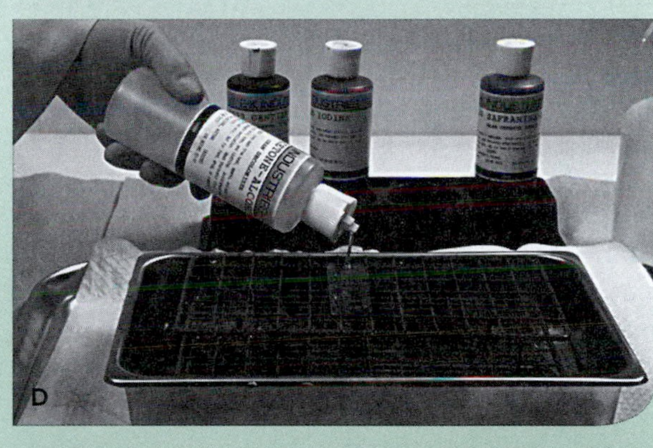

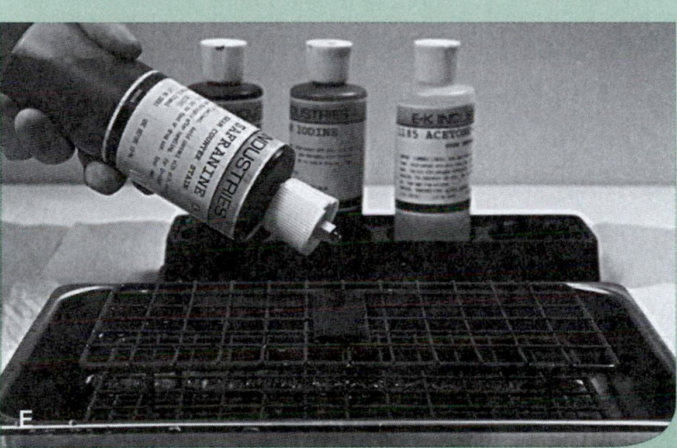

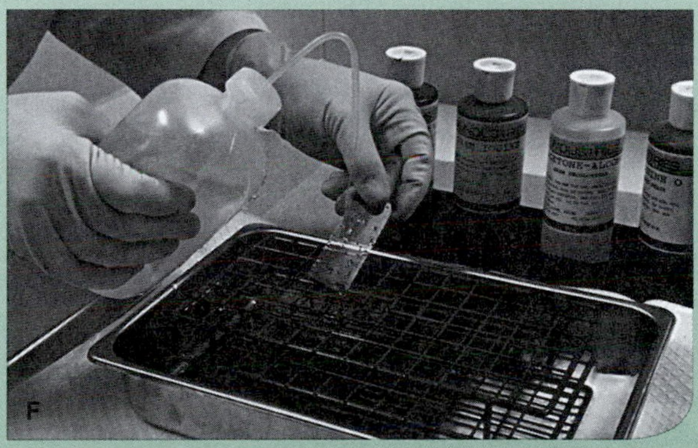

FIGURE 20-29 (A) Pour crystal violet stain over the entire slide and let it stand for one minute. (B) Tilt the slide to drain excess stain and rinse it with water. (C) Pour Gram iodine stain over the entire slide and let it stand for one minute. (D) Gently pour decolorizer with alcohol-acetone all over the slide for 15 seconds or until the blue color stops running. (E) Pour safranine stain over the entire slide and let it stand for 30 seconds. (F) Rinse with water and wipe the back of the slide.

In cases where organisms must be kept alive in order to observe motility and morphology, a wet mount, also known as a *wet prep*, may be necessary. The three methods of preparing a wet mount include the following:

Normal Saline	A drop of saline is mixed into the smear; a slip cover is placed over the specimen, and the specimen is immediately examined. This method is used to identify *Trichomonas vaginalis*.
Potassium Hydroxide	Also known as *KOH* Potassium hydroxide may be added to the specimen smear, left to sit at room temperature for 30 minutes, and then examined. This method is used to identify vaginal yeast infections.
India Ink	After spinal fluid has been centrifuged, a drop of sediment and a drop of India ink are placed together on a slide. This method is used to identify *Cryptococcus neoformans*.

procedure 20-23

PREPARING A WET MOUNT SLIDE

Objective: Prepare a wet mount slide for microscopic examination without error.

EQUIPMENT AND SUPPLIES

- clean, dry slide, frosted
- cover slip
- saline specimen from a Culturette applicator or swab
- paper/pen
- microscope
- gloves

Note: Follow standard precautions and safety guidelines when working with body fluid samples. Take care to avoid splashing or spilling body fluids. Wipe up all spills using the guidelines established by OSHA.

METHOD

1. Perform hand hygiene and apply gloves.
2. Label the dry slide with the patient's name and date.
3. Inoculate the dry slide by rolling a swab containing the specimen across the surface.
4. Place a drop of saline solution on top of the specimen.
5. Place the cover slip on top of the smeared slide.

Note: The following steps would be performed by a physician or laboratory specialist (Figure 20-30).

6. Observe the wet mount slide immediately under the microscope.
7. Special stains may be used to enhance characteristics.
8. Note what is observed, remove the slide, and dispose of it properly.
9. Remove gloves and perform hand hygiene.
10. Chart the findings in the patient's record.

CHARTING EXAMPLE

11/16/XX Wet mount prepared from vaginal swab for physician to examine. .... M. King, CMA (AAMA)

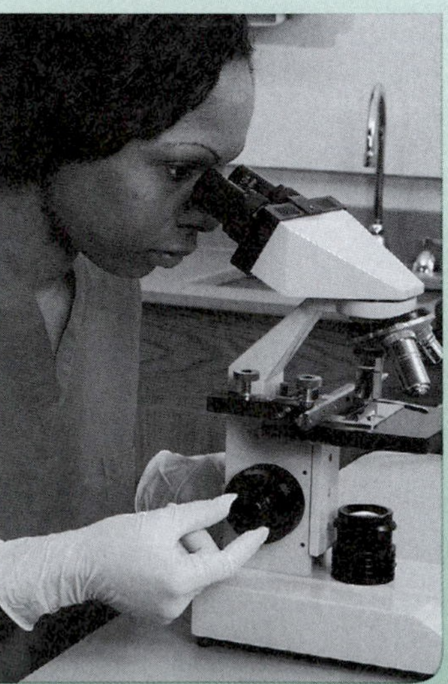

FIGURE 20-30 A medical technician examining a wet mount.

20 APPLICATION

Directions: Select the best answer for each of the following questions. Check your answers in the Answer Key at the end of the book.

1. Hematopoiesis is:
   a. Study of blood and blood-forming tissues
   b. Process that allows neutrophils to surround, swallow, and digest bacteria
   c. Normal formation or development of blood cells
   d. Process whereby worn-out cells and bacteria are destroyed
   e. Abnormal formation and development of blood cells

2. Which of the following best describes white blood cells?
   a. They contain hemoglobin.
   b. They defend against infection.
   c. They are smaller than red blood cells.
   d. They carry oxygen to the lungs.
   e. A and C

3. Platelets are:
   a. Granules in cytoplasm
   b. Largest cells in the blood
   c. Responders to allergies
   d. Smallest cells in the blood
   e. Antibody producers

4. __________ is the reaction that occurs when an antigen clumps together with an antibody.
   a. Immune response
   b. Agglutination
   c. Hematopoiesis
   d. Clotting
   e. Phagocytosis

5. The basic rules for specimen collection include the following:
   a. Screen the patient to determine if the pretest preparation was followed.
   b. Collect a specimen after beginning antibiotic treatment.
   c. Collect a specimen prior to beginning antibiotic treatment.
   d. A and B
   e. A and C

6. The most common site for a capillary puncture is:
   a. The ring finger
   b. The antecubital space
   c. The wrist
   d. The back of the hand
   e. Either C or D

7. When drawing blood by the vacuum tube method, it is important to fill the tubes in order as recommended by the CLSI. Which of the following is the correct order for the first five tubes?
   a. Yellow, light blue, red marbled, red, green
   b. Lavender, red, red marbled, yellow, light blue
   c. Dark blue, light green, green, red, light blue
   d. Yellow, light blue, red, red marbled, green
   e. Green, red marbled, red, light blue, yellow

8. The correct culture process in order for identification of microorganisms is:
   a. Identification, incubation, inoculation, inspection
   b. Inspection, identification, incubation, inoculation
   c. Identification, inspection, incubation, inoculation
   d. Inoculation, incubation, inspection, identification
   e. Incubation, identification, inoculation, inspection

9. A/An ______ separates specimens into layers by spinning.
   a. Photometer
   b. Centrifuge
   c. Hemoglobinometer
   d. Autoclave
   e. Petri dish

10. The best definition of a control sample is:
    a. A sample similar to the testing specimen, previously tested with a known value
    b. A substance required for a chemical reaction
    c. A sample used to measure the accuracy of equipment
    d. A sample taken under the observation of the physician
    e. A sample taken under the observation of the supervising clinical coordinator

11. Which test provides information about red blood cell volume?
    a. Hgb
    b. Hct
    c. Platelet
    d. Coagulation
    e. ESR

12. The normal WBC count for adults is ______.
   a. 6000–12,000
   b. 2000–4500
   c. 3500–4250
   d. 4500–11,000
   e. 5500–13,500

13. For the following question, choose the best answer. A ________ is an opportunistic pathogen that causes disease when the normal balance of flora is upset.
   a. Fungus
   b. Bacterium
   c. Virus
   d. Protozoan
   e. Parasite

14. Regarding quantitative tests, which of the following statements is not true?
   a. Performed to determine whether or not a substance is present
   b. Determines the amount of substance present
   c. Results reported out as either positive or negative
   d. May indicate the level of pregnancy hormone present
   e. Reported out using numerical values

15. Which of the following is not a WBC?
   a. Neutrophil
   b. Eosinophil
   c. Basophil
   d. Thrombocyte
   e. Lymphocyte

16. Which of the following statements best describes eosinophils?
   a. Granules in cytoplasm; combat infection by phagocytosis
   b. Granules in cytoplasm; respond to allergies and inflammation
   c. Granules in cytoplasm; contain histamine
   d. No granules in cytoplasm; produce antibodies against bacteria, viruses and pollens
   e. No granules in cytoplasm; assist in phagocytosis

17. Which of the following is not a standard-sized vacuum tube?
   a. 5 mL
   b. 7 mL
   c. 10 mL
   d. 15 mL
   e. 20 mL

18. Coagulation tests consist of which of the following?
   a. PT/PTT
   b. WBC
   c. RBC
   d. Platelets
   e. ESR

19. When performing a Gram stain, once you have poured the crystal violet over the slide, you should let it set for _______ minute(s) before draining the excess stain and rinsing with water
   a. One
   b. Two
   c. Three
   d. Four
   e. Five

20. For the following question, choose the best answer. When labeling a specimen, which of the following is not required?
   a. Patient's full name
   b. Patient's date of birth
   c. Date of collection
   d. Type of specimen
   e. Your initials

21. Under normal circumstances, when performing a manual capillary puncture, which of the following is not advised?
   a. Select either the ring or great finger on the dominant hand.
   b. After wiping the chosen site with an alcohol sponge, allow the alcohol to evaporate.
   c. Grasp the patient's hand and gently squeeze the finger 1 inch below the chosen site.
   d. Puncture the site using a quick motion.
   e. Wipe away the first drop of blood with a 2 × 2 gauze square.

22. When performing venipuncture using the Vacutainer method, which of the following is the proper angle at which to insert the needle?
   a. 15 to 20 degrees
   b. 30 degrees
   c. 45 degrees
   d. 60 degrees
   e. 90 degrees

23. Which of the following tubes is used for a CBC?
   a. Yellow
   b. Light blue
   c. Red
   d. Lavender
   e. Gray

24. Which of the following lists in correct order how to obtain a throat culture?
   a. Wash hands, identify the patient, apply gloves, remove a sterile swab from the Culturette, depress the tongue, insert the swab and roll it firmly across the back of the patient's throat area where infected, crush the internal vial of transport medium, insert the swab into a plastic vial.
   b. Wash hands, identify the patient, apply gloves, remove a sterile swab from the Culturette, depress the tongue, insert the swab and roll it firmly across the back of the patient's throat and uvula where infected, insert the swab into a plastic vial, crush the internal vial of transport medium to ensure that the swab is saturated.
   c. Wash hands, identify the patient, apply gloves, remove a sterile swab from the Culturette, insert the swab and roll it firmly across the back of the patient's throat and uvula where infected, depress the tongue, insert the swab into a plastic vial, crush the internal vial of transport medium to ensure that the swab is saturated.
   d. Identify the patient, wash hands, apply gloves, remove a sterile swab from the Culturette, depress the tongue, insert the swab and roll it firmly across the back of the patient's throat area where infected, insert the swab into a plastic vial, crush the internal vial of transport medium to ensure that the swab is saturated.
   e. Identify the patient, wash hands, apply gloves, remove a sterile swab from the Culturette, depress the tongue, insert the swab and roll it firmly across the back of the patient's throat area where infected, crush the internal vial of transport medium, insert the swab into a plastic vial.

25. Which of the following microscopes is the most common type found in physicians' offices?
   a. Electron
   b. Fluorescence
   c. Dark field
   d. Phase contrast
   e. Compound

26. When documenting the physical characteristics of urine, specifically its clarity, which of the following descriptions is not appropriate?
   a. Straw
   b. Clear
   c. Slightly cloudy
   d. Cloudy
   e. Turbid

27. When preparing a urine specimen for microscopic examination, how many drops of urine sediment should be placed on the slide?
   a. 1
   b. 2
   c. 3
   d. 4
   e. 5

28. The purpose of a BUN is:
   a. Detection of liver disease or inflammation
   b. Measures the amount of nitrogen in the blood, indicating renal function
   c. Determines how quickly the body is able to filter glucose
   d. Aids in the determination of an MI
   e. Diagnosis of several conditions, including gout

29. Regarding blood cultures, which of the following statements is not true?
   a. You may use either a blood culture medium set or a green-top vacuum tube.
   b. It is best to draw a blood sample during a febrile episode.
   c. One specimen should be drawn from the right arm and one from the left.
   d. Label the specimen(s) with the patient's name, date of draw, time of collection, and your initials.
   e. Blood specimens should be delivered to the lab within two hours.

30. When performing a blood glucose test using a glucometer, which of the following statements is not correct?
   a. Identify the patient and ensure that he or she has been fasting, if required.
   b. Wash hands, apply gloves, and turn the glucometer on.
   c. Perform a capillary puncture using a sterile lancet.
   d. Gently touch the test strip to the first drop of blood that forms on the patient's finger.
   e. Have the patient apply a drop cotton ball to the puncture site, remove gloves, wash hands, and record the results.

21 Medication and Pharmacology

CONTENTS

Applied Math Review

When calculating medication dosages, it is imperative that you have a good understanding of basic math principles. Simple math mistakes can result in incorrect dosages and in turn potentially cause harm to the patient.

MATHEMATICAL RULES AND GUIDELINES

Function	Rules	Example
Adding and Subtracting Fractions	• When adding and subtracting fractions, you must have a common denominator. • Remember to multiply the entire fraction by the correct multiplier necessary to obtain the common denominator. • Add the numerators, while the denominator remains the same. • Reduce the final answer to its simplest terms.	$\frac{1}{8} + \frac{1}{3} =$ Common denominator = 24 ***Steps:*** 1. $\frac{1}{8} \times \frac{3}{3} + \frac{1}{3} \times \frac{8}{8} =$ 2. $\frac{3}{24} + \frac{8}{24} =$ 3. $\frac{11}{24}$ $\frac{3}{5} - \frac{1}{15} =$ Common denominator = 15 ***Steps:*** 1. $\frac{3}{5} \times \frac{3}{3} - \frac{1}{15} =$ 2. $\frac{9}{15} - \frac{1}{15} =$ 3. $\frac{8}{15}$
Multiplying Fractions	• If a numerator and a denominator have a common divisor, you may cancel out those terms. • Multiply all numerators across. • Multiply all denominators across. • Reduce the final answer to its simplest terms.	$\frac{3}{5} \times \frac{10}{18} =$ ***Steps:*** 1. $\frac{(1)\cancel{3}}{(1)\cancel{5}} \times \frac{\cancel{10}^{(2)}}{\cancel{18}_{(6)}} =$ 2. $\frac{1}{1} \times \frac{2}{6} =$ 3. $\frac{2}{6}$ 4. $\frac{1}{3}$
Dividing Fractions	• Invert the second fraction of the equation, finding its reciprocal. • Multiply the numerators of the first fraction and the reciprocal. • Multiply the denominators of the first fraction and the reciprocal. • Reduce the final answer to its simplest terms.	$\frac{2}{3} \div \frac{1}{5} =$ ***Steps:*** 1. $\frac{2}{3} \times \frac{5}{1}$ 2. $\frac{10}{3}$ $\quad 3\overline{)10}^{\,3\frac{1}{3}}$ $\frac{9}{1}$ 3. $3\frac{1}{3}$

(continued)

(Continued)

Function	Rules	Example
Converting an Improper Fraction to a Mixed Number	• An improper fraction is any fraction with a numerator larger than a denominator. • Divide the numerator by the denominator. This becomes the whole number. • The remainder (if any) is then placed over the denominator to form the fractional component of the mixed number. • Reduce the fractional component to its simplest form.	$\frac{14}{6} =$ ***Steps:*** 1. $\frac{14}{6}$ 2. $6\overline{)14}$ = $2\frac{2}{6}$; 12; 2 3. $2\frac{2}{6}$ 4. $2\frac{1}{3}$
Converting a Fraction to a Decimal	• Divide the numerator by the denominator.	$\frac{2}{3} =$ ***Steps:*** $2 \div 3 = 0.67$
Adding and Subtracting Decimals	• Always line up the decimals of every number. • Add zero (0) placeholders to help keep numbers aligned.	$1.9 + 0.33 + 12.344 =$ ***Steps:*** 1.900 0.330 +12.344 14.574
Multiplying Decimals	• Multiply the numbers as normal. • Place zero (0) placeholders as needed. • Count the total number of decimal spaces to the right of the decimal point for both numbers. • Place your decimal point with this many numbers to the right of the decimal.	$12.14 \times 8.2 =$ ***Steps:*** 12.14 × 8.2 1. 2428 97120 99548 2. 99.548 (Decimal point is placed three spaces in from the right, because there are three decimal placeholders in the original equation.)
Dividing Decimals	• If it is not a whole number, move the decimal point of the divisor the necessary number of spaces to make the divisor a whole number. • If the dividend has a decimal, move it to the right the same number of places as you moved the divisor's decimal point. • Add zero (0) placeholders as necessary. • Divide as usual, and then move the decimal directly up in the quotient.	$32.4 \div 8.5 = 3.8$ ***Steps:*** $32.4 \div 8.5$ becomes $8.5\overline{)32.4}$ $8.5\overline{)32.4}$ (decimal moved) The decimal point was moved one place to the right to make 8.5 become 85, so you must move the decimal point of the dividend the same number of places so that it becomes 324 3.811 85) 324 255 690 680 100 85 150 85 Most medications only require carrying out the problem one position past the decimal point. Round up as appropriate

Function	Rules	Example
Converting a Decimal to a Fraction	• Simply place the entire number over the value of the decimal placeholder of the last digit of the number. • Remember to reduce the final answer to its simplest terms.	Convert 0.75 to a fraction. ***Steps:*** $\frac{75}{100}$ • Note that the 5 is located in the hundredths placeholder; thus, 75 is placed over 100.

DECIMAL POINT PLACE VALUES

Ones	Decimal Point	Tenths	Hundredths	Thousandths	Hundred Thousandths
1	.	0.1	0.01	0.001	0.0001

USING ZEROS WITH DECIMALS

Leading Zero	Must be used with decimal numbers less than 1 *Example*: **0**.5 mg
Trailing Zero	*Do not include a zero* after a whole number *Example*: 15.**0** mg is incorrect and should be written as 15 mg

EXAMPLES OF MATHEMATICAL EQUIVALENTS

Fraction	Ratio	Percentage	Decimal
¼	1:4	25 percent	0.25
½	1:2	50 percent	0.50
⅔	2:3	66 percent	0.66
¾	3:4	75 percent	0.75
⅞	7:8	88 percent	0.88
1/100	1:100	1 percent	0.01
1/200	1:200	0.5 percent	0.005
1/1000	1:100	0.1 percent	0.001

Dosage Calculation

WEIGHTS AND MEASURES

Two separate sets of weights and measures are used to calculate doses: the apothecary system and the metric system. Most offices and pharmacies use the metric system; however, it is important that you are familiar with the apothecary system as well.

Apothecary System	Oldest system of measurement Based on dry weight of grain (gr). 1 gr was equal to the weight of 1 grain of wheat. Also includes the following measures: • Dram (dr) • Ounce (oz) • Pound (lb) • Mimim (m) • Fluid dram (fl dr) • Fluid ounce (fl oz) • Pint (pt) • Quart (qt) • Gallon (gal) Roman numerals are used with the apothecary system for numbers 1 through 10, 15, 20, and 30. Arabic numbers are used for amounts other than those listed above. Fractions may also be used with the apothecary system.

ARABIC NUMBERS, ROMAN NUMERALS, AND APOTHECARY NOTATIONS

Arabic Number	Roman Numeral	Apothecary Notation	Arabic Number	Roman Numeral	Apothecary Notation
1	I	i, $\overline{i}$	8	VIII	viii, $\overline{viii}$
2	II	ii, $\overline{ii}$	9	IX	ix, $\overline{ix}$
3	III	iii, $\overline{iii}$	10	X	x, $\overline{x}$
4	IV	iv, $\overline{iv}$	15	XV	xv, $\overline{xv}$
5	V	v, $\overline{v}$	20	XX	xx, $\overline{xx}$
6	VI	vi, $\overline{vi}$	25	XXV	xxv, $\overline{xxv}$
7	VII	vii, $\overline{vii}$	30	XXX	xxx, $\overline{xxx}$

Metric System	Most commonly used system for dosage calculations Doses are written with the number as a decimal first, followed by the unit of measurement (e.g., 2.5 mg).

Metric Prefix	Value
kilo	1000 of a unit
hecto	100 of a unit
deka	10 of a unit
BASE UNIT	
deci	0.1 of a unit
centi	0.01 of a unit
milli	0.001 of a unit
micro	0.0001 of a unit

Figure 21-1 shows how to perform a metric conversion using the place value chart.

Kilo-	Hecto-	Deka-	Numeral w/ base unit (g, l, or m)	Deci-	Centi-	Milli-	Micro-

Example:

Convert 45.2 grams (g) to milligrams (mg).

1. Place 45.2 under the numeral/base unit

Kilo-	Hecto-	Deka-	Numeral w/ base unit (g, l, or m)	Deci-	Centi-	Milli-	Micro-
			45.2				

2. Move the decimal point to the right three times so that the base unit ends in the milli- box:

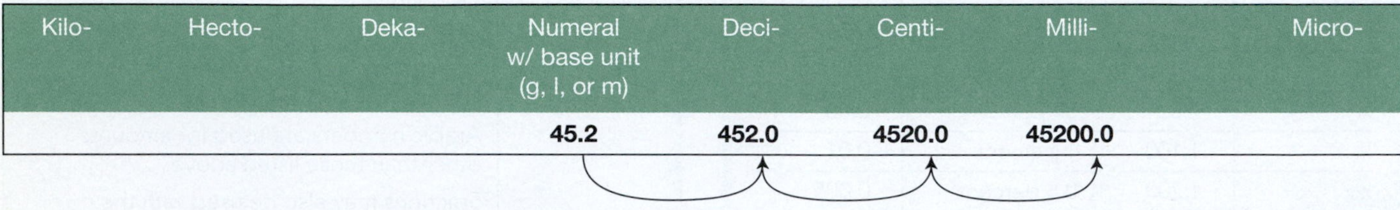

Kilo-	Hecto-	Deka-	Numeral w/ base unit (g, l, or m)	Deci-	Centi-	Milli-	Micro-
			45.2	**452.0**	**4520.0**	**45200.0**	

3. 45.2g = 45,200 mg

FIGURE 21-1 Metric conversion using the place value chart.

COMMON UNITS OF MEASURE IN THE METRIC SYSTEM

Metric Unit	Measures
Liter	Volume
Gram	Weight
Meter	Length

COMMON ABBREVIATIONS FOR WEIGHTS AND MEASURES

Apothecary System		Metric System
Symbol/Abbreviations		**Meaning**
gtt	drop	drop
♏	min	minim
	dr, ʒ	dram
	fl dr, fl ʒ	fluid dram
	oz, ℥	ounce
	fl oz, fl ℥	fluid ounce
O	pt	pint
C	gal	gallon
	gr	grain
Symbol/Abbreviations		**Meaning**
Weights		
kg		kilogram
gm		gram
mg		milligram
mcg		microgram
Symbol/Abbreviations		**Meaning**
Volume		
L		liter
mL		milliliter
cc		cubic centimeter

CALCULATING DOSAGES

Many factors are considered when calculating correct dosages for medications, including the patient's age, weight, current state of health, and other medications the patient is currently taking.

The first step when calculating dosages is to make sure that the weight and measure of the medication on hand are the same as those being prescribed. If not, you must first convert the prescription to the weight/measure you have on hand.

COMMONLY USED EQUIVALENTS FOR THE APOTHECARY AND METRIC SYSTEMS

Measure Apothecary	Equivalent Metric
1 gr	65 mg or 0.065 g
5 gr	325 mg or 0.33 g
10 gr	650 mg or 0.67 g
15 or 16 gr	1 g
15 or 16 m	1 mL or cc
1 dram	4 mL
1 oz	30 cc, 30 mL, 8 tsp, 8 drams, 2 tbsp
1 lb	450 g
1 lb	0.4536 kg
1 minim (♏)	0.06 mL
4 m	0.25 mL
Liquid Measure	
1 fl dr	4 mL
2 fl dr	8 mL
2.5 fl dr	10 mL
4 fl dr	15 mL
1 fl oz	30 mL
3.5 fl oz	100 mL
7 fl oz	200 mL
1 pt	500 mL
1 qt	1000 mL
60 gtts	4 mL

In order to calculate the correct dose for a medication, you must know what has been ordered and what is available. The following formula should be used for dosage calculation:

$$\frac{\text{Available strength}}{\text{Available amount}} = \frac{\text{Ordered Strength}}{\text{Ordered Amount}}$$

Most often the physician will provide the ordered strength and you will need to calculate the ordered amount. For example, the physician may order 25 mg to be given to the patient (ordered strength), and you will need to calculate what the ordered amount will be. This most likely will be in the form of tablets or millileters.

If the available strength is 15 mg/mL and the physician ordered 25 mg, you would need to calculate how many milliliters you would need to give in order to provide the 25 mg ordered. You may calculate the ordered amount using the following formula:

Available	Ordered
15 mg	25 mg
1 mL	?? mL

Multiply the denominator of the available medication and the numerator of the medication ordered.

(1 × 25 = 25)

Available	Ordered
15 mg	25 mg
1 mL	?? mL

Then divide the product by the numerator of the available medication:

(25/15 = 1.7)

The quotient is the amount of medication to be administered.

The math would be like this: 1 × 25 = 25/15 = 1.7

The physician orders 25 mg of a drug, and the available tablets vial contains 12.5 mg per tablet. How many tablets would you administer?

Available	Ordered
12.5 mg	25 mg
1 tablet	?? tablets

a. 1 × 25 = 25

b. 25/12.5 = 2

c. Administer 2 tablets.

The physician orders 1 gram of medication to be administered. You have 500 mg/mL on hand. How many milliliters will you administer?

Available	Ordered
500 mg	1 g
1 mL	??? mL

First, you must convert the amount ordered to the same measurement of the medication available.

1 g = 1000 mg

Available	Ordered
500 mg	1000 mg
1 mL	??? mL

(1 × 1000 = 1000)

Available	Ordered
500 mg	1000 mg
1 mL	??? mL

(1000/500 = 2)

You would administer 2 mL.

Available	Ordered
500 mg	1000 mg
1 mL	2 mL

PEDIATRIC DOSAGES

Pediatric medications and dosages are typically calculated differently than adult medications and dosages. The following table outlines the different methods, when each is used, and how to calculate it.

West's Nomogram (Figure 21-2)	Dosage based on the child's body surface area (BSA), which considers the child's height and weight Can be used for infants and children	See nomogram below To calculate a child's BSA, using a ruler, a straight line is drawn from the child's height in centimeters or inches across the columns to the child's weight in kilograms or pounds and the corresponding number where the line intersects the BSA is the number to be used for the dosage calculation.

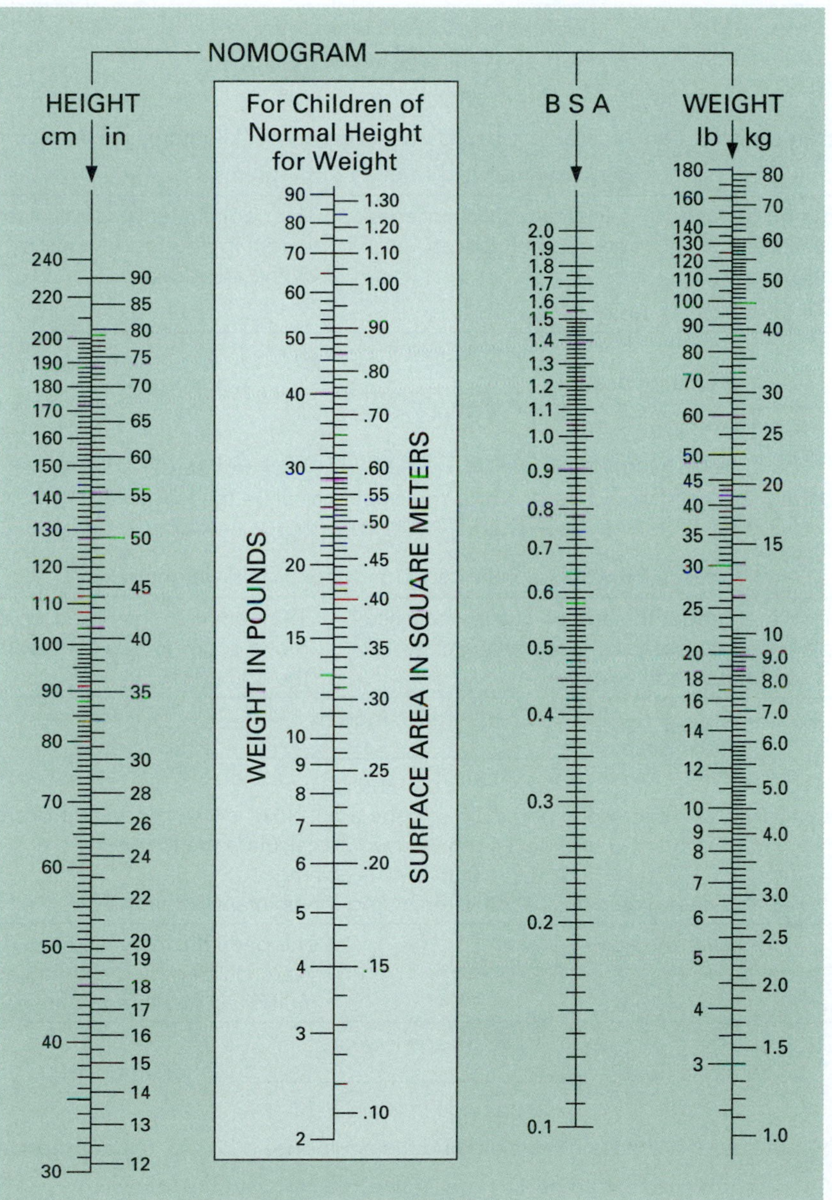

FIGURE 21-2 Nomogram chart.

(continued)

(Continued)

$$\text{Pediatric dose} = \frac{\text{BSA of child}}{\text{1.73 square meters}} \times \text{adult dose}$$

(1.73 m2 is the standard adult BSA)

Based on the nomogram example below, a child who is 74 cm and 12 kg has a BSA of 0.5.

Using this information for an adult dose of 50 mg, you would calculate the following:

0.5/1.73 = 0.29 × 50 = 14.5

In this case, you would administer 14.5 mg for a child with a BSA of 0.5.

Body Weight Method	Medications are most often ordered based on the child's weight, and the body weight method allows you to convert pounds to kilograms.	To convert a child's weight from pounds to kilograms, you must know that 1 kg = 2.2 lb.

Weight in lb/2.2 = weight in kg

A child who weighs 88 lb weighs 40 kg.

88/2.2 = 40

Most pediatric medication dosages are based on milligrams per kilogram, so it is essential that you know the child's weight in kilograms.

Clark's Rule	Most common law used in calculating child dosages because children's weight at the same age can vary significantly. Also based on the child's weight	The pediatric dose is calculated based on the child's weight in pounds, divided by 150 lb and multiplied by the adult dose.

$$\text{Pediatric dose} = \frac{\text{Child's weight in pounds}}{\text{150 lb}} \times \text{adult dose}$$

Using Clark's Rule, if a child weighed 63 lb and the adult dose is 25 mg, the appropriate dose for this child would be 10.5 mg. You would calculate the following:

63/150 = 0.42 × 25 = 10.5 mg

In this case, you would administer 10.5 mg for a child weighing 63 lb.

Fried's Law	Used for children under the age of 1 year. The calculations are based on the assumption that a child 12½ years old can take an adult dose.	The pediatric dose is based on the child's age in months, divided by 150 (months) and multiplied by the adult dose.

$$\text{Pediatric dose} = \frac{\text{Child's age in months}}{\text{150 months}} \times \text{adult dose}$$

Using Fried's Law, if an infant is 9 months old and the adult dose is 40 mg, the appropriate dose for this infant would be 2.4 mg. You would calculate the following:

9/150 = 0.06 × 40 = 2.4 mg

In this case, you would administer 2.4 mg for an infant 9 months old.

Young's Rule	Used for children over the age of 1 year	The pediatric dose is based on the child's age in years, divided by the child's age in years + 12 and multiplied by the adult dose.

$$\text{Pediatric dose} = \frac{\text{Child's age in years}}{\text{Child's age in years} + 12} \times \text{adult dose}$$

Using Young's Rule, if a child is 7 years old and the adult dose is 30 mg, the appropriate dose for this child would be 11.1 mg. You would calculate the following:

7/19 = 0.37 × 30 = 11.1 mg

In this case, you would administer 11.1 mg for a 7-year-old child.

PHARMACOLOGY TERMINOLOGY

Term	Definition
Absorption	Movement of medication from the site of administration into the bloodstream
Adverse Effect	Undesirable and potentially harmful side effect of a drug
Antagonism	Administering two medications together causes the medications to be less effective than if each one is administered separately.
Contraindication	Conditions in which the drug should not be used
Cumulative Effect	Occurs when the next dose of medication is given before the previous dose has had time to be metabolized/excreted
Dependence	Psychological or physiological need to take a particular drug
Distribution	When medication is moved from the bloodstream to the intended body tissue(s)
Drug Action	Drugs cause specific effects on the body by causing changes in cells, either on the surface or within the cells themselves Four main drug actions: • Depressing • Stimulating • Destroying • Replacing
Drug Interaction	Result of medications interacting with other medications or with the diet; can be desirable or undesirable
Efficacy	How well a medication treatment works
Excretion	Removal of waster products. Most medications are excreted through the kidneys and large intestine.
Half-Life	Amount of time required for a medication's concentration to be reduced by 50% once administered
Idiosyncrasy	When the opposite effect of what was intended occurs
Metabolism	Breakdown and conversion of drugs to a water-soluble compound that can be excreted by the body
Over the Counter (OTC)	Medications that can be purchased without a prescription
Pharmacodynamics	Study of the actions of drugs
Pharmacokinetics	Study of drugs during • Absorption • Distribution • Metabolism • Excretion
Pharmacology	Study of medications and drugs
Pharmacy	Preparing and dispensing medications
Placebo	Inactive substance given as a medication but has no pharmacologic effect
Polypharmacy	Concurrent administration of many drugs
Potentiation	Effects of one drug increase the effects of another drug.
Prophylactic	Preventing disease
Synergism	Two drugs administered at the same time produce a more powerful response than if each medication is administered separately.
Teratogens	Drugs that cause birth defects and should not be administered to pregnant women
Therapeutic Effect	The desired or anticipated effect of a medication: the reason the medication is administered
Tolerance	Occurs when larger doses are required to produce the same effects as the normal dose
Toxicology	The study of poisons

COMMONLY USED PHARMACOLOGY ABBREVIATIONS

Abbreviation	Meaning
	at
ā	before
Aa	of each
ac	before meals
ad lib	as desired
alt dieb	alternate days
alt hor	alternate hours
alt noc	alternate nights
am, AM	morning
amt	amount
ante	before
aq	aqueous (water)
ba	barium
bid	twice a day
C	100
c	with
cap(s)	capsule(s)
DC, d/c, and disc	discontinue
dil	dilute
disp	dispense
dr	dram
dx	diagnosis
elix	elixir
emul	emulsion
et	and
ext	extract/external
Fe	iron
fl	fluid
G	gauge
G	gram
gal	gallon
gr	grain
gt	1 drop
gtt	2 or more drops
H	hour/hypodermic
IM	intramuscular
Inj	injection
IV	intravenous
K	potassium
kg	kilogram
L	liter
liq	liquid
mcg	microgram
mg	milligram
mL	milliliter
mm	millimeter
noct	night
non rep	Do not repeat
NPO	Nothing by mouth
NS	normal saline
p̄	after
PR	per rectum
prn	as needed
pt	pint
pulv	powder
q	every
qhs	every night
R	right
Rx	take
s̄	without
Sig.	Label as follows/ directions
SL	under the tongue
SOB	shortness of breath
Sol	solution
ss	one-half
stat	at once/immediately
SubQ	subcutaneous
subling	sublingual
suppos	suppository
susp	suspension
syr	syrup
T, tbsp	tablespoon
Tab	tablet
tid	3 times a day
tinc, tr	tincture
top	apply topically
tsp	teaspoon
ung	ointment
UT	under the tongue
ut dict UD	as directed
wt	weight

Drugs

Drugs are chemical substances that are used in diagnosing, treating, curing, and preventing disease and are derived from plants, animals, minerals, and chemicals.

One medication may be known by three different names: its chemical name; generic, or nonproprietary, name, and its trade, or proprietary name.

TYPES OF MEDICATION NAMES

Chemical Name	Official pharmaceutical name and based on the chemical composition of the drug
Generic or Nonproprietary Name	Also known as the *common name* Never capitalized A pharmaceutical name used by all manufacturers that produce the medication
Trade, Brand, or Proprietary Name	Registered by the manufacturer for use only by that manufacturer First letter is always capitalized

CLASSES

Drug classifications are listed in the following table.

DRUG CLASSIFICATIONS

Classes and Examples	Main Functions
Alzheimer treatment: Cognex, Aricept	Stimulate nerve transmitters as a means of improving memory and behavior.
Analgesics, narcotic: morphine, Demerol, codeine, oxycontin, diladid, Duragesic, Darvon	Relieve severe pain, including postoperative pain, myocardial pain, pain from trauma and terminal illness.
Analgesics, non-narcotic or non-opioid: acetaminophen, aspirin, ibuprofen, naproxen	Relieve minor to moderate pain and chronic pain.
Antiallergic: cromolyn (Intal)	Used prophylactically to prevent asthma attacks and associated bronchospasms, coughing, and wheezing.
Antianxiety: Valium, Xanax, Ativan, Tranxene	Relieve anxiety, some psychosomatic disorders, muscle tension, nausea and vomiting.
Antiarrhythmic agents: atenolol (Tenormin), propanolol (Inderal), verapamil (Isoptin, Calan), Topril	Treat arrhythmias and restore normal heartbeat.
Antibiotics: penicillin (ampicillin, amoxicillin, Staphcillin, Unipen, Geocillin, Pipracil); cephalosporins (Duricef, Keflex, Cecloe, Suprax, Rocephin); aminoglycosides (Amikin, Garamycin, Nebcin); tetracyclines (Vibramycin Terramycin, Minocin); sulfonamide antimicrobials (Sulfonamide, Sulamyd, Gantanol, Gantrisin); macrolides (erythromycin, Zithromax, Biaxin, Dynabac); fluroquinolone antimicrobials (Cipro)	Treat bacterial infections.
Anticoagulants: dicumarol, warfarin sodium (Coumadin), heparin sodium	Prevent or delay blood clots from forming. Also prescribed to treat deep vein thrombosis and other thrombosis conditions.
Anticonvulsants, antiepileptics: Dilantin, Zarontin, Tegretol, phenobarbital, Valium, Depakene, Mysoline, Klonopin, Neurontin, Keppra, Zarontin, Lyrica	Prevent seizures, treat and halt seizures in progress. Barbiturates used in all forms of epilepsy; Dilantin, Keppra, Neurontin for grand mal seizures; Zarontin for petit mal seizures. Neurontin also used to treat post-herpetic neuralgia and some nerve pain.
Antidepressants, tricyclic agents: Elavil, Triavil, Trifanil, Pamelor; **SSRI,** Prozac, Paxil, Zoloft; **MAO inhibitor,** Nardil	Treat depression; often referred to as mood elevators.
Antiemetics: Phenergan, Tigan, Reglan, Compazine, Zofran	Prevent vomiting, relieve nausea.
Antifungal: fluconazole (Diflucan), Monistat 3, Mycelex vaginal tabs, Vagistat-1, griseofulvin (Grisactin), tolnaftate (Tinactin)	Treat candidiasis, coccidiodomycosis, tinea capitis, tinea pedis, and other miscellaneous fungal infections.

(continued)

(Continued)

Classes and Examples	Main Functions
Antihistamines: diphenhydramine (Benadryl), chlorpheniramine (Chlor-Trimeton), clemastine (Tavist), fexofenadine (Allegra), loratadine (Claritin), cetirizine (Zyrtec). (See Histaminic II blockers)	Relieve symptoms of allergic response by blocking histamine reactions in tissue. Often used to treat runny nose and watery eyes connected with hay fever and other allergies.
Antihyperlipidemic or hypolipidemic drugs: simvastin (Zocor), pravastatin (Pravachol), atorvastatin (Lipitor), ezetimibe (Zetia)	Treat hyperlipidema by reducing blood cholesterol levels; statin drugs may reverse some plaque accumulation in blood vessels.
Antihypertensive agents: ramipril (Altace), doxazosin (Cardura), benzothiazepine (Cardizem), clonidine (Catapres), methyldopa (Aldoril)	Treat hypertension. Altace inhibits angiotension-converting enzymes; Cardura dilates vessels.
Anti-inflammatory agents: *NSAIDS:* aspirin, acetaminophen (Tylenol), ibuprofen (Motrin, Advil), naproxen (naprosyn, Aleve), nabumetone (Relafen), celecoxib (Celebrex), valdecoxib (Bextra). *Steroids:* prednisone	Treat conditions caused by inflammation of the muscles and joints.
Antineoplastic agents: fluorouracil (5-FU), cyclophosphamide (Cytoxan), methotrexate (Folex)	Chemotherapy prescribed to treat cancer and inhibit growth of neoplasms. Often used before surgery or radiation to shrink tumors or as adjunct therapy with surgery or radiation.
Antiparasitic: Vermox, Biltricide, Antiminth, Pin-Rid, Mintezol	Treat parasitic worm infections.
Anti-Parkinson's drugs: Symmetrel, Sinemet, Cogentin, Kemadrin, Artane	Treat symptoms of Parkinson's by increasing level of dopamine or dopaminergic activity. Anticholinergic drugs reduce activity of ACH. Goal is to stop or moderate tremors, muscle spasms, and muscle rigidity.
Antipruritic: diphenhydramine (Benadryl), calamine lotion, corticosteroid ointments and creams, hydroxyzine HCl (Atarax), clemastine (Tavist)	Treat itching. Some used directly on skin, others systemic.
Antipsychotic drugs: Thorazine, Haldol, Eskalith, Risperdal, Mellari, Prolixin	Treat symptoms of psychosis and severe neurosis. Lithium levels must be routinely monitored. Eskalith is a lithium preparation used to treat bipolar disorders.
Antipyretic agents: acetaminophen, aspirin, ibuprofen, naproxen	Lower elevated body temperature.
Antispasmodics: atropine, belladonna, Robinul, Pro-Banthine, Bentyl, Zelmac	Treat hypermotility in GI tract.
Antitussive drugs: codeine sulfate, dextromethorphan (Romilar, Robitussin DM, Benylin, Triaminic)	Treat or suppress cough.
Antiulcer treatment: Biaxin, Amozil	Peptic ulcer treatment; eliminates *H. pylori* from stomach
Antivirals: amantadine, rimantadine, ganciclovir, ribravirin, acyclovir, famciclovir, trifluridine, valacuclovir, vidarabine; **for HIV,** didanosine, delavirdine, nelfinavir, nevirapine, zalcitabine	Treat viral infections including influenza, CMV retinitis, RSV syncytial virus infections, herpes zoster, genital herpes, herpes simplex, keratitis, HIV (drugs used to treat HIV are fairly new; success uncertain).
Asthma prophylactics: cromolyn sodium	Used before exposure to allergen to prevent allergic reaction.
Bronchodilators: Proventil, Theo-Dur	Relax smooth muscle in bronchi and slow or stop bronchial spasm.
Cardiac glycosides: digitoxin (Digitoline, Crystodigin), digoxin (Lanoxin)	Slow and strengthen the heartbeat. Used in treatment of congestive heart failure.
Cathartics and laxatives: CoLyte, mineral oil, citrate of magnesia, Dulcolax, castor oil, Surfak, Serutan	Stimulate evacuation of the bowel.

Classes and Examples	Main Functions
Contraceptives: Ovral, Triphasic	Prevent pregnancy.
Decongestants: Afrin, Sudafed	Used to constrict the nasal membrane to open air passageways. Constricts nasal mucosal vessels.
Diuretics: Lasix, Bumex, HydroDIURIL	Used to treat fluid retention, CHF, hypertension.
Expectorants: Robitussin, Organidin	Increases respiratory secretions, liquefies secretions for easier expectoration.
General anesthetics: thiopental Na (Pentothal), midazolam (Versed), methohexital (Brevital)	Produce loss of sensation for surgical, dental, and other procedures. General anesthesia induces loss of consciousness.
Hemostatic/coagulants: menadiol sodium (Synkavite), phytonadione (AquaMEPHYTON, vitamin K)	Increase coagulating ability of blood, treat hemorrhage and excessive or uncontrolled bleeding.
Histaminic II blockers (antagonists): Tagamet, Axid, Zantac, Pepcid	Treat peptic ulcers; also reduce gastric acid secretion by blocking histaminic II receptors.
Hormone replacement therapy: Premarin, Estrace, Provera, Prempro	Treat symptoms of menopause.
Hypoglycemic agents: Glucotrol, Glynase, Diabeta, Glucophage	Stimulate production of insulin by pancreas.
Hypnotics/sedatives: Amytal, Seconal, Noctec, Dalmane, Halcion, Ambien, Restoril, Lunesta	Promote rest and sleep.
Insulin: NPH, Humulin	Replaces insulin not produced by pancreas.
Local anesthetics: lidocaine (Xylocaine), procaine (Novocaine), bupivacaine (Marcaine)	Produce regional or local anesthesia for specific area of body.
Platelet inhibitors: aspirin, dipyridamole (Persantine), clopidogrel (Plavix)	Prevent platelet aggregation. Usually prescribed in combination with aspirin for better effect.
Proton pump inhibitors: Prilosec, Prevacid, Nexium, Aciphex	Treat peptic ulcers; reduce gastric acid secretion by blocking enzyme responsible for secreting hydrochloric acid.
Thrombolytics: alteplase (Activase), streptokinase (Streptase), tenectoplase (tissue plasminogen activator, TPA)	Dissolve blood clots, especially in MIs and CVAs.
Thyroid medications: antithyroid (Tapazole, propylthiouracil) and thyroid replacement (Synthroid)	Inhibit production of thyroid hormone when too much is produced; replacement therapy when inadequate amounts are produced.
Vasoconstrictors: norepinephrine (Levophed), epinephrine (Adrenalin)	Treat shock; primary action is constriction of vessels.
Vasodilators: nitroglycerin (Nitro-stat), isoxsuprine (Isordil), hydralazine (Apresoline), sodium nitroprusside (Nipride)	Treat angina and hypertensive crisis.

Source: Medical Assisting: Foundations and Practices by M. S. Frazier, C. Malone, and C. Morgan, Upper Saddle River, NJ: Pearson Education, Inc., 2010, p. 510. Reprinted with permission.

Drugs with the potential for abuse, such as narcotics, addictive, or habit-forming drugs, and drugs with hallucinogenic capabilities have been identified in the Federal Controlled Substances Act. This act sets forth guidelines for storage, record keeping, and safe keeping of these controlled substances, which are also known as *schedule drugs*.

SCHEDULE FOR CONTROLLED SUBSTANCES

Level	Description	Comment
Schedule I	Highest potential for addiction and abuse Not accepted for medical use *Examples:* cocaine, heroin, LSD	Not prescribed drugs
Schedule II	High potential for addiction and abuse Accepted for medical use in the United States *Examples:* codeine, morphine, opium, and secobarbital	A Drug Enforcement Administration (DEA)–licensed physician must complete the required triplicate prescription forms entirely written in his or her own handwriting. The prescription must be filled within seven days, and it may not be refilled. In an emergency, the physician may order a limited amount of the drug by telephone. These drugs must be stored under lock and key if they are kept on office premises. The law requires that a dispensing record of these drugs be kept on file for two years.
Schedule III	Moderate to low potential for addiction and abuse *Examples:* butabarbital, anabolic steroids, APC with codeine	A DEA number is not required to write a prescription for these drugs, but the physician must handwrite the order. Five refills, which must be indicated on the prescription form, are allowed during a six-month period. Only the physician can give telephone orders to the pharmacist for these drugs.
Schedule IV	Lower potential for addiction and abuse than Schedule III drugs *Examples:* chloral hydrate, phenobarbital, diazepam	A medical assistant may write the prescription order for the physician, but it must be signed by the physician. Five refills are allowed over a six-month period.
Schedule V	Low potential for addiction and abuse *Examples:* low-strength codeine combined with other drugs to form a cough suppressant	Inventory records must be maintained on these drugs.

FORMS

DRUG FORMS AND ROUTES OF ADMINISTRATION

Form	Route
Aerosol	Inhalation
Caplets	Oral
Capsules	Oral
Elixir	Oral
Liniment	Topical
Lotion	Topical
Lozenges	Oral
Ointment	Topical

Form	Route
Pills	Oral
Powders	Topical
Skin patch	Topical
Spansules	Oral
Spray	Oral, topical
Suppository	Rectal, vaginal
Syrup	Oral
Tablet	Oral

USES Medications may be referred to based on how the medication is used. See the following table for examples of these types of terms.

Type of Use	Why Used	Example
Diagnostic	Diagnose disease	Iodine used for radiographic procedures
Palliative	Keep the patient comfortable	Morphine for terminal cancer patients
Preventive	Prevent certain conditions	Vaccines
Replacement	Replace substances that the body is not able to produce at sufficient levels	Synthroid for patients with thyroid disease
Therapeutic	Cure disease	Antibiotics to cure pneumonia

DRUG ACTIONS

The reactions to medications may vary from patient to patient as well as each time a particular patient takes a medication. The factors that contribute to a patient's response to medication are as follows:

- Age
- Size
- Diet
- Sex
- Genetic factors
- Pathological conditions
- Psychological factors
- Route of administration
- Time of administration
- Drug-taking history
- Environment

SIDE EFFECTS

Most medications have some type of side effect; some are desirable and others are undesirable. These effects are different than the desired therapeutic effect of the medication.

DRUG INTERACTIONS

When two or more medications (by prescription or OTC) are taken, there is a possibility that a drug interaction may occur. A drug interaction occurs when the effects of one medication modify those of the other medication(s). The following terms are defined in the pharmacology terms table on page 369 with examples of drug interaction:

- Antagonism
- Potentiation
- Synergism

Most Commonly Used Medications

See Box 21-1 and the table showing the fifty most frequently administered drugs on the next page.

Box 21-1 The Top 50

An excellent way to stay current in pharmacology is to find out which drugs are most commonly prescribed. *Pharmacy Times* publishes a list of the 50 most frequently prescribed drugs in its April issue each year. Peruse the list, check previous years' lists, and see if you can spot any trends. This will give you a snapshot of where drug therapy has been and where it is now.

Source: Medical Assisting: Foundations and Practices by M. S. Frazier, C. Malone, and C. Morgan, Upper Saddle River, NJ: Pearson Education, Inc., 2010, p. 509. Reprinted with permission.

FIFTY FREQUENTLY ADMINISTERED DRUGS

Brand Name	Type
1. Amoxil	antibiotic
2. Lanoxin	cardiotonic
3. Zantac	antiulcer
4. Xanax	tranquilizer
5. Premarin	hormone (estrogen)
6. Cardizem	cardiotonic
7. Ceclor	antibiotic
8. Synthroid	hormone (thyroid)
9. Seldane	antihistamine
10. Tenormin	beta blocker
11. Vasotec	antihypertensive
12. Tagamet	antiulcer
13. Naprosyn	anti-inflammatory (nonsteroidal)
14. Capoten	antihypertensive
15. Ortho-Novum 7/7/7	synthetic hormone
16. Dyazide	diuretic
17. Ortho-Novum	synthetic hormone
18. Proventil	bronchodilator
19. Tylenol with codeine	analgesic (narcotic)
20. Procardia	calcium channel blocker
21. Calan	calcium channel blocker
22. Ventolin	bronchodilator
23. Inderal	beta blocker
24. Halcion	sedative
25. Theo-Dur	bronchodilator
26. Lopressor	beta blocker
27. Lasix	diuretic
28. Voltaren	anti-inflammatory (nonsteroidal)
29. Darvocet-N	analgesic (narcotic)
30. Dilantin	anticonvulsant
31. Monistat	antibiotic (antifungal)
32. Augmentin	antibiotic (penicillin)
33. Micronase	oral hypoglycemic agent
34. Feldene	anti-inflammatory (nonsteroidal)
35. Micro-K	potassium supplement
36. Provera	hormone (progestin)
37. Motrin	anti-inflammatory (nonsteroidal)
38. Mevacor	cholesterol-lowering agent
39. Triphasil	synthetic hormone
40. Prozac	antidepressant
41. Lo/Ovral	synthetic hormone
42. Valium	tranquilizer
43. Retin-A	antiacne agent
44. Cipro	antibiotic
45. E-Mycin	antibiotic
46. Maxzide	diuretic
47. Coumadin	anticoagulant
48. Carafate	antiulcer
49. Timoptic	beta blocker
50. Slow-K	potassium supplement

Reading and Writing a Prescription

The parts of the prescription are listed below and shown in Figure 21-3.

PARTS OF PRESCRIPTION

Superscription	Patient's name, address, age, and date
Inscription	Name of the medication and dosage
Subscription	Directions to the pharmacist on how to mix the drug and how much to provide the patient
Signa (sig)	Instructions on how the patient is to take the medication
Physician's name, address, telephone number, and DEA number	Usually preprinted on the prescription pad
Number of Refills	In addition to the initial amount on the prescription, the number of times the patient may refill the prescription
Dispense as Written (DAW)	My be included if the physicians wants the patient to have a brand-name medication only

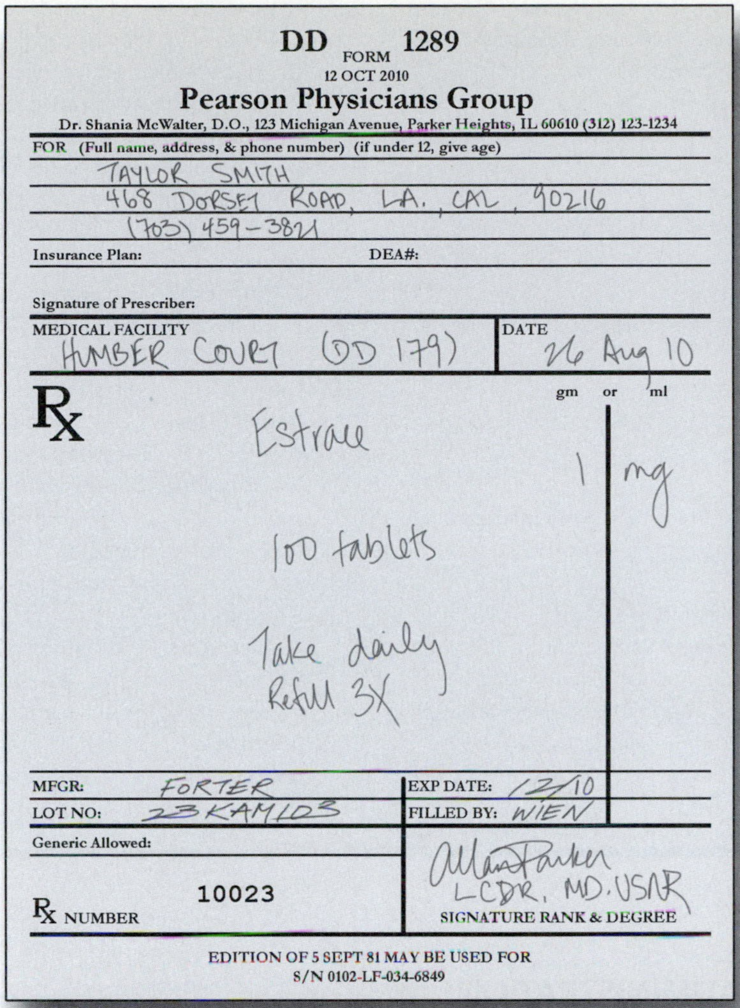

DD FORM 1289
12 OCT 2010
Pearson Physicians Group
Dr. Shania McWalter, D.O., 123 Michigan Avenue, Parker Heights, IL 60610 (312) 123-1234
FOR (Full name, address, & phone number) (if under 12, give age)
TAYLOR SMITH
468 DORSET ROAD, LA., CAL, 90216
(703) 459-3821
Insurance Plan: DEA#:
Signature of Prescriber:
MEDICAL FACILITY HUMBER COURT (DD 179) DATE 26 Aug 10
Rx gm or ml
Estrace 1 mg
100 tablets
Take daily
Refill 3X
MFGR: FORTER EXP DATE: 12/10
LOT NO: 23KAMLO3 FILLED BY: WIEN
Generic Allowed:
Rx NUMBER 10023
Allan Parker LCDR, MD, USAR
SIGNATURE RANK & DEGREE
EDITION OF 5 SEPT 81 MAY BE USED FOR
S/N 0102-LF-034-6849

FIGURE 21-3 The parts of a prescription include the superscription, inscription, subscription and signa.

Preparing and Administering Medications

Box 21-2 Guidelines for Medication Administration

1. Medications/drugs can only be administered to a patient under the supervision of a licensed physician. To do otherwise is considered "practicing medicine without a license." The medication order must be written and signed on the patient's medical record by the physician.
2. The medical assistant acts as the liaison or intermediary between the physician and the patient. Some of his or her duties include ordering, storing, rotating, and checking expiration dates on medications.
3. Medications must be checked three times before administration as follows:
   - Before medication is removed from the medication cabinet
   - Before medication is poured, drawn up into a syringe, or placed in a medication cup
   - Before medication is returned to the cabinet
4. Medications cannot be returned to the container once they have been removed. If they are not administered, they must be discarded.
5. Remember the "ten rights" for administering medications. The first six rights are:
   - Right patient
   - Right medication
   - Right dosage
   - Right route
   - Right time
   - Right documentation

It is recommended that you consider four additional rights of medication administration:

- Right client education
- Right to refuse
- Right assessment
- Right evaluation.

6. Keep a record of all allergies on the patient's medical record. Often these allergies are noted on the front of the medical record as well as within it.
7. The documentation on the patient's medical record must include the following:
   a. Name of medication
   b. Dosage
   c. Route of administration
   d. Site of administration
   e. Signature of the person administering the medication, along with initials designating the person's status (e.g., CMA or RMA (AMT))
8. All narcotics must be documented in a record maintained for that purpose. This is referred to as *logging a narcotic.* Every narcotic must be accounted for fully.
9. Be careful to administer the medication by the correct route. Methods of administration include these:
   a. Oral (by mouth)
   b. Sublingual (under the tongue)
   c. Buccal (in the cheek)
   d. Rectal (inserted into the anal cavity)
   e. Vaginal (inserted into the vaginal canal)
   f. Parenteral (by injection)
   g. Topical (applied to the skin)
   h. Inhalation (by breathing the medication)

   Medical assistants do not administer medications by the following routes:
   a. Intrathecal (into the meningeal space)
   b. Intracavity (into a body cavity)
   c. Intravenous (IV) (into a vein)
10. Medication labels should be clean and readable. If they become soiled or unreadable or fall off the container, they must be discarded.
11. If you are not familiar with a particular medication, you must look it up in the *Physicians' Desk Reference* (*PDR*). Never violate this rule.
12. Know the side effects of the medication you are administering.
13. Always advise the patient to take the complete number of doses ordered in the prescription. This is especially important when using antibiotics.
14. Inform the patient that the medication should be used only by him or her—the person for whom it was prescribed.

NONPARENTERAL ADMINISTRATION

METHODS FOR NONPARENTERAL ADMINISTRATION OF DRUGS

Method	Description
Eardrops	Placed directly into the ear canal to relieve pain or treat infection.
Eyedrops	Placed into the eye to control eye pressure in glaucoma Also administered this way during eye examinations to dilate the pupil of the eye for better examination of the interior of the eye Also used to treat infections
Inhalation	Inhaled directly into the nose and mouth. Aerosol sprays are administered by this route.
Oral	Taken by mouth and swallowed by the patient
Rectal	Introduced directly into the rectal cavity in the form of suppositories or solution. Drugs may have to be administered by this route if the patient is unable to take them by mouth due to nausea, vomiting, or surgery of the mouth.
Sublingual or Buccal	Placed under the lip or tongue (sublingual) or between the cheek and gum (buccal). Nitroglycerin for anginal pain is administered this way.
Topical	Applied directly to the skin or mucous membranes in ointment, cream, or lotion form Used to treat skin infections and eruptions Transdermal patches are also used; examples include Nicotrol, Estraderm, and Nicoderm.
Vaginal	Inserted or spread vaginally to treat vaginal yeast infections and other irritations

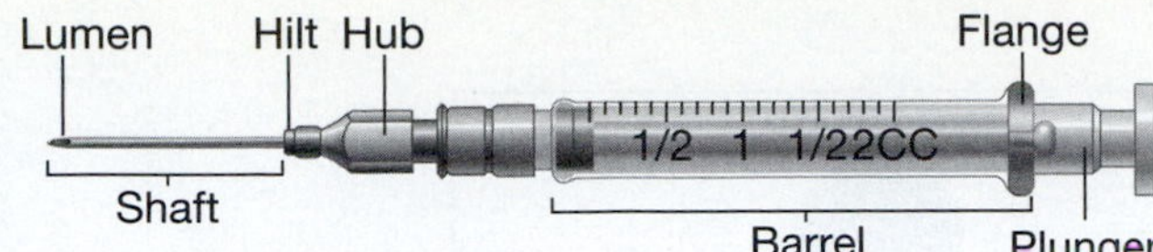

FIGURE 21-4 Parts of a syringe.

Lumen	The bore of the needle Determines the gauge of the needle The higher the gauge, the smaller the lumen.
Shaft	The length of the hollow needle
Hilt	Connects the shaft to the hub
Hub	Connects the needle to the syringe
Barrel	Holds the liquid in the syringe
Flange	Prevents the needle from rolling
Plunger	Expels medication from the syringe when pushed When pulled, allows medication to fill the syringe

PARENTERAL ADMINISTRATION

Medications administered via the parenteral route require the use of a syringe. It is important to understand the parts of the syringe so that it will be used correctly (Figure 21-4). See Tables (on pages 379–382) and Procedure 21-1.

METHODS FOR PARENTERAL ADMINISTRATION OF DRUGS

Method	Description
Intraarticular	Injection into a joint. Corticosteroids are often injected into the joint of the knee or toes.
Intradermal	Also known as an *ID* injection A very shallow injection within the top layer of skin (Figures 21-5 and 21-6). This method is commonly used in skin testing for allergies and tuberculosis.

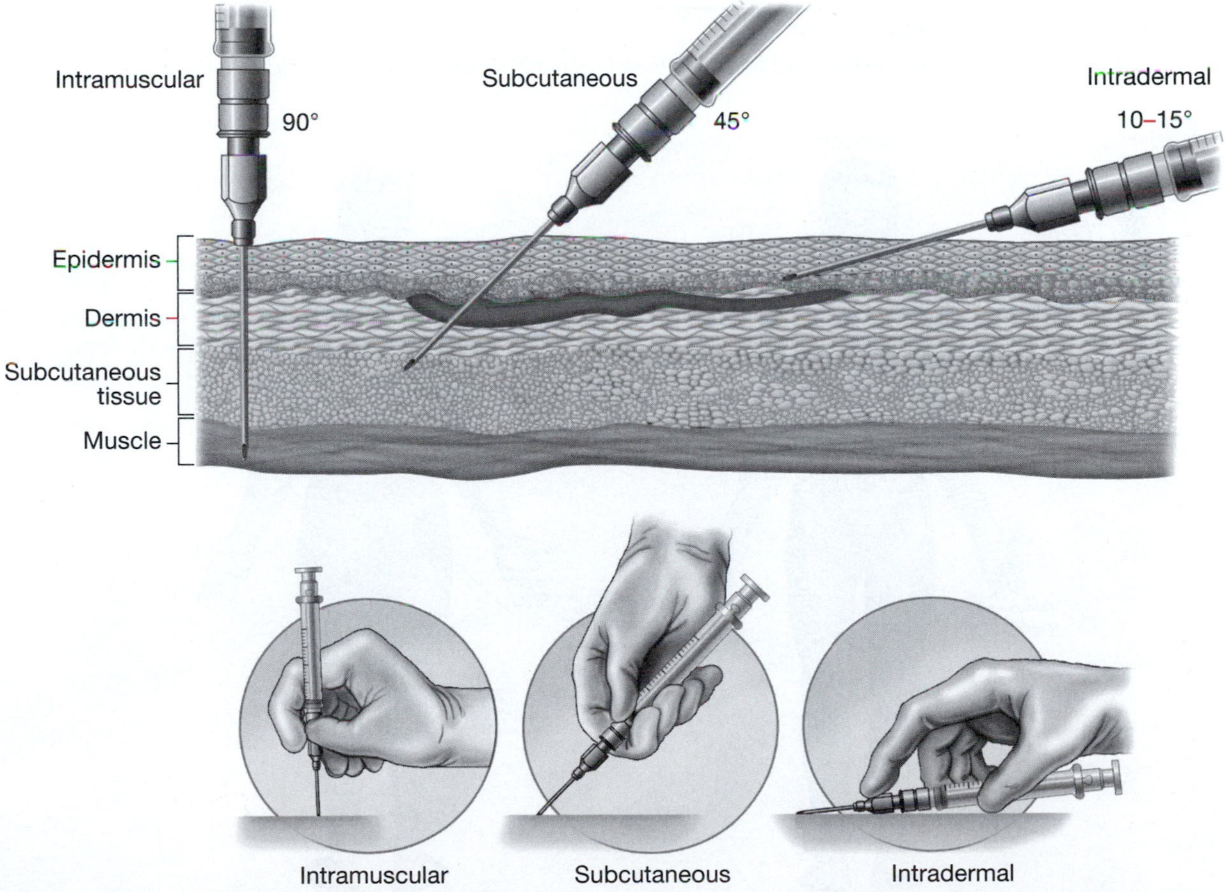

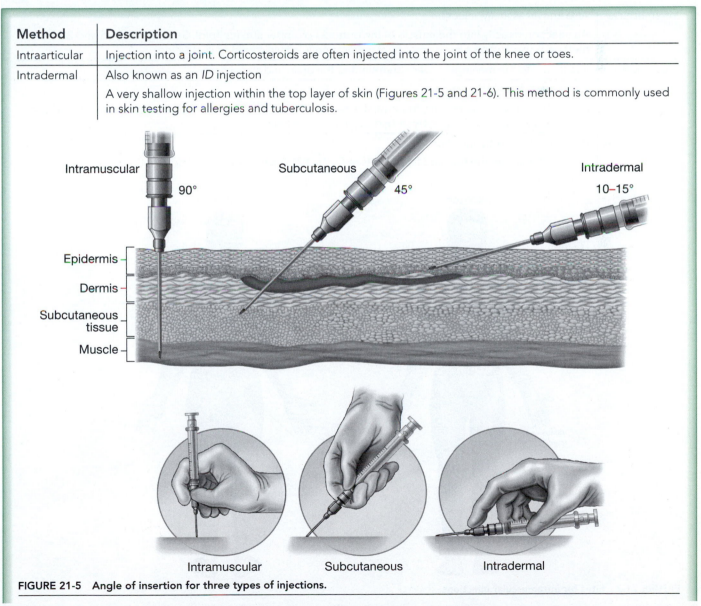

FIGURE 21-5 Angle of insertion for three types of injections.

(continued)

(Continued)

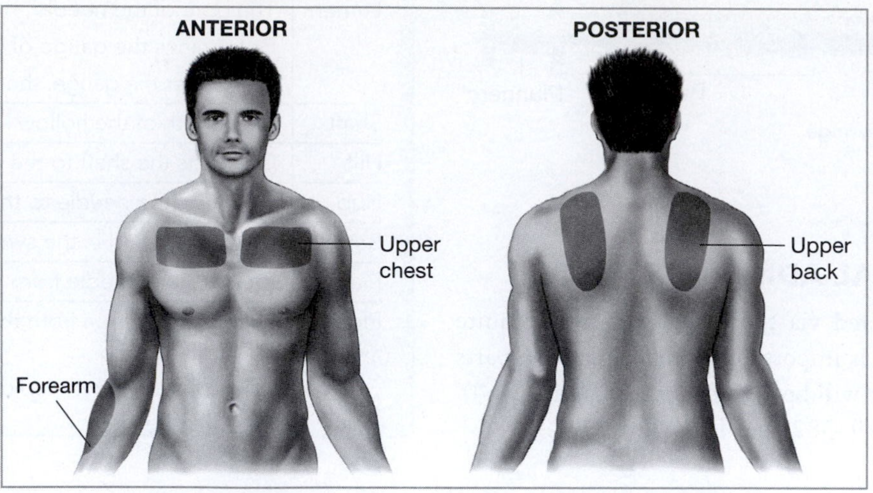

FIGURE 21-6 Intradermal skin injection sites.

Intramuscular	Also known as an *IM* injection An injection directly into the muscle of the buttocks or upper arm (deltoid). See Figures 21-5 and 21-7. This method is used when a large amount of medication is administered or is irritating.
Intrathecal	Injection into the meningeal space surrounding the brain and spinal cord
Intravenous	Also known as an *IV* injection An injection into the veins. This route can be set up so that there is continuous administration of medication, usually after a major surgery or during a major procedure.
Subcutaneous	Also known as an *SC* injection An injection under the skin and fat layers (see Figures 21-5 and 21-8). The middle of the upper, outer arm is usually used.

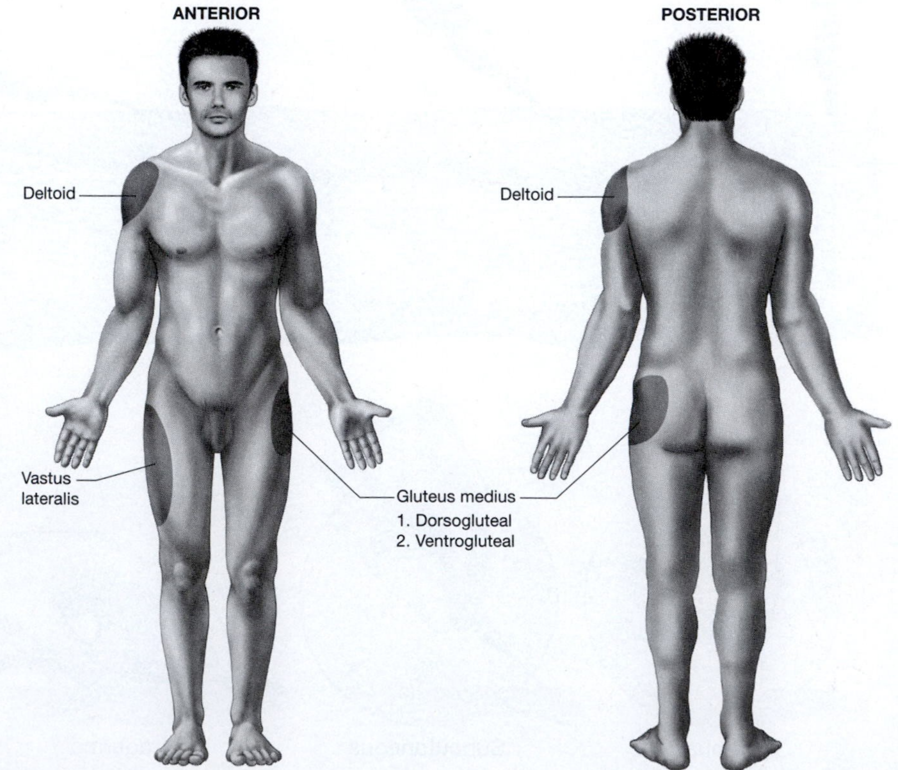

FIGURE 21-7 Sites for intramuscular injections.

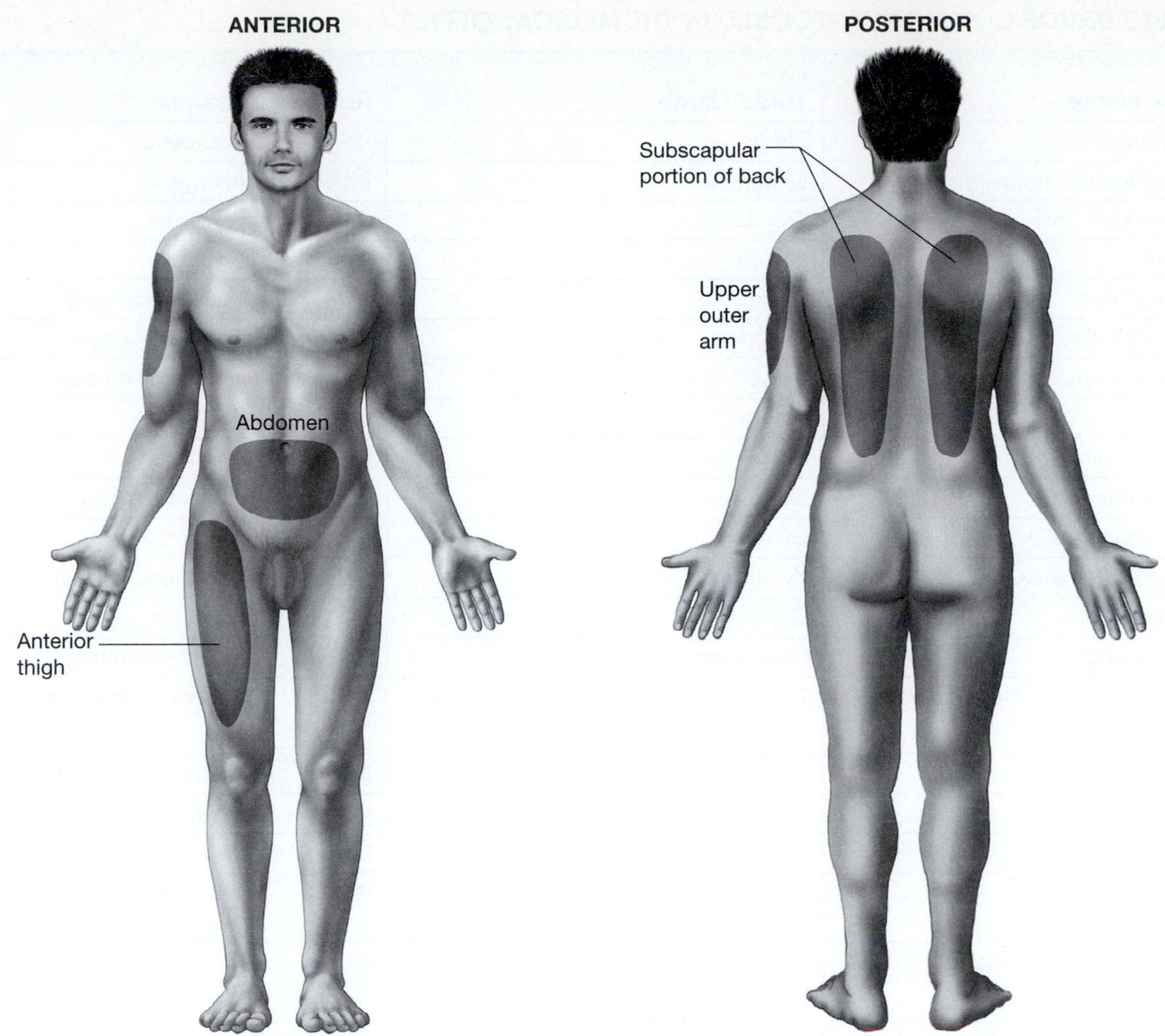

FIGURE 21-8 Sites for subcutaneous injection.

Figure 21-8 shows the angle of sites for subcutaneous injections.

TYPES OF INJECTIONS

	Intradermal	Subcutaneous	Intramuscular
Purpose	Allergy tests and Mantoux testing	Quick bloodstream absorption of medication	Gradual and maximum bloodstream absorption of medication
Sites	Distal to the antecubital space of the anterior aspect of the forearm	Outer aspect of the upper arm, abdomen, and anterior thigh	Dorsal aspect of the gluteus, deltoid, vastus lateralis of the thigh, and ventral aspect of the gluteus
Amount	0.1 to 0.3 ml	Less than 2 ml	2 to 5 ml. Dosages above 4 ml should be divided and administered at two different sites.
Needle Length and Size	1½″ to ⅝″ length, 25 to 27 gauge	⅝″ to 1″ length, 22 to 27 gauge	1½″ to 2″ length, 14 to 22 gauge

Source: Medical Assisting: Foundations and Practices by M. S. Frazier, C. Malone, and C. Morgan, Upper Saddle River, NJ: Pearson Education, Inc., 2010, p. 523. Reprinted with permission.

INJECTABLE DRUGS COMMONLY STOCKED IN THE MEDICAL OFFICE

Generic Name	Trade Name	Route	Usage
amitriptyline HCl	Elavil	IM	Depression
brompheniramine maleate	Dimetane	IM/SC	Allergy
chlorpromazine HCl	Thorazine	IM	Psychosis
diazepam	Valium	IM	Anxiety
dimenhydrinate	Dramamine	IM	Nausea/vomiting
diphenhydramine	Benadryl	IM	Allergic reaction
diphtheria, tetanus toxoid	Same name	IM	Immunization active vaccine
furosemide	Lasix	IM	Edema
gentamicin sulfate	Garamycin	IM	Infection
heparin sodium	Same name	SC	Prevent clotting
hydromorphone HCl	Dilaudid	SC/IM	Severe pain
lidocaine HCl 1 percent, 2 percent	Xylocaine	SC	Anesthetic for minor surgery
prochlorperazine	Compazine	IM	Psychosis
promethazine HCl	Phenergan	IM	Nausea/vomiting
sodium chloride with benzyl alcohol 0.9 percent	Bacteriostatic 0.9% Sodium Chloride	—	Diluent for injection
tetanus and diphtheria toxoids	Same name	IM	Immunization (active vaccine)
tetanus antitoxin	Same name	IM	Prevention (passive vaccine)
tetanus immune globulin	Hyper-Tet	IM	Prevention (passive vaccine)
tetanus toxoid	Same name	IM	Immunization (active vaccine)
tuberculin protein derivative	Tine test	ID	Tuberculin testing
water for injection	Same name		Diluent for injection
Emergency Drugs			
bretylium tosylate	Bretylol	IV	Arrhythmia
epinephrine		IV SC	Cardiac arrest Allergic reaction
norepinephrine	Levophed	IV	Hypotension
sodium bicarbonate		IV	Acidosis
electrolytes/Ringer's 1000 mL		IV	Dehydration

ID, intradermal; IM, intramuscular; IV, intravenous; SC, subcutaneous.
Note: Only physicians and nurses may administer IV medications.

procedure
21-1

ADMINISTERING AN INTRADERMAL INJECTION

Objective: Administer an intradermal injection.

EQUIPMENT AND SUPPLIES

- disposable gloves
- biohazard sharps container
- alcohol sponges
- sterile needle
- sterile syringe
- vial of medication
- medication order signed by physician
- pen

METHOD

I. Preparation

1. Perform hand hygiene.
2. Apply gloves and follow universal blood and body fluid precautions.
3. Select the correct medication using the "three befores." Always double-check the label to make sure that the strength is correct because medications are manufactured with different strengths (e.g., 1:10, 1:100, or 1:1000 dilutions).
4. Gently roll the medication between your hands to mix any medication that may have settled. Refrigerated medication can be rolled between your hands to warm it slightly.
5. Prepare the syringe using the correct technique. Carefully carry the covered needle and syringe to the patient.
6. Greet and identify the patient both by stating his or her name and by examining any printed identification, such as a wrist name band or medical record. Introduce yourself to the patient and ask if he or she has any allergies.
7. Tell the patient the name of the medication and the dosage that you are administering per the physician's order. Explain the process of the PPD skin test. Ask the patient if he or she has any questions prior to receiving the medication.
8. Select the proper site (center of the forearm, upper chest, or upper back). (See Figure 21-5 for intradermal skin injection sites.)
9. Using a circular motion, clean the patient's skin with an alcohol sponge. Wipe the skin with a sweeping motion from the center of the area outward. This prevents recontamination of the injection site by the alcohol sponge.
10. Allow time for the antiseptic on the sponge to dry to reduce the possibility of its reacting with the medication.
11. Check the medication dosage against the patient's order to determine if this is the correct time to administer the dose (one of the "ten rights").
12. Remove the protective covering from the needle, taking care not to touch the needle. If you accidentally touch the needle, then excuse yourself to the patient. Return to your preparation area and change the needle on the syringe. If you are using a self-contained syringe and needle unit that does not come apart, you will have to discard the entire syringe with the medication and start the process again.

II. Injection

13. Hold the syringe between the first two fingers and thumb of your dominant hand, with the palm down and the bevel of the needle up. Figures 21-9A–F illustrate the steps used to perform an intradermal skin test.
14. Hold the skin taut with the fingers of your nondominant hand. If you are using the center of the forearm, then place the nondominant hand under the patient's arm and pull the skin taut. This will allow the needle to slip into the skin more easily.
15. Using a 15-degree angle, insert the needle through the skin to about ⅛ inch. The bevel of the needle will be facing upward and covered with skin. The needle will still show through the skin. Do not aspirate.
16. Slowly inject the medication beneath the surface of the skin. A small elevation of skin or wheal will occur where you have injected the medication.
17. Quickly withdraw the needle. With your other hand, discard the needle into the biohazard sharps container.

III. Patient Follow-Up

18. Do not massage the area.
19. Make sure that the patient is safe before leaving him or her unattended. Observe the patient for any untoward effect, such as an allergic reaction to the medication, for at least 20 to 30 minutes. Tell the patient not to rub the area. Instruct the patient to return to the office within 48 to 72 hours for the reading of the skin test. Make certain that the patient understands the directions and does not have any questions.

20. Correctly dispose of all materials.
21. Remove and discard gloves and perform hand hygiene.
22. Chart the medication administration on the patient's record, noting the time, medication name, dosage, injection site, route, appearance of the intradermal site after injection, and your name.

CHARTING EXAMPLE

2/14/XX 10:00 A.M. Mantoux (PPD) tuberculin test, 0.10 mL ID Right anterior forearm. Instructed to return on 2/16 to have test read. .... M. King, CMA (AAMA)

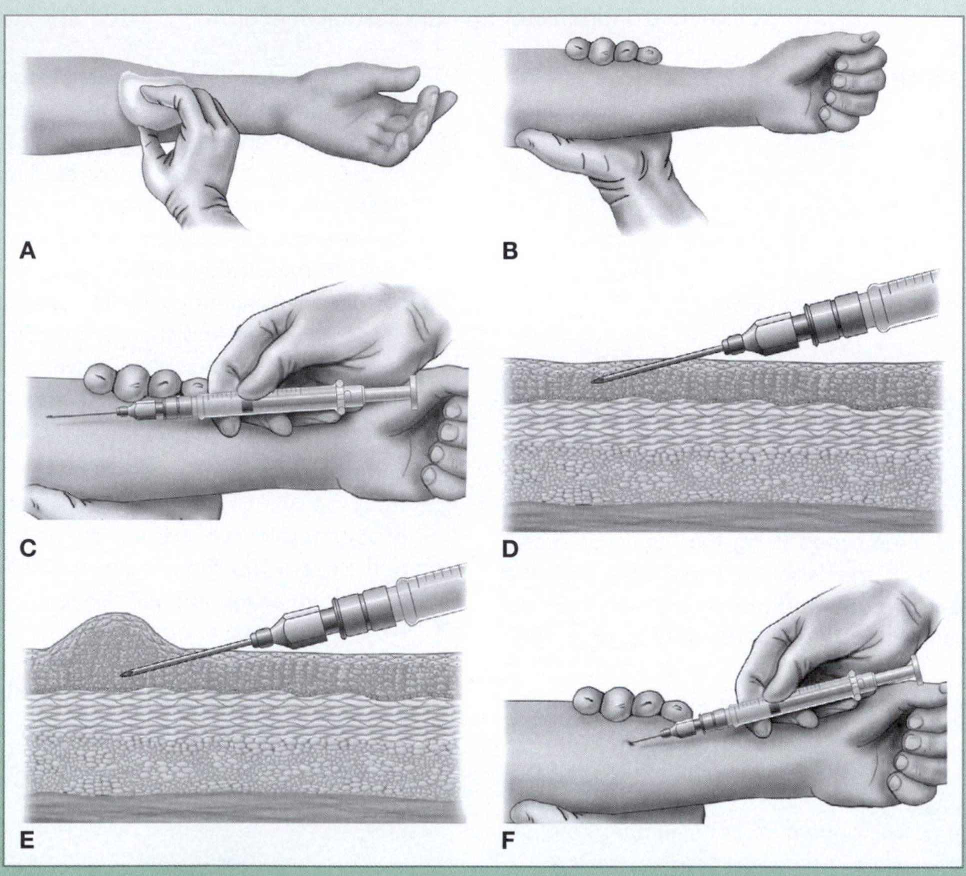

FIGURE 21-9 A–F administering an intradermal skin test.

Immunizations

Figures 21-10 and 21-11 show the immunization schedules for children and adolescents.

Principles of IV Therapy

State practice acts determine which health care professionals may initiate IV fluid therapy and medication administration. Medical assistants must be familiar with the state practice act for the state in which they practice. Some states allow medical assistants with advanced training and physician supervision to start IV fluid therapy.

IV therapy allows medications, solutions, nutritional supplements, blood, and blood products to be directly injected into the bloodstream. Because of the direct access to the bloodstream, it is imperative that the medical assistant is aware of potential adverse reactions that may occur. These reactions may vary from fatal reactions, as a result of a particular medication, to swelling at the IV site caused by giving too many fluids too rapidly or obstruction of the IV line. Any office performing IV fluid therapy must have emergency equipment, emergency access, and appropriate policies and procedures outlining what must occur if a patient experiences an adverse reaction.

Recommended Immunization Schedule for Persons Aged 0 Through 6 Years—United States • 2010

For those who fall behind or start late, see the catch-up schedule

Vaccine ▼ Age ►	Birth	1 month	2 months	4 months	6 months	12 months	15 months	18 months	19–23 months	2–3 years	4–6 years
Hepatitis B[1]	HepB	HepB			HepB						
Rotavirus[2]			RV	RV	RV[2]						
Diphtheria, Tetanus, Pertussis[3]			DTaP	DTaP	DTaP	see footnote[3]	DTaP				DTaP
Haemophilus influenzae type b[4]			Hib	Hib	Hib[4]	Hib					
Pneumococcal[5]			PCV	PCV	PCV	PCV				PPSV	
Inactivated Poliovirus[6]			IPV	IPV	IPV						IPV
Influenza[7]					Influenza (Yearly)						
Measles, Mumps, Rubella[8]						MMR		see footnote[8]			MMR
Varicella[9]						Varicella		see footnote[9]			Varicella
Hepatitis A[10]						HepA (2 doses)				HepA Series	
Meningococcal[11]										MCV	

Range of recommended ages for all children except certain high-risk groups

Range of recommended ages for certain high-risk groups

This schedule includes recommendations in effect as of December 15, 2009. Any dose not administered at the recommended age should be administered at a subsequent visit, when indicated and feasible. The use of a combination vaccine generally is preferred over separate injections of its equivalent component vaccines. Considerations should include provider assessment, patient preference, and the potential for adverse events. Providers should consult the relevant Advisory Committee on Immunization Practices statement for detailed recommendations: **http://www.cdc.gov/vaccines/pubs/acip-list.htm**. Clinically significant adverse events that follow immunization should be reported to the Vaccine Adverse Event Reporting System (VAERS) at **http://www.vaers.hhs.gov** or by telephone, **800-822-7967**.

1. **Hepatitis B vaccine (HepB).** (Minimum age: birth)
   At birth:
   - Administer monovalent HepB to all newborns before hospital discharge.
   - If mother is hepatitis B surface antigen (HBsAg)-positive, administer HepB and 0.5 mL of hepatitis B immune globulin (HBIG) within 12 hours of birth.
   - If mother's HBsAg status is unknown, administer HepB within 12 hours of birth. Determine mother's HBsAg status as soon as possible and, if HBsAg-positive, administer HBIG (no later than age 1 week).

   After the birth dose:
   - The HepB series should be completed with either monovalent HepB or a combination vaccine containing HepB. The second dose should be administered at age 1 or 2 months. Monovalent HepB vaccine should be used for doses administered before age 6 weeks. The final dose should be administered no earlier than age 24 weeks.
   - Infants born to HBsAg-positive mothers should be tested for HBsAg and antibody to HBsAg 1 to 2 months after completion of at least 3 doses of the HepB series, at age 9 through 18 months (generally at the next well-child visit).
   - Administration of 4 doses of HepB to infants is permissible when a combination vaccine containing HepB is administered after the birth dose. The fourth dose should be administered no earlier than age 24 weeks.
2. **Rotavirus vaccine (RV).** (Minimum age: 6 weeks)
   - Administer the first dose at age 6 through 14 weeks (maximum age: 14 weeks 6 days). Vaccination should not be initiated for infants aged 15 weeks 0 days or older.
   - The maximum age for the final dose in the series is 8 months 0 days
   - If Rotarix is administered at ages 2 and 4 months, a dose at 6 months is not indicated.
3. **Diphtheria and tetanus toxoids and acellular pertussis vaccine (DTaP).** (Minimum age: 6 weeks)
   - The fourth dose may be administered as early as age 12 months, provided at least 6 months have elapsed since the third dose.
   - Administer the final dose in the series at age 4 through 6 years.
4. ***Haemophilus influenzae* type b conjugate vaccine (Hib).** (Minimum age: 6 weeks)
   - If PRP-OMP (PedvaxHIB or Comvax [HepB-Hib]) is administered at ages 2 and 4 months, a dose at age 6 months is not indicated.
   - TriHiBit (DTaP/Hib) and Hiberix (PRP-T) should not be used for doses at ages 2, 4, or 6 months for the primary series but can be used as the final dose in children aged 12 months through 4 years.
5. **Pneumococcal vaccine.** (Minimum age: 6 weeks for pneumococcal conjugate vaccine [PCV]; 2 years for pneumococcal polysaccharide vaccine [PPSV])
   - PCV is recommended for all children aged younger than 5 years. Administer 1 dose of PCV to all healthy children aged 24 through 59 months who are not completely vaccinated for their age.
   - Administer PPSV 2 or more months after last dose of PCV to children aged 2 years or older with certain underlying medical conditions, including a cochlear implant. See *MMWR* 1997;46(No. RR-8).
6. **Inactivated poliovirus vaccine (IPV)** (Minimum age: 6 weeks)
   - The final dose in the series should be administered on or after the fourth birthday and at least 6 months following the previous dose.
   - If 4 doses are administered prior to age 4 years a fifth dose should be administered at age 4 through 6 years. See *MMWR* 2009;58(30):829–30.
7. **Influenza vaccine (seasonal).** (Minimum age: 6 months for trivalent inactivated influenza vaccine [TIV]; 2 years for live, attenuated influenza vaccine [LAIV])
   - Administer annually to children aged 6 months through 18 years.
   - For healthy children aged 2 through 6 years (i.e., those who do not have underlying medical conditions that predispose them to influenza complications), either LAIV or TIV may be used, except LAIV should not be given to children aged 2 through 4 years who have had wheezing in the past 12 months.
   - Children receiving TIV should receive 0.25 mL if aged 6 through 35 months or 0.5 mL if aged 3 years or older.
   - Administer 2 doses (separated by at least 4 weeks) to children aged younger than 9 years who are receiving influenza vaccine for the first time or who were vaccinated for the first time during the previous influenza season but only received 1 dose.
   - For recommendations for use of influenza A (H1N1) 2009 monovalent vaccine see *MMWR* 2009;58(No. RR-10).
8. **Measles, mumps, and rubella vaccine (MMR).** (Minimum age: 12 months)
   - Administer the second dose routinely at age 4 through 6 years. However, the second dose may be administered before age 4, provided at least 28 days have elapsed since the first dose.
9. **Varicella vaccine.** (Minimum age: 12 months)
   - Administer the second dose routinely at age 4 through 6 years. However, the second dose may be administered before age 4, provided at least 3 months have elapsed since the first dose.
   - For children aged 12 months through 12 years the minimum interval between doses is 3 months. However, if the second dose was administered at least 28 days after the first dose, it can be accepted as valid.
10. **Hepatitis A vaccine (HepA).** (Minimum age: 12 months)
    - Administer to all children aged 1 year (i.e., aged 12 through 23 months). Administer 2 doses at least 6 months apart.
    - Children not fully vaccinated by age 2 years can be vaccinated at subsequent visits
    - HepA also is recommended for older children who live in areas where vaccination programs target older children, who are at increased risk for infection, or for whom immunity against hepatitis A is desired.
11. **Meningococcal vaccine.** (Minimum age: 2 years for meningococcal conjugate vaccine [MCV4] and for meningococcal polysaccharide vaccine [MPSV4])
    - Administer MCV4 to children aged 2 through 10 years with persistent complement component deficiency, anatomic or functional asplenia, and certain other conditions placing tham at high risk.
    - Administer MCV4 to children previously vaccinated with MCV4 or MPSV4 after 3 years if first dose administered at age 2 through 6 years. See *MMWR* 2009;58:1042–3.

The Recommended Immunization Schedules for Persons Aged 0 through 18 Years are approved by the Advisory Committee on Immunization Practices (**http://www.cdc.gov/vaccines/recs/acip**), the American Academy of Pediatrics (**http://www.aap.org**), and the American Academy of Family Physicians (**http://www.aafp.org**).

Department of Health and Human Services • Centers for Disease Control and Prevention

CS207330-A

FIGURE 21-10 Child Immunization Schedule (0 to 6).

Source: http://www.cdc.gov/vaccines/recs/schedules/downloads/child/2010/10_0-6yrs-schedule-bw.pdf

Recommended Immunization Schedule for Persons Aged 7 Through 18 Years—United States • 2010

For those who fall behind or start late, see the schedule below and the catch-up schedule

Vaccine ▼ Age ►	7–10 years	11–12 years	13–18 years
Tetanus, Diphtheria, Pertussis[1]		Tdap	Tdap
Human Papillomavirus[2]	see footnote 2	HPV (3 doses)	HPV series
Meningococcal[3]	MCV	MCV	MCV
Influenza[4]		Influenza (Yearly)	
Pneumococcal[5]		PPSV	
Hepatitis A[6]		HepA Series	
Hepatitis B[7]		Hep B Series	
Inactivated Poliovirus[8]		IPV Series	
Measles, Mumps, Rubella[9]		MMR Series	
Varicella[10]		Varicella Series	

Range of recommended ages for all children except certain high-risk groups

Range of recommended ages for catch-up immunization

Range of recommended ages for certain high-risk groups

This schedule includes recommendations in effect as of December 15, 2009. Any dose not administered at the recommended age should be administered at a subsequent visit, when indicated and feasible. The use of a combination vaccine generally is preferred over separate injections of its equivalent component vaccines. Considerations should include provider assessment, patient preference, and the potential for adverse events. Providers should consult the relevant Advisory Committee on Immunization Practices statement for detailed recommendations: **http://www.cdc.gov/vaccines/pubs/acip-list.htm**. Clinically significant adverse events that follow immunization should be reported to the Vaccine Adverse Event Reporting System (VAERS) at **http://www.vaers.hhs.gov** or by telephone, **800-822-7967**.

1. **Tetanus and diphtheria toxoids and acellular pertussis vaccine (Tdap).** (Minimum age: 10 years for Boostrix and 11 years for Adacel)
   - Administer at age 11 or 12 years for those who have completed the recommended childhood DTP/DTaP vaccination series and have not received a tetanus and diphtheria toxoid (Td) booster dose.
   - Persons aged 13 through 18 years who have not received Tdap should receive a dose.
   - A 5-year interval from the last Td dose is encouraged when Tdap is used as a booster dose; however, a shorter interval may be used if pertussis immunity is needed.
2. **Human papillomavirus vaccine (HPV).** (Minimum age: 9 years)
   - Two HPV vaccines are licensed: a quadrivalent vaccine (HPV4) for the prevention of cervical, vaginal and vulvar cancers (in females) and genital warts (in females and males), and a bivalent vaccine (HPV2) for the prevention of cervical cancers in females.
   - HPV vaccines are most effective for both males and females when given before exposure to HPV through sexual contact.
   - HPV4 or HPV2 is recommended for the prevention of cervical precancers and cancers in females.
   - HPV4 is recommended for the prevention of cervical, vaginal and vulvar precancers and cancers and genital warts in females.
   - Administer the first dose to females at age 11 or 12 years.
   - Administer the second dose 1 to 2 months after the first dose and the third dose 6 months after the first dose (at least 24 weeks after the first dose).
   - Administer the series to females at age 13 through 18 years if not previously vaccinated.
   - HPV4 may be administered in a 3-dose series to males aged 9 through 18 years to reduce their likelihood of acquiring genital warts.
3. **Meningococcal conjugate vaccine (MCV4).**
   - Administer at age 11 or 12 years, or at age 13 through 18 years if not previously vaccinated.
   - Administer to previously unvaccinated college freshmen living in a dormitory.
   - Administer MCV4 to children aged 2 through 10 years with persistent complement component deficiency, anatomic or functional asplenia, or certain other conditions placing them at high risk.
   - Administer to children previously vaccinated with MCV4 or MPSV4 who remain at increased risk after 3 years (if first dose administered at age 2 through 6 years) or after 5 years (if first dose administered at age 7 years or older). Persons whose only risk factor is living in on-campus housing are not recommended to receive an additional dose. See *MMWR* 2009;58:1042–3.
4. **Influenza vaccine (seasonal).**
   - Administer annually to children aged 6 months through 18 years.
   - For healthy nonpregnant persons aged 7 through 18 years (i.e., those who do not have underlying medical conditions that predispose them to influenza complications), either LAIV or TIV may be used.
   - Administer 2 doses (separated by at least 4 weeks) to children aged younger than 9 years who are receiving influenza vaccine for the first time or who were vaccinated for the first time during the previous influenza season but only received 1 dose.
   - For recommendations for use of influenza A (H1N1) 2009 monovalent vaccine. See *MMWR* 2009;58(No. RR-10).
5. **Pneumococcal polysaccharide vaccine (PPSV).**
   - Administer to children with certain underlying medical conditions, including a cochlear implant. A single revaccination should be administered after 5 years to children with functional or anatomic asplenia or an immunocompromising condition. See *MMWR* 1997;46(No. RR-8).
6. **Hepatitis A vaccine (HepA).**
   - Administer 2 doses at least 6 months apart.
   - HepA is recommended for children aged older than 23 months who live in areas where vaccination programs target older children, who are at increased risk for infection, or for whom immunity against hepatitis A is desired.
7. **Hepatitis B vaccine (HepB).**
   - Administer the 3-dose series to those not previously vaccinated.
   - A 2-dose series (separated by at least 4 months) of adult formulation Recombivax HB is licensed for children aged 11 through 15 years.
8. **Inactivated poliovirus vaccine (IPV).**
   - The final dose in the series should be administered on or after the fourth birthday and at least 6 months following the previous dose.
   - If both OPV and IPV were administered as part of a series, a total of 4 doses should be administered, regardless of the child's current age.
9. **Measles, mumps, and rubella vaccine (MMR).**
   - If not previously vaccinated, administer 2 doses or the second dose for those who have received only 1 dose, with at least 28 days between doses.
10. **Varicella vaccine.**
    - For persons aged 7 through 18 years without evidence of immunity (see *MMWR* 2007;56[No. RR-4]), administer 2 doses if not previously vaccinated or the second dose if only 1 dose has been administered.
    - For persons aged 7 through 12 years, the minimum interval between doses is 3 months. However, if the second dose was administered at least 28 days after the first dose, it can be accepted as valid.
    - For persons aged 13 years and older, the minimum interval between doses is 28 days.

CS207330-A

The Recommended Immunization Schedules for Persons Aged 0 through 18 Years are approved by the Advisory Committee on Immunization Practices (**http://www.cdc.gov/vaccines/recs/acip**), the American Academy of Pediatrics (**http://www.aap.org**), and the American Academy of Family Physicians (**http://www.aafp.org**).

Department of Health and Human Services • Centers for Disease Control and Prevention

FIGURE 21-11 Adolescent Immunization Schedule (7 to 18).

Source: http://www.cdc.gov/vaccines/recs/schedules/downloads/child/2010/10_7-18yrs-schedule-bw.pdf

procedure

21-2

PREPARING AN INTRAVENOUS TRAY

Objective: Prepare an intravenous (IV) tray.

EQUIPMENT AND SUPPLIES

- absorbent disposable sheet
- alcohol prep pads
- Betadine swabs
- disposable tourniquet
- IV setup: IV tubing with attached filter; IV catheter; bag of IV fluid labeled with type and patient's name, date, time; paper tape; syringe; port cap; disposable gloves; gauze (2 × 2 or 4 × 4); IV setup tray; IV pole with pump

METHOD

1. Perform hand hygiene.
2. Apply gloves.
3. Prepare IV fluid administration set:
   a. Inspect the fluid bag to make sure that it contains the desired fluid, that the fluid is clear, and that the bag is free from any leaks and has not expired.
   b. Select the correct administration set (either mini or macro drip) and uncoil the tubing, being careful that the ends of the tubing do not become contaminated.
   c. Close the flow regulator to the fluid bag.
   d. Remove the protective covering from the port of the fluid bag and the protective covering from the spike of the administration set.
   e. Insert the spike of the administration set into the port of the fluid bag with a quick twisting motion, being careful not to puncture yourself.
   f. While holding the fluid bag higher than the drip chamber of the administration set, squeeze the drip chamber once or twice to start the flow of the fluid. Fill the chamber to the marker line. If the chamber is overfilled, quickly lower the bag below the level of the drip chamber and squeeze some of the fluid back into the fluid bag.
   g. Open the flow regulator and allow the fluid to flush all the air from the tubing. A trash can or the wrapper the fluid came in can be used for the overflow of fluid.
   h. Turn off the flow and place the sterile cap back on the end of the administration set (if you had to remove it). Then place this end nearby so that it can be easily reached by the person ready to connect it to the IV catheter in the patient's arm.
4. Place the absorbent disposable sheet on the tray.
5. Assemble the equipment and supplies on the tray in order of use.
6. If you are using an IV pole or pump, hang the IV solution (bag) on the pole; do not set it up or calculate drops in the pump; this will be done by the person starting the IV.
7. Notify the appropriate personnel (registered nurse, licensed vocational nurse, physician) that the IV tray setup is ready for administration.
8. Remove and discard gloves and perform hand hygiene.
9. Document the procedure.
10. Clean the work area and equipment according to the OSHA guidelines.

Once the IV tray has been prepared, use the following steps to start an IV:

1. Select the IV site and appropriate size/type of catheter. Most IVs are started in the arm; however, they may be started at other sites, depending on the situation.
2. Place a tourniquet above the chosen IV site.
3. Working from the intended IV site outward in a circular pattern, cleanse the IV site.
4. Introduce the catheter into the vein to obtain an open blood supply.
5. Release and remove the tourniquet.
6. Advance the plastic cannula into the vein and remove the needle.
7. Reassure the patient that the needle has been removed and that only the plastic cannula remains.
8. Anchor the site with tape.
9. Connect the IV tubing and finish dressing the site.
10. Dispose of all needles and biohazard materials per office policy and OSHA standards

It is important to evaluate the IV site frequently to ensure that the fluids are flowing properly and there is no infiltration. Infiltration occurs when the tip of the IV catheter withdraws from the vein or pokes through the vein, causing the fluid to leak into the surrounding tissue. If this occurs, the IV will need to be replaced.

21 APPLICATION

Directions: Select the best answer for each of the following questions. Check your answers in the Answer Key at the end of the book.

1. Movement of medication from the site of administration into the bloodstream is known as:
   a. Antagonism
   b. Cumulative effect
   c. Absorption
   d. Excretion
   e. Idiosyncrasy

2. "Administering two medications together causes them to be less effective than if they are administered separately" is known as:
   a. Antagonism
   b. Cumulative effect
   c. Absorption
   d. Excretion
   e. Idiosyncrasy

3. When drugs are broken down and converted to a water-soluble compound that can be excreted by the body, this is known as:
   a. Pharmacodynamics
   b. Pharmacokinetics
   c. Synergism
   d. Therapeutic effect
   e. Metabolism

4. Study of the actions of drugs is known as:
   a. Pharmacodynamics
   b. Pharmacokinetics
   c. Synergism
   d. Therapeutic effect
   e. Metabolism

5. If the available medication is 5 mg/2 mL and the physician orders 12 mg, how much medication will be administered?
   a. 4 mL
   b. .4 mg
   c. 4.8 mL
   d. 4.8 mg
   e. 5 mL

6. Using Clark's Rule, the adult dose is 25 mg, and the medication comes in a vial of 25 mg/mL. The child weighs 68 lb; what is the pediatric dose?
   a. 10.8 mL
   b. 11.3 mL
   c. 10.8 mg
   d. 11.3 mg
   e. None of the above

7. Using Young's Rule, the adult dose is 80 mg and the child is 9 years old. What is the appropriate pediatric dose for this child?
   a. 4.8 mg
   b. 4.8 mL
   c. 34.3 mL
   d. 34.3 g
   e. 34.3 mg

8. The common name for a medication is known as the:
   a. Chemical name
   b. Generic name
   c. Trade name
   d. Brand name
   e. Proprietary name

9. Which part of the prescription indicates the name of the medication and the dosage?
   a. Subscription
   b. DAW
   c. Superscription
   d. Inscription
   e. Sig

10. Which portion of the syringe connects the shaft to the hub?
   a. Flange
   b. Barrel
   c. Hilt
   d. Plunger
   e. Lumen

11. Which of the following pediatric dosage calculations is based on the assumption that a child who is 12½ years old could take an adult dose?
   a. Fried's Law
   b. Young's Rule
   c. West's Rule
   d. Clark's Rule
   e. Freud's Rule

12. Which of the following sets of numerals are equal?
   a. 0.5 mg = 00.5 kg
   b. 4 g = 4000 mcg
   c. 6 g = 6 mL
   d. 5.5 mL = 0.0055 L
   e. 20 kg = 200 g

13. 1 fluid oz is the equivalent of ____________ ml.
   a. 4
   b. 8
   c. 10
   d. 15
   e. 30

14. Dyazide is listed as one of the most frequently administered medications. What type of medication is this?
   a. Diuretic
   b. Hormone
   c. Calcium chanel blocker
   d. Beta blocker
   e. Anticoagulant

15. Which of the following is not an antibiotic?
   a. Duricef
   b. Rocephin
   c. Zithromax
   d. Cipro
   e. Reglan

16. Which of the following types of scheduled drugs allows five refills over a six-month period?
   a. Schedule I drugs
   b. Schedule II drugs
   c. Schedule III drugs
   d. Schedule IV drugs
   e. Both C and D

17. Which of the following is not one of the first six rights of medication administration?
   a. Right patient
   b. Right medication
   c. Right to refuse
   d. Right route
   e. Right documentation

18. For a subcutaneous injection, which of the following sites is most often used?
   a. Deltoid
   b. Upper outer portion of the arm
   c. Anterior thigh
   d. Abdomen
   e. Vastus lateralis

19. What gauge needle is typically used for an IM injection?
   a. 22 to 27
   b. 23 to 28
   c. 25 to 27
   d. 14 to 22
   e. 16 to 30

20. Which of the following is the best answer for the angle at which intradermal injections are administered?
   a. 10 degrees
   b. 15 degrees
   c. 10 to 15 degrees
   d. 45 degrees
   e. 90 degrees

21. ____________ occurs when the next dose of medication is given before the previous dose has had time to be metabolized/excreted.
   a. Absorption
   b. Adverse effect
   c. Drug action
   d. Cumulative effect
   e. Antagonism

22. In the metric system, the prefix *kilo* corresponds with what value?
   a. 1000 of a unit
   b. 10 of a unit
   c. 100 of a unit
   d. 0.1 of a unit
   e. 0.001 of a unit

23. __________ is the common unit of measure for volume in the metric system.
   a. Meter
   b. Pound
   c. Gram
   d. Liter
   e. None of the above

24. The Roman numeral VI is equivalent to the Arabic number ______________.
   a. 4
   b. 5
   c. 6
   d. 3
   e. 11

25. *alt dieb* is a pharmacology abbreviation meaning ________________.

   a. Amount
   b. As desired
   c. Alternate hours
   d. Alternate days
   e. Alternate nights

26. Which of the following is not part of a syringe?

   a. Plunger
   b. Barrel
   c. Chamber
   d. Hilt
   e. Shaft

27. Antiemetic drugs are used to:

   a. Prevent vomiting, relieve nausea
   b. Treat parasitic worm infections
   c. Treat itching
   d. Stimulate nerve transmitters
   e. Relieve anxiety

28. All of the following are examples of antiypyretics except:

   a. aspirin
   b. acetaminophen
   c. naproxen
   d. atropine
   e. ibuprofen

29. Antispasmodics are used to treat ________________.

   a. Brain
   b. GI tract
   c. Convulsions
   d. Coughing
   e. Asthma

30. Which schedule of drugs has high potential for addiction and is accepted for medical use in the United States?

   a. Schedule I
   b. Schedule II
   c. Schedule III
   d. Schedule IV
   e. Schedule V

22 Safety and Emergency Practices

CONTENTS

Action Plan

It is important that all employees in the medical office are aware of specific emergency and disaster plans that have been put in place to protect the safety of both the patients and the medical office staff. These emergency plans should be kept in the policy/procedure manual.

All new hires should be trained in all emergency steps within the first days of employment. This training should be documented in writing and kept on file.

Assessment

Even though you are familiar with the medical office where you work, when there is an emergency or a disaster, you must first survey the scene and determine whether it is safe. You should never put yourself in harm's way.

Once you have determined that the scene is safe, you must survey everyone affected and begin to triage, taking care of the most seriously injured patients first.

If the victims are able to talk, gather and document as much information as possible regarding their name, pain (the location and the level of pain), current medications, and allergies.

Emergency Preparedness

It is important that all employees within the medical office know how to respond properly to a natural or human-made disaster. Important rules when dealing with emergencies and disasters are as follows:

- Remain calm.
- Take care of the patients in the office and ensure their safety.
- Notify the appropriate authorities.
- Evacuate if necessary and gather at the designated meeting place.

FIRE

Floor plans showing all exits, fire extinguishers, and stairwells should be placed in conspicuous areas throughout the facility. These plans should clearly show the most direct route out of the building. They should be large enough to be easily read in dim light and from a reasonable distance. During fire drills, it should be determined who will be designated for each area and responsible for making sure that all patients and staff are able to get out of the area safely.

Many offices have adopted the acronym RACE to help employees remember what to do in case of fire.

R	**Rescue** employees and patients from the fire area.
A	**Alert** by calling 911.
C	**Confine** by closing doors and windows.
E	**Extinguish** the fire.

The PASS method is used to operate fire extinguishers (Figure 22-1).

NATURAL DISASTERS

According to the Federal Emergency Management Agency (FEMA), there are six steps in planning for a natural disaster such as an earthquake, tornado, hurricane, or flood:

- Check for hazards around the facility.
- Identify safe places indoors and outdoors.
- Educate the staff.
- Have disaster supplies on hand.
- Develop an emergency communication plan.
- Assist the community in preparing for disasters.

Once the plan for your office has been developed, make sure that everyone knows what his or her particular role is.

TERRORISM

In the event of a bomb threat, remain calm and act quickly. If a bomb threat is called in, notify the police immediately. While the caller is on the telephone, listen carefully for any background noise and gather as much information as possible. Ask the following questions:

- Where is the bomb?
- When will it explode?
- What kind of bomb is it?

First Aid for Common Injuries

When someone has suddenly become ill or injured, you may need to use basic first aid to save his or her life, reduce pain, prevent further injury or damage, or increase the chance of recovery.

In the event of an emergency, as a medical assistant you may be responsible for providing first aid; however, you will never be responsible for diagnosing or providing treatment.

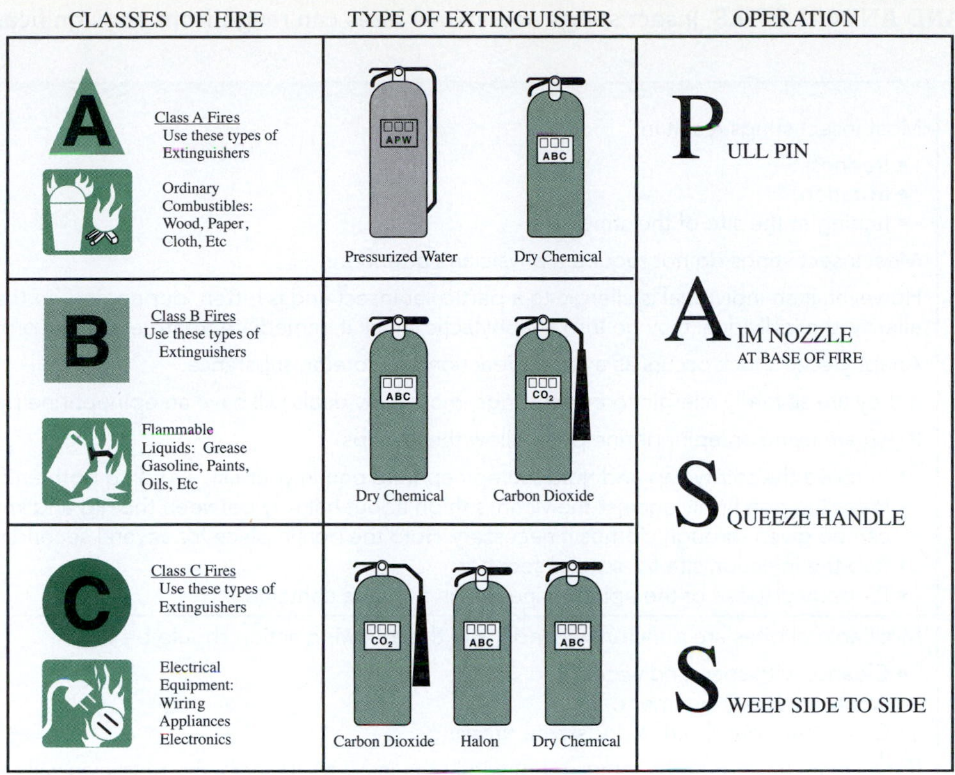

CLASSES OF FIRE
TYPE OF EXTINGUISHER
OPERATION
A
Class A Fires
Use these types of Extinguishers
Ordinary Combustibles: Wood, Paper, Cloth, Etc
APW
ABC
Pressurized Water
Dry Chemical
PULL PIN
B
Class B Fires
Use these types of Extinguishers
Flammable Liquids: Grease Gasoline, Paints, Oils, Etc
ABC
CO2
Dry Chemical
Carbon Dioxide
AIM NOZZLE
AT BASE OF FIRE
SQUEEZE HANDLE
C
Class C Fires
Use these types of Extinguishers
Electrical Equipment: Wiring Appliances Electronics
CO2
ABC
ABC
Carbon Dioxide
Halon
Dry Chemical
SWEEP SIDE TO SIDE

FIGURE 22-1 PASS method of firefighting: Pull the pin, aim at the base of the fire, squeeze the trigger, and sweep from side to side.
From the University of Texas Health Science Center at Houston Environmental Health and Safety Department.

Anytime an emergency occurs in the office, it is important to notify the physician immediately.

Occasionally, there will be an emergency within the office that will require the use of a crash cart. The following items are typically found in the crash cart and/or the emergency medical box:

- Oxygen tank with accompanying tubing, canula, masks
- IV fluids
- Butterfly bandages
- Hemostats
- Tourniquets
- Iodine
- Activated charcoal
- Atropine
- Diphenhydramine (Benadryl)
- Epinephrine
- Instant glucose
- Insulin
- Lidocaine
- Local anesthetics
- Nitroglycerin
- Phenobarbital and diazepam
- Sodium bicarbonate
- Solu-Cortef™
- Spirits of ammonia
- Verapamil

The crash cart and/or medical box must contain a checklist of all the equipment and medications that the cart or box contains. This list should be checked daily and the cart or box restocked as necessary.

INSECT STINGS AND ANIMAL BITES Insect stings and animal bites can range from nonsignificant to life-threatening.

Insect Stings (Box 22-1)	Most insect stings result in: • Redness • Irritation • Itching at the site of the sting *Most* insect stings do not require a physician's attention. However, if an individual is allergic to a particular insect and is bitten, depending on the severity of the allergy, the individual may go into anaphylactic shock if immediate treatment is not provided. Anaphylactic shock occurs as a severe reaction to a foreign substance. If they are severely allergic to insect stings, most individuals will have an epinephrine pen available. If you are using an epinephrine pen, follow these steps: • Remove the safety cap and hold the epinephrine pen in your fist, avoiding both ends. • Press the pen firmly against the victim's thigh about halfway between the hip and knee. The injection can be given through clothes if necessary. Hold the pen in place for several seconds. • Rub the injection site for several seconds. • Properly dispose of the epinephrine pen in a sharps container.
Animal Bites (Box 22-2)	Most animal bites are puncture wounds, and the following action should be taken: • Cleanse with soap and water. • Apply antibiotic ointment. • Cover the wound with a dry, sterile dressing. If the victim has not had a tetanus shot within the last 7 to 10 years, the physician will most likely order it to be administered as well.

Box 22-1 Treating Insect Stings

Insect stings may be insignificant or life-threatening. Some are quite painful, while others cause no pain and the victim is unaware of the sting until itching, redness, or a reaction develops. Help the victim by following these steps.

1. Remove the stinger by scraping across the affected area with a credit card or other rigid object. This is usually the only treatment necessary to remove the stinger.
2. Apply a paste of baking soda and water to the area.
3. If the victim is allergic to certain types of insect stings (bees, wasps, hornets), administer antihistamine or epinephrine, as ordered by the physician.

Source: Medical Assisting: Foundations and Practices by M. S. Frazier, C. Malone, and C. Morgan, Upper Saddle River, NJ: Pearson Education, Inc., 2010, p. 906. Reprinted with permission.

Box 22-2 Animal Bites

Any animal, including humans, can inflict bites. First aid in the medical office involves cleansing the wound with soap and water and covering it with a sterile dressing until the physician assesses it and decides on the next step. Depending on the extent and location of the bite, sutures may be necessary. When children are bitten on the face, arms, and hands, they are often referred to a plastic surgeon for repair with minimal scarring.

Obtain information regarding the animal that inflicted the injury. Contact your local law enforcement agency for the name of the appropriate agency to call. A law enforcement officer may notify the agency for you. In many communities, animal bites are reported to an animal control department. You should familiarize yourself with local guidelines.

Source: Medical Assisting: Foundations and Practices by M. S. Frazier, C. Malone, and C. Morgan, Upper Saddle River, NJ: Pearson Education, 2010, p. 906. Reprinted with permission.

procedure

22-1

RESPONDING TO A PATIENT WHO HAS FAINTED

1. If the patient communicates a faint feeling, help the patient sit, bend forward, and place the head on the knees. If the patient collapses with no warning, do not move the patient. The patient may have sustained a neck or back injury.
2. Immediately notify the physician.
3. Loosen any tight clothing, and cover the patient with a blanket for warmth.
4. If the physician directs, use a footstool to support the patient's legs in a raised position.
5. If the physician directs, call for Emergency Medical Service (EMS).
6. Once the emergency passes, obtain a full set of vital signs and document all activities in the patient's medical record.

SYNCOPE

Syncope, also known as *fainting,* occurs as a result of a brief interruption in the flow of blood to the brain and, in turn, causes a sudden loss of consciousness that typically is very brief. If it becomes apparent that someone is about to faint, try to make sure that he or she is not injured as a result of falling to the ground (Procedure 22-1).

INJURIES CAUSED BY EXTREME TEMPERATURES

Injuries caused by either extreme heat or extreme cold may result in injury to the tissues of the integumentary system or may cause systemic injuries.

Burns may be caused by heat, chemicals, electricity, or radiation and are classified by depth, area involved, and source of the burn.

BURNS ACCORDING TO DEGREE OF INJURY, SYMPTOMS, AND TREATMENT

Burn Type	Symptoms	Treatment
First degree: superficial burns; heal without scarring	Reddened skin; no blisters; painful	Submerge in cool water 2 to 5 minutes. If patient is young or elderly, or if hands, face, feet, or genitals are involved, see physician.
Second degree: partial-thickness burns; heal with very little scarring	Reddened skin; fluid-filled blisters within 48 hours; very painful; white spots possible	Stop the burning. Do not break blisters. If patient is young or elderly, or if hands, face, feet, or genitals are involved, see physician.
Third degree: full-thickness burns; scarring is likely	Gray, black, or charred skin; underlying tissue involved; extremely painful or no pain if nerve endings are damaged	Call EMS. Treat for shock. Physician evaluation is necessary for treatment. Skin grafting may be necessary.

Source: Medical Assisting: Foundations and Practices by M. S. Frazier, C. Malone, and C. Morgan, Upper Saddle River, NJ: Pearson Education, Inc., 2010, p. 896. Reprinted with permission.

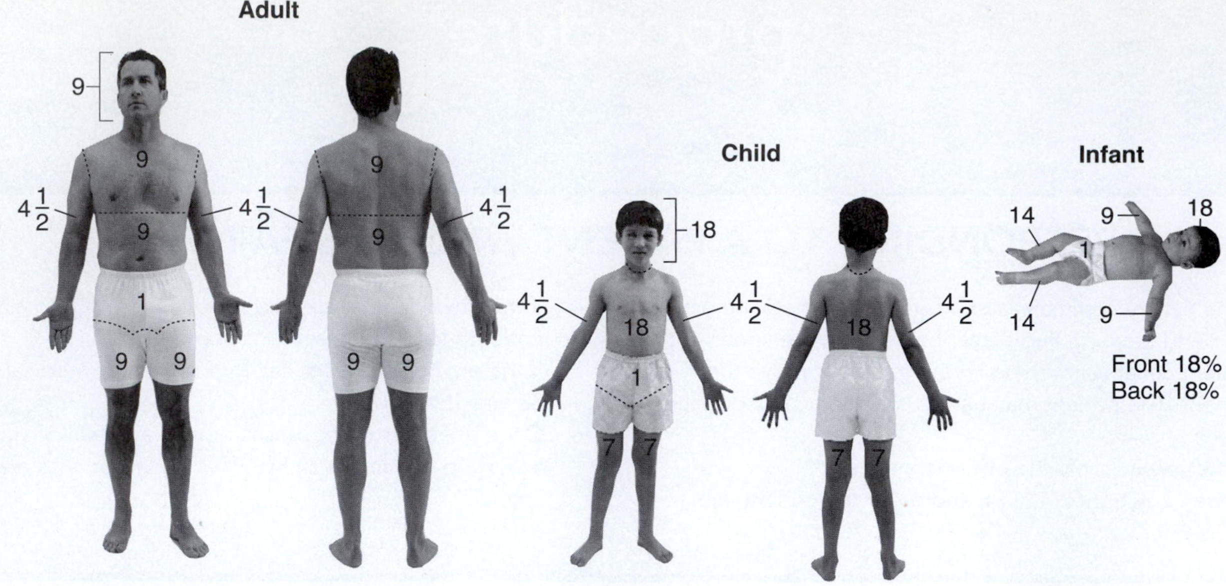

FIGURE 22-2 Rule of Nines.

From *Pearson's Comprehensive Medical Assisting Administrative and Clinical Competencies,* 2nd ed., executive ed. J. Gill, Upper Saddle River, NJ: Pearson Education, Inc., 2011, p. 962. Reprinted with permission.

The Rule of Nines is used to calculate the extent of the burn area (Figure 22-2).

Exposure to extreme cold for extended periods of time can cause frostbite and damage to the integumentary system.

Move the frostbite victim from the cold to a warmer environment so that the tissue can warm slowly. Someone with early frostbite may begin warming by gently blowing on the affected area, placing the hands under the armpits or immersing the affected area in warm water. If the tissue is hard to the touch, call 911. Never rub, squeeze, or massage frozen tissue.

FROSTBITE INJURIES

Injury	Symptoms	Prognosis
Frostnip: involves tips of ears, nose, cheeks, fingers, toes, or chin	Numbness Tingling	Completely reversible
Superficial frostbite: water freezes in upper layers of the skin	Edema Blisters	Reversible
Frostbite: tissue beneath skin is frozen solid	Light skin: redness Dark skin: lightening Small blisters Blanching Numbness No sensation Finally, area all white	Permanent damage may occur

Source: Medical Assisting: Foundations and Practices by M. S. Frazier, C. Malone, and C. Morgan, Upper Saddle River, NJ: Pearson Education, Inc., 2010, p. 898. Reprinted with permission.

THERMAL INSULTS

Insult	Causes	Symptoms	Treatment
Heat stroke	Continued exposure to extremely hot temperatures Failure of the body to cope with excessive heat	Body temperature >105°F Dry, hot, red skin Dry mouth Nausea Vomiting Dizziness Weakness SOB Rapid pulse Decreasing BP Anxiety, confusion Possible seizures	Cool the body rapidly. Pour cool water over the body to bring the core temperature down below 100°F. Transport to an emergency facility.
Heat exhaustion	Continued exposure to extremely hot temperatures Depletion of salt or water in the body	Normal or below normal body temperature Profuse sweating Skin: moist, cool, pale Headache Dizziness Fatigue Nausea Muscle cramps Pulse: weak, rapid Dilated Pupils	Move to a cool place. Apply cool compresses. Elevate the feet. If conscious, give small amounts of liquid.
Hypothermia	Continued exposure to wind, cold, or cold water	Numbness or cold feeling Fatigue Core body temperature <95°F Skin: blue, puffy Pulse: weak, slow Confusion Decreased level of consciousness	Remove wet clothing. Warm the patient by wrapping in warm blankets. Transport to an emergency facility.

Source: Medical Assisting: Foundations and Practices by M. S. Frazier, C. Malone, and C. Morgan, Upper Saddle River, NJ: Pearson Education, Inc., 2010, p. 899. Reprinted with permission.

Systemic injuries include heat exhaustion, hyperthermia, and hypothermia and are caused by continuous exposure to the elements.

BLEEDING

Bleeding may be internal or external. External bleeding occurs when the skin is broken, and internal bleeding occurs when there is tissue damage and the skin remains intact.

EXTERNAL BLEEDING

Arterial Bleeding	Usually abundant, bright red, rapid, and usually spurts in rhythm with the heartbeat. In order to minimize blood loss, arterial bleeding needs to be brought under control as quickly as possible. Applying direct pressure over the wound may halt the flow of blood (Figure 22-3). If direct pressure does not stop the flow of blood, external pressure on the pressure points may need to be used (Figure 22-4).
Venous Bleeding	Slower than arterial bleeding, darker in color, and usually controlled by direct pressure using a sterile dressing over the wound

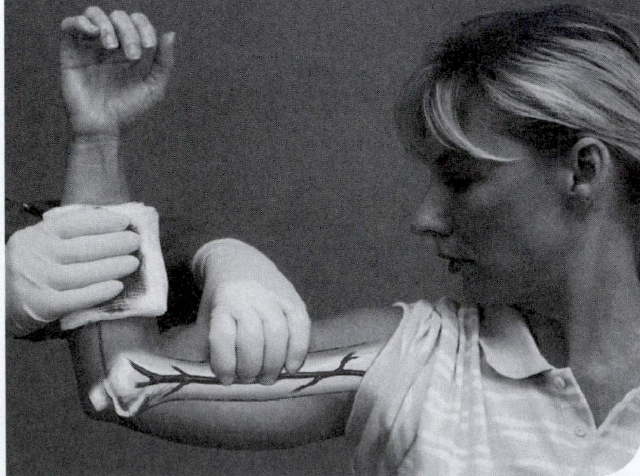

FIGURE 22-3 Applying direct pressure to the wound may halt the flow of blood.

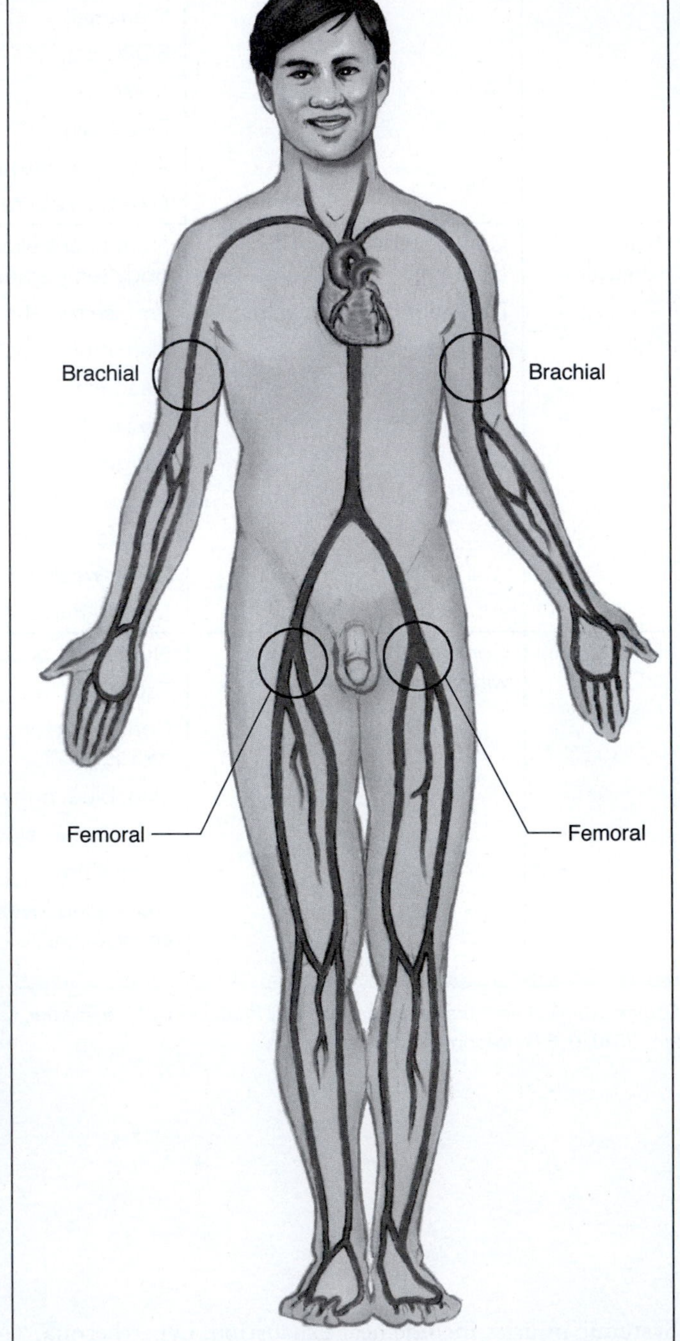

FIGURE 22-4 Brachial and femoral pressure points.

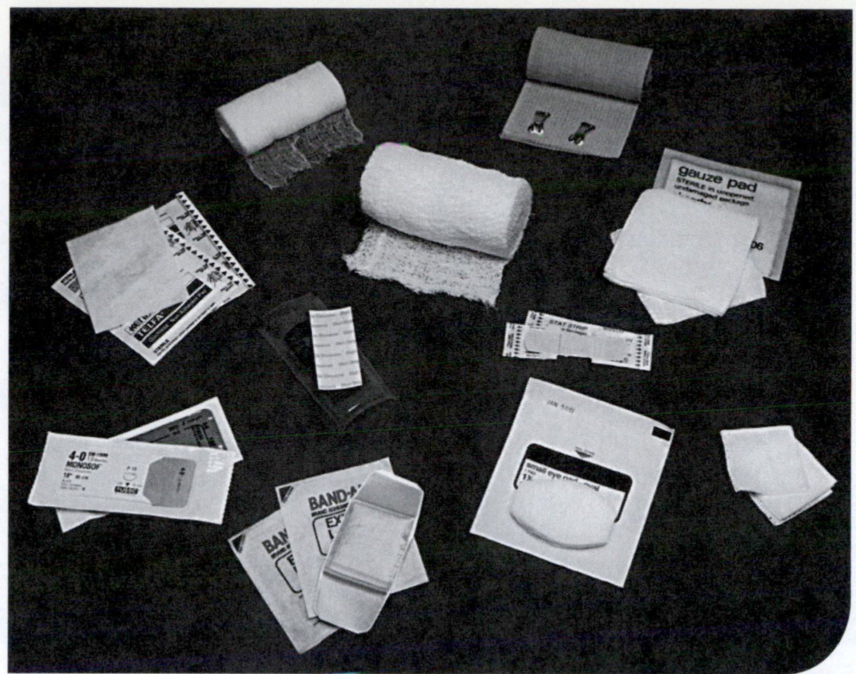

FIGURE 22-5 Types of bandages.

When using pressure points to control bleeding, pressure is applied to the artery where it is close to the skin and can be compressed against an underlying bone. It is important to choose the pressure point that will control bleeding distal to the pressure point.

Signs and symptoms of internal bleeding include bruising, tenderness, and swelling at the site of injury as well as pain in the area of the injury. Call 911 and keep the victim quiet, warm, and lying down, with the feet slightly elevated, until EMS arrives.

Epistaxis

Epistaxis (nosebleed) is usually a non-life-threatening emergency that may occur spontaneously or following a blow to the nose. However, it may also be caused by hypertension and may be a sign of a more serious problem. When a nosebleed occurs, follow these steps:

- Have the patient sit in a chair and tilt the head forward.
- Ask the patient to apply direct pressure by pinching and holding the sides of the nose together. It may take up to 15 minutes for the bleeding to be controlled.
- Once the bleeding is controlled, apply an ice pack.
- Instruct the patient not to blow the nose for several hours after the bleeding has stopped.
- If the bleeding cannot be controlled, call 911.

BANDAGING

Dressing	Sterile covering placed directly over a wound to absorb blood and body fluids
Bandage	Strips of binding material that hold a dressing in place
Pressure Dressing	Compress held in place by an elastic bandage

Different types of bandages are shown in Figure 22-5.

WOUNDS AND FRACTURES

Wounds can either be superficial (affecting only the skin) or deep (affecting the fascia and possibly the structures below the fascia). Figure 22-6 shows the classification of open wounds.

Open wounds are typically not life-threatening unless they penetrate the head, chest, throat, or abdomen. Depending on their severity, most wounds simply require irrigation, debridement, sutures, and antibiotics. Anytime there is an open wound, the status of the victim's last tetanus shot should be noted.

A break in a bone is referred to as a *fracture*. The different types of fractures are discussed in Chapter 5. Treatment of

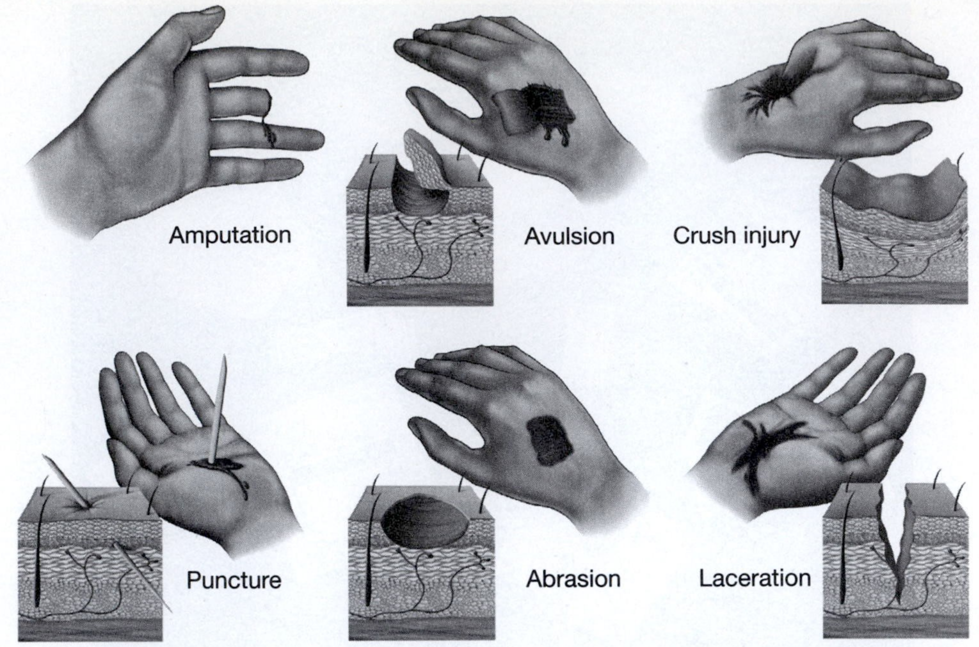

FIGURE 22-6 Classification of open wounds.

fractures requires immobilization of the body area and application of either a splint or a cast.

Splint	Orthopedic device that immobilizes/supports any part of the body May be rigid or flexible
Cast	Rigid dressing made of plaster or fiberglass that is molded to the body

REMOVAL OF FOREIGN BODIES

Foreign bodies may include dirt, rust particles, insects, metal objects, and other small objects. Any foreign object in the eye requires immediate attention. Sterile eyewash may be required. Have the victim turn the head toward the affected side, and allow the eyewash to run from the inner cannula outward.

An insect in the ear can be removed by placing the patient in a dark room and shining a flashlight down the ear canal. If the insect is alive, it will automatically be drawn to the light and come out on its own. If the insect is dead, the ear may need to be irrigated with a solution of 50% hydrogen peroxide and 50% warm water.

ACUTE ABDOMINAL PAIN

Acute abdominal pain of sudden onset is often a sign of a serious underlying medical condition and must be assessed by the physician as soon as possible. The medical assistant should attempt to help make the patient as comfortable as possible. Typically, the patient will be most comfortable sitting with the knees drawn up. Medical assistants are not licensed to diagnose, but pain in certain areas of the abdomen may be indicative of the following conditions:

Pain in the Following Area:	May Indicate the Following Disorder:
Upper Right Quadrant (URQ)	Gallbladder disorders
Lower Right Quadrant (LRQ)	Appendicitis
Back or Flank (Retroperitoneal)	Kidney disorders
Pelvis	Urinary tract infection, pelvic infection, problem in the lower gastrointestinal tract

DIABETIC EMERGENCIES

At times, patients with diabetes may exhibit signs of either hypoglycemia or hyperglycemia. A diabetic with a blood sugar level below 70 mg/dL is said to be *hypoglycemic.* A diabetic with a blood sugar level above 120 mg/dL is said to be *hyperglycemic.*

HYPOGLYCEMIA VERSUS HYPERGLYCEMIA

	Hypoglycemia, Insulin Reaction	Hyperglycemia, Diabetic Coma
Signs and Symptoms	Rapid, abrupt onset Patient complains of hunger Cool, moist skin and profuse perspiration (diaphoresis) Pale, clammy skin Blood glucose level below 70 mg/dl Rapid onset of decreased level of consciousness	Slow, insidious onset Patient complains of intense thirst and dry mouth Dry, warm skin Flushed skin Blood glucose level elevated above normal Increased urine output Rapid and deep respirations Abdominal pain and vomiting Slow onset of decreased level of consciousness Acetone-smelling breath
Treatment	Give patient a simple sugar source such as hard candy, soda, or orange juice. If patient is unable to swallow or is comatose, give dextrose or glucagon by intravenous route.	Give patient insulin by subcutaneous injection, plus fluids and sodium (such as salt) by mouth. If patient is unable to swallow or is comatose, give insulin, fluids, and sodium by intravenous route.

Source: Medical Assisting: Foundations and Practices by M. S. Frazier, C. Malone, and C. Malone, Upper Saddle River, NJ: Pearson Education, Inc., 2010, p. 862. Reprinted with permission.

POISONING

The majority of accidental poisonings occur at home and in children under the age of 5. Symptoms of poisoning include the following:

- Abdominal pain
- Cramping
- Nausea/vomiting
- Diarrhea
- Odor
- Stains/burns around the mouth
- Drowsiness
- Unconsciousness

Poison Control Centers have been established in most areas of the United States and offer emergency advice concerning accidental poisoning and overdose. They will advise the best course of action for the poison ingested. The Poison Control Center's telephone number should be kept close to the telephones in the medical office.

SHOCK

Shock is a life-threatening state that occurs when there is insufficient cardiac output, which in turn causes a decrease in blood supply and nourishment to the tissues and organs.

Type of Shock	Cause
Anaphylactic	Follows an allergic reaction
Cardiogenic	Reduction in cardiac output, such as pulmonary embolism, myocardial infarction, tachycardia, and bradycardia
Hypovolemic	Inadequate intravascular volume Occurs after an injury with major fluid loss
Neurogenic	Severe cerebral trauma or hemorrhage
Septic	Systemic infection that causes vasodilation and decreased vascular resistance

The following table lists the symptoms of shock.

SYMPTOMS OF SHOCK FOLLOWING A CRISIS SITUATION

Weakness	Dizziness	Clammy skin	Disorientation
Rapid heartbeat	Restlessness	Cyanosis	Unresponsiveness
Thirst	Pallor	Confusion	Shallow breathing
Nausea	Cool skin		

In addition to the treatments listed in the following table it is important to have the victim lay on his or her back with the feet above heart level and to keep the victim warm.

TREATMENT FOR SHOCK IN THE MEDICAL OFFICE

Cause	Treatment
Anaphylactic Shock	Epinephrine
Cardiogenic Shock	IV dopamine, immediate transport to the emergency department
Hemorrhagic Shock	Stop bleeding, replace volume, immediate transport to the emergency department
Hypovolemic Shock	Replace volume
Insulin Shock	Give sugar to patient by any means tolerated
Neurogenic Shock	IV dopamine and immediate transport to the emergency department
Poisoning	Consult Poison Control Center for treatment specific to the poison
Respiratory Shock	Intubation and immediate transport to the emergency department
Sepsis	Fluids, IV dopamine, and immediate transport to the emergency department

NEUROLOGICAL EMERGENCIES **Neurologic emergencies include head trauma, seizures, epilepsy, altered level of consciousness, cerebrovascular accident, and transient ischemic attack.**

Altered Level of Consciousness	Also known as altered *LOC* May vary from dizziness/light-headedness to complete loss of consciousness If a patient begins to complain of light-headedness, have the patient sit in a chair with the head between the knees. If the patient feels as if he or she may pass out, lower the patient to the ground in a supine position and elevate the feet and legs about 12 inches.
Seizures	Occur as a result of involuntary muscular contraction Your primary responsibility while helping a seizing victim is to keep him or her safe. Following is a list of actions you should take when caring for someone who is seizing: • Move furniture and other objects out of the way to minimize the risk of injury. • Do not force the victim's mouth open. • Stay with the victim and provide privacy. • Loosen constricting clothing. *Once the seizure stops:* • Make sure that the airway is open. • If mucus and saliva are found in the patient's mouth, turn the head to help facilitate drainage and prevent aspiration. • Note the length of the seizure.

(Continued)

Cerebrovascular Accident	Also known as *CVA* or a *stroke* Occurs when circulation to the brain is compromised Signs and symptoms of stroke may include: • Paralysis on one side of the body • Impaired/slurred speech • Confusion • Dizziness • Facial droop • Arm drift • Loss of balance/coordination • Visual difficulties • Loss of consciousness • Headache Do not leave the victim alone; place him or her in a semisitting position and call 911
Transient Ischemic Attack	Also known as *TIA* or a *mini-stroke* Temporary, but similar in nature to CVA Symptoms similar to those of CVA (except that there is no loss of consciousness) and usually resolve within 24 hours of onset Do not leave the victim alone; place him or her in a semisitting position and call 911.
Head Injury (Figure 22-7)	Severity of injury depends on the following: • Cause of the injury • Force of the offending object • Where within the brain the trauma has occurred Keep the victim quiet and gather information.

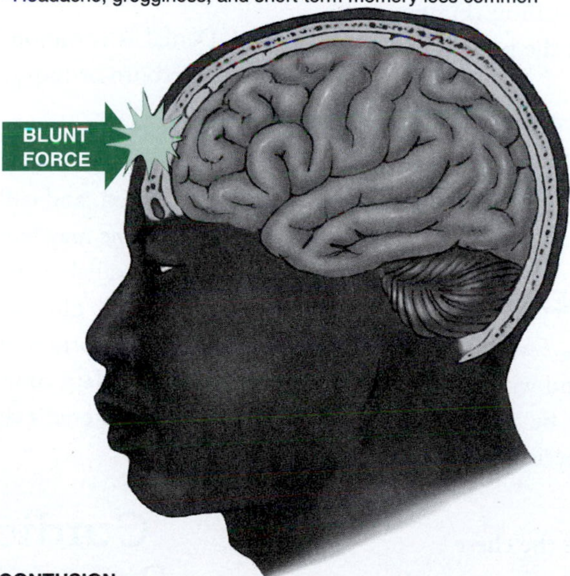
CONCUSSION
• Mild injury, usually with no detectable brain damage
• May have brief loss of consciousness
• Headache, grogginess, and short-term memory loss common
BLUNT FORCE
CONTUSION
• Unconsciousness or decreased level of responsiveness
• Bruising of brain tissue

FIGURE 22-7 Closed head injuries.

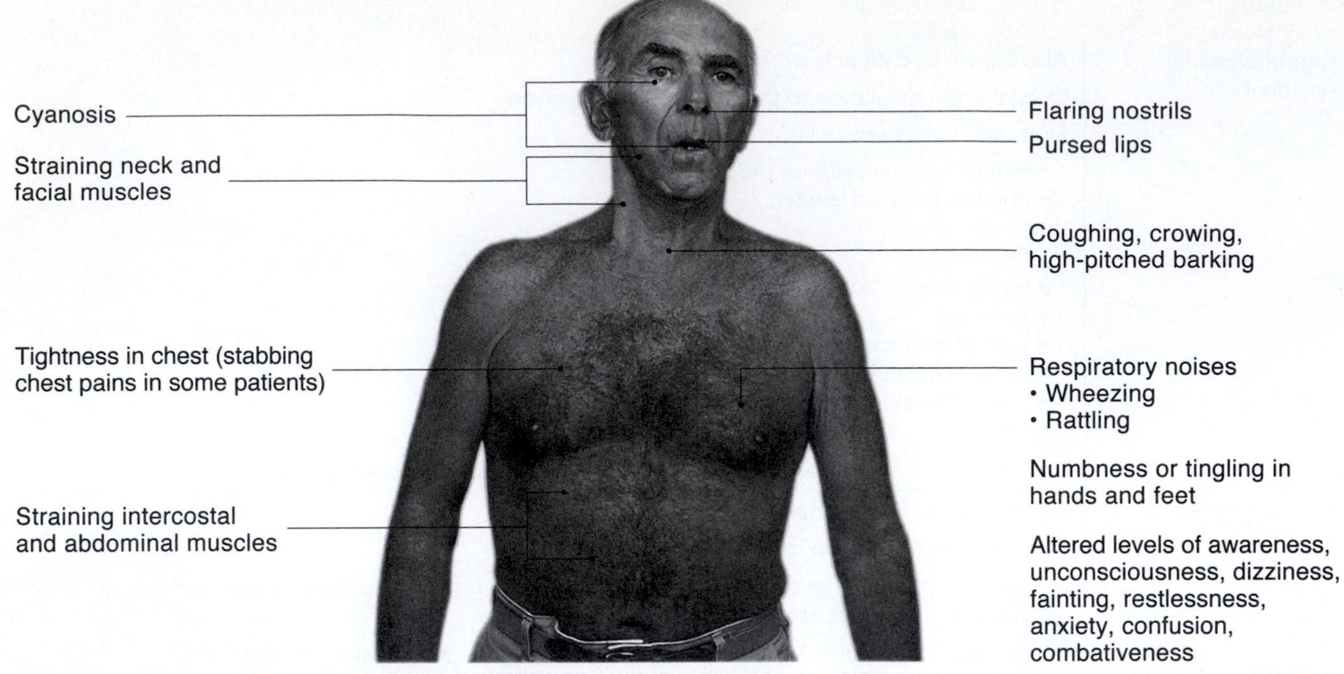

FIGURE 22-8 Signs and symptoms of breathing difficulty.

RESPIRATORY EMERGENCIES

Respiratory emergencies may occur as a result of a long-term illness or disease, such as chronic obstructive pulmonary disease (COPD), asthma, pneumonia, or pulmonary edema, or they may take place in an acute situation.

If a patient is having difficulty breathing (Figure 22-8), notify the physician, call 911, and ask the patient to sit in a chair with his or her feet propped up.

The inability to get enough oxygen may cause extreme anxiety for the patient. Remain calm and provide emotional support. If the patient has an occluded airway, proceed to the choking protocol.

CARDIOVASCULAR EMERGENCIES

Myocardial infarctions, also known as *heart attacks*, are the leading cause of death for both men and women.

The symptoms of chest pain may be very different for different people. Individuals may experience some or all of the following:

- Pain in the middle or left side of the chest
- May be described as sharp, crushing, stabbing, squeezing, or aching pain
- May or may not radiate to the left arm, the back, or up the neck.
- Sometimes occurs suddenly and without explanation; at other times, may occur with exertion
- Nausea
- Weakness
- Shortness of breath (SOB)
- Apprehension
- Skin may be clammy, moist, pale, or cyanotic
- Denial is common, and the pain may be explained as heartburn or indigestion.

If someone is complaining of any of the above symptoms, have the person stop what he or she is doing, sit down with the feet elevated, and call 911. If the person has a history of angina, he or she may have been prescribed nitroglycerin and may have it available. If the person does have nitroglycerin available, apply gloves and insert one tablet under the tongue. It is important that you do not touch the nitroglycerin, as it will dilate your blood vessels as well. Nitroglycerin may be administered every five minutes for a total of three doses.

Cardiopulmonary Resuscitation (CPR)

For individuals experiencing chest pain, loss of consciousness, or respiratory arrest, the CPR protocol should be followed. The guidelines are similar for respiratory arrest, cardiac arrest, and obstructed airway but vary somewhat according to age. Figures 22-9 through 22-11 show hand

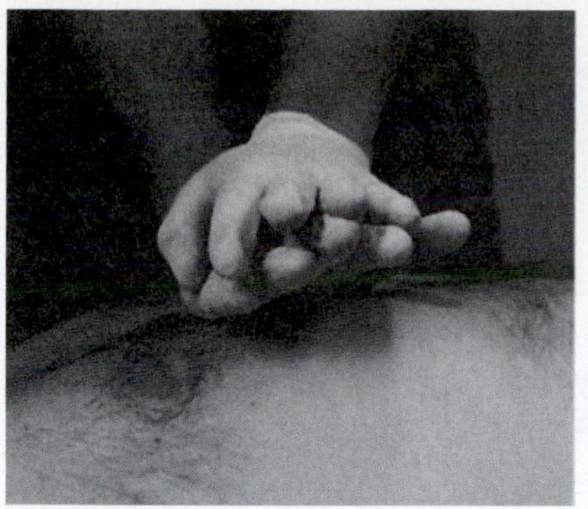
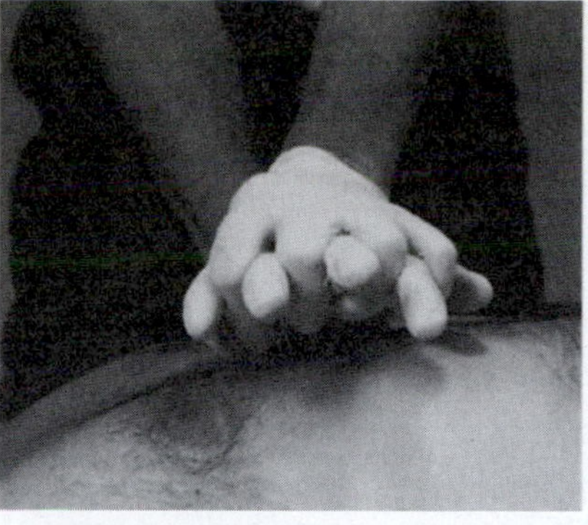
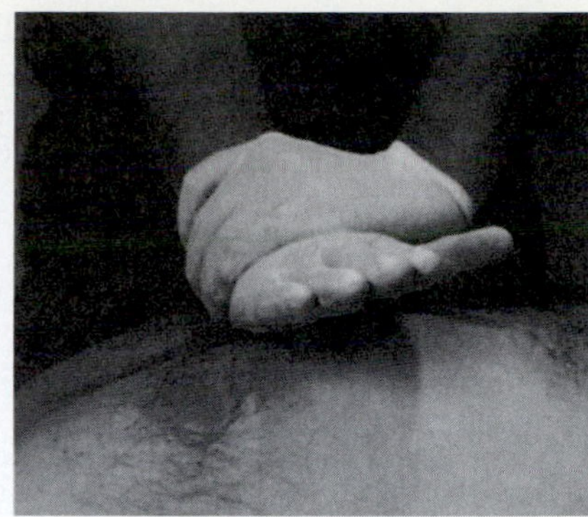

FIGURE 22-9 Hand placement during chest compressions for an adult.

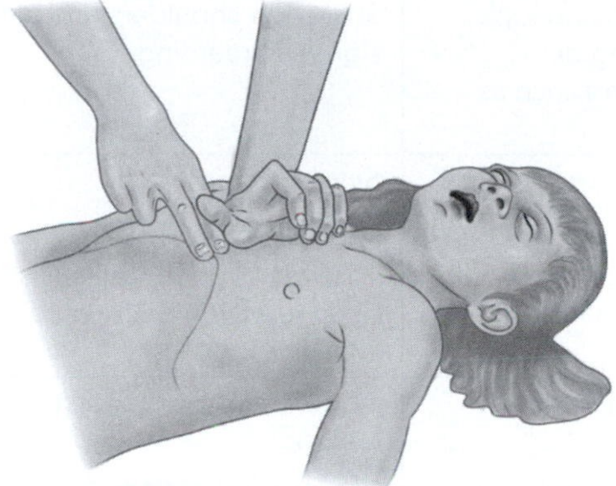

FIGURE 22-10 Hand placement during chest compressions for a child.

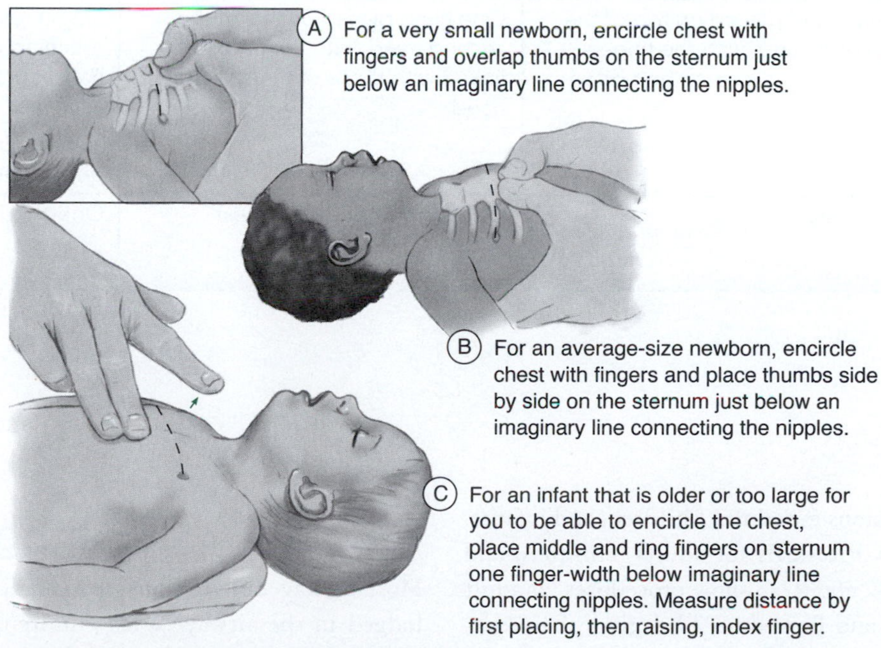

A For a very small newborn, encircle chest with fingers and overlap thumbs on the sternum just below an imaginary line connecting the nipples.
B For an average-size newborn, encircle chest with fingers and place thumbs side by side on the sternum just below an imaginary line connecting the nipples.
C For an infant that is older or too large for you to be able to encircle the chest, place middle and ring fingers on sternum one finger-width below imaginary line connecting nipples. Measure distance by first placing, then raising, index finger.

FIGURE 22-11 Hand placement during chest compressions for an infant.

ADULT, CHILD, AND INFANT CPR SKILLS

It is important to remember C-A-B when performing CPR for an adult, a child and an infant:

C = compressions

A = airway

B = breathing

CPR Skill	Adult	Child: 1 Year to Puberty (approximately 12 to 14 years)	Infant: Under 1 Year
Activate EMS by calling 911 and giving emergency information	If sudden collapse is witnessed, immediately activate EMS and get automated external defibrillator (AED). If asphyxiation (e.g., drowning, injury, overdose) is suspected, first perform CPR for two minutes (or five cycles), then activate EMS.	If sudden collapse is witnessed, immediately activate EMS and get AED. Otherwise, perform two minutes of CPR (five cycles), then activate EMS.	If sudden collapse is witnessed, immediately activate EMS. Otherwise, perform two minutes of CPR (five cycles), then activate EMS.
Assessment of unresponsiveness and breathing	Shake the shoulders and look for signs of breathing or inadequate breathing such as agonal respirations.	Shake the shoulders and look for signs of breathing.	Sharply poke the feet and look for signs of breathing. Do *not* shake the shoulders.
Rescue breathing and chest compression rate	*Single rescuer: 30:2* *Two rescuers:* 30:2 The rate of compressions should be at least 100 per minute.	*Single rescuer:* 30:2 *Two rescuers:* 15:2 The rate of compressions should be at least 100 per minute.	*Single rescuer:* 30:2 *Two rescuers:* 15:2 The rate of compressions should be at least 100 per minute.
Obstructed airway foreign body	Abdominal thrusts if victim is conscious Chest compressions if victim is unconscious	Abdominal thrusts if victim is conscious Chest compressions if victim is unconscious	Back slaps and chest thrusts if victim is conscious Chest compressions if victim is unconscious
Pulse check location	Carotid	Carotid	Brachial or femoral
Compression landmarks	Center of chest, between nipples	Center of chest, between nipples	Center of chest, just below the nipple line
Compression technique	One hand placed on top of the second hand, with the fingers linked with those of the bottom hand	One hand placed on top of the second hand, with the fingers linked with those of the bottom hand	*Single rescuer:* two thumbs touching on the sternum and hand encircling the chest and back *Two rescuers:* two fingertips on sternum
Compression depth	2 inches	One-third of depth of chest	One-third of depth of chest

placement for compressions for adults, children, and infants. The table above lists CPR skills for adults, children, and infants. Procedures 22-2 and 22-3 show procedures for adult and infant/child CPR, and Procedure 22-4 gives the procedure for using an automated external defibrillator.

Choking

Most airway obstructions are caused by a foreign object lodged in the airway. With children, the foreign object is usually food or small toys. With adults, the obstructed airway

procedure

22-2

PERFORM ADULT RESCUE BREATHING AND ONE-RESCUER CPR

Objective: Administer rescue breathing for an adult and one-rescuer CPR for an adult correctly.

EQUIPMENT AND SUPPLIES

- approved mannequin
- gloves
- ventilator mask
- mouth guard

METHOD

1. Assess the victim and determine if help is neeed. Shout "Are you okay?" while gently shaking the victim's shoulders and assessing for adequate breathing.
2. If it is determined that the adult victim is unresponsive, activate EMS immediately by calling 911; then get an AED if available (see Procedure 22-4). Attempt to get another person to call 911.
3. If gloves are available, put them on. If you have a ventilator mask, place it on the victim.

No Breathing, No Pulse

Note: Begin using the AED as soon as it arrives. See Procedure 22-4.

- If it is determined that the victim is not breathing, check for a pulse for at least 5 but no more than 10 seconds (Figure 22-12). If there is no pulse, begin compressions immediately.
- Kneel at the victim's side. Place your hand in the center of the chest between the nipples.
- Place your other hand on top of the first hand, making sure to lift your fingers off the chest, using only the heels of your hands to administer compressions.
- Keeping your shoulders directly over your hands, compress the chest at least 2 inches, allowing the sternum to relax in between compressions. Do not lift your hands off the chest.
- Continue compressing the chest at a rate of 100 compressions per minute for a total of 30 compressions; then administer two breaths.
- If your breaths do not cause the chest to rise, reposition the head using the head-tilt, chin-lift method and make a second attempt to administer breaths.
- If the breath still does not go in, resume compressions. Continue the cycle of 30 compressions and 2 breaths
- If necessary, continue CPR until pulse and breathing return or you are relieved by more advanced medical personnel.

CHARTING EXAMPLE

08/05/XX 7:30 P.M. Patient found collapsed in bathroom and unresponsive. 911 call placed and CPR started. EMS arrived in approximately 10 minutes and took over care. Patient was transferred to Deaconess Medical Center. · · · · V. Nagle, RMA (AMT)

No Breathing, But Pulse Is Present

- Once it is determined that the victim is not breathing, check for a pulse for at least 5 but no more than 10 seconds. If there is a pulse but the victim is not breathing, establish an airway (Figure 22-13) and begin rescue breathing.

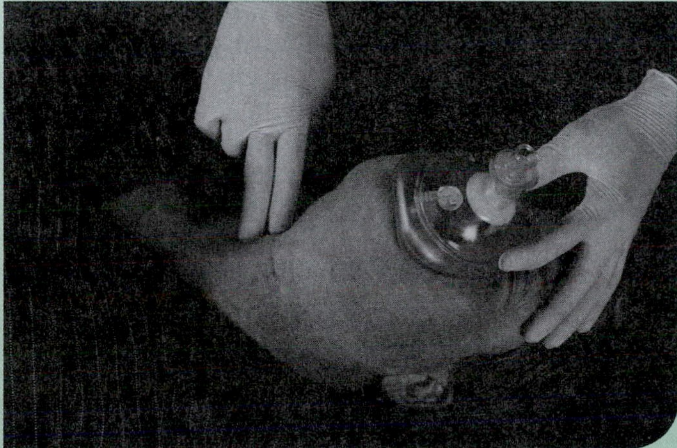

FIGURE 22-12 Assess the victim's circulation by feeling for a pulse at the carotid artery.

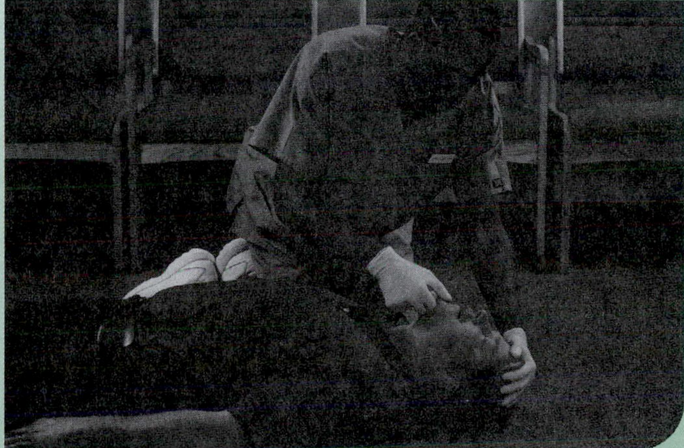

FIGURE 22-13 Establish an open airway.

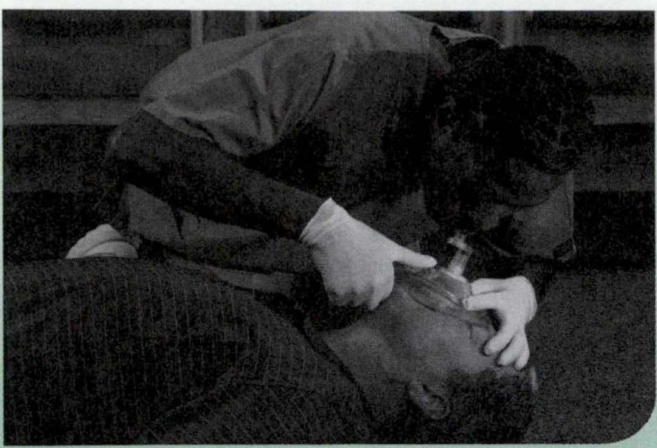

FIGURE 22-14 When performing rescue breathing, administer one breath every five seconds.

- Using a barrier device administer 1 breath every five seconds or 10 to 12 breaths every minute (Figure 22-14). After one minute, reassess the victim for breathing and pulse.
- Wash your hands and document the incident in the patient's chart.

CHARTING EXAMPLE

07/16/XX 2:15 P.M. Patient found collapsed in hallway and unresponsive. 911 call placed and rescue breathing started. EMS arrived in approximately 10 minutes and took over care. Patient was transferred to Deaconess Medical Center. .... V. Nagle, RMA (AMT)

procedure 22-3

PERFORM INFANT OR YOUNG CHILD RESCUE BREATHING AND ONE-RESCUER CPR

Objective: Administer rescue breathing for a child and one-rescuer CPR for an infant.

EQUIPMENT AND SUPPLIES

- approved mannequin
- gloves
- ventilator mask
- mouth guard

METHOD

1. Assess the victim and determine if help is needed. Shout the name of the infant or child and sharply poke at the feet. Never shake an infant.
2. If the infant is determined to be unresponsive and breathing is not present, perform CPR for two minutes prior to activating EMS immediately by calling 911 and then get an AED, if available.
3. Carefully place the victim on the back, being careful not to move the head or allow the neck to twist, especially if a spinal cord injury is suspected.
4. Check the victim's pulse at the brachial artery. If you feel a pulse, begin rescue breathing by administering 1 breath every five seconds or 10 to 12 breaths every minute.
5. If you do not feel a pulse, begin chest compressions. Place two fingers in the center of the chest just below the nipple line. Compressions should be made one-third the depth of the chest. Perform 30 quick compressions.
6. Gently, with two fingers, tilt the victim's head and open the airway.
7. If breathing is absent, place a mouth guard over the victim's mouth and nose. Administer two rescue breaths. If your breaths do not cause the chest to rise, reposition using the head- tilt, chin-lift method and make a second attempt to administer a rescue breath.
8. Continue the sequence of 30 compressions and two breaths.
9. After two minutes, leave the infant and call 911 if you are still alone. Continue compressions and breaths until the infant recovers or EMS arrives.
10. Wash your hands and document the incident in the patient's chart.

CHARTING EXAMPLE

10/09/XX 9:45 A.M. A 10-month-old patient fell in exam room and was not responsive when physician and medical assistant arrived. Called 911 and EMS activated as directed by the physician. Infant CPR was initiated by the physician until EMS arrived. Patient transported to Walters Creek General Hospital. .... M. Cowan, CMA (AAMA)

procedure

22-4

USE AN AUTOMATED EXTERNAL DEFIBRILLATOR

Objective: Use an automated external defibrillator (AED) correctly.

EQUIPMENT AND SUPPLIES

- AED machine
- patient chart

METHOD

1. Place the AED (Figure 22-15) next to the victim's left ear. This position allows the rescuers clear access to the chest and airway for continued rescue measures.
2. Turn the AED on and follow the voice prompts.
3. You will be prompted to attach the electrode pads to the victim's chest on the sternum and at the apex of the heart, following the diagram for correct placement. Use adult-size electrode pads on victims eight years of age and older. Child-size electrode pads are used for infants and victims up to eight years of age or under 55 lb. If child-size electrode pads are not available, adult pads may be used.
4. Next, you will be directed to allow the machine to analyze the heart rhythm to determine if it is a shockable rhythm. CPR should cease while the machine is analyzing.
5. The machine will begin a charging sequence prior to shocking and warn rescuers to stand back. The voice prompt will then tell you to press the SHOCK button to administer the electrical current to the victim.
6. If the machine indicates that "not shock is advised", assess the victim for breathing and circulation. Leave the electrode pads in place and continue CPR as needed until advanced medical personnel arrive.

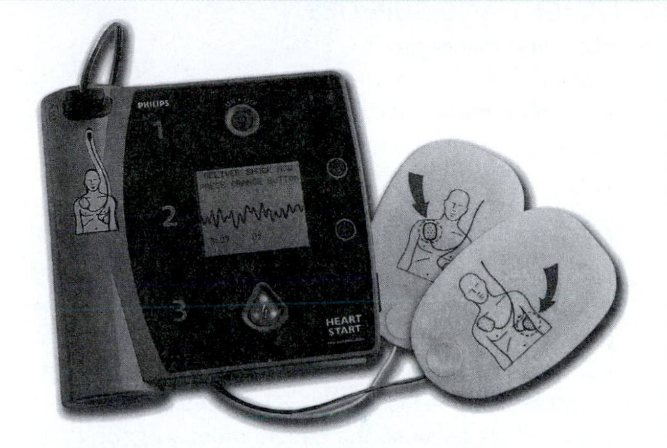

FIGURE 22-15 Automated external defibrillator.

CHARTING EXAMPLE

11/25/XX 3:30 P.M. Patient found in stairwell, unresponsive, with absence of pulse and respirations. 911 protocol initiated with two-rescuer CPR. Third rescuer initiated AED response, and patient was analyzed for shockable rhythm. CPR and AED shocks administered a total of eight cycles prior to arrival of advanced medical support. Patient released to EMS care and transferred to Sacred Heart Medical Center. .... M. Cowan, CMA (AAMA)

may be the result of large pieces of food that have not been properly chewed, talking or laughing too much while eating, drinking alcohol before and during eating, or choking on fluids such as vomit or blood.

It is important to understand that if the victim is able to cough or talk, there is no need to perform the Heimlich maneuver. But it is important to stay close and watch the victim. If he or she loses the ability to cough or talk, ask if you may assist and begin the proper choking procedure.

For someone who is not able to speak or cough and has the hands around the throat, indicating that he or she is choking (Figure 22-16), ask if you may assist and begin the proper choking procedure (Procedure 22-5).

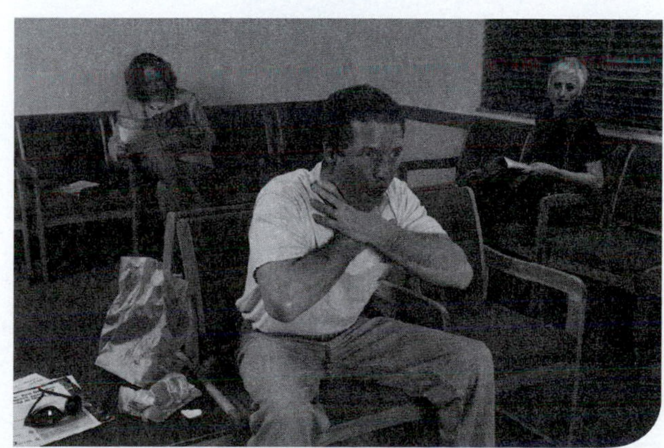

FIGURE 22-16 The universal choking sign.

procedure 22-5

RESPOND TO AN ADULT WITH AN OBSTRUCTED AIRWAY

Objective: Administer the Heimlich maneuver to an adult correctly.

EQUIPMENT AND SUPPLIES

- approved mannequin
- gloves
- ventilation mask with one-way valve for an unconscious patient

METHOD

1. Once it has been established that the patient is choking, with no air exchange, direct someone to call 911 and shout "Are you choking?" or "Can you speak?" If the answer is no—as indicated by a head shake—ask the victim for permission to begin emergency treatment.
2. Stand behind the victim with your feet slightly apart, placing one foot between the patient's feet and one to the outside. This stance will give you greater stability, and if the patient should pass out, you can safely guide the victim to the ground by sliding him or her down your thigh.
3. Place the index finger of one hand at the person's navel or belt buckle to mark that spot. If the victim is a pregnant woman, place your finger above the enlarged uterus.

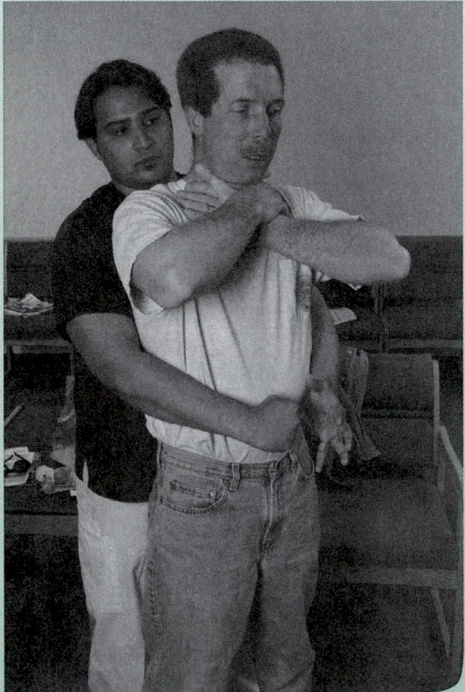

FIGURE 22-17 Delivering abdominal thrusts.

4. Make a fist with your other hand and place it, thumb side to the victim, above your other hand. If the person is very large or far along in pregnancy, you may have to do chest compressions.
5. Place your marking hand over your curled fist and begin to give quick inward and upward thrusts (Figure 22-17).
6. There is no set number of thrusts to give to an adult who remains conscious. Continue to give thrusts until the object is removed or the patient becomes unconscious.
7. If the victim becomes unconscious, gently lower him or her to the ground (Figure 22-18).
8. Activate EMS and put on gloves.
9. Immediately begin CPR with 30 chest compressions and two rescue breaths
10. Before administering the rescue breaths, open the airway with the head-tilt, chin-lift maneuver. Look for a foreign body in the victim's mouth and remove any that is visible. Blind finger sweeps are no longer recommended and should not be performed.
11. Continue with cycles of 30 compressions and two rescue breaths until the foreign body is expelled or advance medical personnel arrive to relieve you.
12. Wash hands and document the event in the patient's chart.

CHARTING EXAMPLE

10/25/XX 11:30 A.M. Jason Jones exhibited signs of choking at lunch. Jason grabbed his throat and was unable to cough or make noise. Tina Muller, RMA, alerted the physician and placed a call to 911. Abdominal thrusts were given until the piece of apple was expelled. EMS arrived and checked Jason for signs of throat irritation and swelling. .... J. Walker, CMA (AAMA)

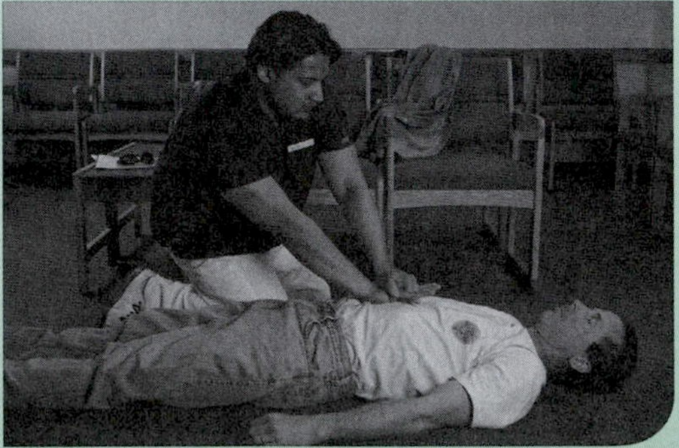

FIGURE 22-18 Administering chest compressions to the unconscious victim

Figure 22-19 shows the procedure to follow for an infant who is choking.

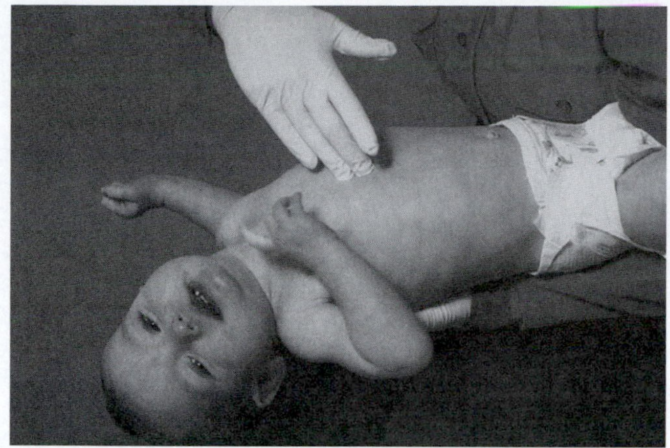

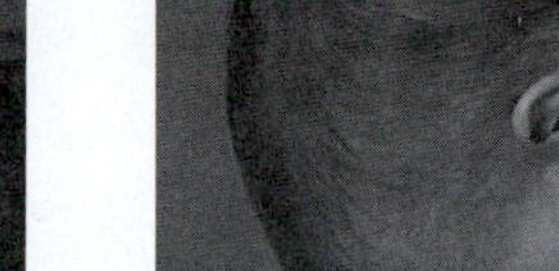

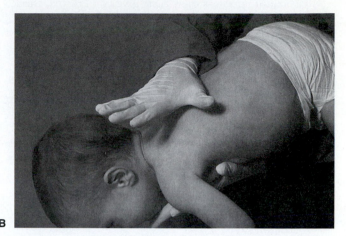

FIGURE 22-19 (A) Administer chest thrusts followed by (B) back blows.

22 APPLICATION

Directions: Select the best answer for each of the following questions. Check your answers in the Answer Key at the end of the book.

1. Which of the following answers lists the proper sequence for performing adult CPR?
   a. Call 911, assess the victim for responsiveness and breathing, assess the CABs, check for a pulse, give 30 compressions, give two breaths, 30 compressions, give two breaths
   b. Call 911, assess the CABs, give two breaths, check for a pulse, give 30 compressions, two breaths, 30 compressions
   c. Assess the victim for responsiveness and breathing, call 911, assess the CABs, check for a pulse, give 30 compressions, give two breaths, give 30 compressions, two breaths, give 30 compressions, two breaths, 30 compressions
   d. Assess the victim call 911, assess the CABs, give two breaths, check for a pulse, give 30 compressions, two breaths, 30 compressions.
   e. Assess the victim for responsiveness and breathing, assess the CABs, give two breaths, check for a pulse, call 911, give 30 compressions, two breaths, 30 compressions

2. Which of the following answers lists the proper sequence for performing infant CPR if sudden collapse was witnessed?
   a. Call 911, assess the victim for responsiveness and breathing, assess the CABs, give two breaths, check for a pulse, give 30 compressions, two breaths, 30 compressions
   b. Call 911, assess the CABs, give two breaths, check for a pulse, give 30 compressions, two breaths, 30 compressions
   c. Assess the victim for responsiveness and breathing, call 911, assess the CABs, check for a pulse, give 30 compressions, give two breaths, give 30 compressions, two breaths
   d. Assess the victim for responsiveness and breathing, call 911, assess the CABs, give two breaths, check for a pulse, give 30 compressions, two breaths, 30 compressions
   e. Assess the victim for responsiveness and breathing, assess the CABs, give two breaths, check for a pulse, call 911, give 30 compressions, two breaths, 30 compressions

3. When using the AED on a child, which of the following statements is not true?
   a. An AED can be used on children ages one to eight.
   b. An AED can be used on children under 55 lb.
   c. Adult-size pads can be used on children nine years old.
   d. You should continue CPR while the AED is analyzing.
   e. If the AED indicates "No shock advised," assess the patient for breathing/circulation and begin CPR.

4. Using the Rule of Nines, the front of each arm equals ________ %.
   a. 4.5
   b. 7
   c. 9
   d. 14
   e. 18

5. When using an epinephrine pen, which of the following statements does not apply?
   a. Remove the safety cap.
   b. Hold the epinephrine pen in your fist, avoiding both ends.
   c. Press the pen firmly against the victim's thigh, close to the hip.
   d. The injection can be given through clothes if necessary.
   e. Rub the injection site for several seconds.

6. What type of shock follows an allergic reaction?
   a. Septic
   b. Neurogenic
   c. Hypovolemic
   d. Cardiogenic
   e. Anaphylactic

7. Regarding a transient ischemic attack, which of the following statements is not true?
   a. Also known as a *mini-stroke*
   b. Similar in nature to CVA
   c. Temporary
   d. Involves loss of consciousness
   e. Characterized by paralysis on one side of the body

8. When performing rescue breathing for a child, which of the following statements is correct?
   a. Give one breath every two to three seconds.
   b. Give one breath every three to five seconds.
   c. Give one breath every five to seven seconds.
   d. Give one breath every six to eight seconds.
   e. Give one breath every seven to nine seconds.

9. Which of the following is not a symptom of shock?
   a. Weakness
   b. Thirst
   c. Cool, clammy skin
   d. Bradycardia
   e. Shallow breathing

10. When a diabetic patient's blood sugar falls below ________ mg/dL, he or she is said to be hypoglycemic.
    a. 50
    b. 60
    c. 70
    d. 100
    e. 120

11. Regarding arterial bleeding, which of the following is incorrect?
    a. Abundant
    b. Dark red
    c. Rapid
    d. Spurts in rhythm with the heartbeat
    e. Needs to be brought under control as quickly as possible

12. Which of the following open wounds leaves a flap of skin?
    a. Avulsion
    b. Abrasion
    c. Laceration
    d. Puncture
    e. Crush injury

13. Which of the following is *not* one of FEMA's six steps in planning for a natural disaster?
    a. Ensure that your insurance paperwork is in order.
    b. Educate the staff.
    c. Have disaster supplies on hand.
    d. Check for hazards throughout the facility.
    e. Develop an emergency communication plan.

14. The Rule of Nines is used to calculate the extent of _____.
   a. Frostbite
   b. A crush wound
   c. A burn area
   d. Open wounds
   e. Animal bites

15. ______ occurs as a brief interruption in the flow of blood to the brain and causes a typical brief loss of consciousness.
   a. Fainting
   b. Stroke
   c. Syncope
   d. A and B but not C
   e. A and C but not B

16. Superficial wounds affect ________________ .
   a. Bones
   b. The skin
   c. The fascia
   d. Ligaments
   e. None of the above

17. If a patient suffers respiratory shock in the medical office, which of the following should be administered?
   a. Intubation and immediate transport to the Emergency Department
   b. Epinephrine
   c. IV dopamine
   d. Sugar given by any means
   e. Replacement volume

18. A ______ is a compress held in place by an elastic bandage.
   a. Dressing
   b. Pressure dressing
   c. Bandage
   d. Compression wrap
   e. None of the above

19. Which of the following statements applies to contusions?
   a. Mild injury
   b. Decreased level of consciousness
   c. No brain damage
   d. Headache
   e. Grogginess

20. Which of the following type of burns is described as a partial-thickness burn?
   a. Sunburn
   b. First degree
   c. Second degree
   d. Third degree
   e. Fourth degree

21. Heat stroke occurs when the body temperature is greater than ___________ F.
   a. 99°
   b. 100°
   c. 102°
   d. 104°
   e. 105°

22. Regarding diabetic coma, which of the following statements is incorrect?
   a. Increased urine output
   b. Flushed skin
   c. Acetone-smelling breath
   d. Rapid onset
   e. Abdominal pain and vomiting

23. What percentage of the body is involved if an individual sustains burns on the front and back of both legs?
   a. 9
   b. 18
   c. 27
   d. 36
   e. 45

24. During the initial assessments prior to administering CPR, you would do all of the following except:
   a. Check for responsiveness
   b. Check breathing
   c. Check for a pulse
   d. Check for a patent airway
   e. Check for AED

25. When someone is having a seizure, you should do all of the following except:
   a. Move furniture and other objects out of the way to minimize the risk of injury
   b. Force the mouth open
   c. Stay with the victim
   d. Provide privacy
   e. Loosen constricting clothing

APPENDIX A
Chapter Questions Answer Key with Rationales

CHAPTER 1

1. E. All of the above

   Rationale: Resumes should be kept between one and two pages long, typed on good-quality white or off-white paper that is 8½ × 11 inches and should contain the following information:

   - Name, address, telephone number, and e-mail address. (Be sure that the voice message for the telephone number listed and the e-mail address listed are professional.)
   - Objective listing your career goal.
   - Educational background, including a summary of the skills learned
   - Relevant work experience, including dates of employment and brief summaries of duties performed
   - Professional organizations and memberships
   - Certifications obtained
   - Reference information

2. E. A and B

   Rationale: The most common mistakes made during an interview are as follows:

   - Inappropriate dress or poor grooming
   - Poor posture
   - Poor eye contact
   - Smoking or chewing gum
   - Lack of enthusiasm
   - Arriving late
   - Use of slang or improper grammar
   - Talking too much
   - Speaking critically of previous employers
   - Inability to ask questions about the organization

3. B.

   Rationale: The applicant shall have been employed in the profession of Medical Assisting for a minimum of five years, no more than two years of which may have been as an instructor in the postsecondary medical assistant program (proof of current work experience and high school education or equivalent is needed). Employment dates must be within the last five years.

4. E. A and B

   Rationale: Some of the duties performed by a medical administrative specialist include:

   - Set appointment times
   - Greet patients
   - File and pull charts
   - Handle insurance information
   - Assist new patients with paperwork
   - Know word processing
   - Know bookkeeping
   - Type medical correspondence
   - Transcribe medical dictation
   - Understand and know insurance coding information
   - Schedule hospital admissions
   - Type case histories
   - Fill out and submit insurance medical forms
   - Collect and record payments
   - Know medical terminology

5. E. All of the above

   Rationale: **Classified ads**—Use local and out-of-town newspapers, professional journals, and trade magazines. Use the local public library's access to national newspapers.

   Employment agencies—Place your name with the agency and career consultants.

   Health care facilities—Contact hospitals, veterans' facilities, extended care facilities, and ambulatory care sites in your area.

   Internet—Use various websites, such as monster.com, careerbuilder.com, or jobs.com.

   Local medical society—Obtain a list of physicians who are looking for help or a list of all the medical practice offices in your area.

   Parents, friends—Network with your own friends and relatives. Make sure they know that you are looking for employment.

   Personal physician—Your own physician may network for you and call his or her colleagues.

   Professional organizations—Use both state and local chapters of any professional associations and allied health groups to which you belong.

Publications—American Association of Medical Assistants and other local professional publications.

School placement service—One of the best sources since the staff know your training and skills well. In many cases, prospective employers will call schools to identify potential new employees.

State employment office—After completing the required application forms, your name will be on file for available.

6. C. AMT

   Rationale: The American Medical Technologists (AMT) award the Registered Medical Assistant (RMA) credential.

7. E. 30

   Rationale: The AMT requires all RMAs (AMT) and CMAS who were initially certified on or after January 1, 2006, to obtain 30 CEUs over a three-year period.

8. E. 60

   Rationale: The AAMA requires that all CMAs (AAMA) remain current in their practice. In addition, in order to maintain the credential, they must complete 60 CEUs (30 of which must be AAMA approved) in the five years following certification, which must be distributed as follows: 10 administrative, 10 clinical, and 10 general. The remaining 30 CEUs can be distributed anywhere among the three areas.

9. D. 34

   Rationale: According to the Bureau of Labor Statistics, U.S. Department of Labor, *Occupational Outlook Handbook, 2010–2011 Edition,* medical assisting is among the fastest-growing occupations and has a projected growth of 34% between 2008 and 2018.

10. B. $95

    Rationale: The nonrefundable application fee for either the computerized or paper-and-pencil version of the RMA (AMT) exam is $95

11. E. $250

    Rationale: Qualified applicants must complete and sign the CMA (AAMA) exam application and send it to the American Medical Assistants along with the exam application fee.

    The application fee is as follows:

    - AMA members and recent CAAHEP/ABHES graduates, $125
    - All others pay $250

12. A. 70

    Rationale: The RMA (AMT) exam's minimum passing score is a scaled score of 70.

13. E. 425

    Rationale: The CMA (AAMA) minimum passing score is 425.

14. B. Include all work experience

    Rationale: Resumes should contain the following information:

    - Name, address, telephone number and e-mail address. (Be sure that the voice message for the telephone number listed and the e-mail address listed are professional.)
    - Objective listing of your career goal
    - Educational background, including a summary of the skills learned
    - Relevant work experience, including dates of employment and brief summaries of duties performed
    - Professional organizations and memberships
    - Certifications obtained
    - Reference information

15. C. Talk about former employees

    Rationale: Arrive 5 to 10 minutes before your scheduled appointment. You may wish to wait outside the facility if you arrive too early. Dress conservatively to project a well-groomed professional appearance. Ask questions about the position and the organization and show enthusiasm.

CHAPTER 2

1. B. Visual

   Rationale: The visual learner: tries to envision the word when spelling it out; dislikes listening for long periods of time; becomes distracted by movement when trying to concentrate; may not remember names but typically will remember faces; prefers face-to-face meetings; prefers to read descriptions when learning new material; likes to look at pictures when learning new material.

2. E. All of the above

   Rationale: Many individuals devise various memory aids to help them while studying, such as rhymes, acronyms, word associations, and flash cards. These memory aids are especially helpful when studying for medical terminology, anatomy, physiology, and pharmacology exams.

3. D. 90

   Rationale: It is estimated that when you are required to teach another individual, you retain approximately 90% of what was taught.

4. E. A and C

   Rationale: Some of the benefits of study groups are as follows:

   - Participants are able to break down complex ideas into understandable bits.
   - Group members depend on your participation, so you are more apt to be prepared.
   - Opportunity to compare study notes with other members. They may have information you missed and vice versa.
   - Studying becomes an interactive activity.
   - Group members become a support system.
   - Opportunity to learn what others do to study and prepare for exams.

5. E. A, B, and D

   Rationale: Have two #2, sharpened pencils with erasers available. You may not have purses, backpacks, cell phones, pagers, calculators, etc. with you. All of these items must be left either outside the exam room or in a designated area within the exam room.

6. D. A and B

   Rationale: Studies have shown that more information is retained when you study in two or three 30- to 45-minute increments than when you study for two hours straight.

7. B. 200 questions, three hours to complete

   Rationale: The CMA (AAMA) exam consists of 200 questions, and you have three hours to complete it. In order to complete the exam within the time allowed, you must answer 67 questions per hour and you must not spend more than an average of 54 seconds on each question.

8. C. Between 200 and 210 questions, two hours to complete

   Rationale: The RMA (AMT) exam consists of between 200 and 210 questions, and you have two hours to complete it. In order to complete the exam within the time allowed, you must answer 105 questions per hour and you must not spend more than an average of 36 seconds on each question.

9. E. A and C

   Rationale: Have two forms of valid identification, including one that includes your photo. Once you have presented your identification, you will be fingerprinted and have your picture taken. The fingerprint will allow you access to and from the testing room.

10. C. Read the directions, read the entire question, determine the correct answer in your head, look for the answer in the choices, mark the correct answer

    Rationale: Read through the directions and make sure that you understand them. As you begin to work through the questions, keep the following in mind:

    - Be sure to read the entire question before answering.
    - After you have read the question, come up with the answer in your head and then look for the corresponding answer in the available choices.

CHAPTER 3

1. D. Diseased

   Rationale: *–pathy* means "diseased."

2. C. Straight

   Rationale: *ortho* means "straight."

3. B. *o*

   Rationale: The most common combining vowel is *o*.

4. E. A and C

   Rationale: The suffix usually provides information about a procedure, condition, disorder, or disease; however, there are several suffixes that merely mean "pertaining to."

5. D. Color

   Rationale: *chromo* means "color."

6. A. Tissue

   Rationale: *histo* means "tissue."

7. E. A and C

   Rationale: Both *veno* and *phlebo* mean "vein."

8. E. *Ventro*

   Rationale: *antero* and *ventro* both mean "toward the front."

9. A. Inflammation of the eyelid

   Rationale: *Blepharo* means "eyelid"; *itis* means "inflammation."

10. B. Removal of a stone in the ureter

    Rationale: *Otomy* means "removal"; *litho* means "stone"; *uretero* means "ureter."

11. A. *–dynia*

    Rationale: *–dynia* means "pain."

12. D. Osteomalacia

    Rationale: *–malacia* means "softening"; *osteo* means "bone."

13. D. Instrument used to view the vagina

Rationale: *–scope* means "an instrument used to view"; *colpo* means "vagina."

14. B. Left and right

Rationale: *Sagittal:* divides the body into right and left sides.

15. C. Proximal

Rationale: *Proximal:* Toward the trunk

16. B *–rrhexis*

Rationale: *–rrhexis* means "rupture."

17. C. Bradycardia

Rationale: *–ia* means "pertaining to"; *cardio* means "heart": *brady–* means "slow."

18. E. A and C

Rationale: Both *endo–* and *intra–* mean "within.

19. B. Scanty urine

Rationale: *–uria* means "urine"; *oligo* means "scanty."

20. C. Gerontologist

Rationale: *–ologist* means "one who studies"; *geronto* means "elderly."

21. E. Gastroenterologist

Rationale: *–ologist* means "one who studies"; *entero* means "intestines"; *gastro* means "stomach"

22. C. ices

Rationale: Singular terms ending in *ax* are converted to *ices* when plural.

23. B. Part of the liver, gallbladder, and intestines

Rationale: The RUQ contains part of the liver, gallbladder, and intestines.

24. E. PRN

Rationale: The abbreviation for "as needed" is PRN.

25. D. Onychomycosis

Rationale: *–osis* means "abnormal condition"; *myco* means "fungus"; *onycho* means "nail."

26. D. oophorectomy

Rationale: *–ectomy* means "surgical removal"; *oophoro* means "ovaries."

27. E. Difficulty breathing

Rationale: *pnea* means "breathing"; *dys–* means "difficult."

28. A. Controlled bleeding

Rationale: *–stasis* means "controlled"; *hemo* means "blood."

29. E. All of the above

Rationale: A prefix provides information about location, number, time, and status.

30. D. Xantho

Rationale: *xantho* means "yellow."

CHAPTER 4

1. B. Cerebellum

Rationale: The cerebellum is located at the back of the head, is the second largest part of the brain, and coordinates voluntary muscle activity.

2. D. All of the above

Rationale: Examples of molecules are sugar, proteins. and water.

3. E. Cranium

Rationale: The maxilla and mandible are found within the cranium.

4. D. Femur

Rationale: The femur is the bone found in the upper leg. It is the longest and strongest of the bones.

5. B. Atom → Molecule → Organelle → Cell → Tissue → Organ → Organ System → Organism

Rationale: Atom → Molecule → Organelle → Cell → Tissue → Organ → Organ System → Organism reflects the organization within the human body. The atom is the smallest and the organism is the largest.

6. B. Extension

Rationale: Extension—the process of straightening a flexed limb and increasing the angle.

7. E. Sternocleidomastoid

Rationale: The sternocleidomastoid pulls the head from side to side and the head to the chest.

8. E. None of the above

Rationale: The large intestine consists of the cecum, colon, rectum, and anus.

9. B. Oxytocin

Rationale: Oxytocin causes uterine contractions and influences milk production. It is also known as *OXT.*

10. A. Sweet

Rationale: The tip of the tongue has taste receptors that are sensitive to sweet substances.

11. C. On the top of the kidneys

Rationale: The adrenal glands are located at the top of each kidney.

12. D. Abduction

Rationale: Abduction is movement of a body part away from the midline.

13. A. Patella

Rationale: The patella (kneecap) is an example of a sesamoid bone.

14. B. Bicuspid valve

Rationale: The bicuspid valve controls the opening between the left atrium and left ventricle, and is also known as the *mitral valve*.

15. E. Dendrites

Rationale: Dendrites are found within neurons. They receive impulses and send them throughout the cell body.

16. B. Connective

Rationale: Connective tissue connects and supports various body structures. Blood, adipose, and osseous tissues are types of connective tissue. Blood is the only liquid tissue in the body.

17. B. Keeps skin oiled and elastic and prevents dry hair and scalp by producing sebum

Rationale: The epidermis is the outermost layer of the skin, acting as a barrier from the outside; therefore, it is protective. It is also a receptor for touch, prevents water loss, and synthesizes vitamin D.

18. C. 206

Rationale: There are 206 bones in the human body.

19. A. Foramen

Rationale: A foramen is an opening in a bone where blood vessels, nerves, and ligaments pass through.

20. D. A and B

Rationale: The appendicular skeleton consists of 126 bones found in the upper extremities (shoulders, arms, forearms, wrists, and hands) and lower extremities (hips, thighs, legs, ankles, and feet).

21. C. Facial nerve

Rationale: Cranial nerve number 7, also known as the *facial nerve,* controls muscle contraction, some taste sensation, and some glandular innervations.

22. D. A and C

Rationale: Cardiac and skeletal muscle tissue is striated (striped).

23. B. Wrist and ankle

Rationale: Short bones are found in the wrist and ankle (carpals and tarsals).

24. B. Origin

Rationale: Muscle attachment to bone at the point that is more fixed is known as the *origin*.

25. A. Large intestine

Rationale: The large intestine is approximately 5 feet long. Digestion and absorption are completed in the large intestine, and vitamin K produced there.

26. A. Epithelial

Rationale: Epithelial tissue is found in the skin and lining of the respiratory, intestinal, and urinary tracts. These tissues protect, absorb, secrete, and excrete.

27. D. Liver

Rationale: The liver produces bile, which breaks down fats, stores proteins, removes excess glucose from blood, and destroys old erythrocytes.

28. A. Left atrium

Rationale: The left atrium receives oxygen-rich blood from the lungs.

29. A. Illium

Rationale: The illium is found in the upper portion of the hip and is wing-shaped.

30. A. **Initiating and establishing the rhythm of the heartbeat**

Rationale: The sinoatrial node is responsible for initiating and establishing the rhythm of the heartbeat, is located in the upper wall of the right atrium, and is also known as the *SA node* and/or *pacemaker.*

31. A. Carpals

Rationale: Carpals are the short bones found within the wrist.

32. C. Thrombocytes

Rationale: Thrombocytes are also known as *platelets* and are responsible for clotting blood.

33. E. Spleen

Rationale: The spleen, located in the left upper quadrant of the abdominal cavity, helps fight infection by killing or weakening bacteria, viruses, cancer cells, and other invaders and destroys damaged red blood cells.

34. C. Internal respiration

Rationale: Internal respiration is the exchange of gases at the cellular level between blood and tissues.

35. B. Spinal nerves

Rationale: The central nervous system (CNS) consists of the following: meninges cerebrospinal fluid, cerebrum, thalamus, hypothalamus, cerebellum, brainstem, and spinal cord.

36. C. Hypothalamus

Rationale: The hypothalamus is located below the thalamus and regulates the following: autonomic nervous activity related to behavior and emotions, hormones, body temperature, hunger sensations, thirst, and the sleep-wake cycle.

37. D. Constricted pupils

Rationale: The sympathetic response may include increased respiration rate, increased heart rate, increased blood flow to muscles, dilated pupils, and dilated bronchioles.

38. D. 12

Rationale: There are 12 vertebrae in the thoracic region.

39. A. Fascia

Rationale: Fascia is a sheet of connective tissue that covers, supports, and separates muscle tissues.

40. E. Iris

Rationale: The iris provides the color of the eye.

41. A. Tympanic membrane

Rationale: The tympanic membrane separates the outer ear from the middle ear and transmits sound waves by vibrating.

42. B. Ureter

Rationale: The ureters are two tubes that allow urine to flow from the kidneys down to the urinary bladder.

43. D. Glans penis

Rationale: The glans penis is the soft, sensitive, bulbous part of the penis and is also known as the *head* of the penis.

44. D. Complication during pregnancy producing hypertension, edema, and proteinuria

Rationale: Preeclampsia is a complication during pregnancy producing hypertension, edema, and proteinuria. It is also known as *toxemia.*

45. D. Prolactin

Rationale: Prolactin promotes female breast development and milk production following childbirth. It also stimulates male sex hormone production.

46. B. Gastrocnemius

Rationale: The gastrocnemius is one of the posterior calf muscles that flexes the foot and aids in pushing the body forward.

47. E. Follicle-stimulating hormone

Rationale: Follicle-stimulating hormones influence the reproductive organs. In females it stimulates secretion of estrogen. In males it stimulates production of sperm. It is also known as *FSH.*

48. E. Behind the knee

Rationale: The popliteal artery is found behind the knee.

49. D. Regulates the transport of glucose to the cells and increases metabolism of carbohydrates

Rationale: Insulin regulates the transport of glucose to the cells, increases metabolism of carbohydrates, and decreases blood sugar.

50. E. Epiphysis

Rationale: The epiphysis is the wide end of a long bone.

51. B. Corpus luteum

Rationale: A corpus luteum is a small mass of cells that form following ovulation.

CHAPTER 5

1. C. The patient's rectum

Rationale: Proctoscopy is viewing of the rectum to detect problems using a proctoscope.

2. B. Impetigo

Rationale: Impetigo is a contagious skin infection usually caused by *Streptococcus* or *Staphylococcus* and is transferred via skin-to-skin contact and by handling contaminated objects.

3. B. Gout

Rationale: Gout is Inflammation of the joints caused by formation of crystals in the joints.

4. E. All of the above

Rationale: Psoriasis is chronic red, raised areas of the skin that are scaly and itchy; it may progress to silver-yellow scales. The condition is hereditary.

5. B. Pneumoconiosis

Rationale: Pneumoconiosis is a disease of the lung caused by chronic inhalation of dust.

6. E. None of the above

Rationale: A Colles fracture is a break in the distal portion of the radius, typically the result of trying to break a fall.

7. C. Cataracts, presbycusis, presbyopia, hyperopia

Rationale: Cataracts, presbycusis, presbyopia, and hyperopia are all common conditions in the aged patient.

8. A. Myxedema

Rationale: Myxedema is a severe, life-threatening form of adult hypothyroidism.

9. B. Urticaria

Rationale: Urticaria is hives or raised wheals caused by an allergic reaction or stress.

10. D. Angina pectoris

Rationale: Angina pectoris is a spasm of the heart muscle due to decreased oxygen to the myocardium, causing pain and later ischemia. It usually results from stress or physical activity.

11. B. Cardiac catheterization

Rationale: During cardiac catheterization, a catheter is inserted through a vein or artery and guided into the heart. It allows visualization of heart activity and measures pressures within the heart's chambers.

12. B. Nocturia

Rationale: Incontinence is defined as the inability to control the flow of urine. All of the following are forms of urinary incontinence: **Stress incontinence**—Most common form of incontinence. Urine may leak when the individual sneezes, coughs, or laughs. **Urge incontinence**—The bladder contracts without warning, which in turn may allow urine to leak. **Overflow incontinence**—Blockage prevents complete emptying of the bladder and in turn bladder overflows. **Enuresis**—Bed wetting. Nocturia is defined as excessive urination at night.

13. C. Oblique

Rationale: An oblique fracture is a fracture that is at an angle.

14. D. Uterine fibroids

Rationale: Uterine fibroids are benign tumors that grow within the wall of the uterus. They are also known as *leiomyomas.*

15. E. All of the above

Rationale: A neoplasm is defined as abnormal tissue that grows more rapidly than normal. It can be either benign (noncancerous) or malignant (cancerous). It is not contagious.

16. A. Atrophy

Rationale: Atrophy occurs when muscles waste away as a result of poor nutrition, lack of use, or lack of nerve impulses.

17. C. Gigantism

Rationale: Gigantism is defined as excessive production of growth hormone, which causes abnormally tall individuals.

18. E. Both A and C

Rationale: Sprain is defined as overstretching or tearing of ligaments that support a joint.

19. B. The telescoping or sliding of one part of the intestine into another

Rationale: Intussusception is defined as the telescoping or sliding of one part of the intestine into another.

20. E. Both A and C

Rationale: Cellulitis is an acute infection of cells or connective tissue that is caused by either *Staphylococcus* or *Streptococcus* bacteria via a cut or lesion on the skin.

21. E. All of the above

Rationale: Scoliosis is an abnormal lateral curvature of the spine. Kyphosis is an exaggerated outward curvature of the spine. Lordosis is an exaggerated inward curvature of the spine.

22. D. Malignancy of red blood cells

Rationale: All of the following pertain to sickle cell anemia: Red blood cells are sickle shaped; the condition is a life-threatening inherited form of anemia; an individual may be a carrier without having the disease; it occurs most often in African Americans.

23. E. Both B and C

Rationale: An electrocardiogram is a record showing a tracing of the heart's electrical activity and rhythm. It is Also known as an *EKG* or *ECG*.

24. C. Inflammation of the lining around the lungs

Rationale: Pleurisy is inflammation of the lining around the lungs (pleura).

25. D. 140/90 or greater

Rationale: Hypertension is defined as blood pressure of 140/90 or greater.

26. D. Thick, dry, sticky mucus clogs organs, mainly the lungs

Rationale: Diphtheria is an acute infection of the throat and upper respiratory tract caused by bacteria. It is a potentially fatal childhood disease.

27. D. Causes destruction of neurons

Rationale: Multiple sclerosis is an autoimmune disorder that causes destruction of the myelin sheath, resulting in episodic tremors, weakness, mood swings, and vision changes. It is also known as *MS*.

28. C. Cerebral palsy

Rationale: Cerebral palsy is defined as brain damage before or during birth resulting in poor muscle control and spasticity.

29. E. Amblyopia

Rationale: Amblyopia occurs when eye muscles are weaker in one eye than the other.

30. A. Emphysema

Rationale: Emphysema is a long-term, progressive disease that causes shortness of breath and occurs when the number of alveoli is decreased and those left are enlarged and unable to function properly.

31. A. Hyperopia

Rationale: Hyperopia is the ability to see faraway objects more clearly than those close by. It occurs most commonly after age 40 and is also known as *farsightedness.*

32. B. Emergency procedure performed to obtain an airway

Rationale: Tracheotomy is an emergency procedure performed to obtain an airway.

33. D. All of the above

Rationale: Ménière's disease is a condition of the inner ear that may cause vertigo, tinnitus, and nerve loss.

34. A. Measuring intraocular pressure to check for glaucoma

Rationale: Tonometry is the measurement of intraocular pressure to check for glaucoma using a tonometer.

35. C. Process of recording brain waves

Rationale: Electroencephalography is the process of recording brain waves. It is also known as *EEG*.

36. E. Both B and C

Rationale: A lumbar puncture is defined as a puncture made with a spinal needle between the L3 and L4 or L4 and L5 vertebrae in which cerebrospinal fluid is aspirated for examination. It is also known as a *spinal tap*.

37. D. Polycystic kidney disease

Rationale: Polycystic kidney disease is an inherited disorder that causes clusters of cysts to form on the kidneys.

38. B. Oval window

Rationale: Otosclerosis is defined as hardening of the oval window, resulting in fusion of the stapes and hearing loss.

39. D. Cryosurgery

Rationale: Cryosurgery is the destruction or elimination of abnormal tissue through extremely cold applications, usually liquid nitrogen.

40. E. Cystitis

Rationale: Cystitis is an inflammation of the bladder that occurs when bacteria infect the lower urinary tract. It is most often caused by *Escherichia coli*.

41. B. Enlargement of the prostate

Rationale: Benign prostatic hypertrophy occurs when there is an enlargement of the prostate. It typically occurs in men over the age of 50 and is also known as *BPH*.

42. C. Difficult and/or painful menstruation

Rationale: Dysmenorrhea is defined as difficult and/or painful menstruation.

43. B. PID

Rationale: Pelvic inflammatory disease is defined as an inflammation of the female reproductive organs, usually as a result of a sexually transmitted infection. It is also known as *PID*.

44. C. Leading cause of PID

Rationale: Trichomoniasis is a common sexually transmitted infection in men and women; however, men typically do not exhibit symptoms. It is caused by the protozoan *Trichomonas vaginalis*.

45. E. Cauterization

Rationale: Cauterization is defined as destruction of abnormal cells or tissue by using either electrical or chemical heat.

46. C. IVP

Rationale: An intravenous pyelogram is an X-ray of the kidneys and ureters after a contrast medium has been injected. It is also known as *IVP*.

47. A. Pinpoint hemorrhages found on the skin

Rationale: Petechiae are pinpoint hemorrhages found on the skin.

48. C. Excess of glucocorticoids

Rationale: Diabetes mellitus is a metabolic disease due to hyperglycemia and glycosuria as a result of poor insulin secretion and/or action.

49. D. All of the above

Rationale: Pathophysiology is the study of the changes that happen to the structures and functions of the body and in turn lead to disease.

50. D. All of the above

Rationale: Acromegaly is a chronic disease of middle-aged adults as a result of excess growth hormone in adulthood. It can result in diabetes mellitus, hypertension, and an increased risk of cardiovascular disease.

51. C. Bacterial function of the hair follicles

Rationale: Decubitus ulcers are caused by lack of blood flow to a bony prominence when a patient lies in the same position too long. They are also known as *bed sores* or *pressure ulcers*.

52. C. Cryptorchidism

Rationale: Cryptorchidism is a condition in which one or both testicles fail to descend into the scrotum.

53. D. Paralysis of both legs and the lower part of the body

Rationale: Paraplegia is defined as paralysis of both legs and the lower part of the body. It is caused by a spinal cord injury.

54. E. Fatigue

Rationale: Hyperthyroidism is defined as excessive thyroid hormone production and thus an increase in metabolic rate, increased sweating, nervousness, and weight loss. Graves' disease is an autoimmune disease characterized by hyperthyroidism, exophthalmos, and goiter. Exophthalmia is the condition of bulging eyes. Goiter is an enlarged thyroid due to lack of iodine.

55. B. Greenstick

Rationale: Greenstick fracture takes place most often in children and occurs when one side of the long bone is broken. The fracture does not go all the way through the bone. It is also known as an *incomplete fracture*.

56. B. Atherosclerosis

    Rationale: Atherosclerosis is a form of arteriosclerosis caused by a reduction of blood flow to the heart muscle in the myocardium due to a buildup of fatty plaques in the coronary arteries.

CHAPTER 6

1. D. Vegetables

   Rationale: The six nutrient classifications are carbohydrates, proteins, fats, vitamins, minerals, and water.

2. B. Vitamin B_{12}

   Rationale: The water-soluble vitamins are vitamin B_2, vitamin B_{12}, vitamin C, and niacin.

3. A. A, D, K

   Rationale: With the exception of vitamins A, D, and K, vitamins cannot be formed within the body, so they must be taken in through the foods that are consumed.

4. E. A, B, and C

   Rationale: A clear liquid diet consists of clear soup and broth, plain gelatin, black coffee, tea, carbonated beverages, and popsicles.

5. B. High-protein diet

   Rationale: Because proteins can promote the healing process, the high-protein diet is often prescribed for those recovering from bone injury. However, it should be combined with fruits and vegetables in order to maintain a balanced diet.

6. D. Bananas

   Rationale: The BRAT diet consists of bananas, rice, applesauce, and toast.

7. C. Between 20 and 30 grams

   Rationale: The low-fat/low-cholesterol diet is recommended for patients with hypercholesterolemia and for those with gallbladder, pancreatic, and liver disease. Daily fat intake should be between 20 and 30 grams.

8. C. Botulism

   Rationale: Botulism is a rare but serious condition caused by the toxins produced by the *Clostridium botulinum* bacterium. This bacterium can survive in environments with little oxygen, such as in canned food. Symptoms typically begin 12 to 36 hours following ingestion of the bacteria and include vision problems, difficulty swallowing, nausea, and vomiting.

9. B. Iodine

   Rationale: Iodine enables the thyroid gland to perform its function of controlling the rate at which foods are oxidized in the cells. Sources include fish (obtained from the sea), some plant foods grown in soils containing iodine, and table salt fortified with iodine (iodized).

10. E. D

    Rationale: Vitamin D enables the growing body to use calcium and phosphorus in a normal way to build bones and teeth. It is provided by vitamin D fortification of certain foods, such as milk and margarine, and by fish-liver oils and eggs. Sunshine is also a source of vitamin D.

CHAPTER 7

1. E. All of the above

   Rationale: **Content**—Address all areas of interest and answer all questions fully. **Conciseness**—Get to the point; say what needs to be said in as few words as possible. **Clarity**—Choose words that accurately and precisely convey your meaning. **Coherence**—Create a logical, easy-to-follow train of thought. **Check**—Ask for feedback or clarification to ensure comprehension.

2. B. Are you in pain?

   Rationale: Questions that can be answered with a simple "yes" or "no" are referred to as *close-ended questions*. For example, "Are you in pain?" is a close-ended question.

3. D. Passive, active, evaluative

   Rationale: Active listening is two-way and requires a response. Passive listening is one-way and does not require a response. Evaluative listening allows you to evaluate the information as it is being disseminated and to form an immediate response and an opinion.

4. C. Open-ended questions

   Rationale: Examples of nonverbal communication are as follows: **facial expressions**—may or may not reflect judgment; **eye contact**—depending on whether eye contact is or is not maintained, it may reflect level of interest, attention, and sensitivity; **gestures**—may be positive or negative; **posture**—may or may not reflect interest and a feeling of self-worth; **therapeutic touch**—may convey empathy and sensitivity, but you must be aware of the recipient's reaction, as not everyone likes to be touched by those they don't know very well.

5. E. A and D

Rationale: Personal space measurements typical in the United States: **intimate distance** (0–18 inches): shows affection, provides comfort and protection; **personal distance** (18 inches to 4 feet): the distance for most communication; **social distance** (4 to 12 feet): less personal, used in social and business encounters; **public distance** (greater than 12 feet): least personal, observed in lectures, religious, and impersonal social encounters.

6. E. All of the above

Rationale: The use of correct words when writing office correspondence includes avoiding the use of the following: technical terms, **gender bias** (indicating either male or female by the type of language used), long sentences and paragraphs, excessive use of the personal pronoun, repetition, and the passive voice.

7. C. Homophones

Rationale: Homophones have similar pronunciations but very different meanings and spellings.

8. A. Drugs

Rationale: The correct plural of *drug* is *drugs.*

9. D. Salutation

Rationale: **Noun**—names a person, place, or thing. **Pronoun**—substitutes for a noun. **Verb**—*helping verb*: comes before main verb; *main verb*: asserts action, being, or state of being. **Adjective**—modifies a noun or pronoun, usually answering the questions "Which one?" "What kind?" or "How many?" **Adverb**—modifies a verb, adjective, or adverb, usually answering the questions "When?" "Where?" "Why?" "How?" "Under what conditions?" or "To what degree?" **Preposition**—indicates the relationship between the noun and pronoun that follows it and another word in the sentence. **Conjunction**—connects words or word groups. **Interjection**—word used to express strong feeling.

10. C. Salutation

Rationale: Basic components of a business letter include: **Salutation**—courteous greeting typed at the left margin; spaced two lines below the inside address. **Body**—contains the purpose of the letter; begins two spaces below the salutation; single-spaced, with a double space between each paragraph. **Complimentary close**—contains courtesy word(s), such as "Sincerely," "Sincerely yours," or "Yours truly"; appears two spaces below the end of the body of the letter. **Signature line**—contains the name and title of the writer; typed four spaces below the complimentary close. **Reference initials**—Indicate who keyed the letter; placed at the lower left margin in lowercase. **Enclosure**—If other documents are included with the letter, a notation is made on the letter indicating that those documents have been enclosed. **Copy notation**—used when a copy of the letter is sent to someone other than the addressee.

11. B. Face the patient

Rationale: Guidelines when working with hearing-impaired patients are as follows: Make sure that you are in a quiet, well-lit room; face the patient; speak slowly and clearly; don't have anything in your mouth, such as gum or candy; Have paper and pen available so that the patient can communicate in writing if desired.

12. A. Demonstration/return demonstration

Rationale: Demonstration/return demonstration means showing patients how to do something and then immediately having them do the same procedure.

13. D. All of the above

Rationale: The following are usually found in the policy manual: Compensation and reimbursement for work-related activities, such as attending conventions and courses (CEU/degree), and for parking fees; Emergency leave, Grievance (complaint) process, Health benefits, Holidays, Jury duty, Overtime policy, Pension plan, Performance review and evaluation, Probationary period, Sick leave, Termination of employment, Vacation, and Work hours, including flex time.

14. E. A, C, and D

Rationale: Patient information booklets should provide information on the following: office hours, payment guidelines, appointment and cancellation policy, telephone answering service, information about the physician(s), after-hours availability, directions to the facility, and parking information.

15. C. The procedure manual

Rationale: The procedure manual, when properly updated, is an excellent reference tool for the new employee since it provides guidelines for performing specific tasks.

16. C. [/]

Rationale: [/] indicates that brackets should be inserted.

17. D. Stimulus

Rationale: The communication cycle includes a source, message, channel, and receiver.

18. B. Active

Rationale: Active listening: the form of listening that is two-way and requires a response. Example: "What brings you to the office today?" requires a response.

19. D. A and C

Rationale: In general, the following rules apply when using numbers in written correspondence. Numbers 1 to 10 are spelled out—one to ten. For numbers greater than ten, it is acceptable to use the number designation, as in 32, 128, or 1020. The only exception to this rule is when the number occurs at the beginning of a sentence. Then it should be spelled out.

20. C. At the lower left margin in lowercase.

Rationale: **Reference initials**—Indicate who keyed the letter; they are placed at the lower left margin in lowercase.

21. C. Aggressive behavior

Rationale: Aggressive behavior—imposing your point of view on others; also known as being "bossy."

22. D. Assertive behavior

Rationale: Assertive behavior—maintaining a positive, yet firm perspective based on your values; being the boss without being "bossy."

CHAPTER 8

1. D. Prepubescent

Rationale: The developmental stages of the life cycle are as follows: **prenatal period**—conception to birth; **infancy**—childbirth to toddler period; **childhood**—early childhood: ages 3 to 5; middle childhood: ages 6 to 11; **adolescence**—early adolescence: ages 12 to 14; late adolescence: ages 15 to 19; **adulthood**—early adulthood: ages 20 to 30s; middle adulthood: ages 40 to 50s; late adulthood: age 60 to death.

2. E. C and D

Rationale: Piaget's theory of cognitive development includes the following stages: sensorimotor, preoperational, concrete operational, and formal operational.

3. E. A and C

Rationale: Adolescence is characterized by the following: operational thinking, sexual maturation, beginning of the desire for independence, and the importance of friendships.

4. C. Oral

Rationale:

Stage	Age
Oral	Birth to 18 months
Anal	18 months to 3 years
Phallic	4 to 6 years
Latency	7 years to puberty
Genital	Puberty to adulthood

5. C. Self-actualization

Rationale: Self-actualization is at the top of Maslow's hierarchy of needs.

6. D. Food, shelter, water

Rationale: At the physiological stage of Maslow's hierarchy of needs is the need for food, water, and shelter.

7. B. 8

Rationale: Erikson believed that individuals go through eight stages of development as they progress through life.

8. A. Inferiority

Rationale:

Conflict	
Positive	**Negative**
Trust	Mistrust
Autonomy	Shame and doubt
Initiative	Guilt
Industry	Inferiority
Identity	Role confusion
Intimacy	Isolation
Generativity	Stagnation
Ego integrity	Despair

9. B. Classical conditioning

Rationale: While studying the digestion process of dogs, Pavlov discovered that the malnourished dogs salivated when his assistants entered the room to feed them. He began to precede the feeding of the dogs with the ringing of a bell. Eventually, the dogs salivated at the sound of the bell. This is known as *classical conditioning*.

10. A. B. F. Skinner

Rationale: B. F. Skinner was a psychologist who worked from the late 1950s to the early 1970s and developed a more complex theory of learning. Operant conditioning is based on voluntary behavior linked to a previous experience and the idea that a response (positive or negative) occurs as a result of a certain behavior.

11. D. Acceptance

Rationale: The five stages are denial, anger, bargaining, depression, and acceptance. Acceptance is the final stage and occurs when there is a sense of peace and calm.

12. C. Fight or flight

Rationale: Compensation, denial, displacement, identification, intellectualization, introjection, minimization, projection, rationalization, reaction formation, regression, repression, sublimation, substitution, and undoing are the defense mechanisms identified by Freud.

13. D. **Neuroses, psychoses, personality disorder**

Rationale: Mental diseases can be divided into three major categories: **neuroses**—mild emotional disturbances that impair judgment; **psychoses**—severe mental disorders that interfere with the individual's perception of reality; **personality disorder**—antisocial reactions, paranoia, and narcissistic behavior.

14. A. Language and symbols

Rationale:

Age	Stage	Focus
2 to 7 years	Preoperational	Language and symbols

15. D. Repression

Rationale: Repression is an unconscious mechanism by which threatening thoughts, feelings, and desires are kept from becoming conscious; the repressed material is denied entry into consciousness. This response protects a person from a traumatic experience until he or she has the resources to cope.

CHAPTER 9

1. B. Each state regulates itself

Rationale: Each state regulates the practice of medicine within that particular state. These medical practice acts establish the requirements for licensure, the duties attached to that license, and the basis for revocation or suspension of the license.

2. C. Endorsement, examination, reciprocity

Rationale: The medical license may be obtained one of three ways: examination, reciprocity, or endorsement. **Examination**—The qualifying examinations accepted for licensure varies from state to state; however, all states accept the United States Medical Licensing Exam (USMLE), which consists of four separate exams broken down into *steps*. **Reciprocity**—In some cases, a physician who holds a current license in one state and wishes to practice medicine in another state may not be required to take that state's licensure exam because the physician's current license requirements are recognized. **Endorsement**—When a physician has successfully completed a nationally recognized examination considered to have high standards, his or her current license and examination scores may be recognized and the physician may not have to take the state examination.

3. B. Misfeasance

Rationale: Misfeasance is defined as performing the correct treatment with errors.

4. E. *Respondeat superior*

Rationale: *Respondeat superior* is a Latin term literally translated as "let the master answer." The physician is liable for the negligent actions of anyone who works for him or her.

5. C. Offer, acceptance, consideration

Rationale: A contract is a voluntary agreement between two parties resulting in benefit for both of them. There are three parts to a contract: **offer**—initiation of the contract; **acceptance**—both parties agree to the terms of the contract; **consideration**—services are provided and a fee is paid.

6. A. Good Samaritan

Rationale: The Good Samaritan Act protects healthcare workers from liability when they provide first aid in emergency situations.

7. E. Shoplifting

Rationale: Intentional tort occurs when someone intentionally injures another individual.

8. A. Battery

Rationale: Battery is actual physical touching of another person without the person's consent; it includes physical abuse. *Example:* taking a patient's temperature against the patient's will.

9. C. Duplicity

Rationale: The four Ds of negligence are duty, dereliction or neglect of duty, direct Cause, and damages.

10. E. A and C

Rationale: A physician's license may be revoked or suspended for one of the following reasons: unprofessional conduct, conviction of a crime, inability to perform due to physical or emotional incapacities.

11. E. A, B, and C

Rationale: The following is included in the Patients' Bill of Rights: information disclosure, choice of providers and plans, access to emergency services, participation in treatment decisions, respect and nondiscrimination, confidentiality of health information, complaints, and appeals.

12. A. First

Rationale: **First degree**—committed the crime (the most serious); **second degree**—was at the scene of the crime and assisted in the crime; **third degree**—assisted in the crime before the crime occurred; **fourth degree**—assisted the person who committed the crime after the fact.

13. D. Torts and contracts

Rationale: Civil law is concerned with the relationships between individuals and between individuals and the government. Civil law includes tort law and contract law.

14. B. Abandonment

Rationale: Abandonment occurs when a healthcare professional initiates care of a patient and leaves the patient without completing the care or finding an acceptable substitute.

15. B. Undue influence

Rationale: Undue influence is an intentional tort that occurs when people are intentionally persuaded to do things they do not want to do.

16. B. Bioethics

Rationale: Ethical decisions as they pertain to life issues are referred to as *bioethics*.

17. E. B and D

Rationale: Genetic engineeing involves altering an individual's genes in order to alter genetic traits and cure or eliminate genetic diseases such as sickle cell anemia. Cloning, genetic testing, gene therapy, and stem cell research involving adult and embryonic stem cells are all examples of genetic engineering.

18. D. Cloning

Rationale: Cloning occurs when one cell is copied to create a genetically identical organism.

19. D. All of the above

Rationale: The legal protocol for terminating a patient's care requires the physician to notify the patient in writing and provide the following information: the physician intends to terminate the relationship and gives the reason; the patient's medical records will be available to transfer to another physician; the physician offers to refer the patient to another physician; and the physician will continue to provide care until a set date (typically 30 days from the time the patient receives the letter).

20. A. Gene therapy

Rationale: Gene therapy consists of altering or eliminating harmful genes or inserting normal genes into defective cells.

21. A. Freedom of choice

Rationale: The AAMA Code of Ethics addresses the following: human dignity, confidentiality, honor, continued study, and responsibility for an improved community. The AMA Principles of Medical Ethics addresses the following: human dignity, honesty, responsibility to society, confidentiality, continued study, freedom of choice, and responsibility to the community.

22. E. Unethical behavior is always unlawful.

Rationale: It is important to understand that unethical behavior is not always unlawful; however, unlawful behavior is always unethical.

CHAPTER 10

1. E. A and B

Rationale: PHI is any information that would identify a patient: name, address, telephone number, date of birth, Social Security number, e-mail address, medical record number, insurance information including the ID and group number, driver's license number, and photos.

2. A. Helps reduce the likelihood that employees will lose their health insurance

Rationale: Title II of the HIPAA law, commonly known as the *privacy rule*, requires providers to notify patients in writing of how the patients' medical information is handled and under what circumstances their PHI may be released. Patients have more control over their health information and over who may have access to that information. Title II safeguards patient information and establishes rules by which healthcare providers must abide. It prevents fraud and abuse. It sets standards and requirements regarding electronic transmission of health information. It requires the use of Employer Identification Numbers (EINs).

3. C. The physician or facility where the physician works

   Rationale: The physician or the facility where the physician works owns the medical record, but the patient has the legal right of *privileged communication* and access to his or her records.

4. B. Parents

   Rationale: Although medical records are confidential, there are times when they can be released without a patient's consent. In special cases, records are released to:

   - Healthcare workers who need the records to care for a patient.
   - Qualified people or organizations that perform services, such as data processing, medical record transcription, microfilming, administrative functions, or other such related services.
   - Qualified people or organizations for approved research and education functions.
   - Certain government authorities, as permitted or required by law, to investigate or regulate health-related issues such as child abuse, communicable diseases, and the use of prescription drugs.
   - Certain lawyers and parties in a lawsuit if a patient's medical condition is an issue in the suit.

5. C. A HIPAA-compliant fax cover sheet

   Rationale: Any faxed documents must have an accompanying HIPAA-compliant fax cover sheet that contains the disclaimer that faxed information cannot be shared with any other party without the patient's written consent.

6. C. Portability of insurance coverage when an employee changes or loses his or her job

   Rationale: Title I of HIPAA is the portion of the law that addresses portability of insurance coverage when the employee changes or loses his or her job.

7. B. A court order or a patient's signed consent

   Rationale: Patient information should never be released without a court order or a patient's signed consent.

8. E. A, B, and C

   Rationale: All persons who have access to patient records are required to have a unique password. HIPAA compliance mandates that computer systems must be in a secured and private space. HIPAA requires healthcare organizations to protect the privacy and security of confidential health information and calls for standard formats of electronic transactions.

9. C. $100 to $25,000

   Rationale: Penalties range from not more than $100 for each violation up to $25,000 for all violations of an identical requirement during a calendar year.

10. E. All of the above

    Rationale: PHI is any information that would identify a patient: name, address, telephone number, date of birth, Social Security number, e-mail address, medical record number, insurance information including the ID and group number, driver's license number, and photos.

CHAPTER 11

1. D. Clear articulation and pronunciation of words

   Rationale: Enunciation is defined as clear articulation and pronunciation of your words.

2. C. UPS next day

   Rationale: First Class, Priority, Second Class, Third Class, Fourth Class, and Express Mail/Next Day Service are the classifications of mail.

3. D. All of the above

   Rationale: When taking a telephone message, it is important to obtain the following information: first and last names of the caller (with spelling verified); telephone number, including the area code, at which he or she can be reached for a callback; the reason for the call; and the name of the person he or she is trying to reach. If the patient is requesting a medication refill, it is important to also document the name of the pharmacy the patient uses, as well as the pharmacy's telephone number and fax number.

4. E. 8½ × 11″

   Rationale:

Stationery	Stationery Dimensions	Corresponding Envelope	Envelope Dimensions	Commonly Used For:
Standard	8½ × 11″	No. 10	9½ × 4⅛″	Most office correspondence

5. A. No. 10

Rationale:

Stationery	Stationery Dimensions	Corresponding Envelope	Envelope Dimensions	Commonly Used For:
Standard	8½ × 11″	No. 10	9½ × 4⅛″	Most office correspondence

6. B. 2

Rationale: State abbreviations contain two letters.

7. A. Registered mail

Rationale: Registered mail is the safest way to send first-class or priority mail.

8. D. All of the above

Rationale: Examples of the types of documents that should be sent via certified mail are contracts, mortgages, birth certificates, deeds, and checks.

9. A. A document that demonstrates proof that mail was posted

Rationale: A document that demonstrates proof that mail was posted is useful for mailing items such as tax returns, which need to be received by a certain date.

10. C. 108 inches

Rationale: The maximum size for mail is no more than 108 inches—in length and girth combined.

11. D. Medical record

Rationale: The medical record contains all the written documentation that relates to the patient's health care.

12. D. Insurance plan

Rationale: The four parts of the POMR are as follows: **database**—the physical examination, the patient history, and the results of baseline laboratory or diagnostic procedures; **problem list**—list of patient problems kept at the front of the chart, much like a table of contents; each problem the patient has experienced is titled and numbered; **plan**—a written plan for each numbered problem identified on the problem list; **progress notes**—consists of several sections, with the first initial spelling out the word SOAP (also known as *SOAP notes*).

13. B. 10

Rationale: The American Medical Association recommends keeping medical records for 10 years.

14. E. Indefinitely

Rationale: Patients' immunization records should be kept indefinitely in case they need them in the future.

15. D. B and C

Rationale: The types of scheduling systems are specified time scheduling, **wave scheduling, modified wave scheduling,** scheduling by grouping procedures, double-booking patients, and the open office hours system.

16. D. MI

Rationale: The postal abbreviation for Michigan is MI.

17. E. A and C

Rationale: According to the alphabetic filing rules, initials come before a full name and names are filed by last name, first name, and middle name. For all of the rules, see page 160, "Rules for Alphabetic Filing."

18. D. Both A and B

Rationale: Subjective information is the same as the chief complaint and is provided by the patient.

19. E. Both A and C

Rationale: Patients who have been seen within the past three years and are currently being treated are considered to have active records.

20. B. Terminal digit filing

Rationale: Terminal digit filing is based on the last six digits of the ID number.

21. A. Three

Rationale: The appointment book is considered a legal document and should be treated as such. Old appointment books should be kept for at least three years.

22. E. All of the above

Rationale: The appointment schedule should show the periods of time blocked out on the daily schedule when appointments are unavailable due to physicians' meetings, surgery time, vacation, and hospital rounds. The periods of time the physician is unavailable is known as the *matrix*.

23. D. All are required.

Rationale: All of the following are required when answering the telephone: smiling, answering the telephone quickly, using clear speech, using the correct volume, speaking at a normal rate, and identifying the caller.

24. A. It is easy to determine a true emergency when talking with someone over the telephone.

Rationale: When someone calls in with an emergency, you should try to get as much information as possible, and it is acceptable to ask the patient specific questions. See Box 11-2, "Questions to Ask When Handling a Telephone Emergency." A call reporting premature labor is an example of an emergency telephone call.

25. C. Privacy Manager

Rationale: The privacy manager allows patients to block access to their home telephones. You will be asked to state the location from which you are calling. Once you have given this information, unless you are cleared, you'll be directed to a voice mail system, where you will leave a message

CHAPTER 12

1. C. Memory

Rationale: **Memory** makes it possible for a computer to temporarily store data and programs.

2. D. Scanner and keyboard

Rationale: Input devices, such as the keyboard and scanners, feed data and instructions into a computer.

3. D. A and C

Rationale: **USB**—A USB, also known as a *jump drive, thumb drive,* or *flash drive,* is a small portable storage device that can hold up to 64 GB or more of data.

4. A. C Drive

Rationale: Computers are based on hard-disk drive technology; the hard-disk drive is usually called the *C drive.*

5. B. Ctrl + V

Rationale: Ctrl + V is the keyboard command for "paste."

6. E. Both B and C

Rationale: The World Wide Web (WWW), or the Web, is a system of Internet servers.

7. C. The password

Rationale: The security code is a group of characters that allows an authorized computer operator access to certain programs or features; also known as a *password.*

8. E. Disk drive

Rationale: The disk drive is a container that holds a read/write head, an access arm, and a magnetic disk for storage.

9. B. Directs the computer's activities and sends electronic signals to the right place at the right time

Rationale: The CPU directs the computer's activities and sends electronic signals to the right place at the right time.

10. A. Feed data and instructions into the computer

Rationale: **Input** devices, such as the keyboard and scanners, feed data and instructions into a computer.

CHAPTER 13

1. B. Cashier's checks

Rationale: A cashier's check is written using the bank's own check or form. It is issued by the bank, which guarantees that the money is available. There is usually a charge for this service

2. C. Interest

Rationale: Interest is money earned and paid to the depositor by the financial institution for allowing the use of the depositor's money (interest-earning savings/checking account).

3. E. A and C

Rationale: The following is true about deposit slips: A deposit slip is completed every time a deposit is made into a bank account. The slip indicates the total dollar amounts of cash and checks being deposited. Entries on the slip should be printed in black ink. Currency (coins and bills) is totaled separately from checks. Each check must be entered on a different line, either noting the payer's name, the check number, or the ABA number, depending on the bank's preferred method. If there are more checks than lines provided, the excessive checks can be entered on the back of the deposit slip. The currency and coin totals and check totals are added together. Then this amount, the total for the deposit, is entered on the bottom line of the deposit slip.

4. A. The day sheet

Rationale: The day sheet is a component of the pegboard system and is used to list or post each day's financial transactions: charges, payments, adjustments, and credits. The day sheet, one for each day of the month, must be balanced at the end of each day.

5. D. Accounting formula

Rationale: The accounting formula is Assets = Liabilities + Net Worth.

6. A. Liability

Rationale: Liabilities are monies the medical practice owes to its creditors, such as money owed for medical supplies to a vendor (supplier).

7. C. W-2 form

Rationale: W-2 forms must be completed at the end of each year and provided to every employee. By law, employers must mail or hand deliver W-2 forms by January 31 of the year immediately following the upcoming tax reporting season.

8. E. All of the above

Rationale: Government regulations require that records must be maintained for each employee relating to the following payroll items: amount of gross pay; Social Security number of the employee; number of exemptions of each employee (taken from the W-4 form completed by the employee at the time of hire); deductions for Social Security, federal, state, and city taxes, state disability insurance, and unemployment tax, where applicable; any pretax deductions such as 401(K) contributions.

9. D. A and C

Rationale: The W-2 form includes gross wages and federal income tax withheld. For a listing of all the items included in the W-2 form, see Figure 13-8.

10. C. Truth in Lending Act of 1969

Rationale: The Truth in Lending Act of 1969 requires full written disclosure concerning the payment of any fee that will be collected in more than four installments. Also referred to as Regulation Z of the Consumer Protection Act.

11. B. Office supplies and rent

Rationale: Accounts payable (AP) is money the physician owes to others for supplies, equipment, and services that have not yet been paid. Examples of AP expenditures in a medical office are office supplies, such as paper goods, day sheets, appointment cards, scheduling books; medical supplies and equipment; equipment repair and maintenance, including housekeeping; utilities such as telephone and electricity; taxes; payroll; and rent.

12. B. Customary

Rationale: Customary—fee charged for the same procedure by the majority of physicians with the same or similar training to perform that procedure.

13. A. Accounts receivable

Rationale: Accounts receivable (AR) is money owed to the practice by insurance companies and patients who have not yet paid.

14. E. A and B

Rationale: The bank statement includes withdrawals, deposits, and cleared checks. To see everything that is included in a bank statement, see Figure 13-1.

15. D. Reconciliation

Rationale: Reconciliation is a comparison of the figures on the bank statements with the banking records maintained in the medical office and adjustment of those banking records so that both are in agreement.

16. A. Located in the bottom left corner of a printed check

Rationale: The American Banker's Association (ABA) number is located in the upper right corner of a printed check. It is printed as a fraction on a business check or as a straight series of numbers (1–109/210) on a personal check. This number identifies the bank and the area where the bank issuing the check is located.

17. D. Payment at time of service

Rationale: Payment at the time of service is the preferred method of payment because it significantly reduces the cost of billing, including the generation of bills, postage fees, and the use of human resources.

18. A. Entered as a debit on the day sheet because it is a discount

Rationale: An adjustment occurs when a change is entered into the account record such as a discount, a write-off, or an amount not allowed by an insurance company (disallowance). A discount is entered as a credit since this amount will be subtracted from the total amount owed.

19. D. Designated amount is usually $100 to $200

Rationale: Petty cash is available for incidentals such as reimbursements, postage due, or other miscellaneous expenses within the medical office. Petty cash must be tracked and recorded in a daily financial log. A designated amount of cash is usually placed in a drawer or box at the beginning of each month for this purpose. This amount will vary from office to office, depending on the needs of the office, and usually ranges from $50 to $100.

20. E. Restrictive

Rationale: A restrictive endorsement specifies to whom money should be paid and the money's purpose, such as "For Deposit Only." You can rubber-stamp the physician's signature. It is considered the safest endorsement.

CHAPTER 14

1. C. Allowed charge

   Rationale: The allowed charge is the highest amount that third-party payers will make for services.

2. B. Crossover claim

   Rationale: A crossover claim is a patient claim that is eligible for both Medicare and Medicaid. It is also called Medi/Medi.

3. D. A subscriber

   Rationale: The subscriber is the person who holds a health benefit plan/contract/policy. This plan, contract, or policy may include other family members.

4. E. A and D

   Rationale: Medicare is health insurance for the elderly that is provided by the U.S. government.

   - Operated by the Social Security Administration
   - Paid for largely through Social Security funds
   - Designed for persons 65 years old and older and for the severely disabled
   - Covers approximately 32 million elderly citizens as well as 2 million permanently disabled persons.

   Eligible patients are issued a Medicare card after applying for services.

5. E. B and C

   Rationale: Medicare Part D

   - Voluntary participation
   - Prescription drugs covered under a separate medical policy
   - Implemented in 2006
   - Is offered as a supplemental plan for Medicare recipients to purchase
   - Covers a predetermined list of prescription drugs at participating pharmacies.

   For those Medicare recipients who choose Medicare Part D, there are annual deductibles, applicable copayments, or coinsurance and maximum benefits that apply.

6. D. U.S. Department of Defense's healthcare program for active duty and retired uniformed services members and their families

   Rationale: TRICARE is the U.S. Department of Defense's worldwide health care program for active duty and retired uniformed services members and their families.

7. A. Referral

   Rationale: A referral occurs when a patient is sent to another provider for a specific plan of care.

8. E. A and D

   Rationale: The following is the definition of self-insured: organizations that are large enough to fund their own insurance programs OR Individuals who purchase insurance directly through the insurance company without going through a group plan.

9. E. Prepaid plan

   Rationale: A prepaid plan is defined as follows: a group of physicians or other healthcare providers who have a contractual agreement to provide services to subscribers on a negotiated fee-for-service or capitated basis (also called a *managed care plan*).

10. B. CMS-1500

    Rationale: The CMS-1500 (previously known as the HCFA 1500) is the most common health insurance claim form and is used to file claims for physicians' services.

11. D. All of the above

    Rationale: All of the following pertains to worker's compensation:

    - Worker's compensation is government-mandated insurance for injuries directly related to work.
    - Payment of premiums is the employer's responsibility; the employee pays nothing.
    - Providers must enroll with their states' worker's compensation plan before they can agree to accept cases.
    - In worker's compensation cases, the provider of services must complete a report called a Doctor's First Report and must submit further reports at predetermined intervals.
    - A patient's records related to his or her worker's compensation case must be kept in a separate file from his or her regular record kept by the physician.

12. C. Capitation rate

    Rationale: The capitation rate is defined as follows: The provider is paid a predetermined amount every month regardless of the number of times the patient is seen within the month. Also known as *prospective payment*.

13. A. A claim

    Rationale: A claim is a written and documented request for reimbursement of an eligible expense under an insurance plan.

14. D. B and C

    Rationale: Two important components of an HMO are as follows:

    - All medical services are provided based on a predetermined (per capita) fee and not on a fee-for-service basis. If the actual cost of services exceeds the predetermined (or capitation) amount, then the provider must absorb the excess costs. This provides the incentive for the provider to control costs.

- A member patient must use the providers and hospitals that are identified by the HMO. The HMO will pay for any covered services that are provided by designated providers, hospitals, durable medical equipment, and pharmacies. Therefore, preapproval must be granted through the primary care provider (PCP) when and if a patient has to seek consultation or medical services outside of the network. The exception to this is a recognized emergency.

15. A. PPO members are not restricted to certain designated providers or hospitals

Rationale: PPO members are not restricted to certain designated providers or hospitals; HMO members are restricted certain providers or hospitals.

CHAPTER 15

1. A. 3

Rationale: ICD-9 includes the following volumes: Volume I-, Also known as the Tabular List Volume II, also known as the Alphabetic Index; and Volume III, which deals with inpatient diagnosis and treatment.

2. A. Volume II

Rationale: Volume II contains an index of poisoning and adverse effects of chemicals and drugs and an index of injuries caused by external efforts, such as accidents.

3. C. Locate the diagnosis in the patient's medical chart

Rationale: The first step in diagnostic coding is to locate the diagnosis in the patient's medical chart.

4. E. A and D

Rationale: V codes may be used in the following ways:

- To add supportive information to a patient, family, or personal history.
- As a primary code to describe a person who may not have a current illness but who is seeing the physician for well-baby care, birth control advice, pregnancy test, or immunizations.

V codes are used as supportive information when some circumstance or problem is present, such as an allergy to penicillin.

5. B. E codes

Rationale: E codes (E930–E949) are mandatory when coding the use of drugs.

6. D. All of the above

Rationale: Adoption of the ICD-10 code sets is expected to support value-based purchasing and Medicare's antifraud and abuse activities by accurately defining services and providing specific diagnosis and treatment information; support comprehensive reporting of quality data; ensure more accurate payments for new procedures, fewer rejected claims, improved disease management, and harmonization of disease monitoring and reporting worldwide; and allow the United States to compare its data with international data to track the incidence and spread of disease and treatment outcomes because the United States is one of the few developed countries that does not use ICD-10.

7. D. CPT

Rationale: The ***Current Procedural Terminology*** (CPT) manual provides a comprehensive list of procedure and service codes that is used to convert the narrative descriptions into a numerical code.

8. A. 99213

Rationale: E and M codes are strictly numerical, begin with "9," and consist of five digits without any decimals.

9. C. The complexity of the examination and the history of the patient

Rationale: E/M (E and M), as it is referred to, is based on the following criteria:

- The history of the patient
- The complexity of the examination
- The degree of difficulty in medical decision making

10. E. A and C

Rationale: The following are basic components of an effective compliance plan:

- Conducting periodic audits of billing and coding practices
- Developing written standards and procedures for compliance
- Training and educating staff members on procedures
- Investigating violations and disclosing incidents to appropriate government agencies
- Discussing in staff meetings how to avoid erroneous or fraudulent conduct

11. C. •

Rationale: • indicates a new code in ICD-9.

12. E. Extremely complex

Rationale: There are four levels of decision making with E/M: straightforward, low complex, moderate complex, and high complex.

13. E. A and C

Rationale: To report services and procedures for Medicaid and Medicare patients, the Healthcare Common Procedure Coding System (HCPCS) is used.

14. A. The codes available are the same as those in the CPT

Rationale: All of the following is true regarding HCPC's Level II: it has codes that are not available in the CPT; includes 22 sections; uses five-digit alphanumeric codes; used for items that Medicare covers, such as durable medical equipment (DME), materials, supplies, and injections. Level II codes begin with a letter, followed by four numbers. HCPCS modifiers consist of two letters and can be used in addition to CPT modifiers.

15. B. Billing separately for multiple services that would normally be covered with one code

Rationale: Unbundling is defined as billing separately for multiple services that would normally be covered under one code and one charge.

CHAPTER 16

1. B. Pathogens

Rationale: Pathogens are disease-causing organisms that are transmitted in a variety of ways, including skin-to-skin contact, airborne droplet nuclei, body fluids, and blood.

2. D. All of the above

Rationale: In order for microorganisms to grow, they must have all of the following: food, moisture, suitable temperature, and darkness.

3. D. Infected reservoir host, portal of exit, means of transmission, portal of entry into new host, susceptible new host

Rationale: The chain of infection is as follows: infected reservoir host, portal of exit, means of transmission, portal of entry into new host, susceptible new host.

4. C. Acquired by having the disease

Rationale: Active acquired natural immunity is defined as immunity acquired by having the disease, which results in production of antibodies and "memory cells" that respond when the antigen reappears again.

5. C. Hepatitis and AIDS

Rationale: Hepatitis and AIDS are among the most common blood-borne pathogens.

6. B. Liver

Rationale: Hepatitis affects the liver.

7. B. High-level disinfection

Rationale: High-level disinfection kills all microorganisms except bacterial spores. It is used on items that may come in contact with mucous membranes, such as sigmoidoscopes and glass thermometers.

8. E. C and D

Rationale: Seventy percent isopropyl alcohol and chlorine bleach are acceptable disinfection methods for certain surfaces.

9. B. 15 minutes

Rationale: Fifteen minutes is the minimum sterilization time for glassware.

10. B. Sterilization

Rationale: Sterilization is defined as being free of all microorganisms. Items must be sanitized and/or disinfected prior to being sterilized.

11. C. Fever

Rationale: Redness, heat, swelling, pain, and stiffness are the cardinal signs of infection.

12. D. Low temperatures kill bacteria growth.

Rationale: Bacteria grow best in moist areas: skin, mucous membranes, wet dressings, wounds, and dirty instruments. Bacteria thrive at body temperature (98.6°F). Low temperatures (32°F and below) retard, but do not kill, bacterial growth. Aerobic bacteria require an oxygen supply to live. Anaerobic bacteria can survive without oxygen. Darkness favors the growth of most bacteria. Some bacteria will die if exposed to direct sunlight or light.

13. C. First mild signs and symptoms appear; a highly contagious period

Rationale: During the prodromal period, the first mild signs and symptoms appear; this is a highly contagious period.

14. D. Vector transmission

Rationale: Vector transmission: Parasitic insects carry disease via animals. An example is Lyme disease, which is carried by a tick commonly found on deer.

15. E. Gloves, mask, eye/face shield, lab coat, and gown

Rationale: If you anticipate that you may be sprayed with blood and the likelihood of gross contamination is high, you should wear the following: gloves, mask, eye/face shield, lab coat, and gown.

CHAPTER 17

1. B. Open-ended

Rationale: Open-ended questions require more than a "yes" or "no" answer. Example: "Mr. Thompson, how would you describe your pain?"

2. E. A and D

Rationale: The patient's past history should include the following: dates of major illnesses, surgeries, and hospitalizations; medications (prescription and over-the- counter); childhood diseases; allergies; immunizations; and the date of the last examination.

3. A. Childhood diseases

Rationale: The social history should include the following: smoking, drinking, recreational drug use, occupation, marital status, sexual preference, and lifestyle, including diet, exercise, and sleep habits.

4. D. Endocrine

Rationale: During the endocrine portion of the ROS, the following are considered: growth and development, goiter, excessive thirst, intolerance to temperature change, hormone therapy, diabetes symptoms, irregular menses, and symptoms of thyroid disorders.

5. B. Comprehensive

Rationale: The six Cs of charting are as follows: client's own words, clarity, completeness, conciseness, chronological, and confidentiality.

6. E. Weight

Rationale: Temperature (T), pulse (P), respiration (R), and blood pressure (BP) measurements are considered vital signs because they measure some of the body's most vital functions and may provide important information about the body's overall state of health.

7. D. 99.6

Rationale: The normal rectal temperature for an adult is 99.6°F.

8. B. Phase 2

Rationale: During the second Korotkoff phase, you will hear a swishing or whooshing sound.

9. E. 10 minutes

Rationale: When measuring a child's temperature using the axillary method, the thermometer should be placed in the child's armpit and held there by folding the child's arm across the chest for the required 10 minutes.

10. E. Oral

Rationale: Oral temperature is the preferred method.

11. E. 50–65 bpm

Rationale: The average pulse rate for an older adult is 50–65 beats per minute.

12. B. The patient's arm should be at least at waist level with the palm down

Rationale: The patient's arm should be at chest level with the palm down.

13. D. Behind the knee

Rationale: The popliteal pulse may be located behind the knee.

14. D. 30–50

Rationale: The normal number of respirations for a newborn is 30–50/minute.

15. B. 120/80 to 139/89

Rationale: Blood pressure readings between 120/80 and 139/89 are considered prehypertensive.

16. D. Primary hypertension of unknown cause

Rationale: Primary hypertension of unknown cause is known as *essential hypertension.*

17. B. If the patient's arm is below heart level, the BP reading will be lower than normal.

Rationale: If the patient's arm is below heart level, the BP reading will be higher than normal.

18. D. 70 bpm

Rationale: The pulse rate in a normal, healthy adult is approximately 70 bpm. A pulse rate above 100 bpm is considered tachycardia and one below 60 bpm is considered bradycardia.

19. A. 16 to 20

Rationale: From 16 to 20 respirations per minute is considered normal.

20. D. Rhonchi

Rationale: Rhonchi (gurgles)—rattling or whistling sound in the throat.

21. D. The patient should move toward the walker and then move the walker to the side.

Rationale: The patient should move the walker and then move toward the walker.

22. B. If one testicle is slightly larger or lies somewhat behind (lower than) the other, this is considered abnormal.

Rationale: If one testicle is slightly larger or lies somewhat lower than the other, this is considered normal.

23. E. Right crutch forward, left foot forward, left crutch forward, right foot forward

Rationale: The proper procedure for a four-point gait is right crutch forward, left foot forward, left crutch forward, right foot forward.

24. E. Contains approximately 300 doses of premeasured medication

Rationale: Metered-dose inhalers (MDIs) contain approximately 200 doses.

25. A. 5

Rationale: A patient using a nebulizer should have his or her pulse monitored every 5 minutes.

CHAPTER 18

1. C. Unwrapped sterile items must be removed with clean transfer forceps.

   Rationale: Unwrapped items must be removed using sterile transfer forceps and must be placed on a sterile field or in a sterile storage area.

2. B. Otoscope

   Rationale: An otoscope is an instrument used to examine the ears. Light is focused through a speculum into the outer ear and onto the tympanic membrane. Additional speculums may be used to view other structures such as the nose.

3. C. Binarual

   Rationale: Binaurals are rigid small metal tubes that connect the tubing to the earpieces.

4. A. Diaphragm

   Rationale: The diaphragm is a disclike sound sensor that picks up both low- and high-pitched sound frequencies.

5. A. Increases circulation to the area for greater comfort and healing

   Rationale: Cryotherapy constricts blood vessels; slows circulation to the affected area; reduces swelling, inflammation, and pain; and decreases body temperature.

6. C. Endoscope

   Rationale: An endoscope is an instrument used to look into a hollow organ or body cavity. It is employed to examine the larynx, bladder, colon, sigmoid colon, stomach, abdomen, and some joints.

7. D. Lighter than synthetic casts

   Rationale: Plaster casts are applied wet around a stockinette liner with cotton padding over the limb. They use a wet bandage roll impregnated with calcium sulfate. They are heavier than synthetic casts. They may soften or crumble with moisture. They can crack or break. They are easily molded to the body part, so immobilization is more effective. They are less expensive than synthetic casts.

8. E. Fixative spray

   Rationale: Fixative spray is used to preserve slides.

9. C. Aneroid

   Rationale: Aneroid sphygmomanometers have a round dial that contains a scale calibrated in millimeters and a needle to register the reading.

10. C. Aural

    Rationale: Tympanic thermometer, also known as an *aural thermometer*. It detects heat waves within the ear canal near the eardrum.

11. E. 24–36 hours

    Rationale: Elevate the casted limb above heart level for the first 24–36 hours to prevent swelling and reduce pain.

12. B. Urine specimen, blood specimen, vital signs, weight and height, EKG, X-ray

    Rationale: The correct sequence of physical exam procedures is urine specimen, blood specimen, vital signs, weight and height, EKG, X-ray.

13. C. Manipulation

    Rationale: Manipulation is the process of passively assessing the range of motion (ROM) in a joint.

14. C. Palpation

    Rationale: Palpation is the process of using the hands to feel the skin and accessible underlying organs and tissues.

15. D. Dorsal recumbent position

    Rationale: The dorsal recumbent position is a supine position with the knees bent.

16. B. Instruments with ratchets should be stored closed in order to maintain their good working condition.

    Rationale: Instruments with ratchets should be stored open to maintain their good working condition. Check all instruments for defects before sterilizing.

17. B. 3-0

    Rationale: 3-0 suture is used most often on muscle.

18. B. Open sterile packets toward you to avoid contaminating the packet.

    Rationale: Sterile packets should be opened away from you to avoid contaminating the packet by touching your clothing.

19. E. B and C

    Rationale: Absorbable suture is typically used for the following: internal organs, subcutaneous tissue, tying off blood vessels.

20. A. Vicryl

    Rationale: Absorbable suture is also known as *catgut* or Vicryl.

21. C. Forceps

    Rationale: Forceps are used to grasp and/or clamp.

CHAPTER 19

1. D. 0.20

   Rationale: Each 5 × 5 mm square equals 0.20 second.

2. D. Red

   Rationale: The left leg limb lead is red.

3. A. P wave

Rationale: The P wave reflects the contraction of the atria via firing of the SA node.

4. B. Poor sensor contact with skin

Rationale: Poor sensor contact with the skin may cause a wandering baseline artifact.

5. D. The fourth intercostal space to the right of the sternum

Rationale: The V2 EKG precordial lead is placed at the fourth intercostal space to the right of the sternum.

6. C. 14–16 inches

Rationale: The adult should hold the Jaeger card 14–16 inches away from him- or herself.

7. E. Residual volume

Rationale: Residual volume is the measurement of air left in the lungs after forced expiration.

8. B. Posterioanterior

Rationale: Posterioanterior positioning allows the X-ray beam to be directed from back to front.

9. D. Ultrasound

Rationale: Ultrasound may require either a full bladder or the use of laxatives.

10. C. Red and green

Rationale: Red and green are the most common color vision defects.

11. C. Three

Rationale: Three leads are required in order for the electrical activity to be transmitted to the EKG machine.

12. A. 20/70

Rationale: When performing a vision test using the Snellen chart, you should ask the patient to begin by reading the 20/70 line.

13. E. 30 inches

Rationale: When screening for color vision acuity, the card/page should be 30 inches from the patient.

14. B. Expiratory reserve volume

Rationale: Expiratory reserve volume is the maximum volume of air left that can be exhaled after normal expiration.

15. E. Axial

Rationale: An axial view is one in which the X-ray tube is angled to direct a ray along the axis of the body or body part.

16. D. Ultrasound

Rationale: The patient does not have to be NPO for an ultrasound exam.

17. D. Patient may smoke up to 1 hour prior to the study

Rationale: The patient should be instructed not to smoke since this can stimulate gastric secretions.

18. E. Whitish stools may be present for 7 to 10 days after the procedure.

Rationale: Whitish stools may be present for 1 or 2 days after the procedure.

19. E. 25

Rationale: A properly calibrated EKG machine will move the paper at a speed of 25 mm/second.

CHAPTER 20

1. C. Normal formation or development of blood cells

Rationale: Hematopoiesis is normal formation or development of blood cells.

2. B. They defend against infection.

Rationale: WBCs defend against infection.

3. D. Smallest cells in the blood

Rationale: Platelets, also known as *thrombocytes,* are the smallest cells in the blood.

4. B. Agglutination

Rationale: Agglutination is the reaction that occurs when an antigen clumps together with an antibody.

5. E. A and C

Rationale: You should screen the patient prior to collecting the specimen to ensure that the patient followed pretest preparation procedures, and the specimen should be collected prior to beginning antibiotic treatment.

6. A. Ring finger

Rationale: The most common site for a capillary puncture is the ring finger, preferably on the non-dominant hand.

7. D. Yellow, light blue, red, red-marbled, green

Rationale: The correct order of draw is: yellow, light blue, red, red marbled, green.

8. D. Inoculation, incubation, inspection, identification

Rationale: Inoculation, incubation, inspection, and identification is the correct order for culture processing.

9. B. Centrifuge

Rationale: A centrifuge separates specimens into layers by spinning.

10. A. A sample similar to the testing specimen, previously tested with a known value

Rationale: A control sample is a sample similar to the testing specimen, previously tested with a known value.

11. B. Hct

Rationale: The hematocrit (Hct) provides information about RBC volume.

12. D. 4,500–11,000

Rationale: The normal white blood cell count for an adult is 4,500–11,000

13. A. Fungus

Rationale: A fungus is an opportunistic pathogen that causes disease when the normal balance of flora is upset.

14. C. Results reported out as either positive or negative

Rationale: Qualitative test results are reported out as either positive or negative.

15. D. Thrombocyte

Rationale: A thrombocyte is not a WBC.

16. B. Granules in cytoplasm that respond to allergies and inflammation

Rationale: Eosinophils can be described as granules in cytoplasm that respond to allergies and inflammation.

17. E. 20 mL

Rationale: A 20 mL vacuum tube is not a standard size.

18. A. PT/PTT

Rationale: PT/PTT tests are coagulation tests.

19. A. One

Rationale: When performing a Gram stain, once you have poured the crystal violet over the slide, you should let it set for 1 minute before draining the excess stain and rinsing with water.

20. B. Patient's date of birth

Rationale: The patient's date of birth is not required when labeling a specimen.

21. A. Select either the ring finger or great finger on the dominant hand.

Rationale: Under normal circumstances, when performing a manual capillary puncture, you should select either the ring finger or the great finger on the nondominant hand.

22. A. 15 to 20 degrees

Rationale: The proper angle for insertion when performing venipuncture using the vacutainer method is 15 to 20 degrees.

23. D. Lavender

Rationale: A lavender tube is used for CBCs

24. D. Identify the patient, wash hands, apply gloves, remove sterile swab from the Culturette, depress the tongue, insert the swab and roll it firmly across the back of the patient's throat area where infected, insert the swab into a plastic vial, crush the internal vial of transport medium, ensuring that the swab is saturated.

Rationale: The correct order for obtaining a throat culture is as follows: Identify the patient, wash hands, apply gloves, remove a sterile swab from the Culturette, depress the tongue, insert the swab and roll it firmly across the back of the patient's throat area where infected, insert the swab into a plastic vial, and crush the internal vial of transport medium, ensuring that the swab is saturated.

25. E. Compound

Rationale: Compound microscopes are most commonly found in physicians' offices.

26. A. Straw

Rationale: *Straw* is a descriptor for the color of urine, not for its clarity.

27. A. One

Rationale: One drop of urine sediment should be placed on the slide.

28. B. Measures the amount of nitrogen in the blood, indicating renal function

Rationale: BUN measures the amount of nitrogen in the blood, indicating renal function.

29. A. You may use either a blood culture media set or a green-top vacuum tube.

Rationale: If the physician has ordered a blood culture, you need to either use a blood culture media set or a yellow-top vacuum tube.

30. D. Gently touch the test strip to the first drop of blood that forms on the patient's finger.

Rationale: The first drop of blood should be wiped away.

CHAPTER 21

1. C. Absorption

Rationale: Absorption is the movement of medication from the site of administration into the bloodstream.

2. A. Antagonism

Rationale: Antagonism is defined as administering two medications together, causing both medications to be less effective than if administered separately.

3. E. Metabolism

Rationale: Metabolism occurs when drugs are broken down and converted to a water-soluble compound that can be excreted by the body.

4. A. Pharmacodynamics

Rationale: Pharmacodynamics is the study of the actions of drugs.

5. C. 4.8 mL

   Rationale: 4.8 mL would be administered.

6. D. 11.3 mg

   Rationale: 11.3 mg is the pediatric dose.

7. E. 34.3 mg

   Rationale: 34.3 mg is the pediatric dose for this child.

8. B. Generic

   Rationale: The generic name is the common name for a medication.

9. D. Inscription

   Rationale: The inscription indicates the name of the medication and the dosage.

10. C. Hilt

    Rationale: The hilt connects the shaft to the hub.

11. A. Fried's Law

    Rationale: Fried's Law is based on the assumption that a child 12½ years old can take an adult dose of medication.

12. D. 5.5 mL = 0.0055 L

    Rationale: 5.5 mL is the equivalent of 0.0055 L.

13. E. 30

    Rationale: 1 fl oz equals 30 mL.

14. A. Diuretic

    Rationale: Dyazide is a diuretic.

15. E. Reglan

    Rationale: Reglan is an antiemetic.

16. E. Both C and D

    Rationale: Schedule III and IV drugs allow up to five refills over a 6-month period.

17. C. Right to refuse

    Rationale: The firs six rights of medication administration are as follows: right patient, right medication, right dosage, right route, right time, and right documentation.

18. B. Upper outer portion of the arm

    Rationale: The most frequently used site for a subcutaneous injection is the upper outer portion of the arm.

19. D. 14 to 22

    Rationale: A 14 to 22 gauge needle is typically used for an intramuscular injection.

20. C. 10 to 15 degrees

    Rationale: Intradermal injections are administered at an angle of 10 to 15 degrees.

21. D. Cumulative effect

    Rationale: A cumulative effect occurs when the next dose of medication is given before the previous dose has had time to be metabolized/excreted.

22. A. 1000 of a unit

    Rationale: A kilo equals 1000 of a unit.

23. D. Liter

    Rationale: The liter is the common unit of measure for volume in the metric system.

24. C. 6

    Rationale: VI equals 6.

25. D. Alternate days

    Rationale: *Alternate days* is abbreviated *alt dieb.*

26. C. Chamber

    Rationale: The chamber is not part of a syringe.

27. A. Prevent vomiting, relieve nausea

    Rationale: Antiemetics are used to prevent vomiting and relieve nausea.

28. D. Atropine

    Rationale: Atropine is an antispasmodic.

29. B. GI tract

    Rationale: Antispasmodics are used to treat the GI tract.

30. B. Schedule II

    Rationale: Schedule II drugs have high potential for addiction and are accepted for medical use in the United States.

CHAPTER 22

1. D. Assess the patient, call 911, assess the CABs, give 30 compressions, two breaths, 30 compressions

   Rationale: The proper sequence for performing adult CPR is as follows: Assess the patient, call 911, assess the CAPs, give 30 compressions, two breaths, 30 compressions.

2. E. Assess the patient, assess the CABs, give 15 compressions and two breaths, repeating compressions and breaths for 2 minutes, and then call 911

   Rationale: The proper sequence for performing infant CPR if collapse was witnessed is as follows: Assess the patient, assess the CABs, give 15 compressions and two breaths, repeating compressions and breaths for 2 minutes, and then call 911.

3. D. You should continue CPR while the AED is analyzing

   Rationale: When the AED is analyzing, you should not touch the victim.

4. A. 4½

   Rationale: Each arm equals 4½%.

5. C. Press the pen firmly against the victim's thigh close to the hip

Rationale: The pen should be pressed firmly against the victim's thigh about halfway between the hip and knee.

6. E. Anaphylactic

   Rationale: Anaphylactic shock follows an allergic reaction.

7. D. Loss of consciousness

   Rationale: Symptoms are similar to those of CVA (except that there is no loss of consciousness).

8. B. One breath every 3–5 seconds

   Rationale: Rescue breathing for a child requires giving one breath every 3–5 seconds.

9. D. Bradycardia

   Rationale: The symptoms of shock are weakness, cool skin, rapid heartbeat, clammy skin, thirst, cyanosis, nausea, confusion, dizziness, disorientation, restlessness, unresponsiveness, pallor, and shallow breathing.

10. C. 70

    Rationale: When a diabetic patient's blood sugar falls below 70 mg/dL, the patient is said to be hypoglycemic.

11. B. Dark red

    Rationale: Arterial bleeding is usually abundant, bright red, and rapid, and usually spurts in rhythm with the heartbeat.

12. A. Avulsion

    Rationale: An avulsion leaves a flap of skin.

13. A. Ensure that your insurance paperwork is in order

    Rationale: According to FEMA, the six steps in planning for a natural disaster are as follows: check for hazards around the facility, identify safe places indoors and outdoors, educate the staff, have disaster supplies on hand, develop an emergency communication plan, and assist the community in preparing for disasters.

14. C. Burn area

    Rationale: The Rule of Nines is used to calculate the extent of a burn area.

15. E. A and C but not B

    Rationale: Fainting and syncope occur as a result of a brief interruption in the flow of blood to the brain, causing a typical brief loss of consciousness.

16. B. The skin

    Rationale: Superficial wounds affect the skin.

17. A. Intubation and immediate transport to the Emergency Department

    Rationale: If a patient suffers a respiratory shock in the medical office, the patient should be intubated and immediately transported to the Emergency Department.

18. B. Pressure dressing

    Rationale: A pressure dressing is a compress held in place by an elastic bandage.

19. B. Decreased level of consciousness

    Rationale: Contusions cause a decreased level of consciousness.

20. C. Second degree

    Rationale: A second-degree burn is considered a partial-thickness burn.

21. E. 105

    Rationale: Heat stroke occurs when the body temperature is greater than 105°F.

22. D. Rapid onset

    Rationale: In patients with hyperglycemia, diabetic coma has a slow, insidious onset.

23. D. 36

    Rationale: If a person has sustained burns on the front and back of both legs, 36% of the body is involved.

24. E. Check for AED

    Rationale: During the initial assessment prior to administering CPR, you should check for responsiveness, for breathing, for a pulse, and for a patent airway.

25. B. Force the mouth open

    Rationale: When someone is having a seizure, you should not force the mouth open.

APPENDIX B
Practice Exam

GENERAL MEDICAL ASSISTING

1. Blood, adipose, and osseous tissues are examples of what type of tissue?
   A. Epithelial
   B. Connective
   C. Muscle
   D. Nervous
   E. None of the above
2. Which of the following is not a muscle tissue?
   A. Adipose
   B. Smooth
   C. Cardiac
   D. Skeletal
   E. All are muscle tissues
3. Which layer of the skin secretes and produces sebum to keep the skin oiled and elastic?
   A. Epidermis
   B. Dermis
   C. Subcutaneous
   D. A and B
   E. None of the above
4. Cyanosis is used to describe what skin color?
   A. Yellow
   B. Redness
   C. Splotchy
   D. Blue
   E. None of the above
5. The skeletal system is made up of different types of bones and two divisions, the axial skeleton and the appendicular skeleton. These two divisions combined consist of how many bones?
   A. 189
   B. 201
   C. 206
   D. 176
   E. None of the above
6. A kneecap is what type of bone?
   A. Long
   B. Short
   C. Flat
   D. Irregular
   E. Sesamoid
7. Which structure of skeletal muscles is described as "connective tissue that attaches muscle to bone?"
   A. Tendons
   B. Muscle fiber
   C. Fascia
   D. Aponeurosis
   E. None of the above
8. The zygomaticus muscle is found where?
   A. Hand
   B. Wrist
   C. Arm
   D. Face
   E. Chest
9. The iliacus muscle is found where?
   A. Foot
   B. Leg
   C. Arm
   D. Hand
   E. None of the above
10. The large intestine is how long?
    A. 1 foot
    B. 2 feet
    C. 3 feet
    D. 4 feet
    E. 5 feet
11. What major organ of the digestive system is also shared with the respiratory system?
    A. Esophagus
    B. Stomach
    C. Pharynx
    D. A and C
    E. None of the above
12. The outer layer of the heart is known as the ___________.
    A. Pericardium
    B. Endocardium
    C. Exocardium
    D. Myocardium
    E. None of the above

13. What does the left atrium of the heart do?
    A. Receives oxygen-poor blood from tissues
    B. Receives oxygen-rich blood from the lungs
    C. Pumps oxygen-poor blood to the pulmonary artery and then out to the lungs
    D. Pumps oxygen-rich blood through the aorta and then out to the body
    E. None of the above

14. Which paranasal sinus is located just above the eyebrows in the frontal bone?
    A. Maxillary sinus
    B. Ethmoid sinus
    C. Frontal sinus
    D. Sphenoid sinus
    E. None of the above

15. Which structure filters and traps bacteria, viruses, cancer cells, and other invaders?
    A. Thymus
    B. Tonsils
    C. Spleen
    D. A and B
    E. None of the above

16. How many pairs of cranial nerves are there?
    A. 8
    B. 11
    C. 31
    D. 15
    E. 12

17. Which lobe of the brain controls eyesight?
    A. Frontal
    B. Parietal
    C. Occipital
    D. Temporal
    E. None of the above

18. Which unit funnels urine from within the kidney into the ureter?
    A. Renal pelvis
    B. Glomerulus
    C. Urethra
    D. Urinary bladder
    E. None of the above

19. Which organ is a long, coiled tube located on the upper part of each testicle and running the length of each testicle?
    A. Seminal vesicle
    B. Epididymis
    C. Bulbourethral glands
    D. Vas deferens
    E. None of the above

20. What is the narrow lower portion of the uterus that extends to the vagina?
    A. Endometrium
    B. Perineum
    C. Cervix
    D. Corpus luteum
    E. None of the above

21. Which hormone stimulates ovulation in females?
    A. Adrenocorticotropic hormone
    B. Prolactin
    C. Follicle-stimulating hormone
    D. Thyroid-stimulating hormone
    E. Luteinizing hormone

22. Which hormone controls secretion of certain hormones from the adrenal cortex?
    A. Adrenocorticotropic hormone
    B. Prolactin
    C. Follicle-stimulating hormone
    D. Thyroid-stimulating hormone
    E. Luteinizing hormone

23. Which of the following hormones influences metabolism, protein synthesis, and maturation of the nervous system?
    A. Calcitonin
    B. Oxytocin
    C. Triiodothyronine
    D. Antidiuretic hormone
    E. None of the above

24. Which hormone works with calcitonin and increases blood calcium and decreases blood phosphate?
    A. Aldosterone
    B. Parathormone
    C. Glucagon
    D. Melatonin
    E. None of the above

25. How many muscles make eye movement possible?
    A. Six
    B. Five
    C. Four
    D. Three
    E. Two

26. Benign neoplasia is best described by which word(s)?
    A. Not progressive
    B. Invasive
    C. Noncancerous
    D. Cancerous
    E. A and C

27. Malignant neoplasia is best described by which word(s)?
    A. Not progressive
    B. Invasive
    C. Noncancerous
    D. Cancerous
    E. B and D

28. Neoplasm of the connective tissue is known as what?
   A. Sarcoma
   B. Carcinoma
   C. Hyperplasia
   D. Metastasis
   E. Carcinoma in-situ

29. What disease is characterized as "a contagious skin infection usually caused by *Streptococcus* or *Staphylococcus*"?
   A. Measles
   B. Impetigo
   C. Herpes simplex
   D. Pediculosis
   E. None of the above

30. What common disease is known as lice?
   A. Pediculosis
   B. Cellulitis
   C. Dermatitis
   D. Petechiae
   E. None of the above

31. Which skeletal system disease is caused by crystals forming in the joints?
   A. Bursitis
   B. Osteomalacia
   C. Ankylosing spondylitis
   D. Gout
   E. Carpal tunnel syndrome

32. Which skeletal system disease is characterized by softening of the bone?
   A. Osteoperosis
   B. Osteomalacia
   C. Ankylosing spondylitis
   D. Gout
   E. Carpal tunnel syndrome

33. Paralysis of all four extremities is known as what?
   A. Torticollis
   B. Myasthenia gravis
   C. Paraplegia
   D. Fibromyalgia
   E. Quadriplegia

34. What is cirrhosis?
   A. Chronic liver cell destruction
   B. Protrusion of the stomach upward into the mediastinal cavity
   C. Inflammation of the colon
   D. Inflammation of the GI tract, usually the small intestine
   E. None of the above

35. An accumulation of fluid in the legs and ankles due to improper drainage is known as what?
   A. Mononucleosis
   B. Hypertension
   C. Bradycardia
   D. Lymphedema
   E. Tachycardia

36. Thick, dry, sticky mucus that clogs organs, mainly the lungs, is known as what?
   A. Influenza
   B. Cystic fibrosis
   C. Pharyngitis
   D. Diphtheria
   E. None of the above

37. Abnormal electrical impulses within the brain that cause bursts of excitement and may result in seizures are known as what?
   A. Hydrocephalus
   B. Encephalitis
   C. Neuralgia
   D. Epilepsy
   E. Sciatica

38. Enuresis is a form of what condition?
   A. Hypospadias
   B. Incontinence
   C. Cystitis
   D. Epispadias
   E. None of the above

39. Difficult and/or painful menstruation is known as what?
   A. Dysmenorrhea
   B. Endometriosis
   C. Salpingitis
   D. Vaginitis
   E. Hydrocele

40. A severe life-threatening form of adult hypothyroidism is known as what?
   A. Tetany
   B. Acromegaly
   C. Gigantism
   D. Myxedema
   E. Dwarfism

41. Which of the following is not an example of positive communication?
   A. Smiling
   B. Empathy
   C. Mumbling
   D. Listening carefully
   E. Being friendly

42. All of the following are part of the five Cs of better communication except ______________.
A. Content
B. Check
C. Clarity
D. Conciseness
E. All are examples of the five Cs of better communication.

43. What is the most commonly used channel of communication?
A. Face-to-face discussion
B. Written notes
C. E-mail
D. Telephone conversations
E. None of the above

44. Which of the following is an example of an open-ended question?
A. Are you in pain?
B. Can you please describe your pain?
C. Where is the pain coming from?
D. B and C
E. All of the above

45. Listening to the news is an example of what type of listening?
A. Evaluative listening
B. Passive listening
C. Active listening
D. All of the above
E. None of the above

46. "The form of listening that is two-way and requires a response" is a definition of what?
A. Active listening
B. Passive listening
C. Evaluative listening
D. All of the above
E. None of the above

47. Which of the following is an example of nonverbal communication?
A. Facial expressions
B. Eye contact
C. Posture
D. Gestures
E. All of the above

48. Most communication in the United States occurs at this distance:
A. Intimate distance
B. Personal distance
C. Social distance
D. Public distance
E. None of the above

49. Which of the following statements is an example of aggressive behavior?
A. This medication works best when it is taken on a daily basis.
B. Let me find someone who can answer that question for you.
C. Why did you do that? That was stupid.
D. Your behavior is inappropriate.
E. Knocking on the door and then coming into an exam room to say, "Excuse me, Dr. Thompson. You are needed on the telephone."

50. Which of the following statements about professionalism is not true?
A. It is exhibited by treating everyone, including patients, co-workers, supervisors, and those from outside the office, in a courteous, conscientious, and businesslike manner.
B. All forms of communication should be delivered with a positive attitude.
C. All forms of communication should be delivered in a respectful manner and should be appropriate for the intended receiver.
D. Maintaining professionalism is of the utmost importance, whether communicating verbally, nonverbally, or by written means.
E. None of the above

51. Which of the following is not part of the communication cycle?
A. Source
B. Message
C. Channel
D. Receiver
E. All are part of the communication cycle.

52. Examples of a professional appearance are:
A. Careful grooming and good hygiene
B. Excessive makeup
C. Facial piercings and tattoos
D. Appropriate dress
E. A and D

53. When communicating with a hearing-impaired patient who has an interpreter, it is important to do what?
A. Maintain eye contact and speak directly to the patient.
B. Don't have anything in your mouth, such as gum or candy.
C. Have paper and pen available so that the patient can communicate in writing if desired.
D. Make sure that you are in a quiet, well-lit room.
E. All of the above

54. When communicating with visually impaired patients, what do you not have to do?
   A. Raise the volume of your voice.
   B. Face the patient.
   C. Explain in detail any procedures the patient may have performed.
   D. Have large-print patient education material available.
   E. All are required.

55. For the following question, choose the best answer. When communicating with non-English-speaking patients in a culturally diverse area, it is important to do what?
   A. Have an interpreter at your office.
   B. Have a list of interpreters available to call when needed.
   C. Use nonverbal communication initially.
   D. A and sometimes C
   E. B and sometimes C

56. The developmental stage of the life cycle that includes the following characteristics is what?

   "Linguistic, physical, and cognitive skills develop. The concept of self begins to develop."
   A. Early adolescence
   B. Infancy
   C. Middle adulthood
   D. Early childhood
   E. Early adulthood

57. According to Elizabeth Kübler-Ross, which of the following best describes the order in which people grieve?
   A. Depression, anger, bargaining, denial, acceptance
   B. Denial, anger, bargaining, depression, acceptance
   C. Denial, acceptance, bargaining, depression, anger
   D. Depression, anger, bargaining, denial, acceptance
   E. Denial, depression, bargaining, anger, acceptance

58. Recognize the defense mechanism that is being displayed in the following example:

   A husband and wife are fighting, and the husband becomes so angry that he hits a door instead of his wife.
   A. Displacement
   B. Denial
   C. Compensation
   D. Minimization
   E. Projection

59. Who was the individual responsible for developing the theory based on the following experiment?

   While conducting a study on the digestive process of dogs, he discovered that the malnourished dogs salivated when his assistants entered the room to feed them. He began to precede the feeding of the dogs with the ringing of a bell. Eventually, the dogs salivated at the sound of the bell.
   A. B. F. Skinner
   B. Carl Jung
   C. Ivan Pavlov
   D. Jean Piaget
   E. Sigmund Freud

60. Which of the following persons developed the theories of personal unconscious, collective unconscious, extroversion, and introversion, which are based on the human unconscious and personality types?
   A. B. F. Skinner
   B. Sigmund Freud
   C. Abraham Maslow
   D. Eric Erickson
   E. Carl Jung

61. Match the following legal terminology definition with its correct term:

   "Presenting testimony at a trial to prove either guilt or innocence."
   A. Guardian ad litem
   B. Burden of proof
   C. *Locum tenens*
   D. Subpoena
   E. *Res judicata*

62. Libel is defined as ____________.
   A. Written defamation
   B. Performing an incorrect treatment
   C. Contributing to the commission of a crime
   D. Spoken defamation
   E. Agreement to a procedure through actions only

63. Which of the following is not one of the four Ds of negligence?
   A. Dereliction or neglect of duty
   B. Damages
   C. Duty
   D. Direct cause
   E. Dysfunction

64. Which legislation provided protection for the patient and the physician and also provided guidance for the patient's caregiver to make decisions based on the wishes of the patient?
   A. Health Insurance Portability and Accountability Act of 1996 (HIPAA)
   B. Patients' Bill of Rights
   C. Patient Self-Determination Act
   D. Good Samaritan Act
   E. Controlled Substance Act of 1970

65. Which of the following Latin terms means "performing the correct treatment with errors"?
A. *malfeasance*
B. *locum tenens*
C. *qui tam*
D. *misfeasance*
E. *nonfeasance*

66. Which of the following is not considered protected health information (PHI)?
A. Address
B. Telephone number
C. E-mail address
D. Photos
E. All are PHI

67. Who can authorize the release of a patient's medical record?
A. Patient
B. Legal guardian
C. Significant other
D. A and B
E. A and C

68. Fax machines must be kept where?
A. In an area of the office not accessible to patients
B. In the waiting room
C. In the exam room
D. In the hallway
E. Doesn't matter where they're kept

69. If a person knowingly and in violation of HIPAA regulations uses a unique health identifier or causes it to be used, what is the punishment?
A. A fine of not more than $250,000, imprisonment for not more than 10 years, or both
B. A fine of not more than $50,000, imprisonment for not more than one year, or both
C. A fine of not more than $100,000, imprisonment for not more than five years, or both
D. A and B
E. None of the above

70. What was the intention of HIPAA when it was created?
A. Improve portability and continuity within group and individual insurance
B. Simplify health insurance information
C. Promote the use of medical savings accounts (MSAs)
D. Improve access to long-term care services and coverage
E. All of the above

71. The basic meaning of a medical term is contained in the:
A. Prefix
B. Suffix
C. Root word
D. Combining form
E. None of the above

72. The word part that usually provides information about a body part is the:
A. Prefix
B. Suffix
C. Root word
D. Combining form
E. None of the above

73. Which of the following is the most common combining vowel?
A. *a*
B. *e*
C. *i*
D. *o*
E. *u*

74. Which of the following is not a true statement?
A. The suffix usually provides information about a disease.
B. The suffix usually provides information about a disorder.
C. The suffix usually provides information about a condition.
D. The suffix usually provides information about location.
E. The suffix usually provides information about a procedure.

75. The root word *albino* means:
A. Black
B. Gray
C. Yellow
D. White
E. Blue

76. The root word *leuko* means:
A. Black
B. Gray
C. Yellow
D. White
E. Blue

77. The root word *xantho* means:
A. Black
B. Gray
C. Yellow
D. White
E. Blue

78. The opposite of *disto* is:
A. *proximo*
B. *ventro*
C. *postero*
D. *medio*
E. *latero*

79. The root word *karyo* means:
   A. Gland
   B. Tissue
   C. Cell
   D. Nucleus
   E. Mucous

80. *Veno* means "vein"; what other root word also means "vein"?
   A. *arterio*
   B. *cardio*
   C. *thrombo*
   D. *phlebo*
   E. *hemo*

81. Which root word means "plaque"?
   A. *arterio*
   B. *athero*
   C. *cardio*
   D. *aorto*
   E. *thrombo*

82. Which of the following medical terms means "nail fungus"?
   A. *onychocryptosis*
   B. *mycosis*
   C. *xeroderma*
   D. *onychomycosis*
   E. *rhytidosis*

83. Which of the following root words means "ovaries"?
   A. *colpo*
   B. *orcho*
   C. *oophoro*
   D. *metro*
   E. *hysteron*

84. Which of the following root words means "ureter"?
   A. *urethra*
   B. *uretero*
   C. *reno*
   D. *nephro*
   E. *litho*

85. The suffix *-algia* means "pain." What other suffix also means "pain"?
   A. *-dynia*
   B. *-blast*
   C. *-malacia*
   D. *-pathy*
   E. *-phagia*

86. What is the proper medical term for drooping of the eyelid?
   A. *cephalgia*
   B. *presbyopia*
   C. *diplopia*
   D. *dysphagia*
   E. *blepharoptosis*

87. Which of the following root words means "pus"?
   A. *pyo*
   B. *pyro*
   C. *carcino*
   D. *crypto*
   E. *kerato*

88. Which term correctly describes the process of recording a hearing test?
   A. *audiogram*
   B. *tympanogram*
   C. *audiography*
   D. *audiograph*
   E. None of the above

89. The prefix *-ecto* means "within." Which prefix(es) below mean the opposite?
   A. *-endo*
   B. *-intra*
   C. *-inter*
   D. Both A and B
   E. Both A and C

90. Which of the following body plane definitions is incorrect?
   A. *Frontal:* divides the body into front and back
   B. *Sagittal:* divides the body into equal right and left sides
   C. *Transverse:* divides the body (at the waist) into superior and inferior
   D. *Coronal:* divides the body into anterior and posterior
   E. *Midsagittal:* divides the body into equal right and left sides

91. Another term for "inferior" is:
   A. *cephalic*
   B. *ventral*
   C. *dorsal*
   D. *caudal*
   E. *proximal*

92. The abbreviation that means "after meals" is:
   A. a.c.
   B. p.c.
   C. p.o.
   D. q.i.d
   E. gtt

93. The abbreviation that means "before meals" is:
   A. a.c.
   B. p.c.
   C. p.o.
   D. q.i.d
   E. gtt

94. Which of the following is the correct root word meaning "heat"?
   A. *pyo*
   B. *pyro*
   C. *carcino*
   D. *crypto*
   E. *kerato*

95. Which of the following medical terms means "dry skin"?
   A. *onychocryptosis*
   B. *mycosis*
   C. *xeroderma*
   D. *onychomycosis*
   E. *rhytidosis*

96. The correct word part for "vein" is:
   A. *veno*
   B. *hemo*
   C. *phlebo*
   D. A and B
   E. A and C

97. Disease of the bone is known as:
   A. *osteopathy*
   B. *osteophage*
   C. *osteonecrosis*
   D. *osteomalacia*
   E. *osteodynia*

98. Colonoscope is defined as which of the following?
   A. Visual examination of the colon
   B. Instrument used to view the colon
   C. Visual examination of the vagina
   D. Instrument used to view the vagina
   E. None of the above

99. The suffix meaning "to suture" is:
   A. *-rrhaphy*
   B. *-rrhexis*
   C. *-rrhagia*
   D. *-rrhea*
   E. *-rrhectomy*

100. Dysphagia is defined as:
   A. Abnormality in the color of the skin
   B. Difficulty swallowing
   C. Disturbance of the normal sleep pattern
   D. Difficulty urinating
   E. Difficulty breathing

ADMINISTRATIVE MEDICAL ASSISTING

1. Which of the following proofreader's marks means "move to the right?"
   A.]
   B. [
   C. [/]
   D. >
   E. <

2. Which of the following proofreader's marks means "straighten type (horizontally)?"
   A. =/
   B. ;/
   C. =
   D. →
   E. None of the above

3. Words that have similar pronunciations but very different meanings and spellings are called what?
   A. Similes
   B. Metaphors
   C. Homophones
   D. Onomatopoeia
   E. None of the above

4. Which of the following homophones has the correct meaning matched with the word?
   A. *they're:* belonging to them
   B. *there:* the place or position
   C. *complement:* an expression of admiration; to praise
   D. *here:* to sense by the ear
   E. None are correct.

5. Of the following times, which one is in the proper form for correspondence in writing?
   A. 10:00 A.M.
   B. 11 A.M.
   C. 10:30 A.M.
   D. A and C
   E. B and C

6. Which of the following is a verb?
   A. *them*
   B. *office*
   C. *why?*
   D. *hooray*
   E. None of the above

7. Match the following example with the common grammatical error:

   "I did good on that exam."
   A. Adjective used as an adverb
   B. Noun/verb mismatch
   C. Run-on sentence
   D. Sentence that ends with a preposition
   E. None of the above

8. Which of the following is a basic component of a business letter?
   A. Salutation
   B. Reference initials
   C. Enclosure
   D. Copy notation
   E. All of the above

9. The two most commonly used letter styles in the medical office are what?
   A. Block and modified block with indentations
   B. Block and modified block
   C. Modified block and modified block with indentations
   D. Indented block and modified block
   E. None of the above

10. Interoffice memoranda, also called *memos,* may be used to inform office personnel about which of the following?
    A. News items
    B. General changes that affect all employees, such as a change in office hours
    C. Meetings
    D. Special projects
    E. All of the above

11. When should patient education occur?
    A. At the beginning of a visit
    B. At the end of a visit
    C. It may occur at any time
    D. Before the visit
    E. After the visit

12. Which of the following patient teaching methods is matched with its correct description?
    A. Contracting: Teaching a close relative/friend the same information the patient receives
    B. Case problem: Applies information to real situations
    C. Lecture: Setting up goals with clear behaviors and responsibilities for the patient
    D. Use of the significant other: Short play in which the learner participates in "playing out" the story
    E. All are incorrect

13. What are the primary functions of a policies and procedures manual?
    A. List the tasks to be performed within the office, including equipment needed in order to complete the procedure.
    B. Standardize the procedure for each task.
    C. Describe job responsibilities and titles.
    D. All of the above.
    E. None of the above.

14. In the personnel policy manual, also known as the *employee handbook,* what information is typically not included?
    A. Emergency leave
    B. Performance review and evaluation
    C. Jury duty
    D. Health benefits
    E. All information listed above is included.

15. Patient information booklets can help do what?
    A. Reduce the number of questions by telephone from patients
    B. Provide fees
    C. Provide a back-line telephone number
    D. All of the above
    E. None of the above

16. Personal characteristics and appearance of a receptionist are important. Which of the following does a receptionist not have to be mindful of?
    A. Good oral care
    B. Clean, well-pressed clothing
    C. Use of a deodorant without a strong scent
    D. Use of clear nail polish
    E. A receptionist should be mindful of all the things listed.

17. Which of the following is not a duty of the receptionist?
    A. Reporting lab results
    B. Closing the office
    C. Opening the office
    D. Collecting co-payments
    E. All are duties of the receptionist.

18. Which of the following is a duty of the receptionist?
    A. Escorting patients to exam rooms
    B. Handling incoming calls
    C. Managing reception area disturbances
    D. B and C
    E. All are duties of the receptionist.

19. The individual responsible for opening the office should arrive how far in advance of the start of office hours?
    A. Two hours
    B. One and a half hours
    C. One hour
    D. 15–30 minutes
    E. Right when office hours start

20. Which of the following is not a responsibility of the individual who opens the office?
    A. Check the security alarm and disengage it.
    B. Prepare all exam rooms for the day.
    C. Turn on all lights and check the general status of the reception room.
    D. Turn on all office machines.
    E. Add paper to the copier, fax machines, and any printers in the office.

21. It is important to speak clearly on the telephone. Which of the following terms is associated with the following statement: "Clear articulation and pronunciation of your words."
    A. Clarity
    B. Enunciation
    C. Inflection
    D. Pitch
    E. None of the above

22. When identifying a caller, which of the following would be helpful information?
    A. First and last names
    B. Date of birth
    C. Date of last visit
    D. A and B
    E. All of the above

23. Triage is a process of determining the order in which patients should be treated. What criteria help to determine who is seen first?
    A. Least severely ill patients are seen first.
    B. The order in which patients sign in
    C. Most severely ill patients are seen first.
    D. Random order
    E. None of the above

24. Which of the following is not considered an emergency?
    A. Broken bone
    B. Inability to breathe (or difficulty breathing)
    C. Profuse bleeding
    D. High temperature
    E. All can be considered emergencies.

25. When receiving an emergency telephone call, it is critical to get what information immediately?
    A. Caller's name
    B. Name of the insurance carrier
    C. Telephone number
    D. A and C
    E. All of the above

26. Which of the following types of information is not important to obtain when taking a telephone message?
    A. First and last names of the caller (with spelling verified)
    B. Telephone number, including the area code at which he or she can be reached for a callback
    C. The reason for the call
    D. The name of the person he or she is trying to reach
    E. All answers are necessary information.

27. All telephone messages regarding a patient should be kept where?
    A. The patient's chart
    B. A filing cabinet with other calls from the same day
    C. On the doctor's desk
    D. A and C
    E. None of the above

28. What needs to be placed on each piece of mail on arrival?
    A. Date of arrival
    B. Time of arrival
    C. Initials of the person who accepted the mail
    D. A and B
    E. All of the above

29. Which of the following is a typical use of baronial stationery?
    A. Physicians may use this for social correspondence.
    B. Brief letters and memoranda
    C. Most office correspondence
    D. Information sent to insurance companies
    E. None of the above

30. Put the following steps to folding a number 6¾ envelope in order so that the contents can remain confidential and be easily removed:
    1. Fold the right edge one-third the width of the paper and press a crease at this fold.
    2. Bring the bottom edge up to ⅜ inch from the top edge.
    3. Fold the left edge to ⅜ inch from the previous crease and insert this edge into the envelope first.
    4. Make a crease at the fold.

    A. 1, 2, 3, 4
    B. 2, 1, 3, 4
    C. 2, 4, 1, 3
    D. 4, 3, 2, 1
    E. 3, 2, 1, 4

31. When typing an address on an envelope, what must the last line of the address contain?
    A. State two-digit code
    B. ZIP code
    C. City
    D. A and B
    E. All of the above

32. According to the USPS, what is the maximum weight for anything mailed?
    A. 70 pounds
    B. 60 pounds
    C. 50 pounds
    D. 40 pounds
    E. 30 pounds

33. Postage meters are used by what size offices?
    A. Offices that have small mailings
    B. Offices that have medium mailings
    C. Offices that have large mailings
    D. A and B
    E. All of the above

34. What piece of office equipment would be ideal for reading text and graphic files and transferring them to a usable computer document?
    A. Copier
    B. Scanner
    C. Fax machine
    D. Color laser printer
    E. None of the above

35. Which of the following is not one of the six Cs of charting?
   A. Clarity
   B. Completeness
   C. Constructive
   D. Confidentiality
   E. Conciseness

36. Which of the following does not fall under the category of patient registration of a medical record?
   A. Nutrition
   B. Patient's full name
   C. Social Security number
   D. Date of the visit
   E. Medical insurance information

37. A consultation report contains which of the following?
   A. Patient's name and medical record number
   B. Medical transcriptionist's name
   C. Referring physician's name
   D. Physical and laboratory evaluations
   E. All of the above

38. Which of the following is not part of a problem-oriented medical record (POMR)?
   A. Database
   B. Plan
   C. Progress notes
   D. Problem list
   E. All are part of the POMR.

39. Which type of numeric filing is based on the last six digits of the ID number?
   A. Straight numeric filing
   B. Terminal digit filing
   C. Middle digit filing
   D. Unit numbering
   E. Serial numbering

40. In which type of numeric filing does the patient receive a different medical record number for each hospital visit?
   A. Straight numerical filing
   B. Terminal digit filing
   C. Middle digit filing
   D. Unit numbering
   E. Serial numbering

41. In which type of numeric filing is a number assigned to the patient the first time he or she is seen and the same number is used for all subsequent visits?
   A. Straight numerical filing
   B. Terminal digit filing
   C. Middle digit filing
   D. Unit numbering
   E. Serial numbering

42. When making corrections to handwritten medical records, what should be used to correct the problem?
   A. A single line through the error
   B. Correction fluid over the error
   C. A double line through the error
   D. Blacking out the error with a pen
   E. None of the above

43. The American Medical Association recommends that medical records be kept for how long?
   A. One year
   B. Two years
   C. Five years
   D. 10 years
   E. None of the above

44. An appointment book should be kept for at least _____.
   A. One year
   B. Two years
   C. Three years
   D. Four years
   E. Five years

45. What type of scheduling system provides built-in flexibility to accommodate unforeseen situations?
   A. Specified time scheduling
   B. Wave scheduling
   C. Double booking patients
   D. Open office hours system
   E. None of the above

46. The period of time that the physician is unavailable is known as what?
   A. The blackout period
   B. The grace period
   C. The matrix
   D. The closed office hours
   E. None of the above

47. A CPU is/does what?
   A. Directs the computer's activities and sends electronic signals to the right place at the right time
   B. Data storage system that allows data to be stored on a compact disc
   C. Small, portable storage device that can hold up to 64 GB or more of data
   D. An internal storage area in the computer where data have been recorded. Once the data are recorded, they cannot be removed, only read
   E. None of the above

48. Scanners and digital cameras are examples of what?
   A. Hardware
   B. Software
   C. Peripherals
   D. Drivers
   E. None of the above

49. Electronic medical records are an example of what?
 A. Hardware
 B. Software
 C. Peripherals
 D. Drivers
 E. None of the above

50. *DOS* stands for what?
 A. Data output system
 B. Database operating system
 C. Disk operating system
 D. Disk output system
 E. None of the above

51. Match the following definition with the proper term: "A printed copy of data in a file."
 A. GIGO
 B. Batch
 C. Hard copy
 D. Write-protect
 E. None of the above

52. Match the following definition with the proper term: "List of all files stored on a storage device."
 A. Batch
 B. GIGO
 C. File maintenance
 D. Database
 E. None of the above

53. A basic computer command is Ctrl + Y. What does it mean?
 A. Redo
 B. Underline
 C. Paste
 D. Save
 E. Undo

54. A basic computer command is Ctrl + Alt + Del. What does it do?
 A. Copy
 B. Cut
 C. Paste
 D. Restart the system
 E. Bold

55. An electronic signature is what?
 A. A mathematical process
 B. A set of numbers
 C. A set of alphabetical characters
 D. A and B
 E. None of the above.

56. What must be provided for patients who pay with cash?
 A. The office telephone number
 B. The patient's next appointment date
 C. A receipt
 D. All of the above
 E. A and B

57. Which check type has the following characteristics?

 Written on the payer's own check form. Guarantees that the money is available. Bank teller verifies the check by placing an official stamp directly on the check.
 A. Certified check
 B. Limited check
 C. Money order
 D. Voucher check
 E. Stale

58. In order to be a negotiable instrument, a check must:
 A. Be written and signed by an authorized payer of the check
 B. State the sum of money to be paid
 C. Be payable on demand or at a fixed date in the future
 D. Be payable to the holder (payee) of the check
 E. All of the above

59. Which of the following is not included in a bank statement?
 A. Checks and debits
 B. Tax ID (usually the Social Security number of the physician)
 C. Average collected balance
 D. Service charges
 E. All are included in a bank statement.

60. On the deposit ticket, what should be totaled separately?
 A. Coins and bills
 B. Coins and bills separately from checks
 C. Checks and bills separately from coins
 D. Bills separately from coins and checks
 E. None of the above

61. What type of account requires a minimum balance of $500 to $5000, depending on the institution?
 A. Savings account
 B. Checking account
 C. Money market savings account
 D. A and B
 E. None of the above

62. How often must the day sheet be balanced?
 A. Daily
 B. Weekly
 C. Biweekly
 D. Monthly
 E. Quarterly

63. What is the definition of *accounts receivable*?
 A. Money the physician owes to others for supplies, equipment, and services that have not yet been paid
 B. Everything owned by the medical practice, such as cash, bank accounts, money owed to the physician, equipment, and real estate
 C. The difference between the debit (money owed) and the credit (money paid)
 D. Money owed to the practice by insurance companies and patients that has not yet been paid
 E. None of the above

64. In accounting, what is a debit?
   A. Indicates that a charge has been entered and added to the account balance
   B. Indicates that a payment has been received on an account
   C. Used by the office so that insurance payments are made directly to the physician
   D. Indicates that overpayment has occurred
   E. None of the above

65. Which of the following is not an acceptable use of petty cash?
   A. Reimbursements
   B. Postage due
   C. Payment to a creditor
   D. Lunch for office personnel
   E. Emergency purchase of pens

66. Which of the following are examples of accounts payable expenditures?
   A. Medical supplies, such as paper goods, day sheets, appointment cards, and scheduling books
   B. Equipment repair and maintenance, including housekeeping
   C. Payroll
   D. Rent
   E. All of the above

67. Which payroll schedule would involve 26 pay periods a year?
   A. Weekly
   B. Biweekly
   C. Semimonthly
   D. Monthly
   E. None of the above

68. Typically, the largest AP account in the medical office is what?
   A. Payroll
   B. Rent
   C. Taxes
   D. Medical supplies and equipment
   E. Equipment repair and maintenance, including housekeeping

69. Which of the following must be included in the W-4 form?
   A. Employee's name and current address
   B. Social Security number
   C. Number of exemptions to be claimed
   D. All of the above
   E. A and C

70. Federal unemployment tax is calculated how often?
   A. Weekly
   B. Biweekly
   C. Monthly
   D. Quarterly
   E. Annually

71. Match the following definition with the correct term:
   "The provider is paid a predetermined amount every month, regardless of the number of times the patient is seen within the month."
   A. Co-payment
   B. Capitation rate
   C. Benefit period
   D. Allowed charge
   E. None of the above

72. Match the following definition with the correct term:
   "Services that are not covered under the insured's health plan."
   A. Exclusions
   B. Fee-for-service
   C. Point-of service plan
   D. Prepaid plan
   E. None of the above

73. Match the following definition with the correct term:
   "Individuals who purchase insurance directly through the insurance company without going through a group plan."
   A. Indemnity plan
   B. Guarantor
   C. Closed-panel HMO
   D. Third-party payer
   E. None of the above

74. The HMO concept was started to control what?
   A. Patient treatment
   B. Costs
   C. Doctor's negligence
   D. All of the above
   E. None of the above

75. Which of the following is not true about a PPO?
   A. Physicians and hospitals are reimbursed for each medical service they provide.
   B. Members or enrollees are not restricted to certain designated providers or hospitals.
   C. Members may receive care from a non-PPO provider; however, they will generally have to pay more out-of-pocket expenses when they do this.
   D. A PPO is a prepayment program.
   E. All are true about a PPO.

76. Which MCO best describes the following characteristics?
   - The primary network is HMO-like.
   - The secondary network is often a PPO network.
   - Members have more choices with less expense than with a PPO.
   - Out-of-pocket expenses are lower within the primary network and higher when using the secondary network.

   A. EPO
   B. PPO
   C. HMO
   D. POS
   E. None of the above

77. __________ patients covered by Medicare must sign an advance beneficiary notice (ABN) prior to receiving covered services that may be denied by Medicare.
   A. Adult
   B. Special needs
   C. Minor
   D. All
   E. None of the above

78. Which part of Medicare is offered by private insurance companies?
   A. Part A
   B. Part B
   C. Part C
   D. Part D
   E. Part E

79. Under which part of Medicare must a patient apply to receive Medicare benefits from the Social Security Administration?
   A. Part A
   B. Part B
   C. Part C
   D. Part D
   E. Part E

80. Regarding diagnosis-related groups (DRGs), which of the following statements is incorrect?
   A. DRGs were developed in the late 1960s.
   B. Payment rates based on DRGs have now been established as the basis for a hospital's Medicare reimbursements.
   C. DRGs are used to calculate payments made to outpatient providers.
   D. DRGs were implemented with the intention of providing a means of monitoring the quality of care.
   E. DRGs were implemented with the intention of providing a means of monitoring the utilization of services.

81. Which of the following statements regarding Medicaid is incorrect?
   A. Medicaid was designed for the medically indigent.
   B. Medicaid was designed for persons without funds.
   C. Medicaid is a direct federal program.
   D. Patients must qualify for benefits on a monthly basis
   E. Medicaid rules for eligibility and payment vary from state to state.

82. TRICARE is the U.S. Department of Defense's worldwide health care program for whom?
   A. Active duty service members
   B. Retired service members
   C. Families of active duty and retired service members
   D. All of the above
   E. None of the above.

83. Which of the following is not a basic guideline for completing the CMS-1500?
   A. Use all capital letters.
   B. Use eight-digit dates
   C. No erasures, overtyping or whiteout are allowed.
   D. Use punctuation.
   E. All are correct.

84. Only small providers are allowed to file paper claims. What designates a "small provider?"
   A. Institutional organizations with fewer than 25 full-time employees
   B. Physicians with fewer than 10 full-time employees
   C. Physicians with 10 to 15 full-time employees
   D. A and B
   E. Any service provider can be considered a small provider.

85. Which of the following is not a method of sending electronic claims to an insurance carrier or clearinghouse?
   A. Dial-up modem
   B. Direct data entry
   C. Over the Internet
   D. Paper
   E. All are correct.

86. To find the numeric code for a disease or injury, what volume of the ICD-9 would you look in?
   A. Volume I
   B. Volume II
   C. Volume III
   D. None of the above
   E. All of the above

87. A patient may have hypertension and is seen for an acute problem such as otitis media. Which one(s) is the primary diagnosis?
   A. Otitis media
   B. Hypertension
   C. Both are the primary diagnosis.
   D. It's up to the insurance company to decide.
   E. None of the above

88. Which of the following is an acceptable use of a V code?
   A. Used as supportive information when some circumstance or problem is present, such as an allergy to penicillin
   B. To add supportive information to the patient, family, or personal history
   C. May be used as a primary code to describe a person who may not have a current illness but is seeing the physician for well-baby care, birth control advice, a pregnancy test, or immunizations.
   D. All of the above
   E. A and B but not C

89. Which of the following is an acceptable use of an E code?
   A. On-duty military personnel activity
   B. Civilian activity done for income or pay
   C. Coding the use of drugs
   D. Off-duty military personnel activity
   E. All of the above

90. Which of the following abbreviations or symbols is not matched with its correct meaning?
   A. [] = encloses synonyms, alternative terminology, or explanatory phrases
   B. **Boldface** type = used for all codes and titles in the Tabular List
   C. ( ) = encloses a series of terms, each of which is modified by the statement appearing to the right side of the parentheses
   D. • = indicates a new code
   E. All are correct.

91. Put the following steps for procedural coding in the correct order:
   1. Using the code in the alphabetic index, verify that it is correct by looking in the tabular index.
   2. Once you know what service was provided or procedure performed, look for the appropriate level of service or procedural term in the alphabetic index. Note the code associated with the narrative description of the service provided or procedure performed.
   3. Look through the list of modifiers to determine if one is needed.
   4. Record the service or procedure code on the insurance claim form.
   5. To the highest level of certainty, begin by identifying what service was provided or what procedure was performed. You will find this information documented in the patient's chart.

   A. 1, 2, 3, 4, 5
   B. 5, 2, 3, 1, 4
   C. 2, 1, 5, 3, 4
   D. 5, 2, 4, 1, 3
   E. 5, 2, 1, 3, 4

92. Which of the following allows patients to block access to their home telephones?
   A. Voice messaging
   B. Call forwarding
   C. Caller ID
   D. Privacy manager
   E. None of the above

93. For optimal efficiency of OCR scanning, which of the following is not recommended?
   A. Address must be typed on the envelope using single spacing
   B. Address must be typed on the envelope using all capital letters
   C. Address must be typed on the envelope with no punctuation
   D. Address numbers must be spelled out on the envelope
   E. None of the above

94. Which of the following is not part of the physical exam component of the medical record?
   A. Allergies
   B. Nutrition
   C. Blood pressure
   D. General appearance
   E. Lymphadenopathy

95. The appointment matrix should reflect which of the following?
   A. Times the physician is available to see patients
   B. Physician surgery time
   C. Physician meetings
   D. Physician vacation
   E. All of the above

96. When you file each record sequentially based on its assigned number, this is known as:
   A. Terminal digit filing
   B. Unit numbering
   C. Serial numbering
   D. Straight numerical filing
   E. None of the above

97. When using SOAP to chart, the "S," or subjective information, is:
   A. Gathered from the patient
   B. The same as the chief complaint
   C. Data gathered during the visit
   D. Both A and B
   E. Both B and C

98. Items that should be sent via certified mail include:
   A. Contracts and deeds
   B. Mortgages and contracts
   C. Deeds and birth certificates
   D. All of the above
   E. None of the above

99. Certain commands for Microsoft Windows can be executed using two or more keys on the keyboard instead of the mouse. The keyboard command for "paste" is:
   A. Ctrl + P
   B. Ctrl + V
   C. Ctrl + P + S
   D. Ctrl + Alt + Delete
   E. There is no keyboard command for "paste."

100. "Written on the payer's own check form" and "Bank withdraws the money from the payer's account" describe which type of check?
   A. Limited checks
   B. Cashier's checks
   C. Certified checks
   D. Traveler's checks
   E. Voucher checks

CLINICAL MEDICAL ASSISTING

1. All of the following are one of the six nutrient classifications except:
   A. Sweets
   B. Proteins
   C. Carbohydrates
   D. Fats
   E. Water

2. Which of the following is a water-soluble vitamin?
   A. Vitamin A
   B. Vitamin D
   C. Vitamin B_2
   D. Vitamin E
   E. Vitamin K

3. The dietary guidelines are developed by which organization?
   A. U.S. Department of Agriculture
   B. U.S. Department of Health and Human Services
   C. OIG
   D. A and C
   E. A and B

4. Which of the following is part of the clear liquid diet?
   A. Ice cream
   B. Creamed or strained soup
   C. Custard
   D. Black coffee
   E. Orange juice

5. Anorexia nervosa is ____________.
   A. An eating disorder that occurs when an individual frequently consumes large amounts of food
   B. Caused by the toxins produced by the *Clostridium botulinum* bacterium
   C. Most commonly caused by *Salmonella* bacteria, *Clostridium perfringens*, or *Staphylococcus*.
   D. A type of roundworm infection that may occur when raw or undercooked meat from an infected animal is eaten
   E. An eating disorder characterized by dangerously low body weight, poor body image, and fear of becoming overweight

6. In order for microorganisms to grow, which of the following is not necessary?
   A. Food
   B. Sunlight
   C. Moisture
   D. Suitable temperature
   E. Darkness

7. Put the following steps into the proper sequence in order for an infection to occur.
   1. Means of transmisson
   2. Susceptible new host
   3. Portal of exit
   4. Portal of entry into new host
   5. Infected reservoir host
   A. 5, 3, 1, 4, 2
   B. 2, 1, 5, 3, 4
   C. 4, 5, 2, 3, 1
   D. 1, 2, 3, 4, 5
   E. 5, 4, 3, 2, 1

8. For which of the blood-borne pathogens is a vaccine available?
   A. Hepatitis A
   B. Hepatitis G
   C. Hepatits C
   D. Hepatits D
   E. Hepatitis B

9. After which of the following actions are you not required to wash your hands?
   A. Performing procedures
   B. Physical contact with patients
   C. Breaks
   D. Eating
   E. All require you to wash your hands afterward.

10. Which of the following falls under the category of high-level disinfection?
   A. Kills mycobacteria and most viruses and bacteria
   B. Used on exam tables, countertops, and walls
   C. Kills all microorganisms except bacterial spores
   D. Used on items that come in contact with skin but not with mucous membranes
   E. Kills most bacteria and viruses.

11. Autoclaving is also known as ____________.
   A. Dry heat sterilization
   B. Chemical sterilization
   C. Light sterilization
   D. Steam and pressure sterilization
   E. Laser sterilization

12. Which of the following is not needed in an exposure control plan?
    - A. Postexposure evaluation and follow-up
    - B. Exposure determination
    - C. Method of compliance
    - D. All of the above
    - E. All are to be included in an exposure control plan.
13. All of the following are considered personal protective equipment except ________.
    - A. Glasses
    - B. Gowns and lab coats
    - C. Mask
    - D. Gloves
    - E. Eye/face shield
14. The history of the present illness (HPI) will provide more information regarding ____________.
    - A. Onset
    - B. Duration
    - C. Intensity
    - D. A and B
    - E. All of the above
15. Social history questions should not include which of the following?
    - A. Family illness
    - B. Sexual preference
    - C. Smoking
    - D. Drinking
    - E. Recreational drug use
16. For every encounter with a patient, there should be timely documentation of the interaction and exchange of information that occurs. The following is not a guideline for proper documentation:
    - A. Give the date and time of every entry.
    - B. Permanent blue ink should be used.
    - C. Be concise.
    - D. Sign every entry.
    - E. Ensure that your handwriting is legible.
17. A normal body temperature for adults is 99.6°F using which method of measuring temperature?
    - A. Oral
    - B. Rectal
    - C. Axillary
    - D. Aural
    - E. Temporal artery
18. What is the average pulse rate for someone 11–16 years old?
    - A. 80–120 bpm
    - B. 80–100 bpm
    - C. 70–90 bpm
    - D. 60–80 bpm
    - E. 50–65 bpm
19. What is the normal respiratory rate for an adult?
    - A. More than 40 per minute
    - B. Less than 12 per minute
    - C. 12 to 16 per minute
    - D. 16 to 20 per minute
    - E. None of the above
20. Which of the following is part of the wellness guidelines?
    - A. Keep a positive attitude.
    - B. Challenge your mind.
    - C. Forgive and forget.
    - D. Soothe your fears.
    - E. All are part of the wellness guidelines.
21. Once nonhealthy habits have been identified, you can provide educational information in the form of __________.
    - A. Brochures
    - B. Videos
    - C. Internet Web sites
    - D. A and C
    - E. All of the above
22. Meter-dosed inhalers (MDIs) consist of a pressurized container that contains approximately how many doses?
    - A. 200
    - B. 175
    - C. 150
    - D. 125
    - E. 100
23. In an outpatient or home setting, oxygen is usually delivered via nasal cannula and is prescribed for which primary reason?
    - A. Decrease the work of breathing
    - B. Decrease the work of the heart
    - C. Reverse or prevent low blood oxygen levels
    - D. A and C
    - E. All of the above
24. Which instrument is described by the following?

    It is used to examine the ears.
    Light is focused through a speculum into the outer ear and into the tympanic membrane.
    Additional speculums may be used to view other structures, such as the nose.
    - A. Oximeter
    - B. Otoscope
    - C. Ophthalmoscope
    - D. Endoscope
    - E. None of the above
25. Which of the following is not a component of the sphygmomanometer?
    - A. Manometer
    - B. Inflatable rubber bladder
    - C. Diaphragm
    - D. Bulb
    - E. Cuff

26. Which instrument is described by the following?

It is used to look into a hollow organ or body cavity. It is used to examine the larynx, bladder, colon, sigmoid colon, stomach, abdomen, and some joints.

A. Oximeter
B. Otoscope
C. Ophthalmoscope
D. Endoscope
E. None of the above

27. The temperature in an autoclave must remain at 250°F for at least how long to kill all bacterial spores and microorganisms?

A. 15 minutes
B. 20 minutes
C. 10 minutes
D. 25 minutes
E. None of the above

28. Which type of thermometer has the following description?

It is also known as an *aural thermometer*. It detects heat waves within the ear canal near the eardrum.

A. Nonmercury
B. Electronic
C. Tympanic membrane
D. Temporal artery
E. Chemical disposable

29. When restocking supplies, it is important to use the first in, first out (FIFO) rule. What does this mean?

A. Older supplies should be used first.
B. Older supplies should be used last.
C. Newer supplies should be used first.
D. It doesn't matter which supplies are used first.
E. None of the above

30. What is the process of listening to the sounds within the body, such as those made by the heart, lungs, stomach, and bowels?

A. Palpatation
B. Percussion
C. Auscultation
D. Manipulation
E. Mensuration

31. If a patient is in the stirrups at an obstetric-gynecologic practice, which examination position is she in?

A. Trendelenberg position
B. Fowler position
C. Dorsal recumbent position
D. Sims position
E. Lithotomy position

32. Which type of cast has the following description?

It extends from the fingers to the axilla, with a bend at the elbow. It is used for a fracture of the upper arm.

A. Short arm cast
B. Long arm cast
C. Medium arm cast
D. A or B
E. None of the above

33. Which of the following materials is not needed for casting?

A. Rubber gloves
B. Stockinette
C. Bandage roll or tape
D. Webril
E. All are needed for casting.

34. Scissors fall under which category of instruments?

A. Curettage
B. Dissecting
C. Grasping and clamping
D. Dilating and probing
E. None of the above

35. Which type of surgical needle requires a holder?

A. Straight needle
B. Curved needle
C. Swaged needle
D. A and B
E. None of the above

36. Which of the following is not an example of a nonabsorbable suture?

A. Silk
B. Nylon
C. Steel
D. Polyester
E. All are examples of nonabsorbable sutures.

37. What is/are the most common sterilization indicator(s) for an autoclave machine?

A. Litmus paper
B. Autoclave tape
C. Indicator strips
D. B and C
E. All of the above

38. Who should record the patient history?

A. Receptionist
B. Medical assistant
C. Laboratory technician
D. A and B
E. None of the above

39. Which of the following occurs prior to a patient's endoscopic/colonoscopy exam?

A. The physician will order a cathartic to be administered at different intervals during the day before the procedure.
B. The physician will provide additional information relating to the procedure(s) performed during the colonoscopy.
C. The physician will order a high intake of fluids to prevent dehydration, unless there is a medical contradiction.
D. B and C
E. None of the above

40. Which of the following therapies improves joint flexibility, muscle tone, and mobility?
   A. Exercise therapy
   B. Cryotherapy
   C. Hydrotherapy
   D. Thermotherapy
   E. Massage

41. A trocar falls under which surgical instrument category?
   A. Cutting
   B. Visualizing
   C. Dissecting
   D. Grasping and clamping
   E. Dilating and probing

42. Regarding sterile fields and instruments, which of the following is not true?
   A. A sterile item can only touch another sterile item.
   B. A sterile item on a sterile field must be within your field of vision and above your waist.
   C. Airborne microorganisms contaminate sterile fields.
   D. The edges of a sterile field are contaminated.
   E. All answers are true.

43. Specialized standard graph paper is needed for EKG machines. Every 5 × 5 mm square on the EKG paper is equivalent to___________.
   A. 1 second
   B. 0.5 second
   C. 0.25 second
   D. 0.20 second
   E. None of the above

44. What color is the limb lead for the right arm on an EKG machine?
   A. White
   B. Black
   C. Green
   D. Red
   E. None of the above

45. Which wave type represents a repolarization of the ventricles?
   A. P wave
   B. PR interval wave
   C. QRSs complex wave
   D. ST segment wave
   E. T wave

46. When a patient complains of having difficulty ___________, near vision acuity tests are performed.
   A. Reading a book
   B. Threading a needle
   C. Reading a computer screen
   D. A and C
   E. All of the above

47. What is the most common color vision defect?
   A. Blue and green
   B. Red and green
   C. Blue and red
   D. Yellow and green
   E. None of the above

48. Pulmonary function tests (PFTs) are performed to evaluate ___________.
   A. Lung volume
   B. Lung capacity
   C. Lung strength
   D. A and B
   E. All of the above

49. Peak flow meters are used to measure the patient's ability to ___________.
   A. Move air into and out of the lungs
   B. Breathe through the nose
   C. Process food
   D. A and B
   E. None of the above

50. Anyone working in the medical field who is around radiation should use a/an ___________ apron.
   A. Steel
   B. Lead
   C. Aluminum
   D. Copper
   E. Iron

51. Which of the following are characteristic of quantitative testing?
   A. Results reported out as either positive or negative
   B. Results reported out using numerical values
   C. Performed to determine whether or not a substance is present and the amount of the substance
   D. B and C
   E. All of the above

52. What is the proper description of hematopoiesis?
   A. Levels of oxygen and carbon dioxide in the blood
   B. Process that allows neutrophils to surround, swallow, and digest bacteria
   C. Study of blood and blood-forming tissues
   D. Process by which cells destroy worn-out cells and bacteria
   E. Normal formation and development of blood cells

53. Which of the following are not white blood cells?
   A. Erythrocytes
   B. Lymphocytes
   C. Monocytes
   D. Leukocytes
   E. Eosinophils

54. What is agglutination?
   A. Study of serum based on antibody/antigen reactions
   B. Antigen/antibody reaction that occurs when an antigen clumps together with an antibody
   C. Plasma without fibrinogen
   D. Study of blood serum and antigen/antibody reactions
   E. Study of the body's reaction to antigens

55. What are the largest cells in the blood?
   A. Eosinophils
   B. Monocytes
   C. Thrombocytes
   D. Leukocytes
   E. Erythrocytes

56. When labeling a patient's specimen that has just been collected, which of the following is not required?
   A. Antibiotic treatment used, if any
   B. Date
   C. Time of collection
   D. Type of specimen.
   E. All are required.

57. What is the fastest and most efficient system for performing venipuncture?
   A. Evacuation tube system
   B. Sterile lancet
   C. Butterfly needle
   D. Needle and syringe
   E. None of the above

58. The most common venipuncture site is the antecubital space, and the vein of choice is the median cephalic. Where is it located?
   A. The top of the hand
   B. The wrist
   C. The forearm
   D. The triangular area below the bend of the elbow
   E. The bicep

59. When explaining to a patient how to collect a clean-catch urine specimen, it is important to tell the patient to start collecting the specimen when?
   A. At the start of the stream
   B. In midstream
   C. At the end of the stream
   D. It doesn't matter when the patient starts collecting.
   E. None of the above

60. When obtaining a stool sample, which of the following equipment is not needed?
   A. Tongue depressors
   B. Sterile applicator sticks
   C. Sterile stool collection container
   D. Bedpan or container
   E. All are needed.

61. What might a low hemoglobin (Hgb) reading indicate?
   A. Iron-deficiency anemia
   B. Polycythemia
   C. Dehydration
   D. Pregnancy
   E. Leukemia

62. A normal red blood cell count for an adult female is________.
   A. 1.5–2.5 million per mm^3
   B. 2.0–3.5 million per mm^3
   C. 3.5–4.5 million per mm^3
   D. 4.5–6.0 million per mm^3
   E. 6.0–7.5 million per mm^3

63. A low platelet level may indicate _______.
   A. Anemia
   B. Use of chemotherapy
   C. Polycythemia
   D. A and B
   E. B and C

64. A normal level of C-reactive protein (CRP) is _______.
   A. 4
   B. 1
   C. 0
   D. 2
   E. 3

65. _______ are formed by urinary salts when pH, temperature, or concentration changes occur.
   A. Crystals
   B. Casts
   C. Reagents
   D. Agars
   E. Antigens

66. $\frac{3}{8} + \frac{1}{3} = ?$
   A. $\frac{4}{11}$
   B. $\frac{17}{24}$
   C. $\frac{4}{24}$
   D. $\frac{3}{11}$
   E. None of the above

67. $\frac{1}{2} \times \frac{1}{5} = ?$
   A. $\frac{1}{7}$
   B. $\frac{2}{7}$
   C. $\frac{2}{10}$
   D. $\frac{1}{10}$
   E. $\frac{2}{5}$

68. Convert the following fraction into a decimal: $\frac{7}{8}$
   A. 0.875
   B. 0.125
   C. 0.67
   D. 0.44
   E. 0.33

69. Which of the following pharmacology abbreviations is not matched with its proper term?
A. K = potassium
B. kg = kilogram
C. Tab = tablespoon
D. DC = discontinue
E. ante = before

70. The definition of *cumulative effect* is __________.
A. An undesirable and potentially harmful side effect of a drug
B. Administering two medications together, which causes both medications to be less effective than if each was administered separately
C. The opposite effect of what was intended occurs.
D. The effects of one drug increase the effects of another drug.
E. The next dose of medication is given before the previous dose has had time to be metabolized/excreted.

71. Match the following definition with its term: "Movement of medication from the site of administration into the bloodstream."
A. Absorption
B. Contraindication
C. Potentiation
D. Teratogen
E. Efficacy

72. What is the correct controlled substance level for the following description?

"High potential for addiction and abuse. Accepted for medical use in the United States. Examples include codeine, morphine, opium, and secobarbital."
A. Schedule I
B. Schedule II
C. Schedule III
D. Schedule IV
E. Schedule V

73. Which of the following is not a method for parenteral administration of drugs?
A. Sublingual
B. Intravenous
C. Intradermal
D. Subcutaneous
E. Intraarticular

74. What is the hilt of a syringe?
A. The bore of the hollow needle
B. Prevents the needle from rolling on flat surfaces
C. Connects the needle to the syringe
D. Holds the liquid in the syringe
E. Connects the shaft to the hub

75. A proper amount for an intramuscular injection is how much?
A. 0.1 to 0.3 mL
B. 0.3 to 1 mL
C. 2 to 5 mL
D. 1 to 1.5 mL
E. 5 mL and higher

76. The angle of insertion for an intradermal injection is __________.
A. 90 degrees
B. 60 degrees
C. 45 degrees
D. 30 degrees
E. 10–15 degrees

77. Tagamet is what type of drug?
A. Antiulcer
B. Bronchodilator
C. Beta blocker
D. Cholesterol-lowering
E. None of the above

78. Provera is what type of drug?
A. Diuretic
B. Antihypertensive
C. Analgesic
D. Sedative
E. Hormone

79. Dilantin is what type of drug?
A. Anticoagulant
B. Antibiotic
C. Synthetic hormone
D. Anticonvulsant
E. Cardiotonic

80. Ceclor is what type of drug?
A. Diuretic
B. Antibiotic
C. Tranquilizer
D. Anti-inflammatory
E. None of the above

81. Xanax is what type of drug?
A. Calcium channel blocker
B. Diuretic
C. Tranquilizer
D. Analgesic
E. Beta blocker

82. What is the minimum age for giving the rotavirus vaccine (RV)?
A. Birth
B. Six weeks
C. 12 weeks
D. 18 weeks
E. 24 weeks

83. Administration of morphine for terminal cancer patients is which type of drug use?
   A. Diagnostic
   B. Palliative
   C. Preventive
   D. Replacement
   E. Therapeutic

84. Vaccines are an example of which type of drug?
   A. Diagnostic
   B. Palliative
   C. Preventive
   D. Replacement
   E. Therapeutic

85. The administration of antibiotics to cure pneumonia is which type of drug use?
   A. Diagnostic
   B. Palliative
   C. Preventive
   D. Replacement
   E. Therapeutic

86. Which of the following is not a factor that contributes to the patient's response to medication?
   A. Age
   B. Diet
   C. Genetic factors
   D. Time of administration
   E. All contribute to a patient's response to medication.

87. A drug in the form of liniment is administered through which route?
   A. Oral
   B. Topical
   C. Inhalation
   D. Rectal
   E. None of the above

88. A drug in spray form is administered through which route?
   A. Oral
   B. Topical
   C. Inhalation
   D. Rectal
   E. A and B

89. Which of the following should be done when treating an animal bite?
   A. Cleanse with soap and water.
   B. Apply antibiotic ointment.
   C. Cover the wound with a dry sterile dressing.
   D. All of the above
   E. A and B

90. Which of the following symptoms is not indicative of a frostbite injury?
   A. Numbness
   B. Area all black
   C. Area all white
   D. Blisters
   E. Tingling

91. What is the cause of anaphylactic shock?
   A. An allergic reaction
   B. Reduction in cardiac output, such as caused by pulmonary embolism, myocardial infarction, tachycardia, or bradycardia.
   C. Inadequate intravascular volume; occurs after an injury with major fluid loss
   D. Severe cerebral trauma or hemorrhage
   E. Systemic infection that causes vasodilation and decreased vascular resistance

92. The guidelines for CPR are similar to those for respiratory arrest, cardiac arrest, and obstructed airway but vary slightly according to what?
   A. Height
   B. Weight
   C. Sex
   D. Age
   E. None of the above

93. The first thing that needs to be done when performing infant or young child rescue breathing is:
   A. Place the patient on the back.
   B. Gently tilt the patient's head and open the airway.
   C. Shake the young child.
   D. Secure a mouth guard over the patient's mouth and nose.
   E. Assess the patient and determine if help is needed.

94. An obstructed airway in an adult cannot be caused by which of the following?
   A. Large pieces of food that have not been properly chewed
   B. Talking or laughing too much while eating
   C. Drinking too much soda during a meal
   D. Drinking alcohol before and during eating
   E. Choking on fluids such as vomit or blood

95. Which of the following is the correct procedure for delivering abdominal thrusts while performing the Heimlich maneuver?
   A. Gentle thrusts into the victim's abdomen with an upward movement
   B. Firm thrusts into the victim's abdomen with an upward movement
   C. Gentle thrusts into the victim's abdomen with a downward movement
   D. Firm thrusts into the victim's abdomen with a downward movement
   E. None of the above.

96. Using Clark's Rule, the adult dose is 25 mg and the medication comes in a vial of 25 mg/mL. The child weighs 68 lb; what is the pediatric dose?
    A. 10.8 mL
    B. 11.3 mL
    C. 10.8 mg
    D. 11.3 mg
    E. None of the above

97. If the available strength of a medication on hand is 15 mg/mL and the physician orders 75 mg, how much will you administer?
    A. 0.2 mL
    B. 2.0 mg
    C. 5 mg
    D. 5 mL
    E. 75 mL

98. The physician orders 1 g of medication to be administered. You have 500 mg/mL on hand. How many liters/milliliters will you administer?
    A. 1 L
    B. 2 L
    C. 2 mL
    D. 1.5 mL
    E. 1000 mL

99. Which of the following scheduled drugs allows five refills over a six-month period?
    A. Schedule I
    B. Schedule II
    C. Schedule III
    D. Schedule IV
    E. Schedule V

100. Regarding the Human papillomavirus vaccine (HPV), which of the following statements is not true?
    A. Prevents cervical, vaginal and vulvar cancers (in females)
    B. Prevents genital warts (in females and males)
    C. Administer the first dose to females at age 11 or 12
    D. Administer the second dose 3 months after the first dose
    E. Administer the third dose 6 months after the first dose

APPENDIX C
Practice Exam Answer Key with Rationales

GENERAL MEDICAL ASSISTING

1. B. Connective

   Rationale: Connective tissue connects and supports various body structures. Blood, adipose, and osseous tissues are types of connective tissue.

2. A. Adipose

   Rationale: There are three types of muscle tissue—skeletal, smooth, and cardiac.

3. B. Dermis

   Rationale: The dermis keeps skin oiled and elastic and prevents dry hair and scalp by producing sebum.

4. D. Blue

   Rationale: *Cyanosis* is used to describe blue skin.

5. C. 206

   Rationale The skeletal system is made up of different bones and two divisions, the axial skeleton and the appendicular skeleton. These two divisions combined consist of 206 bones.

6. E. Sesamoid

   Rationale A kneecap is a sesamoid bone.

7. A. Tendons

   Rationale: Tendons are connective tissues that attach muscle to bone.

8. D. Face

   Rationale: A zygomaticus muscle is found in the face. It pulls the corner of the mouth up.

9. B. Leg

   Rationale: An iliacus muscle is found in the leg. It flexes the thigh.

10. E. 5 feet

    Rationale: The large intestine is 5 feet long.

11. C. Pharynx

    Rationale: The pharynx is also known as the *throat* and is shared with the respiratory system.

12. A. Pericardium

    Rationale: The outer layer of the heart is the pericardium.

13. B. Receives oxygen-rich blood from the lungs

    Rationale: The left atrium of the heart receives oxygen-rich blood from the lungs.

14. C. Frontal sinus

    Rationale: The frontal sinus is located just above the eyebrows in the frontal bone.

15. A. Thymus

    Rationale: The thymus filters and traps bacteria, viruses, cancer cells, and other invaders.

16. E. 12

    Rationale: There are 12 pairs of cranial nerves.

17. C. Occipital

    Rationale: The occipital lobe controls eyesight.

18. A. Renal pelvis

    Rationale: The renal pelvis funnels urine from within the kidney into the ureter.

19. B. Epididymis

    Rationale: The epididymis is a long, coiled tube located on the upper part of each testicle and runs the length of each testicle.

20. C. Cervix

    Rationale: The narrow lower portion of the uterus that extends to the vagina is the cervix.

21. E. Luteinizing hormone

    Rationale: Luteinizing hormone stimulates ovulation in females.

22. A. Adrenocorticotropic hormone

    Rationale: Adrenocorticotropic hormone controls secretion of certain hormones from the adrenal cortex.

23. C. Triiodothyronine

    Rationale: Triiodothyronine influences metabolism, protein synthesis, and maturation of the nervous system.

24. B. Parathormone

    Rationale: Parathormone works with calcitonin and increases blood calcium and decreases blood phosphate.

25. A. Six

    Rationale: Six muscles make eye movement possible.

26. E. A and C

    Rationale: Neoplasia is defined as growth of cells that may be either benign (not progressive and noncancerous) or malignant (invasive and cancerous).

27. E. B and D

Rationale: Neoplasia is defined as growth of cells that may be either benign (not progressive and noncancerous) or malignant (invasive and cancerous).

28. A. Sarcoma

Rationale: Sarcoma is a neoplasm of the connective tissue.

29. B. Impetigo

Rationale: Impetigo is a contagious skin infection usually caused by *Streptococcus* or *Staphylococcus*.

30. A. Pediculosis

Rationale: Pediculosis is also known as *lice*.

31. D. Gout

Rationale: The skeletal system disease that is caused by crystals forming in the joints is gout.

32. B. Osteomalacia

Rationale: The skeletal system disease that is characterized by softening of the bone is osteomalacia.

33. E. Quadriplegia

Rationale: Quadriplegia is paralysis of all four extremities. It is caused by a spinal cord injury.

34. A. Chronic liver cell destruction

Rationale: Cirrhosis is chronic liver cell destruction.

35. D. Lymphedema

Rationale: Lymphedema is an accumultaion of fluid in the legs and ankles due to improper draining.

36. B. Cystic fibrosis

Rationale: Thick, dry, sticky mucus that clogs organs, mainly the lungs, is cystic fibrosis.

37. D. Epilepsy

Rationale: Epilepsy is the result of abnormal electrical impulses within the brain that cause bursts of excitement and may result in seizures.

38. B. Incontinence

Rationale: Incontinence is the inability to control the flow of urine. Nocturnal incontinence is also known as *bedwetting*.

39. A. Dysmenorrhea

Rationale: Difficult and/or painful menstruation is dysmenorrhea.

40. D. Myxedema

Rationale: Myxedema is a severe life-threatening form of adult hypothyroidism

41. C. Mumbling

Rationale: Mumbling is an example of negative communication.

42. E. All are examples of the five Cs of better communication

Rationale: The five Cs of better communication are content, conciseness, clarity, coherence, and check.

43. A. Face-to-face discussion

Rationale: The most commonly used channel of communication is face-to-face discussion.

44. D. B and C

Rationale: "Can you please describe the pain?" and "Where is the pain coming from?" are both examples of open-ended questions because they require more than a yes or no response.

45. B. Passive listening

Rationale: Listening to the news is an example of passive listening because a response is not required.

46. A. Active listening

Rationale: Active listening is the form of listening that is two-way and requires a response.

47. E. All of the above

Rationale: Facial expressions, eye contact, posture, and gestures are all examples of nonverbal communication.

48. B. Personal distance

Rationale: Most communication in the United States takes place at a personal distance of 18 inches to 4 feet.

49. C. Why did you do that? That was stupid.

Rationale: Saying "Why did you do that? That was stupid" is an example of aggressive behavior.

50. E. None of the above

Rationale: All of the statements about professionalism are true.

51. E. All are part of the communication cycle

Rationale: The communication cycle includes a source, message, channel, and receiver.

52. E. A and D

Rationale: Careful grooming, good hygiene, and appropriate dress are examples of a professional appearance.

53. E. All of the above

Rationale: When communicating with hearing-impaired patients, it is important to make sure that you are in a quiet, well-lit room; face the patient; speak slowly and clearly; don't have anything in your mouth, such as gum or candy; and have paper and a pen available so that the patient can communicate in writing if desired.

54. A. Raise the volume of your voice

Rationale: You do not have to raise the volume of your voice; remember that they are visually impaired, not hearing impaired.

55. E. B and sometimes C

Rationale: If you are working in a culturally diverse area, it is best to have a list of interpreters available to call when needed. If a patient is being cared for within the practice and nobody within the practice is familiar with his or her language, you may need to rely on nonverbal communication initially; however, this can be dangerous, as there are many opportunities for error when neither of the communicating parties is absolutely sure of what is being communicated by the other.

56. D. Early childhood

Rationale: In early childhood, ages three to five, the following characteristics are displayed: Linguistic, physical, and cognitive skills develop. The concept of self begins to develop.

57. B. Denial, anger, bargaining, depression, acceptance

Rationale: The order that best describes the way that people grieve is: denial, anger, bargaining, depression, and acceptance.

58. A. Displacement

Rationale: Displacement allows feelings to be expressed with less dangerous objects or people.

59. C. Ivan Pavlov

Rationale: Ivan Pavlov was responsible for the classical conditioning theory.

60. E. Carl Jung

Rationale: Carl Jung developed the personal unconscious, collective unconscious, extroversion, and introversion theories.

61. B. Burden of proof

Rationale: Burden of proof is defined as "presenting testimony at a trial to prove either guilt or innocence."

62. A. Written defamation

Rationale: Libel is defined as "written defamation."

63. E. Dysfunction

Rationale: The four Ds of negligence are duty, dereliction or neglect of duty, direct cause, and damages.

64. C. Patient Self-Determination Act

Rationale: The Patient Self-Determination Act provides protection for the patient and the physician and also provides guidance for the patient's caregiver to make decisions based on the wishes of the patient. Documents include a living will, a durable power of attorney, and a uniform anatomical gift act.

65. D. *Misfeasance*

Rationale: *Misfeasance* means "performing the correct treatment with errors."

66. E. All are PHI

Rationale: PHI is any information that would identify a patient. This includes the patient's name, address, telephone number, date of birth, Social Security number, e-mail address, medical record number, insurance information including ID and group number, driver's license number, and photos.

67. D. A and B

Rationale: Generally, only a patient can authorize the release of his or her own medical records. However, there are some exceptions to the rule, and generally the following can sign a release: parents of minor children, a legal guardian, or an agent (someone the patient selects to act on his or her behalf in a health care power of attorney).

68. A. Area of the office not accessible to patients

Rationale: In order to maintain patient confidentiality, fax machines must be kept in areas of the office that are not accessible to patients.

69. B. A fine of not more than $50,000, imprisonment for not more than one year, or both.

Rationale: A person who knowingly and in violation of HIPAA regulations uses a unique health identifier or causes it to be used shall be punished by a fine of not more than $50,000, imprisoned for not more than one year, or both.

70. E. All of the above

Rationale: The intention of HIPAA was to do the following: improve portability and continuity within group and individual insurance; combat waste, fraud, and abuse in health insurance and within the health-care delivery system; promote the use of medical savings accounts (MSAs); improve access to long-term care services and coverage; simplify health insurance information; and provide a way to pay for reform and related initiatives.

71. C. Root word

Rationale: *Root:* the basic meaning of the word.

72. C. Root word

Rationale: Root words usually provide information about the body part.

73. D. *o*

Rationale: *O* is the most common combining vowel.

74. D. The suffix usually provides information about location.

Rationale: The suffix usually provides information about a procedure, condition, disorder, or disease; however, there are several suffixes that merely mean "pertaining to."

75. D. White

Rationale: *albino* means "white."

76. D. White

Rationale: *leuko* means "white."

77. C. Yellow

Rationale: *xantho* means "yellow."

78. A. *proximo*

Rationale: *disto* means "away from the trunk"; *proximo* means "toward the trunk."

79. D. nucleus

Rationale: The root word *karyo* means "nucleus."

80. D. *phlebo*

Rationale: *veno* and *phlebo* both mean "vein."

81. B. *athero*

Rationale: *athero* means "plaque."

82. D. Onycomycosis

Rationale: *onycho* = nail, *myco* = fungus, *osis* = abnormal condition.

83. C. *oophoro*

Rationale: *oophoro* means "ovaries."

84. B. *uretero*

Rationale: *uretero* means "ureter."

85. A. *-dynia*

Rationale: Both *-algia* and *-dynia* mean "pain."

86. E. *blepharoptosis*

Rationale: *blepharo* means "eyelid" and *optosis* means "drooping."

87. A. *pyo*

Rationale: The root word *pyo* means "pus."

88. C. *audiography*

Rationale: *audio* means "hearing" and *graphy* means "the process of recording."

89. E. Both A and C

The prefixes *-endo* and *-inter* both mean "within."

90. B. *Sagittal:* divides the body into equal right and left sides

Rationale: *Sagittal:* divides the body into right and left sides; they are not equal. Equal division is *midsagittal*.

91. D. *caudal*

Rationale: Inferior (caudal): lower, below.

92. B. p.c.

Rationale: The abbreviation meaning "after meals" is p.c.

93. A. a.c.

Rationale: The abbreviation meaning "before meals" is a.c.

94. B. *pyro*

Rationale: The root word *pyro* means "heat."

95. C. Xeroderma

Rationale: *xero* = dry, *derma* = skin

96. E. A and C

Rationale: Both *veno* and *phlebo* refer to vein.

97. A. Osteopathy

Rationale: *osteo* = bone, *-pathy* = disease

98. B. Instrument used to view the colon

Rationale: *colono* = colon, *-scope* = instrument used to view

99. A. *-rrhaphy*

Rationale: *-rrhaphy* means "to suture."

100. B. Difficulty swallowing

Rationale: *dys* = difficulty, *-phagia* = swallowing

ADMINISTRATIVE MEDICAL ASSISTING

1. A.]

Rationale:] = move to the right.

2. C. =

Rationale: = means straighten type (horizontally).

3. C. Homophones

Rationale: Words that have similar pronunciations but very different meanings and spellings are homophones.

4. B. *there:* the place or position

Rationale: *there* means "the place or position."

5. E. B and C

Rationale: Do not use zeros when writing on-the-hour time. Use A.M. and P.M. with the time designation.

6. E. None of the above

Rationale: Verbs assert action, being, or state of being.

7. A. Adjective used as an adverb

Rationale: The word *well* should replace *good*.

8. E. All of the above

Rationale: The basic components of the business letter are the salutation, body, complimentary close, signature line, reference initials, enclosure, and copy notation.

9. B. Block and modified block

Rationale: Block and modified block are the forms most commonly used in the medical office.

10. E. All of the above

Rationale: Memos may be used to inform office personnel about the following: meetings and general changes that affect all employees, such as a change in office hours, special projects, and new items.

11. C. It may occur at any time

Rationale: Patient education may occur at any point during the visit as well as before and after the visit.

12. B. Case problem: applies information to real situations

Rationale: The case problem method of patient teaching is described as "applying information to real situations."

13. D. All of the above

Rationale: The primary functions of a policies and procedures manual are as follows: list the tasks to be performed within the office, including equipment needed in order to complete the procedure; standardize the procedure for each task; describe job responsibilities and titles.

14. E. All information listed is included.

Rationale: In the personnel policy manual, the following information is available:

compensation and reimbursement for work-related activities, such as attending conventions and courses and paying parking fees, emergency leave, grievance process, health benefits, holidays, jury duty, overtime policy, pension plan, performance review and evaluation, probationary period, sick leave, termination of employment, vacation, and work hours, including flex time.

15. A. Reduce the number of questions by telephone from patients

Rationale: Patient information booklets can help reduce the number of questions by telephone from patients, enhance the office's image, and reduce the number of patients who fail to remember instructions.

16. E. A receptionist should be mindful of all things listed.

Rationale: Receptionists need to be mindful of the following: careful grooming, good hygiene, appropriate dress, good hygiene including daily bathing, use of a deodorant without a strong scent, good oral care, and clean, well-pressed clothing. Makeup, hairstyles, and jewelry worn by male and female receptionists should reflect professionalism. Accessories should be conservative and minimal, generally limited to one finger ring, a watch with a second hand, a name tag, and a professional association pin. Long hair should be worn tied back and off the shoulders. Nails should be well trimmed, and only clear polish should be used. Name pins/tags should be visible at all times.

17. A. Reporting of lab results

Rationale: Reporting of lab results is not a duty of the receptionist.

18. E. All are duties of the receptionist.

Rationale: Escorting patients to exam rooms, handling incoming calls, and managing reception area disturbances are all duties of the receptionist.

19. D. 15–30 minutes

Rationale: The individual responsible for opening the office should arrive 15–30 minutes prior to the start of office hours.

20. B. Prepare all exam rooms for the day

Rationale: The individual responsible for opening the office must do the following: check the security alarm and disengage it; turn on all lights and check the general status of the reception room; check to make sure that all paper charts are pulled and prepared for that day's patients; have charge slips printed in advance for the day, with any balances due highlighted; make sure that all office machines are turned on and ready for use; add paper to the copier, fax machines, and any printers in the office.

21. B. Enunciation

Rationale: Enunciation is "clear articulation and pronunciation of your words."

22. D. A and B

Rationale: Steps must be taken to protect patient information. Ask the caller for identifying information such as his or her first and last names, Social Security number, and/or date of birth.

23. C. Most severely ill patients seen first

Rationale: The severity of the patient's illness or injury determines the order of treatment.

24. E. All can be considered emergencies.

Rationale: Broken bones, inability to breathe, profuse bleeding, and a high temperature are all considered emergencies

25. D. A and C

Rationale: When receiving an emergency telephone call, it is critical to get the caller's name and telephone number in case you are disconnected.

26. E. All answers are necessary information.

Rationale: When taking a telephone message, it is important to obtain the following information: the first and last names of the caller (with spelling verified); the telephone number, including the area code, at which he or she can be reached for a callback; and the name of the person he or she is trying to reach.

27. A. The patient's chart

Rationale: All telephone messages regarding a patient should be placed in the patient's chart as documentation of an interaction that occurred between the office and the patient.

28. D. A and B

Rationale: Place a current date and time of arrival on each piece of mail.

29. B. Brief letters and memoranda

Rationale: Baronial stationary is commonly used for brief letters and memoranda.

30. C. 2, 4, 1, 3

Rationale: 2. Bring the bottom edge up to ⅜ inch from the top edge. 4. Make a crease at the fold. 1. Fold the right edge one-third of the width of the paper and press a crease at this fold. 3. Fold the left edge to ⅜ inch from the previous crease and insert this edge into the envelope first.

31. E. All of the above

Rationale: The last line in the address must include the city, the state two-digit code, and the ZIP code. It cannot exceed 27 characters in length.

32. A. 70 pounds

Rationale: Maximum weight for anything mailed is 70 pounds. Maximum size for mail is no more than 108 inches in length and girth combined.

33. C. Offices that have large mailings

Rationale: Postage meters are used by offices with large mailings to stamp envelopes and packages.

34. B. Scanner

Rationale: Scanners "read" text and graphic files and transform them into a usable computer document.

35. C. Constructive

Rationale: The six Cs of charting are: client's words, clarity, completeness, conciseness, chronological, and confidentiality.

36. A. Nutrition

Rationale: Patient registration includes the following: patient's full name; address; contact information, including the home phone, work phone and cell phone; e-mail address, if applicable; date of the visit; patient's age; date of birth; Social Security number; driver's license number, if applicable; medical insurance information; person responsible for payment.

37. E. All of the above

Rationale: The consultation report will include the patient's name and medical record number; date of the consultation; medical transcriptionist's name; referring physician; reason for the consultation; physical and laboratory evaluations; consulting physician's impression and recommendations.

38. E. All are part of the POMR.

Rationale: The four parts of the POMR are the database, problem list, plan, and progress notes.

39. B. Terminal digit filing

Rationale: Terminal digit filing is based on the last six digits of the ID number.

40. E. Serial numbering

Rationale: With serial numbering, the patient receives a different medical record number for each hospital visit.

41. D. Unit numbering

Rationale: With unit numbering, a number is assigned to the patient the first time he or she is seen, and the same number is used for all subsequent visits.

42. A. A single line through the error

Rationale: To correct handwritten entries, simply draw a single line through the error so that the original entry can still be seen, initial above the single line, date it, and write "error." Once this is complete, write in the correction.

43. D. 10 years

Rationale: The American Medical Association recommends keeping medical records for 10 years.

44. C. Three years

Rationale: The appointment book is considered a legal document and should be treated as such. Old appointment books should be kept for at least three years.

45. B. Wave scheduling

Rationale: Wave scheduling provides built-in flexibility to accommodate unforeseen situations.

46. C. The matrix

Rationale: The periods of time the physician is unavailable are known as the *matrix*.

47. A. Directs the computer's activities and sends electronic signals to the right place at the right time

Rationale: A CPU (central processing unit) directs the computer's activities and sends electronic signals to the right place at the right time.

48. C. Peripherals

Rationale: Scanners and digital cameras are examples of peripherals. Peripherals are the extras that can be attached to hardware to expand the computer's capability.

49. B. Software

Rationale: Electronic medical records are software.

50. C. Disk operating system

Rationale: *DOS* stands for *disk operating system*.

51. C. Hard copy

Rationale: Hard copy is defined as a printed copy of data in a file.

52. E. None of the above

Rationale: A list of all files stored on a storage device is a catalog.

53. A. Redo

Rationale: The computer command Ctrl + Y performs the function "redo."

54. D. Restart the system

Rationale: The computer command Ctrl + Alt + Del restarts the system.

55. D. A and B

Rationale: Traditional signatures found on paper documents can now be converted into a mathematical process (or a set of numbers) to create an electronic number.

56. C. Receipt

Rationale: Receipts must be given for all cash payments.

57. A. Certified check

Rationale: A certified check has the following characteristics: written on the payer's own check form; guarantees that the money is available; bank teller verifies the check by placing an official stamp directly on the check; bank withdraws the money from the payer's account when it certifies the check.

58. E. All of the above

Rationale: A negotiable instrument permits the transfer of money to another person. In order to be a negotiable instrument, the check must be written and signed by an authorized payer of the check; state the sum of money to be paid; be payable on demand or at a fixed date in the future; be payable to the holder (payee) of the check.

59. E. All are included in a bank statement.

Rationale: The following are included in a bank statement: account number, average collected balance, minimum balance, tax ID number (usually the Social Security number of the physician) beginning balance, deposit history including credit card transaction deposits, interest/credits, checks and debits, service charges, ending balance.

60. B. Coins and bills separately from checks

Rationale: Currency (coins and bills) is totaled separately from checks.

61. C. Money market savings account

Rationale: A money market savings account requires a minimum balance of $500 to $5000, depending on the institution.

62. A. Daily

Rationale: The day sheet, one for each day of the month, must be balanced at the end of each day.

63. D. Money owed to the practice by insurance companies and patients that has not yet been paid

Rationale: Accounts receivable is the money owed to the practice by insurance companies and patients that has not yet been paid.

64. A. Indicates that a charge has been entered and added to the account balance

Rationale: A debit in accounting indicates that a charge has been entered and added to the account balance.

65. C. Payment to a creditor

Rationale: Petty cash is available for incidentals such as reimbursements, postage due, or other miscellaneous expenses within the medical office.

66. E. All of the above

Rationale: Accounts payable are the amounts the physician owes to others for supplies, equipment, and services that have not yet been paid.

67. B. Biweekly

Rationale: Biweekly payroll schedules have 26 pay periods a year. Employees are paid every two weeks.

68. A. Payroll

Rationale: Typically, the largest AP account in the medical office is payroll.

69. D. All of the above

Rationale: The W-4 form must include the following: employee's name and current address; Social Security number; marital status; number of exemptions to be claimed.

70. D. Quarterly

Rationale: Federal unemployment tax (FUTA) is calculated quarterly.

71. Capitation rate

Rationale: The capitation rate is defined as follows: the provider is paid a predetermined amount every month, regardless of the number of times the patient is seen within a month.

72. A. Exclusions

Rationale: Exclusions are services that are not covered under the insured's health plan.

73. E. None of the above

Rationale: An individual policy is defined as a policy purchased by an individual directly from the insurance company without participating in a group plan.

74. B. Cost

Rationale: The HMO concept was started to control the cost explosion in healthcare as a result of overutilization of services.

75. D. A PPO is a prepayment program.

Rationale: A PPO is a fee-for-service program; it is not based on prepayment.

76. D. POS

Rationale: A POS has the following characteristics: hybrid of HMO and PPO networks; members may choose from a primary or secondary network; the primary network is HMO-like; the secondary network is often a PPO network; out-of-pocket expenses are lower within the primary network and higher when the secondary network is used; members have more choices with less expense than with a PPO.

77. D. All

Rationale: All patients covered by Medicare must sign an advance beneficiary notice (ABN) prior to receiving covered services that may be denied by Medicare.

78. C. Part C

Rationale: Medicare Part C is offered by private insurance companies.

79. A. Part A

Rationale: Under Medicare Part A, the patient must apply to receive Medicare benefits from the Social Security Administration.

80. C. DRGs are used to calculate payments made to outpatient providers.

Rationale: While DRGs have an effect on hospital reimbursements, they are not used to calculate payments made to outpatient providers.

81. C. Medicaid is a direct federal program.

Rationale: Medicaid was designed for the medically indigent, or persons without funds, and even though it is not a direct federal program, it qualifies as government insurance. Funding for each state's Medicaid program comes from state funds, with some federal money to offset costs. The program is administered by individual states, and the rules for eligibility and payment vary from state to state. Patients must qualify for benefits on a monthly basis.

82. D. All of the above

Rationale: TRICARE is the U.S. Department of Defense's worldwide healthcare program for active duty and retired uniformed service members and their families.

83. D. Use punctuation.

Rationale: When completing the CMS-1500, no punctuation is to be used.

84. D. A and B

Rationale: Only small providers (institutional organizations with fewer than 25 full-time employees and physicians with fewer than 10 full-time employees) may file paper claims.

85. D. Paper

Rationale: Electronic claims are sent to an insurance carrier or clearinghouse via dial-up modem, direct data entry, or over the Internet rather than on paper.

86. B. Volume II

Rationale: Volume II lists diseases and injuries in alphabetical order and the associated numerical code afterward.

87. A. Otitis media

Rationale: Otitis media would be the primary diagnosis because it is the reason for the visit.

88. D. All of the above

Rationale: The following are acceptable uses of V codes: They add supportive information to the patient, family, or personal history. They may be used as a primary code to describe a person who may not have a current illness but who is seeing the physician for well-baby care, birth control advice, a pregnancy test, or immunizations. They may be used as supportive information when some circumstance or problem is present, such as an allergy to penicillin.

89. Coding the use of drugs

Rationale: E codes (E930–E949) are mandatory when coding the use of drugs.

90. C. ( ) = encloses a series of terms, each of which is modified by the statement appearing to the right side of the parentheses.

Rationale: Parentheses enclose supplementary words, (nonessential modifiers) that may be present in the narrative description of a disease without affecting the code assignment.

91. B. 5, 2, 3, 1, 4

Rationale: The following is the correct sequence for procedural coding: 5. To the highest level of certainty, begin by identifying what service was provided or what procedure was performed. You will find this information documented in the patient's chart. 2. Once you know what service was provided or procedure performed, look for the appropriate level of service or procedural term in the alphabetic index. Note the code associated with the narrative description of the service provided or procedure performed. 3. Look through the list of modifiers to determine if one is needed. 1. Using the code in the alphabetic index, verify that it is correct by looking in the tabular index. 4. Record the service or procedure code on the insurance claim form.

92. D. Privacy manager

Rationale: The privacy manager allows patients to block access to their home telephones. Patients will be asked to state the location from which they are calling. Once they have given this information, unless they are cleared, they'll be directed to a voice mail system, where they will leave a message.

93. D. Address numbers must be spelled out on the envelope.

Rationale: For optimal efficiency of OCR scanning, the address must be typed on the envelope, using single spacing and all capital letters with no punctuation.

94. A. Allergies

Rationale: All of the following are physical exam components of the medical record: patient's general appearance; nutrition; blood pressure; head—an eyes, ears, nose, and throat examination (EENT), including the mouth, and scalp; results of neck and thyroid examinations; results of thorax and breast examinations; lymphadenopathy; results of examinations of the heart and lungs, abdomen, pelvic, genital and rectal areas, and skin; overall impression; treatment plan.

95. E. All of the above

Rationale: The appointment schedule should show the periods of time blocked out on the daily schedule when appointments are unavailable due to the physician's meetings, surgery time, vacation, and hospital rounds. The periods of time the physician is unavailable is known as the *matrix*.

96. D. Straight numerical filing

Rationale: In straight numerical filing, each record is filed sequentially based on its assigned number.

97. D. Both A and B

Rationale: Subjective information is gathered from the patient and is the same as the chief complaint.

98. D. All of the above

Rationale: Mail that is not valuable in itself, but would be difficult to replace if lost, should be sent as certified mail. Examples include contracts, mortgages, birth certificates, deeds, and checks.

99. B. Ctrl + V

Rationale: The command for paste is Ctrl + V.

100. C. Certified checks

Rationale: A certified check is written on the payer's own check form. It guarantees that the money is available. The bank teller verifies the check by placing an official stamp directly on the check. The bank withdraws the money from the payer's account when it certifies the check.

CLINICAL MEDICAL ASSISTING

1. A. Sweets

Rationale: The six nutrient classifications are carbohydrates, proteins, fats, vitamins, minerals, water.

2. C. Vitamin B_2

Rationale: The water-soluble vitamins are vitamin B_1, vitamin B_2, vitamin B_{12}, vitamin C, and niacin.

3. E. A and B

Rationale: Dietary guidelines are developed by the U.S. Department of Agriculture and the Department of Health and Human Services.

4. D. Black coffee

Rationale: The clear liquid diet consists of the following: clear soup and broth, plain gelatin, black coffee, tea, carbonated beverages, and popsicles.

5. E. An eating disorder characterized by dangerously low body weight, poor body image, and fear of becoming overweight

Rationale: Anorexia nervosa is an eating disorder characterized by dangerously low body weight, poor body image, and fear of becoming overweight.

6. B. Sunlight

Rationale: In order for microorganisms to grow, they must have all of the following: food, moisture, suitable temperature, and darkness.

7. A. 5, 3, 1, 4, 2

Rationale: In order for infection to occur, the following must be available: an infected reservoir host, a portal of exit, a means of transmission, a portal of entry into a new host, and a susceptible new host.

8. E. Hepatitis B

Rationale: Hepatitis B is the only form of hepatitis for which a vaccine is available.

9. E. All require you to wash your hands afterward.

Rationale: All of the actions require you to wash your hands afterward.

10. C. Kills all microorganisms except bacterial spores

Rationale: High-level disinfection kills all microorganisms except bacterial spores.

11. D. Steam and pressure sterilization

Rationale: Autoclaving is also known as *steam and pressure sterilization.*

12. E. All are to be included in an exposure control plan.

Rationale: An exposure control plan must include the following: exposure determination, method of compliance, postexposure evaluation, and follow-up.

13. A. Glasses

Rationale: Personal protective equipment items are gloves, masks, eye/face shields, gowns, and lab coats.

14. E. All of the above

Rationale: The history of the present illness (HPI) will provide information regarding onset, duration, and intensity.

15. A. Family illness

Rationale: Social history questions should consist of the following: smoking, drinking, recreational drug use, occupation, marital status, sexual preference, and lifestyle including, diet, exercise, and sleep habits.

16. B. Permanent blue ink should be used.

Rationale: The following are guidelines for proper documentation: give the date and time of the entry; use legible handwriting; use permanent black ink; use proper terminology, correct spelling, and correct grammar; document in sequence as the visit occurred; be concise; correct errors by drawing a single line through the incorrect entry and initialing it; then record the correct entry; sign every entry.

17. B. Rectal

Rationale: A normal body temperature for a rectal body temperature measurement is 99.6°F.

18. C. 70–90 bpm

Rationale: The average pulse rate for someone 11–16 years old is 70–90 bpm.

19. D. 16 to 20 per minute

Rationale: A normal respiratory rate is 16 to 20 per minute.

20. E. All are part of the wellness guidelines.

Rationale: Keeping a positive attitude, challenging your mind, forgiving and forgetting, and soothing your fears are all part of the wellness guidelines.

21. E. All of the above

Rationale: Once nonhealthy habits have been identified, you can provide educational information in the form of brochures, videos, and Internet Web sites that the patient may visit.

22. A. 200

Rationale: The MDI consists of a pressurized canister that contains approximately 200 doses.

23. E. All of the above

Rationale: In an outpatient or home setting, oxygen is usually delivered via nasal cannula and is prescribed for three primary reasons: to decrease the work of breathing, decrease the work of the heart, and reverse or prevent low blood oxygen levels.

24. B. Otoscope

Rationale: An otoscope is used to examine the ears. Light is focused through a speculum into the outer ear and into the tympanic membrane. Additional speculums may be used to view other structures, such as the nose.

25. C. Diaphragm

Rationale: The four components of the sphygmomanometer are the manometer, inflatable rubber bladder, bulb, and cuff.

26. D. Endoscope

Rationale: An endoscope is used to look into a hollow organ or body cavity. It is used to examine the larynx, bladder, colon, sigmoid colon, stomach, abdomen, and some joints.

27. A. 15 minutes

Rationale: A temperature in an autoclave must remain at 250°F for a minimum of 15 minutes to kill all bacterial spores and microorganisms.

28. C. Tympanic membrane

Rationale: A tympanic membrane thermometer is also known as an *aural thermometer*. It detects heat wave within the ear canal near the eardrum.

29. A. Older supplies should be used first.

Rationale: The FIFO rule means that older supplies should be used first.

30. C. Auscultation

Rationale: Auscultation is the process of listening to the sounds within the body, such as those made by the heart, lungs, stomach, and bowels.

31. E. Lithotomy position

Rationale: If a patient is in the stirrups at an obstetric-gynecologic practice, she is in the lithotomy position.

32. B. Long arm cast

Rationale: A long arm cast extends from the fingers to the axilla, with a bend at the elbow. Long arm casts are used for fractures of the upper arm.

33. E. All are needed for casting.

Rationale: The following materials are needed for casting: bandage roll or tape, container of warm water, stockinette, Webril™ (sheer wadding), padding rolls, bandage scissors, rubber gloves, and sponge rubber.

34. B. Dissecting

Rationale: Scissors are an example of a tool that falls under the dissecting category.

35. B. Curved needle

Rationale: A curved needle allows the surgeon to go into and out of tissue when there is not enough room to suture using a straight needle. It requires a needle holder.

36. E. All are examples of nonabsorbable sutures.

Rationale: The following are examples of non-absorbable sutures: silk, nylon, steel, polyester, and cotton.

37. D. B and C

Rationale: The most common indicators are autoclave tape and sterilization indicator strips.

38. D. A and B

Rationale: A receptionist or medical assistant should record the patient's history.

39. B. The physician will provide additional information relating to the procedure(s) performed during the colonoscopy.

Rationale: Following the colonoscopy, the physician will provide additional information relating to the procedure(s) performed during the colonoscopy.

40. A. Exercise therapy

Rationale: Exercise therapy improves joint flexibility, muscle tone, and mobility. It should be monitored by a physician or physical therapist.

41. E. Dilating and probing

Rationale: A trocar is a dilating and probing instrument.

42. E. All answers are true.

Rationale: All answers are true. A sterile item can only touch another sterile item. A sterile item on a sterile field must be within your field of vision and above your waist. Airborne microorganisms contaminate sterile fields. The edges of a sterile field are contaminated.

43. D. 0.20 second

Rationale: The paper is divided into squares of 5 × 5 mm. Each 5 × 5 mm square is the equivalent of 0.20 second and is made up of smaller 1 × 1 mm squares. Each 1 × 1mm square is the equivalent of 0.04 second.

44. A. White

Rationale: The right arm limb lead for an EKG machine is white.

45. E. T wave

Rationale: A T wave represents repolarization of the ventricles.

46. E. All of the above

Rationale: Near vision acuity tests are performed when the patient complains of having difficulty reading or performing other close tasks such as threading a needle.

47. B. Red and green

Rationale: The most common color vision defect is the inability to distinguish between red and green.

48. D. A and B

Rationale: Pulmonary function tests (PFTs) are performed to evaluate lung volume and capacity.

49. A. Move air into and out of the lungs

Rationale: Peak flow meters are used to measure the patient's ability to move air into and out of the lungs.

50. B. Lead

Rationale: In order to help protect personnel, anyone in the medical field working around radiation should use a lead apron.

51. D. B and C

Rationale: Quantitative tests are performed to determine whether or not a substance is present and the amount of the substance. Results are reported out using numerical values.

52. E. Normal formation and development of blood cells

Rationale: Hematopoiesis is the normal formation and development of blood cells.

53. A. Erythrocytes

Rationale: Erythrocytes are red blood cells.

54. B. Antigen/antibody reaction that occurs when an antigen clumps together with an antibody

Rationale: Agglutination is an antigen/antibody reaction that occurs when an antigen clumps together with an antibody.

55. Monocytes

Rationale: The largest cells in the blood are monocytes.

56. E. All are required.

Rationale: The antibiotic treatment in use, date, time of collection, and type of specimen are all required when labeling a patient's specimen.

57. A. Evacuation tube system

Rationale: The fastest and most efficient system for performing venipuncture is an evacuation tube system.

58. D. The triangular area below the bend of the elbow

Rationale: The most common venipuncture site is the antecubital space, which is the triangular area just below the end of the elbow.

59. B. Midstream

Rationale: A clean-catch urine specimen should be collected in midstream.

60. E. All are needed.

Rationale: All of the equipment listed is needed to obtain a stool sample.

61. A. Iron-deficiency anemia

Rationale: A low Hgb may indicate iron-deficiency anemia.

62. D. 4.5–6.0 million per mm^3

Rationale: A normal red blood cell count for females is 4.5–6.0 million per mm^3.

63. D. A and B

Rationale: A low platelet level may indicate anemia or leukemia.

64. C. 0

Rationale: Normally, the level of C-reactive protein (CRP) detected in the blood is 0.

65. A. Crystals

Rationale: Crystals are formed by urinary salts when pH, temperature, or concentration changes occur.

66. B. $\frac{17}{24}$

Rationale: $\frac{3}{8} + \frac{1}{3} = \frac{17}{24}$

67. D. $\frac{1}{10}$

Rationale: $\frac{1}{2} \times \frac{1}{5} = \frac{1}{10}$

68. A. .875

Rationale: $\frac{7}{8} = 0.875$

69. C. Tab = tablespoon

Rationale: The proper abbreviation for *tablespoon* is T or tbsp.

70. E. The next dose of medication is given before the previous dose has had time to be metabolized/excreted.

Rationale: A cumulative effect occurs when the next dose of medication is given before the previous dose has had time to be metabolized/excreted.

71. A. Absorption

Rationale: Absorption is the movement of medication from the site of administration into the bloodstream.

72. B. Schedule II

Rationale: Schedule II drugs are described as having a high potential for addiction and abuse. They are accepted for medical use in the United States. Examples include codeine, morphine, opium, and secobarbital.

73. A. Sublingual

Rationale: The methods for parenteral administration of drugs are intraarticular, intradermal, intramuscular, intrathecal, intravenous, and subcutaneous.

74. E. Connects the shaft to the hub

Rationale: The hilt of a syringe connects the shaft to the hub.

75. C. 2 to 5 mL

Rationale: The proper amount for an intramuscular injection is 2 to 5 mL. Dosages above 5 mL should be divided and administered at two different sites.

76. E. 10 to 15 degrees

Rationale: The angle of insertion for an intradermal injection is 10 to 15 degrees.

77. A. Antiulcer

Rationale: Tagamet is an antiulcer drug.

78. E. Hormone

Rationale: Provera is a hormone (progestin) drug.

79. D. Anticonvulsant

Rationale: Dilantin is an anticonvulsant.

80. B. Antibiotic

Rationale: Ceclor is an antibiotic drug.

81. C. Tranquilizer

Rationale: Xanax is a tranquilizer.

82. B. Six weeks

Rationale: The minimum age for giving the rotavirus vaccine (RV) is six weeks.

83. B. Palliative

Rationale: Administration of morphine for terminal cancer patients is a palliative use of the drug. It is used to keep the patient comfortable.

84. C. Preventive

Rationale: Vaccines are used as a preventive measure.

85. E. Therapeutic

Rationale: Antibiotics used to cure pneumonia are therapeutic drugs.

86. E. All contribute to a patient's response to medication.

Rationale: The factors that contribute to a patient's response to medication include age, size, diet, sex, genetic factors, pathological condition, psychological factors, route of administration, time of administration, drug-taking history, and environment.

87. B. Topical

Rationale: A liniment is administered topically.

88. E. A and B

Rationale: A drug in spray form is administered either orally or topically.

89. D. All of the above

Rationale: Most animal bites are puncture wounds, and the following action should be taken: cleanse with soap and water, apply antibiotic ointment, and cover the wound with a dry sterile dressing.

90. B. Area all black

Rationale: Numbness, tingling, edema, blisters, light skin: redness, dark skin: lightening, small blisters, blanching, no sensation; finally, area all white.

91. A. An allergic reaction

Rationale: Anaphylactic shock is caused by an allergic reaction.

92. D. Age

Rationale: The guidelines are similar for respiratory arrest, cardiac arrest, and obstructed airway but vary somewhat according to age.

93. E. Assess the victim and determine if help is needed.

Rationale: Assess the victim and determine if help is needed. Shout the name of the infant or child and sharply poke the feet. Never shake an infant.

94. C. Drinking too much soda during a meal

Rationale: An obstructed airway in an adult may be the result of failing to chew properly large pieces of food, talking or laughing too much while eating, drinking alcohol before and during eating, or choking on fluids such as vomit or blood.

95. B. Firm thrusts into the victim's abdomen with an upward movement

Rationale: Abdominal thrusts are delivered with a firm thrust into the victim's abdomen with an upward movement.

96. D. 11.3 mg

Rationale:

$$\text{Pediatric dose} = \frac{\text{Child's weight in pounds}}{150\text{ lb}} \times \text{adult dose}$$

97. D. 5 mL

Rationale: $75 \div 15 = 5$. You would administer 5 mL.

98. C. 2 mL

Rationale: You must first convert the grams to milligrams. 1 gram equals 1000 mg. On hand is 500 mg/mL. $1000 \div 500 = 2$. You would administer 2 mL.

99. D. Schedule IV

Rationale: Schedule IV drugs may have up to five refills over a six-month period.

100. D. The second dose should be administered 1 to 2 months after the first dose

Note: If this information needs to be verified within a chapter, please see Chapter 21, page 386, Figure 21-11.

INDEX